Biosystems & Biorobotics

Volume 19

Aims & Scope

Biosystems & Biorobotics publishes the latest research developments in three main areas: 1) understanding biological systems from a bioengineering point of view, i.e. the study of biosystems by exploiting engineering methods and tools to unveil their functioning principles and unrivalled performance; 2) design and development of biologically inspired machines and systems to be used for different purposes and in a variety of application contexts. The series welcomes contributions on novel design approaches, methods and tools as well as case studies on specific bioinspired systems; 3) design and developments of nano-, micro-, macrodevices and systems for biomedical applications, i.e. technologies that can improve modern healthcare and welfare by enabling novel solutions for prevention, diagnosis, surgery, prosthetics, rehabilitation and independent living.

On one side, the series focuses on recent methods and technologies which allow multiscale, multi-physics, high-resolution analysis and modeling of biological systems. A special emphasis on this side is given to the use of mechatronic and robotic systems as a tool for basic research in biology. On the other side, the series authoritatively reports on current theoretical and experimental challenges and developments related to the "biomechatronic" design of novel biorobotic machines. A special emphasis on this side is given to human-machine interaction and interfacing, and also to the ethical and social implications of this emerging research area, as key challenges for the acceptability and sustainability of biorobotics technology.

The main target of the series are engineers interested in biology and medicine, and specifically bioengineers and bioroboticists. Volume published in the series comprise monographs, edited volumes, lecture notes, as well as selected conference proceedings and PhD theses. The series also publishes books purposely devoted to support education in bioengineering, biomedical engineering, biomechatronics and biorobotics at graduate and post-graduate levels.

About the Cover

The cover of the book series Biosystems & Biorobotics features a robotic hand prosthesis. This looks like a natural hand and is ready to be implanted on a human amputee to help them recover their physical capabilities. This picture was chosen to represent a variety of concepts and disciplines: from the understanding of biological systems to biomechatronics, bioinspiration and biomimetics; and from the concept of human-robot and human-machine interaction to the use of robots and, more generally, of engineering techniques for biological research and in healthcare. The picture also points to the social impact of bioengineering research and to its potential for improving human health and the quality of life of all individuals, including those with special needs. The picture was taken during the LIFEHAND experimental trials run at Università Campus Bio-Medico of Rome (Italy) in 2008. The LIFEHAND project tested the ability of an amputee patient to control the Cyberhand, a robotic prosthesis developed at Scuola Superiore Sant'Anna in Pisa (Italy), using the tf-LIFE electrodes developed at the Fraunhofer Institute for Biomedical Engineering (IBMT, Germany), which were implanted in the patient's arm. The implanted tf-LIFE electrodes were shown to enable bidirectional communication (from brain to hand and vice versa) between the brain and the Cyberhand. As a result, the patient was able to control complex movements of the prosthesis, while receiving sensory feedback in the form of direct neurostimulation. For more information please visit http://www.biorobotics.it or contact the Series Editor.

More information about this series at http://www.springer.com/series/10421

Giorgio Sandrini · Volker Homberg
Leopold Saltuari · Nicola Smania
Alessandra Pedrocchi
Editors

Advanced Technologies for the Rehabilitation of Gait and Balance Disorders

Springer

Editors
Giorgio Sandrini
Department of Brain and Behavioural Sciences, University of Pavia
C. Mondino National Neurological Institute
Pavia
Italy

Volker Homberg
SRH Gesundheitszentrum
Bad Wimpfen
Germany

Leopold Saltuari
Department of Neurology
Hospital Hochzirl
Zirl
Austria

Nicola Smania
Department of Neurological, Biomedical and Movement Sciences
Verona University
Verona
Italy

Alessandra Pedrocchi
Department of Electronics, Information and Bioengineering
Politecnico di Milano
Milan
Italy

ISSN 2195-3562 ISSN 2195-3570 (electronic)
Biosystems & Biorobotics
ISBN 978-3-319-72735-6 ISBN 978-3-319-72736-3 (eBook)
https://doi.org/10.1007/978-3-319-72736-3

Library of Congress Control Number: 2017962982

Printed on acid-free paper

This Springer imprint is published by Springer Nature
The registered company is Springer International Publishing AG
The registered company address is: Gewerbestrasse 11, 6330 Cham, Switzerland

Preface

Gait and balance disorders can occur in all the major neurological diseases dealt with by rehabilitation specialists, and they often impact significantly on the autonomy, and thus the quality of life, of affected patients. Moreover, the consequences of falls, which are frequently associated with these disorders, and measures for their prevention have very high social and healthcare costs.

The European Federation of Neurorehabilitation Societies, in its Congresses, has always given particular prominence to these issues.

With the intention of building on the success of the 'European Summer School on Gait and Balance Rehabilitation in Neurological Diseases', held in Pavia a few years ago, we decided to propose a book that summarises the main issues related to the management of gait and balance disorders.

This book looks at all the major issues related to rehabilitation of these disorders, starting with an analysis of the pathophysiological mechanisms and the most important clinical and instrumental assessment methods.

Several chapters focus on the integrated approach to major neurological diseases, which takes into account the full range of problems presented by neurological patients with impaired balance and gait.

Much of the book is devoted to the use of new advanced technologies in diagnostics, but above all to the treatment of these disorders.

The arrival of these advanced technologies (robotics, virtual reality rehabilitation, neuromodulation, etc.) on the market has greatly altered the approach to rehabilitation of gait and balance disorders in neurological patients, which is an increasingly rich field that sees new developments every day.

For this reason, we felt it would be valuable to compile a book that, in addition to providing a summary of the main knowledge on this subject, also offers an update on the use of advanced technologies for rehabilitation in this setting.

Pavia, Italy	Giorgio Sandrini
Bad Wimpfen, Germany	Volker Homberg
Zirl, Austria	Leopold Saltuari
Verona, Italy	Nicola Smania
Milan, Italy	Alessandra Pedrocchi

Contents

Part I
Assessment of Gait and Balance Disorders

An Overview of the Physiology and Pathophysiology of Postural Control

Antonio Nardone and Anna Maria Turcato

1 Introduction

The postural control system consists of the combined activity of the sensorimotor, integrative and musculoskeletal components involved in the production of postural tone, postural stability and postural orientation [94]. Postural tone corresponds to the active and passive muscle tone of extensor muscles aimed at counteracting gravity; postural stability refers to balance, the condition in which the projection of the center of mass is contained within the boundaries of the base of support, while postural orientation is the positioning of the body segments with respect both to each other and the environment. Disease can affect the postural control system, thus preventing or severely impairing both quiet stance and coordinated voluntary movements.

An exhaustive review of postural control and its relationship with disease is beyond the scope of this chapter. We confine ourselves to summarizing the physiology of the postural control system, and providing some examples of the pathophysiology of postural disorders in common neurological diseases. We will deal here with balance during quiet stance, postural perturbations and posturo-kinetic coordination, but do not look at the role of computerized dynamic posturography platforms since this is dealt with elsewhere in the book.

A. Nardone (✉)
Centro Studi Attività Motorie, ICS Maugeri SPA SB, Institute of Pavia, IRCCS, 27100 Pavia, Italy
e-mail: antonio.nardone@icsmaugeri.it

A. Nardone
Department of Clinical-Surgical, Diagnostic and Pediatric Sciences, University of Pavia, 27100 Pavia, Italy

A. M. Turcato
Posture and Movement Laboratory, Division of Physical Medicine and Rehabilitation, ICS Maugeri SPA SB, Institute of Veruno, IRCCS, 28010 Veruno, NO, Italy

G. Sandrini et al. (eds.), *Advanced Technologies for the Rehabilitation of Gait and Balance Disorders*, Biosystems & Biorobotics 19,
https://doi.org/10.1007/978-3-319-72736-3_1

2 Postural Control System

The body consists of a chain of bone segments connected by muscles, tendons and ligaments. During quiet stance, the knee, hip and shoulder are situated anterior to the frontal plane passing through the ankles. Thus, gravitational torques tend to extend the knee and hip [220], which in turn are stabilized through passive viscoelastic forces produced by muscles, tendons and ligaments. In order to stabilize the body, low-level tonic EMG activity in the antigravity foot muscles [185, 182, 186] and soleus is necessary [79], as well as in the biceps femoris, erectores spinae and neck muscles, while other muscles are not active or only negligibly so [199]. As a consequence, the energy expenditure to maintain upright stance of the human body is low [97].

Human upright stance is an unstable condition. Two-thirds of body mass is located at two-thirds of body height above the ground [218]. The body can be envisaged as an inverted pendulum that moves around the ankle (the so-called ankle strategy) or as two linked pendulums that move around the hip (the so-called hip strategy) [91]. Actually, under most conditions of daily life, postural perturbations are counteracted by a continuum of segmental movements up and down the body [179]. Gravity acts continuously on the body, challenging balance. However, in healthy subjects, the postural control system ensures that falls do not occur. The interplay that occurs between the external forces acting on the body and the functioning of the control system means that subjects do not stand completely still during upright stance, but sway. However, body sway recorded with a force platform during quiet stance is very small, corresponding to about the width of a 10-cent euro coin.

Balance during upright stance is maintained through the action of sensorimotor systems. Sensory inputs (proprioceptive, visual and vestibular inputs and cutaneous inputs from the sole of the foot) ([99]; see Chiba et al. [38], for a recent review) provide information about the orientation of the body in space and the environmental conditions. Integration of afferent information at the level of the central nervous system means that postural responses can be selected according to prior experience, the degree of postural stabilization, and the environment. Postural responses are mediated by the spinal and supraspinal centers (which include several areas of the cortex) (see Bolton [23]; Takakusaki et al. [209]). Postural control works best if both the inputs and outputs, as well as the sensorimotor integration, are not affected by disease. However, thanks to a redundancy of sensory input, it is still possible to preserve balance even when one or two afferent inputs are lost [133].

3 Sensory Inputs Involved in Postural Control

3.1 *Visual Input*

Visual stabilization of posture is obtained through the detection of a displacement of the retinal target during head movements [204]. Visual sensory input can be modified easily by opening and closing the eyes or altering the quality or type of visual input available, which results in a decrease of postural stability [94]. Simply closing the eyes during quiet upright stance (Romberg test) can increase body sway even in healthy subjects, and progressive reduction of visual acuity causes linearly increasing postural instability under static [203] and dynamic conditions [189]. Unsurprisingly, the reduction of visual acuity and contrast sensitivity that occurs with aging affects body sway [119]. The role of central and peripheral vision in the maintenance of upright stance is debated in the literature, but it is plausible that central and peripheral vision [7] play a complementary role in the control of posture [3, 163]. The optimal working range of vision for detecting body sway is below 1 Hz, i.e. higher than the threshold required for labyrinthine activation but lower than that required for muscle proprioception [46, 52, 66]. Interestingly, as shown by comparisons of static or dynamic stability in persons with congenital blindness and in healthy subjects with eyes closed, deprivation of vision from birth does not prevent normal postural control [190]. Therefore, blind subjects do not take advantage of other sensory inputs for controlling balance, which suggests that long-term absence of visual information cannot be substituted by other sensory inputs.

3.2 *Somatosensory Input*

The somatosensory system is made up of mechanoreceptors, their sensory innervations and central pathways (see Shaffer and Harrison [194], for a review on aging of the somatosensory system and implications for balance control).

Muscle spindles are mechanoreceptors that detect velocity and length of muscle stretch. Stretch velocity is detected by spindle primary endings innervated by large afferent fibers (group Ia), whilst stretch length is detected by secondary endings, innervated by smaller afferent fibers (group II) in addition to Ia ones. Spindles contribute to the perception of joint movement (kinesthesia) and to joint position sense. The Golgi tendon organs are located at the muscle-tendon interface and transduce information about active tension generated by the muscle at this interface [103, 121, 171]. Joint receptors discharge signals in response to a deformation of the joint capsule and ligaments. Together, muscle spindles, Golgi tendon organs and joint receptors provide so-called proprioceptive sensation.

In upright standing, movements between the feet and the base of support generate shearing and vertical forces that can activate cutaneous mechanoreceptors [165]. Cutaneous input appears to detect body sway occurring at a low frequency, as during quiet stance [60]. In addition, the input from these receptors provides information about body orientation with respect to the ground [99].

Experiments using vibration of the foot sole [108] and lateral translation of the supporting platform [137] have shown that vibration affects postural responses even though cutaneous input per se plays a negligible role in evoking postural responses to balance perturbations [60, 187]. Also, any effect of foot sole skin vibration is lesser in standing than in sitting conditions [134]. Cooling the plantar surface has a very small effect on postural control despite the anesthetic effects identified in each study reviewed [84]. Overall, these findings suggest that any hypoesthesia of the foot sole induced by disease would not play a major role in the postural instability observed in some patients.

Light contact of the finger on a stationary frame induces a marked reduction of body sway during quiet stance (see Sozzi et al. [200]). In addition, it decreases the amplitude of leg muscle responses to a perturbation [130, 183]. This occurs even before the hand touches the frame, suggesting that the command to touch the frame and the reduction of the postural responses are closely associated [184]. It has been suggested that an external point of contact provides a reference for the vertical posture [80]. In this context, light finger touch of a stationary surface has been shown to suppress the disorientation provoked by neck muscle vibration [28]. If, on the other hand, subjects are required to touch a moving plate, this can enhance their postural sway [104]. This finding suggests that subjects combine cutaneous input from the finger and proprioception from the arm to stabilize upright posture.

Proprioception gives us information about the static and dynamic components of joint position and orientation (see Proske and Gandevia [170], for a review) and plays a major role in defining the sense of verticality [10, 83]. Information about lower limb and ankle orientation is especially important for posture control. Proprioception, and consequently body orientation, can be altered through the vibration of muscles such as the soleus in standing subjects (see Roll et al. [178], for a review), which induces trains of action potentials in the primary endings innervated by the group Ia afferent fibers. This input produces a false signal of triceps surae lengthening [32, 178] and a backward sway of the body [64, 107]. On the other hand, vibration of the dorsal neck muscles produces body sway forwards [120]. Proprioceptive input from leg muscles contributes to the low-level balance-related ankle stiffness regulation required to counteract gravity during quiet stance [136]. However, proprioceptive information is not crucial during quiet stance: in fact, under this condition no relationship can be found between changes in activity of the triceps surae and its lengthening induced by body sway, suggesting that balance corrections do not strictly depend on stretch reflexes evoked by ankle muscle lengthening [81].

3.3 Vestibular Input

The vestibular system is involved in balance and motor control as well as in spatial self-motion perception [58, 202]. Afferents from the otolith organs and the semicircular canals converge with optokinetic, somatosensory and motor-related signals in the vestibular nuclei, which are reciprocally interconnected with the vestibulo-cerebellar cortex and deep cerebellar nuclei (see Green and Angelaki [77], for a review). The reflexes relayed through the vestibular nuclei are strongly involved in balance and movement, and are grouped into three categories. The vestibulo-spinal reflex regulates muscle tone of the limb and trunk muscles, while the vestibulo-collic reflex is involved in head and neck posture and movement, and the vestibulo-ocular reflex regulates the position of the eyes in the orbits in order to compensate for movements of the head.

3.4 Neck Input

The mechanoreceptors in the neck have important connections with the vestibular and visual apparatus and with several regions of the central nervous system. These connections explain the importance of neck input for postural stability. In particular, neck receptors play a key role in the control of postural orientation, perception of motion and locomotion (see Treleaven [215], and Pettorossi and Schieppati [167], for reviews). For example, input from the neck feeds the central nervous system with information about the position of the head relative to the trunk. This makes it possible to integrate vestibular input with whole body motion.

As in the case of leg muscles, mentioned earlier, vibratory stimulation has been used to assess the involvement of neck proprioceptive input in postural control. When vibrating either the lateral or dorsal aspect of the neck in a standing subject, the body sways in the opposite direction to the stimulated site [29, 120]. Thus, neck input contributes to the construction of body orientation, together with signals from the vestibular system, eye and limb muscles. The effects of neck muscle vibration are strongly reduced during light touch of a stationary surface, suggesting the existence of a strong central interaction of inputs from neck receptors and finger skin receptors [28].

4 Central Integration of Sensory Inputs

4.1 Cerebellum

The cerebellum is intimately involved in the control of various kinds of motor activity, including limb movements, balance and motor learning (see Synofzik and

Ilg [207]; Taylor and Ivry [210]). Colnaghi et al. [41] have recently shown that functional inactivation of the cerebellar vermis by theta-burst stimulation is associated with increased sway. Since the cerebellum regulates movements but does not generate them, any cerebellar damage does not lead to paresis, as in the case of damage to the descending motor pathways (e.g. in stroke), but to abnormal sensorimotor integration [125] and discoordination of movements, so-called ataxia (see Akbar and Ashizawa [4], for a recent review). Ataxia affects postural control, and is a risk factor for falls [68].

4.2 Basal Ganglia

The basal ganglia are involved in the planning, initiation and control of voluntary movements. The basal ganglia and dopamine system form the critical neural substrates for changing the 'set', i.e. the preparatory state of the nervous system, which is influenced by context, e.g. instructions for postural configuration [169]. Therefore, the basal ganglia control anticipatory postural adjustments and the interplay between posture and gait [36]. The basal ganglia have important projections to the upper brainstem nuclei (the mesencephalic locomotor region); these nuclei control trunk and proximal musculature for balance and gait through their projections to the brainstem and spinal cord via bilateral midline descending pathways [160].

4.3 Sensorimotor Integration in the Central Nervous System

The integration of sensory information produces an internal representation (or internal model) of the position and movements of the body (kinesthesia). The sensory inputs converge in the spinal cord, vestibular nuclei, brainstem, thalamus, cerebellum and cerebral cortex, and can therefore interact [125]. For example, proprioceptive information must be integrated with visual and vestibular information to interpret complex sensory environments. In a well-lit environment with a firm support base, healthy persons rely mainly on somatosensory, less on vestibular, and least of all on visual information [166]. In the event of impairment of one sensory channel, the sensory redundancy phenomenon allows for compensation, i.e. sensory reweighting, in order to maintain standing balance in spite of the disease-related deterioration of afferent input. However, once compensation fails, balance may become impaired, increasing the potential for falls [164].

The parietal, temporal and insular cortex seem to be essential for sensory integration during postural tasks and are involved in the changing postural responses that occur with alterations in cognitive state or in initial sensorimotor conditions, in the presence of prior experience, and with prior warning of a perturbation [86, 101], all representing changes in the 'central set' [169]. The cerebellar-cortical loop seems to be responsible for adapting postural responses on the basis of prior experience [85] and the basal ganglia-cortical loop for pre-selecting and optimizing postural responses according to the current context [20, 183].

Sensorimotor integration can be affected by higher cognitive processes such as attention or emotions. It should be emphasized that maintaining postural stability is not an attention-free task [195, 212]. Several studies have demonstrated a decrease in cognitive performance as the demands of a concurrent postural task increase. In turn, attentional demands increase as the balance requirements of a task increase: there is a progressive increase in the attentional demands when moving from sitting to standing to walking [212]. In addition, the emotional context may play a role in postural control. In fact, body sway is reduced under the threat of a fall from an elevated surface [35]. Under this condition, healthy young and older adults typically adopt a postural stiffening strategy. These changes are accompanied by increased gain of the proprioceptive and vestibular reflexes [96, 95, 138] that may lead to an altered perception, with subjects at a certain height perceiving themselves to be swaying more than they actually are.

4.4 Feedback and Feed Forward Postural Control

The central nervous system is informed of deviation from equilibrium by sensory signals coming from two modalities of feedback control: continuous and discontinuous [131]. The continuous modality applies in the conditions of quiet stance and unpredictable continuous perturbations of the supporting platform [113]. However, it has been suggested that during quiet stance an individual does not rely only on feedback to control balance. In fact, initially, when there is no feedback for postural control, open-loop control is used [37, 40]. Then, after approximately 1 s, open-loop control changes to closed-loop control, and thereafter the individual uses continuous feedback for postural control.

The other control modality consists of discontinuous feedback, which comes into play when upright stance is perturbed by external forces. These forces trigger phasic postural reactions that can be experimentally induced by surface translation: they are direction-specific and show a distal-to-proximal sequence of muscle activation [91]. These postural responses are evoked by stretching of the muscles. They occur with early and late latency of onset and are mediated respectively by spindle group Ia afferent fibers (corresponding to the monosynaptic stretch reflex) and spindle group II fibers. The latter responses are relayed through a spinal oligosynaptic pathway (see Schieppati et al. [186]; Nardone et al. [143]; Schieppati and Nardone [187, 185]; Nardone and Schieppati [147]; Bove et al. [30]; Grey et al. [78]).

Group II fiber conduction velocity has been estimated to be about 21 m/s, i.e. less than half the value of Ia fibers (51 m/s) [147].

Postural responses can be affected by changes of posture: prior leaning affects the latency and particularly the amplitude of EMG responses to postural perturbation [90, 186]. Also repetition of perturbation affects postural responses, inducing habituation. Repetition of toe-up rotations of a supporting platform induces a rapid attenuation of postural responses in the triceps surae between the first and second perturbation, followed by slower habituation across the subsequent trials [82]. This adaptation has also recently been shown in the case of balance perturbations delivered by repeated sinusoidal translations of the support base [153, 201]. Within the framework of a reproducible general pattern, a broad range of variability has been observed for successive cycles of the same perturbation, suggesting flexibility of dynamic postures [181]. Clear-cut differences in balancing behavior have been observed according to the presence or absence of vision [31, 45, 72, 188]. For instance, when vision is gradually degraded experimentally, good visual acuity strongly reinforces a 'head-fixed-in-space' behavior, while poor vision and no vision instead produce a 'head-moving-with-platform' displacement [190, 189]. Balancing behavior is fairly resistant to abnormal proprioceptive noise obtained by means of postural muscle vibration [157], which points to a significant intervention of feed-forward mechanisms.

Voluntary movement performed by a subject during upright stance is in itself destabilizing. In this case, the central nervous system cannot rely on a feedback mode of postural control since the muscle responses would occur too late to be effective in maintaining balance. On the contrary, the central nervous system must generate anticipatory postural adjustments (APAs) before the onset of the perturbation induced by the voluntary movement. Postural control is thus regulated in a feed-forward manner to generate the APAs necessary for appropriate postural control [131]. This occurs, for example, when a subject performs a fast voluntary upper limb movement [42]. Under this condition, APAs displace body segments in the direction opposite to that in which they can be expected to be displaced by the forces generated by the forthcoming movement. In this way, APAs maintain the center of mass over the base of support [27, 197].

It has recently been shown that the basic APA patterns during a forward reaching task, consisting of an initial posterior shift of the center of pressure (CoP) and tibialis anterior muscle activation, change with repetition of the task [117] to feature earlier muscle onsets and larger anticipatory CoP displacements. As a result, smaller peak center of mass displacements are observed after the voluntary perturbation, indicating greater postural stability [106]. Reaching training induces not only improvements in motor performance, but also changes in the APAs [102]. The latter are correlated with and occur earlier than improvements in motor performance. These results suggest that changes in APAs contribute to improvement in motor performance [180].

APAs are subject to modulation according to the individual's stability. Light touch has been shown to decrease the APAs associated with voluntary arm movement [198]. This phenomenon might depend on the fact that the subject can estimate the current position of the center of mass with higher precision [116]. Furthermore, the APAs in the leg are reduced in magnitude or completely absent when the postural threat is reduced [71, 156, 114]. Finally, APAs are decreased or absent when an external support is available or when the subject is inclined forward [211], suggesting, as indicated above, that the occurrence of APAs is affected by the initial stability condition of the subject.

5 Diseases Affecting Postural Control

5.1 Skeletal Muscle Conditions

Since the skeletal muscles are the 'end effectors' of the chain of events leading to postural stabilization, lower extremity weakness is a risk factor for falls [214]. It has been shown that body sway is increased in boys with Duchenne muscular dystrophy, which is characterized by muscle weakness mainly affecting the lower limbs [12]. In patients previously affected by polio, lower-limb strength is strongly associated with postural sway while standing on a compliant surface [118]. However, postural instability cannot be fully explained by muscle weakness since a functional link has been shown to exist between contractile and sensory muscular processes [33].

5.2 Peripheral Neuropathy

Fall risk is increased in patients with peripheral neuropathy [214]. Patients with diabetic polyneuropathy show increased body sway during quiet stance [26, 75, 148, 196]. Interestingly, these patients have increased body sway not only with eyes closed but also with eyes open, suggesting that vision cannot compensate completely for the somatosensory impairment [148]. Body sway is not necessarily increased in other types of neuropathy. For example, sway is little affected in patients with Charcot-Marie-Tooth disease type 1A (CMT1A) [150, 151]. This is because CMT1A shows axonal demyelination and loss of large-diameter myelinated nerve fibers, which include Ia afferent fibers [63, 192]. Conversely, diabetic patients may develop sensorimotor distal symmetric polyneuropathy involving small- and medium-size afferent fibers in addition to the large ones [15]. Therefore, it is plausible that the increased body sway observed during quiet stance in diabetic patients is connected to the involvement of medium-size spindle group II afferent fibers in addition to group Ia ones [144]. This suggests that the input coming from the length-sensitive spindle secondary endings is better able than that from the spindle primary endings to detect the slow changes in leg muscle lengths due to displacements of the body's center of mass during quiet stance. Contrary to these findings, increased sway has also been reported in patients with CMT1A [115], but this phenomenon might be due to the severity of the demyelination and axonal loss that, in its late stage, might also have involved the smaller afferent fibers [150]. Patients with neuropathy show delayed latency of muscle responses to a postural perturbation [98, 148]; also, they were found to be impaired in their ability to scale the torque magnitude of postural responses to the velocity and amplitude of perturbation [98].

Patients affected by a loss of sensory neurons in the dorsal root ganglia (sensory neuron disease, SND) are severely ataxic [193]. These patients are severely unstable during quiet stance not only with eyes closed, as is to be expected in cases of sensory ataxia, but also with eyes open [141]. This finding highlights the role of sensory integration and suggests that somatosensory input is an enabling condition for optimal use of vision in balance control. These patients also show delayed latency of postural responses to stance perturbation, particularly of the long-loop, presumably supraspinal, responses. This suggests that balance impairment in these patients can be ascribed mainly to the loss of the central projections of the afferent fibers. Indeed, in patients with SND, postural instability is far more severe than in patients with peripheral neuropathy. Patients with myelopathy due to cervical spondylosis show large increases in body sway during quiet stance [139] and increased latency of onset of late responses to postural perturbations [2]. This can be considered a sign of abnormal functioning of spinal pathways transmitting sensory inputs to supraspinal centers and it may play a role in the postural instability of these patients.

Patients with diabetic peripheral neuropathy show largely normal anterior-posterior body displacement when subjected to predictable platform perturbations, in spite of their increased body sway during quiet stance [144]. This unexpected finding may be explained by their capacity to exploit APAs under dynamic conditions. It could also be related to their increased reliance on vestibular input for producing APAs [89]. On the contrary, patients with SND fail to show good balance when standing on a predictably moving platform. The reason for this impairment could lie in the abnormality of the long-loop pathways [141].

5.3 Vestibular Deficit

Patients with chronic bilateral vestibular deficit do not show abnormalities in their postural responses to perturbations of upright stance [16, 52, 85, 92, 154]. Therefore, vestibular inputs are not considered crucial for triggering postural responses to body displacement. Allum and Pfaltz [6] showed that even in patients with complete bilateral vestibular deficit, an upward tilt of the supporting platform could still induce activation of ankle and neck muscle activity during the first 150 ms following backward tilt of the subject. In these patients, the latency of postural reflexes is normal but the amplitude is reduced [52]. These findings suggest that vestibulospinal input is not necessary for triggering a postural response but plays a role in modulating its amplitude.

In spite of the fact that the vestibulospinal system gain is normally very low when standing on a firm surface [66], patients with acute unilateral lesions show body sway mainly directed towards the affected labyrinth [48, 52]. The cause of this instability is the imbalance of labyrinthine inputs from the right and left inner ears to the vestibular nuclei, leading to impairment of the vestibulo-spinal reflexes [5, 52]. The instability could also depend on the fact that impairment of vestibular inflow to the central nervous system leads to abnormal information about head movements, preventing the correct interpretation of visual and somatosensory inputs to orientation [17, 25].

When patients with unilateral vestibular deficit undergo predictable balance perturbations induced by a platform continuously moving in an anterior-posterior direction, their body displacement is greater than that of healthy subjects [44]. However, under both eyes open and eyes closed conditions the overall pattern of body displacements is similar to that observed in healthy subjects [45]. This finding points to a major role of APAs in this task [181] and suggests that the integrity of vestibular input is not necessary for producing appropriate APAs.

Patients with bilateral vestibular deficit adapt to their impairment by increasing the somatosensory loop gain [18, 205]. This is an example of compensation for lost input through exploitation of the remaining ones. In spite of this, patients can become unstable when other sensory inputs are manipulated [17, 52, 155, 174], and under different motor tasks or postures of daily life, e.g. when adopting unusual postures [11] or during head or body movements [110, 161].

5.4 Stroke

Many patients with stroke have sensorimotor deficits that affect balance. In turn, balance impairment strongly affects independence in activities of daily living (ADL) and gait [22, 67, 109], and is an important risk factor for falls [214]. During quiet stance, patients present both an abnormality of posture, since they often stand asymmetrically with the position of the CoP shifted towards the non-paretic leg [140], and postural instability, since their body sway is larger than that of healthy subjects [142]. Neither abnormality of posture nor postural instability are always linked to the side of lesion [126, 142]. However, patients with right cortical hemispheric lesions are said to be more unstable than those with left-sided lesions [124] and less able to voluntarily shift body weight onto their non-paretic leg [100].

In relation to their abnormality of posture, stroke patients unsurprisingly have difficulty maintaining a weight shift onto their paretic leg [8] and this is reflected in gait performance. In fact, gait, during both linear [142] and curved trajectories [76], is affected by the asymmetry of weight distribution. This asymmetry is associated with a decrease in the strength of the paretic leg muscles [21, 142]. However, this is not its sole cause. Distortion of vertical perception (perceived as a contralesional tilt), for example, is another possible cause of asymmetry of weight distribution. This distortion induces patients to align towards the ipsilesional (non-paretic) leg [172]. In addition, experiments with galvanic vestibular stimulation suggest that disruption of corticobulbar projections to the brainstem output pathways involved in the vestibular control of balance also plays a role in these patients' postural abnormalities [129].

As far as postural instability is concerned, the increase in sway seems to depend on sensorimotor and cognitive impairments rather than on spasticity itself. In fact, patients with amyotrophic lateral sclerosis and patients with spastic paraparesis do not show increased body sway during quiet stance in spite of the spasticity of their lower limb muscles [140]. Postural instability in stroke might depend on impaired integration of sensory inputs [127] as well as on an abnormal perception of verticality during upright stance [173]. But the connection between the increased body sway and asymmetry of weight distribution is not a simple one, as no relationship could be found between sway and a medial-lateral position of the CoP [142]. The increased body sway in these patients can also be linked to the finding that, due to the reduced sensory inputs from the paretic limb, their visual dependence for the control of postural sway velocity is, compared with controls, greater in the medial-lateral, but not anterior-posterior direction [126]. In keeping with this finding, during quiet stance there is more postural sway when loading the paretic compared with the non-paretic leg [73].

During postural perturbations delivered by a movable platform, patients with stroke show delayed latencies of onset and a reduced amplitude of postural responses in the paretic leg [51, 217]. Furthermore, the proximal and distal muscles of the paretic leg are co-activated, whilst the timing of muscle activation of the non-paretic leg is normal (i.e. in this leg, the sequence of activation is first in the distal and then in the proximal muscles) [65]. This asymmetric activation of the muscles of the two limbs might play a role in the increased fall risk of these patients [214]. The early postural response to stretch, corresponding to the monosynaptic stretch reflex, is increased [140], in keeping with the hyperexcitability of the tendon reflexes observed on physical examination. Conversely, the late responses to stretch, mediated by the spindle group II afferent fibers [187], are depressed [59, 50]. This suggests that the late responses are subject to a different descending control from that of the early responses [43].

Patients with stroke also show abnormalities in posturo-kinetic coordination. When they flex an arm while standing, APAs are delayed on both sides of the body [87]. Also the task of rising on tiptoes is not performed correctly. Healthy subjects activate the tibialis anterior before the soleus muscle in order to shift the body forwards before rising on tiptoes, in order to avoid falling backwards [146]. Instead, patients with stroke activate the tibialis anterior of the paretic side later than that of the non-paretic side. Hence, they do not have enough time to shift the body forwards, and imbalance may ensue as they attempt to rise on tiptoes [51].

5.5 Cerebellar Diseases

Postural control is affected to different extents, both qualitatively and quantitatively, following lesions in different regions of the cerebellum. In spite of the fact that lesions of the lateral hemisphere can induce severe ataxia of the upper limb, their effects on posture are negligible [47]. Instead, lesions of the vestibulocerebellum affect body orientation with respect to the vertical axis, and patients may show a slow drift away from the vertical [53]. Indeed, a selective relationship between body sway and vermian but not lateral cerebellar volume can be found [206, 216]. When the damage to the brainstem and the cerebellum is diffuse [176], as in the case of patients with spinocerebellar ataxia type 1, balance is globally impaired with a greater instability in the anterior-posterior than medial-lateral direction [135].

Ataxia may be the consequence of an excessive gain of inter-segmental postural reflexes no longer inhibited by the cerebellar output from the Purkinje cells [53]. In addition, the postural responses in cerebellar ataxia are not modulated in amplitude by the velocity of perturbation, and they are constantly enlarged with respect to those of healthy subjects [85]. Abnormal body sway may be absent in patients with eyes open, but asking patients to close their eyes and/or perturbing posture through an upward rotation of the supporting platform can provoke pathological sway [48].

It has long been known that posturo-kinetic coordination is lost in patients with cerebellar disease [9]. In fact, it seems that the cerebellum regulates the time course and modulates the amplitude of motor activity. When cerebellar patients are required to perform rapid arm flexion during stance, the timing and amplitude of the APAs are abnormal; in particular, muscle activity is hypermetric, i.e. its amplitude is excessively large [54, 56, 85]. During the task of rising on tiptoes, different aspects of the motor sequence are disturbed in cerebellar patients, suggesting that the cerebellum contributes to the regulation of amplitude and duration of both the anticipatory and the focal motor activity, as well as to the regulation of their temporal relationship [55]. The feed-forward control of motor activity is deranged in these patients not only when they perform a voluntary movement but also when they undergo predictable postural perturbations. In fact, at variance with healthy subjects, cerebellar patients do not scale postural responses to predictable perturbations of different amplitudes [85]. In general, defective coordination in these patients may be due to impaired anticipation of the muscle activations needed to compensate for body dynamics (see Marquer et al. [128], for a recent review).

5.6 Parkinson's Disease

Disturbances of postural control in Parkinson's disease (PD) are highly disabling motor symptoms since they are poorly controlled by dopaminergic therapy. After the onset of the disease, posture can soon become stooped, with hip and knee flexion [62]. In the late stages of the disease, when postural reactions begin to be impaired, patients also manifest postural instability (for a recent review of the underlying mechanisms of balance dysfunction in PD, see Rinalduzzi et al. [175]) with a consequent increased risk of falling [168]. Balance control can be affected asymmetrically in mild to moderate PD [74, 112]. Subtle balance impairments, such as an increased body sway, have been detected in 'de novo' patients [36, 122]. Patients with early PD are more unstable when required to stand with eyes closed than with eyes open, suggesting that a visual deprivation task could help identify subclinical postural instability [162]. However, it is not clear whether increased body sway during quiet stance is a predictor of postural instability in patients with PD, since increased sway is not always a hallmark of the most unstable patients [91, 183]. Indeed, static posturography seems to discriminate between PD fallers and healthy subjects but not between PD fallers and PD non-fallers [105, 144].

Patients with PD have increased postural stiffness [213], especially of the axial rather than the appendicular muscles [34, 132]. This increase is most prominent in the neck and is related to impaired performance during gross motor tasks, e.g. walking a figure of eight and performing a supine rolling task [70]. The smaller levodopa effect on axial than on appendicular tone suggests that axial and appendicular muscle tone is controlled by separate neural circuits [221].

When patients are required to lean forwards or backwards approaching their stability limits, it has been shown that the anterior-posterior limits are markedly reduced [182]. The main impairment is observed in the sagittal plane, in which ankle joint control plays a major role in postural stability [219]. The reduction of the stability limits is more marked in more severely affected patients [182] and when patients are in the off-phase rather than on-phase [123].

Part of the balance impairment observed in patients with PD could be related to impairment of proprioception or its integration with other sensory systems [1, 111, 208]. In this context, it should be emphasized that administration of levodopa and dopamine agonists in PD patients can induce a worsening of proprioception regarding joint position of the upper limb [159]. Contrary to what is seen in cerebellar patients [85], when patients with PD undergo platform perturbations delivered at different velocities and amplitudes, they are capable of scaling their postural responses [88]. However, their torque responses, especially to the largest displacement amplitudes, are smaller than those of healthy subjects [88]. Administration of levodopa, besides decreasing the tonic activity of leg muscles during quiet stance, further reduces these patients' torque and postural responses to perturbations. This results in less resistance to external displacements and thus faster center of mass displacements, leading to imbalance, suggesting a counterproductive effect of levodopa.

In keeping with the propensity of PD patients to lose their balance when perturbed in the backward direction, their postural responses to an upward tilt of the supporting platform are abnormal. In fact, responses in the stretched soleus muscle show increased amplitude but responses in the shortened tibialis anterior are reduced and/or delayed [14, 20, 19, 57, 191], thus provoking a backward displacement of the body. These changes are clearer in the off-phase [14] whilst amplitude of the responses in medicated patients in the on-phase is similar to that of healthy subjects [14, 183]. When patients undergo postural perturbations in different directions, the direction of maximum activation for each leg and trunk muscle is similar to that of healthy subjects, suggesting that the basal ganglia are not critical for generating postural responses. However, antagonist muscle activation occurs earlier and is larger in patients, resulting in coactivation and stiffening of the body [61]. These abnormalities may play a role in the increased fall risk of PD patients.

Patients with PD exhibit set-changing difficulties in many types of activities; for example, they have difficulty modulating balance responses to perturbations according to postural stabilization [39, 93, 183]. In particular, these patients' ability to decrease the amplitude of stretch-related tibialis anterior responses to downward tilt of the supporting platform when standing and holding onto a frame has been shown to be impaired [183]. This impairment correlates significantly with the severity of the disease but can already be present in early PD [145].

Patients with PD also show impaired coordination between posture and movement, the APAs being reduced [13, 49]. However, this might be an adaptive response. In fact, since voluntary movements in PD are performed at a slower speed, the consequent postural disturbances are smaller and it is possible that APAs are no longer required [177]. Patients show reduced magnitudes and delayed timing of the postural and voluntary components of the rise-to-toes task, as though they have difficulty turning off the postural, tibialis anterior component, and initiating the voluntary, gastrocnemius component [69]. Dopamine improves the relative timing, as well as the magnitude of both the postural and the voluntary components of the rise-to-toes task, suggesting that APAs are under dopaminergic control. Patients with PD show greater asymmetry in both anticipatory and reactive balance control compared with healthy subjects. This suggests that asymmetric reactive balance control during bipedal stance may share a common pathophysiology with asymmetries in APAs [24].

In order to test their APA capabilities, patients with PD have been studied with the use of a movable platform, delivering anterior-posterior predictable perturbations. This test does not help separate fallers from non-fallers when performed with eyes open [149]. However, with eyes closed, fallers show larger body displacements, a sign of impaired APA generation. Interestingly, body displacement increases with levodopa equivalent dose, indicating that medication tends to worsen balance capacity whilst improving patients' motricity [132].

Finally, the ability to adapt to predictable balance perturbations delivered by repeated anterior-posterior sinusoidal translations of the support base [201] has also been assessed in patients with PD [152]. It was shown that adaptation of tibialis anterior EMG activity occurs within the first few cycles of perturbation in healthy subjects, whereas it is slowed down in patients. Body displacement during perturbations was larger in patients than healthy subjects and also its adaptation was slowed down. These abnormalities may partly depend on the known impairment of set-shifting capabilities in PD [158, 169].

6 Conclusions

The postural control system is of the utmost importance in enabling people to interact with and navigate within the environment. Various diseases, affecting either the central or the peripheral nervous system, can affect the postural control system, thus preventing or severely impairing the capacity to produce adequate postural tone, and worsening postural stability and postural orientation. Growing research has shed light on the spinal and supraspinal pathways involved in the normal function of postural control, as well as the functional changes of these pathways in disease. The aim of these studies is not only to increase knowledge, but also to promote the design of new evidence-based rehabilitation strategies. These strategies are the main topic of other chapters in this book.

References

1. Abbruzzese G, Berardelli A. Sensorimotor integration in movement disorders. Mov Disord. 2003;18(3):231–40.
2. Ackermann H, Diener HC, Dichgans J. Changes in sensorimotor functions after spinal lesions evaluated in terms of long-latency reflexes. J Neurol Neurosurg Psychiatry. 1987;50(12):1647–54.
3. Agostini V, Sbrollini A, Cavallini C, Busso A, Pignata G, Knaflitz M. The role of central vision in posture: postural sway adaptations in Stargardt patients. Gait Posture. 2016;43:233–8.
4. Akbar U, Ashizawa T. Ataxia. Neurol Clin. 2015;33(1):225–48.
5. Allum JHJ, Keshner EA, Honegger F, Pfaltz CR. Indicators of the influence a peripheral vestibular deficit has on vestibulo-spinal reflex responses controlling postural stability. Acta Otolaryngol Stockh. 1988;106:252–63.
6. Allum JHJ, Pfaltz CR. Visual and vestibular contributions to pitch sway stabilization in the ankle muscles of normals and patients with bilateral vestibular deficit. Exp Brain Res. 1985;58:82–94.
7. Amblard B, Carblanc A. Role of foveal and peripheral visual information in maintenance of postural equilibrium in man. Percept Motor Skills. 1980;51:903–12.
8. van Asseldonk EH, Buurke JH, Bloem BR, Renzenbrink GJ, Nene AV, van der Helm FC, van der Kooij H. Disentangling the contribution of the paretic and non-paretic ankle to balance control in stroke patients. Exp Neurol. 2006;201(2):441–51.
9. Babinski J. De l'asynergie cérébelleuse. Rev Neurol. 1899;7:806–16.
10. Barbieri G, Gissot AS, Fouque F, Casillas JM, Pozzo T, Pérennou D. Does proprioception contribute to the sense of verticality? Exp Brain Res. 2008;185(4):545–52.
11. Barin K, Seitz CM, Welling DB. Effect of head orientation on the diagnostic sensitivity of posturography in patients with compensated unilateral lesions. Otolaryngol Head Neck Surg. 1992;106:355–62.
12. Barrett R, Hyde SA, Scott OM, Dubowitz V. Changes in center of gravity in boys with Duchenne muscular dystrophy. Muscle Nerve. 1988;11(11):1157–63.
13. Bazalgette F, Zattara M, Bathien N, Bouisset S, Rondot P. Postural adjustments associated with rapid voluntary arm movements in patients with Parkinson's disease. Adv Neurol. 1986;45:371–4.
14. Beckley DJ, Bloem BR, Remler MP. Impaired scaling of long latency postural reflexes in patients with Parkinson's disease. Electroenceph Clin Neurophysiol. 1993;89:22–8.

15. Behse F, Buchthal F, Carlsen F. Nerve biopsy and conduction studies in diabetic neuropathy. J Neurol Neurosurg Psychiatry. 1977;40:1072–82.
16. Black FO, Troost BT, Sufit RL, O'Leary DP. Quantitative analysis for the Romberg test (Posturography) in evaluation of peripheral vestibulopathy, acoustic neuroma and posterior fossa lesions. Neurology. 1978;28:409–10.
17. Black FO, Wall C III, Nashner LM. Effects of visual and support surface orientation references upon postural control in vestibular deficient subjects. Acta Otolaryngol. 1983;55:199–210.
18. Bles W, Vianney de Jong JMB, de Wit G. Somatosensory compensation for loss of labyrinthine function. Acta Oto-Laryngol. 1984;97:213–21.
19. Bloem BR, Beckley DJ, van Dijk JG, Zwinderman AH, Remler MP, Roos RAC. Influence of dopaminergic medication on automatic postural responses and balance impairment in Parkinson's disease. Mov Disord. 1996;11:509–21.
20. Bloem BR, Beckley DJ, Remler MP, Roos RA, van Dijk JG. Postural reflexes in Parkinson's disease during 'resist' and 'yield' tasks. J Neurol Sci. 1995;129(2):109–19.
21. Bohannon RW. Is the measurement of muscle strength appropriate in patients with brain lesions? A special communication. Phys Ther. 1989;69:225–36.
22. Bohannon RW, Leary KM. Standing balance and function over the course of acute rehabilitation. Arch Phys Med Rehabil. 1995;76:994–6.
23. Bolton DA. The role of the cerebral cortex in postural responses to externally induced perturbations. Neurosci Biobehav Rev. 2015;57:142–55 Review.
24. Boonstra TA, van Kordelaar J, Engelhart D, van Vugt JP, van der Kooij H. Asymmetries in reactive and anticipatory balance control are of similar magnitude in Parkinson's disease patients. Gait Posture. 2016;43:108–13.
25. Borel L, Lopez C, Péruch P, Lacour M. Vestibular syndrome: a change in internal spatial representation. Neurophysiol Clin. 2008;38:375–89.
26. Boucher P, Teasdale N, Courtemance R, Bard C, Fleury M. Postural stability in diabetic polyneuropathy. Diabetes Care. 1995;18:638–45.
27. Bouisset S, Zattara M. Biomechanical study of the programming of anticipatory postural adjustments associated with voluntary movement. J Biomech. 1987;20:735–42.
28. Bove M, Bonzano L, Trompetto C, Abbruzzese G, Schieppati M. The postural disorientation induced by neck muscle vibration subsides on lightly touching a stationary surface or aiming at it. Neuroscience. 2006;143:1095–103.
29. Bove M, Courtine G, Schieppati M. Neck muscle vibration and spatial orientation during stepping in place in humans. J Neurophysiol. 2002;88:2232–41.
30. Bove M, Nardone A, Schieppati M. Effects of leg muscle tendon vibration on group Ia and group II reflex responses to stance perturbation in humans. J Physiol (Lond). 2003;550: 617–30.
31. Buchanan JJ, Horak FB. Emergence of postural patterns as a function of vision and translation frequency. J Neurophysiol. 1999;81:2325–39.
32. Burke D, Hagbarth KE, Löfstedt L, Wallin BG. The responses of human muscle spindle endings to vibration of non-contracting muscles. J Physiol. 1976;261:673–93.
33. Butler AA, Lord SR, Rogers MW, Fitzpatrick RC. Muscle weakness impairs the proprioceptive control of human standing. Brain Res. 2008;1242:244–51.
34. Carpenter MG, Allum JH, Honegger F, Adkin AL, Bloem BR. Postural abnormalities to multidirectional stance perturbations in Parkinson's disease. J Neurol Neurosurg Psychiatry. 2004;75(9):1245–54.
35. Carpenter MG, Frank JS, Silcher CP, Peysar GW. The influence of postural threat on the control of upright stance. Exp Brain Res. 2001;138(2):210–8.
36. Chastan N, Debono B, Maltête D, Weber J. Discordance between measured postural instability and absence of clinical symptoms in Parkinson's disease patients in the early stages of the disease. Mov Disord. 2008;23(3):366–72.
37. Chiari L, Cappello A, Lenzi D, Della Croce U. An improved technique for the extraction of stochastic parameters from stabilograms. Gait Posture. 2000;12:225–34.

38. Chiba R, Takakusaki K, Ota J, Yozu A, Haga N. Human upright posture control models based on multisensory inputs; in fast and slow dynamics. Neurosci Res. 2016;104:96–104.
39. Chong RK, Horak FB, Woollacott MH. Parkinson's disease impairs the ability to change set quickly. J Neurol Sci. 2000;175(1):57–70.
40. Collins J, De Luca LC. Open-loop and closed-loop control of posture: a random-walk analysis of center-of-pressure trajectories. Exp Brain Res. 1993;95:308–18.
41. Colnaghi S, Honeine JL, Sozzi S, Schieppati M. Body sway increases after functional inactivation of the cerebellar vermis by cTBS. Cerebellum. 2016 Jan 16. [Epub ahead of print].
42. Cordo PJ, Nashner LM. Properties of postural adjustments associated with rapid arm movements. J Neurophysiol. 1982;47:287–302.
43. Corna S, Grasso M, Nardone A, Schieppati M. Selective depression of medium-latency leg and foot muscle responses to stretch by an alpha 2-agonist in humans. J Physiol. 1995;484(Pt 3):803–9.
44. Corna S, Nardone A, Prestinari A, Galante M, Grasso M, Schieppati M. Comparison of Cawthorne-Cooksey exercises and sinusoidal support surface translations to improve balance in patients with unilateral vestibular deficit. Arch Phys Med Rehabil. 2003;84(8): 1173–84.
45. Corna S, Tarantola J, Nardone A, Giordano A, Schieppati M. Standing on a continuously moving platform: is body inertia counteracted or exploited? Exp Brain Res. 1999;124: 331–41.
46. Dichgans J, Brandt T. Visual-vestibular interaction: effects on self-motion perception and postural control. Perception. Berlin: Springer; 1978. p. 755–804.
47. Dichgans J, Diener HC. Different forms of postural ataxia in patients with cerebellar diseases. Disorders of posture and gait. Amsterdam: Elsevier; 1986. p. 756–804.
48. Dichgans J, Mauritz KH, Allum JH, Brandt T. Postural sway in normals and atactic patients: analysis of the stabilising and destabilizing effects of vision. Agressologie. 1976;17(C Spec No): 15–24.
49. Dick JP, Rothwell JC, Berardelli A, Thompson PD, Gioux M, Benecke R, Day BL, Marsden CD. Associated postural adjustments in Parkinson's disease. J Neurol Neurosurg Psychiatry. 1986;49:1378–85.
50. Diener HC, Ackermann H, Dichgans J, Guschlbauer B. Medium- and long-latency responses to displacements of the ankle joint in patients with spinal and central lesions. Electroenceph Clin Neurophysiol. 1985;60:407–16.
51. Diener HC, Bacher M, Guschlbauer B, Thomas C, Dichgans J. The coordination of posture and voluntary movement in patients with hemiparesis. J Neurol. 1993;240:161–7.
52. Diener HC, Dichgans J. On the role of vestibular, visual and somatosensory information for dynamic postural control in humans. Prog Brain Res. 1988;76:252–61.
53. Diener HC, Dichgans J, Guschlbauer B, Bacher M. Quantification of postural sway in normals and patients with cerebellar diseases. Electroencephalogr Clin Neurophysiol. 1984;57:134–42.
54. Diener HC, Dichgans J, Guschlbauer B, Bacher M, Langerbach P. Disturbances of motor preparation in basal ganglia and cerebellar disorders. Prog Brain Res. 1989;80:481–8.
55. Diener HC, Dichgans J, Guschlbauer B, Bacher M, Rapp H, Klockgether T. The coordination of posture and voluntary movement in patients with cerebellar dysfunction. Mov Disord. 1992;7:14–22.
56. Diener HC, Dichgans J, Guschlbauer B, Bacher M, Rapp H, Langenbach P. Associated postural adjustments with body movement in normal subjects and patients with parkinsonism and cerebellar disease. Rev Neurol. 1990;146:555–63.
57. Diener HC, Horak FB, Stelmach G, Guschlbauer B, Dichgans J. Direction and amplitude precuing has no effect on automatic posture responses. Exp Brain Res. 1991;84:219–23.
58. Dieterich M, Brandt T. The bilateral central vestibular system: its pathways, functions, and disorders. Ann N Y Acad Sci. 2015;1343:10–26.

59. Dietz V. Human neuronal control of automatic functional movements: interaction between central programs and afferent input. Physiol Rev. 1992;72:33–69.
60. Dietz V, Mauritz K-H, Dichgans J. Body oscillations in balancing due to segmental stretch reflex activity. Exp Brain Res. 1980;40:89–95.
61. Dimitrova D, Horak FB, Nutt JG. Postural muscle responses to multidirectional translations in patients with Parkinson's disease. J Neurophysiol. 2004;91(1):489–501.
62. Doherty KM, van de Warrenburg BP, Peralta MC, Silveira-Moriyama L, Azulay JP, Gershanik OS, Bloem BR. Postural deformities in Parkinson's disease. Lancet Neurol. 2011;10(6):538–49.
63. Dyck PJ, Chance P, Lebo R, Carney JA. Hereditary motor and sensory neuropathies. In: Dyck PJ, Thomas PK, Griffin JW, Low PA, Poduslo JF, editors. Peripheral neuropathy. Philadelphia: WB Saunders Co.; 1993. p. 1094–136.
64. Eklund G. General features of vibration-induced effects on balance. Ups J Med Sci. 1972;77:112–24.
65. Di Fabio RP, Badke MB, Duncan PW. Adapting human postural reflexes following localized cerebrovascular lesion: analysis of bilateral long latency responses. Brain Res. 1986;363:257–64.
66. Fitzpatrick RC, McCloskey DI. Proprioceptive, visual and vestibular thresholds for perception of sway during standing in humans. J Physiol. 1994;478:173–86.
67. Fong KN, Chan CC, Au DK. Relationship of motor and cognitive abilities to functional performance in stroke rehabilitation. Brain Inj. 2001;15:443–53.
68. Fonteyn EM, Schmitz-Hübsch T, Verstappen CC, Baliko L, Bloem BR, Boesch S, Bunn L, Giunti P, Globas C, Klockgether T, Melegh B, Pandolfo M, Schöls L, Timmann D, van de Warrenburg BP. Prospective analysis of falls in dominant ataxias. Eur Neurol. 2013; 69(1):53–7.
69. Frank JS, Horak FB, Nutt J. Centrally initiated postural adjustments in parkinsonian patients on and off levodopa. J Neurophysiol. 2000;84(5):2440–8.
70. Franzén E, Paquette C, Gurfinkel VS, Cordo PJ, Nutt JG, Horak FB. Reduced performance in balance, walking and turning tasks is associated with increased neck tone in Parkinson's disease. Exp Neurol. 2009;219:430–8.
71. Friedly WG, Hallett M, Simon SR. Postural adjustments associated with rapid voluntary arm movements. 1. Electromyographic data. J Neurol Neurosurg Psychiat. 1984;47:611–22.
72. Fujiwara K, Toyama H, Kiyota T, Maeda K. Postural muscle activity patterns during standing at rest and on an oscillating floor. J Electromyogr Kinesiol. 2006;16:448–57.
73. Genthon N, Rougier P, Gissot AS, Froger J, Pélissier J, Pérennou D. Contribution of each lower limb to upright standing in stroke patients. Stroke. 2008;39(6):1793–9.
74. Geurts AC, Boonstra TA, Voermans NC, Diender MG, Weerdesteyn V, Bloem BR. Assessment of postural asymmetry in mild to moderate Parkinson's disease. Gait Posture. 2011;33(1):143–5.
75. Giacomini PG, Bruno E, Monticone G, Di Girolamo S, Magrini A, Parisi L, Menzinger G, Uccioli L. Postural rearrangement in IDDM patients with peripheral neuropathy. Diabetes Care. 1996;19:372–4.
76. Godi M, Nardone A, Schieppati M. Curved walking in hemiparetic patients. J Rehabil Med. 2010;42(9):858–65.
77. Green AM, Angelaki DE. Internal models and neural computation in the vestibular system. Exp Brain Res. 2010;200(3–4):197–222.
78. Grey MJ, Ladouceur M, Andersen JB, Nielsen JB, Sinkjaer T. Group II muscle afferents probably contribute to the medium latency soleus stretch reflex during walking in humans. J Physiol. 2001;534(Pt 3):925–33.
79. Gurfinkel VS. Physical foundations of stabilography. Aggressologie. 1973;20:9–14.
80. Gurfinkel VS, Ivanenko YP, Levik YS, Babakova IA. Kinesthetic reference for human orthograde posture. Neuroscience. 1995;68:229–43.

81. Gurfinkel VS, Lipshits MI, Mori S, Popov KE. Interaction of the central program for postural control and inherent reflex mechanisms such as the stretch reflex during standing. Aggressologie. 1983;24:63–4.
82. Hansen PD, Woollacott MH, Debu B. Postural responses to changing task conditions. Exp Brain Res. 1988;73:627–36.
83. Hlavacka F, Mergner T, Schweigart G. Interaction of vestibular and proprioceptive inputs for human self-motion perception. Neurosci Lett. 1992;138(1):161–4.
84. Hoch MC, Russell DM. Plantar cooling does not affect standing balance: a systematic review and meta-analysis. Gait Posture. 2016;43:1–8.
85. Horak FB, Diener HC. Cerebellar control of postural scaling and central set in stance. J Neurophysiol. 1994;72(2):479–93.
86. Horak FB, Diener HC, Nashner LM. Influence of central set on human postural responses. J Neurophysiol. 1989;62(4):841–53.
87. Horak FB, Esselman P, Anderson ME, Lynch MK. The effects of movement velocity, mass displaced, and task certainty on postural adjustments made by normal and hemiplegic individuals. J Neurol Neurosurg Psychiatry. 1984;47:1020–8.
88. Horak FB, Frank J, Nutt J. Effects of dopamine on postural control in parkinsonian subjects: scaling, set, and tone. J Neurophysiol. 1996;75:2380–96.
89. Horak FB, Hlavacka F. Somatosensory loss increases vestibulospinal sensitivity. J Neurophysiol. 2001;86:575–85.
90. Horak FB, Moore SP. The effects of prior learning on human postural responses. Gait Posture. 1993;1:203–10.
91. Horak FB, Nashner LM. Central programming of postural movements: adaptation to altered support-surface configurations. J Neurophysiol. 1986;55(6):1369–81.
92. Horak FB, Nashner LM, Diener HC. Postural strategies associated with somatosensory and vestibular loss. Exp Brain Res. 1990;82:167–77.
93. Horak FB, Nutt JG, Nashner LM. Postural inflexibility in parkinsonian subjects. J Neurol Sci. 1992;111(1):46–58.
94. Horak FB, Macpherson JM. Postural orientation and equilibrium. In: Smith JL, editors. Handbook of physiology: section 12. Exercise: regulation and integration of multiple systems. Oxford: Oxford University Press; 1996. pp. 255–92.
95. Horslen BC, Dakin CJ, Inglis JT, Blouin JS, Carpenter MG. Modulation of human vestibular reflexes with increased postural threat. J Physiol. 2014;592(16):3671–85.
96. Horslen BC, Murnaghan CD, Inglis JT, Chua R, Carpenter MG. Effects of postural threat on spinal stretch reflexes: evidence for increased muscle spindle sensitivity? J Neurophysiol. 2013;110(4):899–906.
97. Houdijk H, Fickert R, van Velzen J, van Bennekom C. The energy cost for balance control during upright standing. Gait Posture. 2009;30(2):150–4.
98. Inglis JT, Horak FB, Shupert CL, Jones-Rycewicz C. The importance of somatosensory information in triggering and scaling automatic postural responses in humans. Exp Brain Res. 1994;101(1):159–64.
99. Inglis JT, Kennedy PM, Wells C, Chua R. The role of cutaneous receptors in the foot. Adv Exp Med Biol. 2002;508:111–7.
100. Ishii F, Matsukawa N, Horiba M, Yamanaka T, Hattori M, Wada I, Ojika K. Impaired ability to shift weight onto the non-paretic leg in right-cortical brain-damaged patients. Clin Neurol Neurosurg. 2010;112(5):406–12.
101. Jacobs JV, Horak FB. Cortical control of postural responses. J Neural Transm (Vienna). 2007;114(10):1339–48.
102. Jagdhane S, Kanekar N, Aruin AS. The effect of a four-week balance training program on anticipatory postural adjustments in older adults: a pilot feasibility study. Curr Aging Sci; 2016 Apr 13. [Epub ahead of print].
103. Jami L. Functional properties of the Golgi tendon organs. Arch Int Physiol Biochim. 1988;96(4):A363–78 Review.

104. Jeka JJ, Ribeiro P, Oie K, Lackner JR. The structure of somatosensory information for human postural control. Mot Control. 1998;2:13–33.
105. Johnson L, James I, Rodrigues J, Stell R, Thickbroom G, Mastaglia F. Clinical and posturographic correlates of falling in Parkinson's disease. Mov Disord. 2013;28(9):1250–6.
106. Kanekar N, Aruin AS. Improvement of anticipatory postural adjustments for balance control: effect of a single training session. J Electromyogr Kinesiol. 2015;25(2):400–5.
107. Kavounoudias A, Gilhodes JC, Roll R, Roll JP. From balance regulation to body orientation: two goals for muscle proprioceptive information processing? Exp Brain Res. 1999;124(1): 80–8.
108. Kavounoudias A, Roll R, Roll JP. The plantar sole is a 'dynamometric map' for human balance control. Neuroreport. 1998;9:3247–52.
109. Keenan MA, Perry J, Jordan C. Factors affecting balance and ambulation following stroke. Clin Orthop 1984;(182):165–71.
110. Kleiber M, Horstmann GA, Dietz V. Body sway stabilization of human posture. Acta Otolaryngol Stockh. 1990;110:168–74.
111. Konczak J, Corcos DM, Horak F, Poizner H, Shapiro M, Tuite P, Volkmann J, Maschke M. Proprioception and motor control in Parkinson's disease. J Mot Behav. 2009;41(6):543–52 Review.
112. van der Kooij H, van Asseldonk EH, Geelen J, van Vugt JP, Bloem BR. Detecting asymmetries in balance control with system identification: first experimental results from Parkinson patients. J Neural Transm. 2007;114(10):1333–7.
113. van der Kooij H, de Vlugt E. Postural responses evoked by platform perturbations are dominated by continuous feedback. J Neurophysiol. 2007;98(2):730–43.
114. Lajoie Y, Teasdale N, Bard C, Fleury M. Attentional demands for static and dynamic equilibrium. Exp Brain Res. 1993;97:139–44.
115. van der Linden MH, van der Linden SC, Hendricks HT, van Engelen BG, Geurts AC. Postural instability in Charcot-Marie-Tooth type 1A patients is strongly associated with reduced somatosensation. Gait Posture. 2010;31(4):483–8.
116. Lipshits MI, Mauritz K, Popov KE. Quantitative analysis of anticipatory postural components of a complex voluntary movement. Fiziol Chelov. 1981;7:411–9.
117. Liu WY, Lin YH, Lien HY, Hsu LY, Tsai YJ, Liao CF, Tang SF. Within-session acquisition of anticipatory postural adjustments during forward reaching task. Clin Neurol Neurosurg. 2015;129(Suppl 1):S53–7.
118. Lord SR, Allen GM, Williams P, Gandevia SC. Risk of falling: predictors based on reduced strength in persons previously affected by polio. Arch Phys Med Rehabil. 2002;83(6): 757–63.
119. Lord SR, Clark RD, Webster IW. Visual acuity and contrast sensitivity in relation to falls in an elderly population. Age Ageing. 1991;20(3):175–81.
120. Lund S. Postural effects of neck muscle vibration in man. Experientia. 1980;36:1398.
121. Macefield VG. Physiological characteristics of low-threshold mechanoreceptors in joints, muscle and skin in human subjects. Clin Exp Pharmacol Physiol. 2005;32(1–2):135–44 Review.
122. Mancini M, Horak FB, Zampieri C, Carlson-Kuhta P, Nutt JG, Chiari L. Trunk accelerometry reveals postural instability in untreated Parkinson's disease. Parkinsonism Relat Disord. 2011;17(7):557–62.
123. Mancini M, Rocchi L, Horak FB, Chiari L. Effects of Parkinson's disease and levodopa on functional limits of stability. Clin Biomech. 2008;23:450–8.
124. Manor B, Hu K, Zhao P, Selim M, Alsop D, Novak P, Lipsitz L, Novak V. Altered control of postural sway following cerebral infarction: a cross-sectional analysis. Neurology. 2010;74(6):458–64.
125. Manzoni D. The cerebellum and sensorimotor coupling: looking at the problem from the perspective of vestibular reflexes. Cerebellum. 2007;6(1):24–37.
126. Marigold DS, Eng JJ. The relationship of asymmetric weight-bearing with postural sway and visual reliance in stroke. Gait Posture. 2006;23(2):249–55.

127. Marigold DS, Eng JJ, Tokuno CD, Donnelly CA. Contribution of muscle strength and integration of afferent input to postural instability in persons with stroke. Neurorehabil Neural Repair. 2004;18:222–9.
128. Marquer A, Barbieri G, Pérennou D. The assessment and treatment of postural disorders in cerebellar ataxia: a systematic review. Ann Phys Rehabil Med. 2014;57(2):67–78.
129. Marsden JF, Playford DE, Day BL. The vestibular control of balance after stroke. J Neurol Neurosurg Psychiatry. 2005;76(5):670–8.
130. Martinelli AR, Coelho DB, Magalhães FH, Kohn AF, Teixeira LA. Light touch modulates balance recovery following perturbation: from fast response to stance restabilization. Exp Brain Res. 2015;233(5):1399–408.
131. Massion J. Movement, posture and equilibrium: interaction and coordination. Prog Neurobiol. 1992;38(1):35–56 Review.
132. Maurer C, Mergner T, Xie J, Faist M, Pollak P, Lücking CH. Effect of chronic bilateral subthalamic nucleus (STN) stimulation on postural control in Parkinson's disease. Brain. 2003;126(Pt 5):1146–63.
133. Mauritz KH, Dietz V. Characteristics of postural instability induced by ischemic blocking of leg afferents. Exp Brain Res. 1980;38:117–9.
134. Mildren RL, Strzalkowski ND, Bent LR. Foot sole skin vibration perceptual thresholds are elevated in a standing posture compared to sitting. Gait Posture. 2016;43:87–92.
135. Mohan G, Pal PK, Sendhil KR, Thennarasu K, Usha BR. Quantitative evaluation of balance in patients with spinocerebellar ataxia type 1: a case control study. Parkinsonism Relat Disord. 2009;15:435–9.
136. Morasso PG, Schieppati M. Can muscle stiffness alone stabilize upright standing? J Neurophysiol. 1999;83:1622–6.
137. Mouchnino L, Blouin J. When standing on a moving support, cutaneous inputs provide sufficient information to plan the anticipatory postural adjustments for gait initiation. PLoS ONE. 2013;8(2):e55081.
138. Naranjo EN, Allum JH, Inglis JT, Carpenter MG. Increased gain of vestibulospinal potentials evoked in neck and leg muscles when standing under height-induced postural threat. Neuroscience. 2015;293:45–54.
139. Nardone A, Galante M, Grasso M, Schieppati M. Stance ataxia and delayed leg muscle responses to postural perturbations in cervical spondylotic myelopathy. J Rehab Med. 2008;40:539–47.
140. Nardone A, Galante M, Lucas B, Schieppati M. Stance control is not affected by paresis and reflex hyperexcitability: the case of spastic patients. J Neurol Neurosurg Psychiatry. 2001;70:635–43.
141. Nardone A, Galante M, Pareyson D, Schieppati M. Balance control in sensory neuron disease. Clin Neurophysiol. 2007;118:538–50.
142. Nardone A, Godi M, Grasso M, Guglielmetti S, Schieppati M. Stabilometry is a predictor of gait performance in chronic hemiparetic stroke patients. Gait Posture. 2009;30:5–10.
143. Nardone A, Grasso M, Giordano A, Schieppati M. Influence of body height on the latency of leg and foot muscle EMG responses to perturbation of stance in humans. Neurosci Lett. 1996;206:89–92.
144. Nardone A, Grasso M, Schieppati M. Balance control in peripheral neuropathy: are patients equally unstable under static and dynamic conditions? Gait Posture. 2006;23:364–73.
145. Nardone A, Pasetti C, Schieppati M. Spinal and supraspinal stretch responses of postural muscles in early Parkinsonian patients. Exp Neurol. 2012;237(2):407–17.
146. Nardone A, Schieppati M. Postural adjustments associated with voluntary contraction of leg muscles in standing man. Exp Brain Res. 1988;69:469–80.
147. Nardone A, Schieppati M. Medium-latency response to muscle stretch in human lower limb: estimation of conduction velocity of group II fibres and central delay. Neurosci Lett. 1998;249:29–32.
148. Nardone A, Schieppati M. Group II spindle fibres and afferent control of stance. Clues from diabetic neuropathy. Clin Neurophysiol. 2004;115:779–89.

149. Nardone A, Schieppati M. Balance in Parkinson's disease under static and dynamic conditions. Mov Disord. 2006;21:1515–20.
150. Nardone A, Tarantola J, Miscio G, Pisano F, Schenone A, Schieppati M. Loss of large diameter spindle afferent fibres is not detrimental to the control of body sway during upright stance: evidence from neuropathy. Exp Brain Res. 2000;135:155–62.
151. Nardone A, Turcato AM, Schieppati M. Effects of balance and gait rehabilitation in cerebellar disease of vascular or degenerative origin. Restor Neurol Neurosci. 2014;32(2): 233–45.
152. Nardone A, Schieppati M, Arcolin I, Godi M, Grasso M, Guglielmetti S, Morlino P. Continuous and predictable perturbation of balance in Parkinson's disease: a way of testing reflex and anticipatory responses of leg muscles and of training balance. Congress on Neurorehabilitation and Neural Repair, Maastricht, The Netherlands, pp. 126–7, 21–22 May 2015.
153. Nardone A, Schieppati M, Crisafulli O, Sozzi S. Adaptation of reflex and anticipatory leg muscle activity during continuous and predictable perturbation of balance. Congress on Neurorehabilitation and Neural Repair, Maastricht, The Netherlands, pp. 119–120, 21–22 May 2015.
154. Nashner LM, Black FO, Wall C III. Adaptation to altered support and visual conditions during stance: patients with vestibular deficits. J Neurosci. 1982;2:536–44.
155. Norré ME. Sensory interaction testing in platform posturography. J Laryngol Otol. 1993;107:496–501.
156. Nouillot P, Bouisset S, Do MC. Do fast voluntary movements necessitate anticipatory postural adjustments even if equilibrium is unstable? Neurosci Lett. 1992;147:1–4.
157. De Nunzio AM, Nardone A, Schieppati M. Head stabilization on a continuously oscillating platform: the effect of a proprioceptive disturbance on the balancing strategy. Exp Brain Res. 2005;165:261–72.
158. De Nunzio AM, Schieppati M. Time to reconfigure balancing behaviour in man: changing visual condition while riding a continuously moving platform. Exp Brain Res. 2007;178: 18–36.
159. O'Suilleabhain P, Bullard J, Dewey RB. Proprioception in Parkinson's disease is acutely depressed by dopaminergic medications. J Neurol Neurosurg Psychiatry. 2001;71(5): 607–10.
160. Pahapill PA, Lozano AM. The physiology of the pedunculopontine nucleus. Brain. 2000;123:1767–83.
161. Panosian MS, Paige GD. Nystagmus and postural instability after headshake in patients with vestibular dysfunction. Otolaryngol Head Neck Surg. 1995;112:399–404.
162. Panyakaew P, Anan C, Bhidayasiri R. Visual deprivation elicits subclinical postural inflexibilities in early Parkinson's disease. J Neurol Sci. 2015;349(1–2):214–9.
163. Park DJ. Effect of visual stimulus using central and peripheral visual field on postural control of normal subjects. J Phys Ther Sci. 2016;28(6):1769–71.
164. Pasma JH, Engelhart D, Schouten AC, van der Kooij H, Maier AB, Meskers CG. Impaired standing balance: the clinical need for closing the loop. Neuroscience. 2014;16(267):157–65.
165. Perry SD, McIlroy WE, Maki BE. The role of plantar cutaneous mechanoreceptors in the control of compensatory stepping reactions evoked by unpredictable, multi-directional perturbation. Brain Res. 2000;877:401–6.
166. Peterka RJ. Sensorimotor integration in human postural control. J Neurophysiol. 2002; 88(3):1097–118.
167. Pettorossi VE, Schieppati M. Neck proprioception shapes body orientation and perception of motion. Front Hum Neurosci. 2014;8:895.
168. Pickering RM, Grimbergen YA, Rigney U, Ashburn A, Mazibrada G, Wood B, Gray P, Kerr G, Bloem BR. A meta-analysis of six prospective studies of falling in Parkinson's disease. Mov Disord. 2007;22(13):1892–900.
169. Prochazka A. Sensorimotor gain control: a basic strategy of motor systems? Prog Neurobiol. 1989;33(4):281–307.

170. Proske U, Gandevia SC. The proprioceptive senses: their roles in signaling body shape, body position and movement, and muscle force. Physiol Rev. 2012;92(4):1651–97.
171. Proske U, Gregory JE. Signalling properties of muscle spindles and tendon organs. Adv Exp Med Biol. 2002;508:5–12 Review.
172. Pérennou D, Piscicelli C, Barbieri G, Jaeger M, Marquer A, Barra J. Measuring verticality perception after stroke: why and how? Neurophysiol Clin. 2014;44(1):25–32.
173. Rao N, Nashner L, Aruin AS. Perceived body position in standing individuals with recent stroke. Clin Neurophysiol. 2010;121(11):1934–8.
174. Redfern MS, Furman JM. Postural sway of patients with vestibular disorders during optic flow. J Vest Res. 1994;4:221–30.
175. Rinalduzzi S, Trompetto C, Marinelli L, Alibardi A, Missori P, Fattapposta F, Pierelli F, Currà A. Balance dysfunction in Parkinson's disease. Biomed Res Int. 2015;2015:434683.
176. Robitaille Y, Lopes-Cendes I, Becher M, Rouleau G, Clark AW. The neuropathology of CAG repeat diseases: review and update of genetic and molecular features. Brain Pathol. 1997;7:901–26.
177. Rogers MW, Kukulka CG, Soderberg GL. Postural adjustments preceding rapid arm movements in parkinsonian patients. Neurosci Lett. 1987;75:246–51.
178. Roll JP, Vedel JP, Ribot E. Alteration of proprioceptive messages induced by tendon vibration in man: a microneurographic study. Exp Brain Res. 1989;76:213–22.
179. Runge CF, Shupert CL, Horak FB, Zajac FE. Ankle and hip postural strategies defined by joint torques. Gait Posture. 1999;10(2):161–70.
180. Saito H, Yamanaka M, Kasahara S, Fukushima J. Relationship between improvements in motor performance and changes in anticipatory postural adjustments during whole-body reaching training. Hum Mov Sci. 2014;37:69–86.
181. Schieppati M, Giordano A, Nardone A. Variability in a dynamic postural task attests ample flexibility in balance control mechanisms. Exp Brain Res. 2002;144:200–10.
182. Schieppati M, Hugon M, Grasso M, Nardone A, Galante M. The limits of equilibrium in young and elderly normal subjects and in parkinsonians. Electroencephalogr Clin Neurophysiol. 1994;93:286–98.
183. Schieppati M, Nardone A. Free and supported stance in Parkinson's disease. The effect of posture and 'postural set' on leg muscle responses to peturbation, and its relation to the severity of the disease. Brain. 1991;114:1227–44.
184. Schieppati M, Nardone A. Time-course of 'set'-related changes in muscle responses to stance perturbation in humans. J Physiol (Lond). 1995;487:787–96.
185. Schieppati M, Nardone A. Medium-latency stretch reflexes of foot and leg muscles analyzed by cooling the lower limb in standing humans. J Physiol (Lond). 1997;503:691–8.
186. Schieppati M, Nardone A, Siliotto R, Grasso M. Early and late stretch responses of human foot muscles induced by perturbation of stance. Exp Brain Res. 1995;105:411–22.
187. Schieppati M, Nardone A. Group II spindle afferent fibers in humans: their possible role in the reflex control of stance. In: Binder MD, editors. Progress in brain research, vol. 123. Amsterdam. Elsevier Science BV; 1999. pp. 461–72.
188. Schmid M, Bottaro A, Sozzi S, Schieppati M. Adaptation to continuous perturbation of balance: progressive reduction of postural muscle activity with invariant or increasing oscillations of the center of mass depending on perturbation frequency and vision conditions. Hum Mov Sci. 2011;30:262–78.
189. Schmid M, Casabianca L, Bottaro A, Schieppati M. Graded changes in balancing behavior as a function of visual acuity. Neuroscience. 2008;153:1079–91.
190. Schmid M, Nardone A, De Nunzio AM, Schmid M, Schieppati M. Equilibrium during static and dynamic tasks in blind subjects: no evidence of cross-modal plasticity. Brain. 2007;130:2097–107.
191. Scholz E, Diener HC, Noth J, Friedemann HH, Dichgans J, Bacher M. Medium and long latency EMG responses in leg muscles: Parkinson's disease. J Neurol Neurosurg Psychiat. 1987;50:66–70.

192. Sereda M, Griffiths I, Puhlhofer A, Stewart H, Rossner MJ, Zimmerman F, Magyar JP, Schneider A, Hund E, Meinck HM, Suter U, Nave KA. A transgenic rat model of Charcot-Marie-Tooth disease. Neuron. 1996;16:1049–60.
193. Sghirlanzoni A, Pareyson D, Lauria G. Sensory neuron diseases. Lancet Neurol. 2005; 4(6):349–61.
194. Shaffer SW, Harrison AL. Aging of the somatosensory system: a translational perspective. Phys Ther. 2007;87(2):193–207.
195. Shumway-Cook A, Woollacott MH, Kerns KA, Baldwin M. The effects of two types of cognitive tasks on postural stability in older adults with and without a history of falls. J Gerontol. 1997;52:M232–40.
196. Simmons RW, Richardson C, Pozos R. Postural stability of diabetic patients with and without cutaneous sensory deficit in the foot. Diab Res Clin Pract. 1997;36:153–60.
197. Slijper H, Latash ML. The effects of instability and additional hand support on anticipatory postural adjustments in leg, trunk, and arm muscles during standing. Exp Brain Res. 2000;135:81–93.
198. Slijper H, Latash ML. The effects of muscle vibration on anticipatory postural adjustments. Brain Res. 2004;1015(1–2):57–72.
199. Soames RW, Atha J. The role of the antigravity musculature during quiet standing in man. Eur J Appl Physiol Occup Physiol. 1981;47:159–67.
200. Sozzi S, Do MC, Monti A, Schieppati M. Sensorimotor integration during stance: processing time of active or passive addition or withdrawal of visual or haptic information. Neuroscience. 2012;14(212):59–76.
201. Sozzi S, Nardone A, Schieppati M. Calibration of the leg muscle responses elicited by predictable perturbations of stance and the effect of vision. Front Hum Neurosci. 2016; 30(10):419.
202. St George RJ, Fitzpatrick RC. The sense of self-motion, orientation and balance explored by vestibular stimulation. J Physiol. 2011;589(Pt 4):807–13.
203. Straube A, Krafczyk S, Paulus W, Brandt T. Dependence of visual stabilization of postural sway on the cortical magnification factor of restricted visual fields. Exp Brain Res. 1994;99:501–6.
204. Straube A, Paulus W, Brandt T. Influence of visual blur on object-motion detection, self-motion detection and postural balance. Behav Brain Res. 1990;40(1):1–6.
205. Strupp M, Arbusow V, Pereira CB, Dieterich M, Brandt T. Subjective straight-ahead during neck muscle vibration: effect of ageing. Neuroreport. 1999;10:3191–4.
206. Sullivan EV, Rose J, Pfefferbaum A. Effect of vision, touch and stance on cerebellar vermian-related sway and tremor: a quantitative physiological and MRI study. Cereb Cortex. 2006;16:1077–86.
207. Synofzik M, Ilg W. Motor training in degenerative spinocerebellar disease: ataxia-specific improvements by intensive physiotherapy and exergames. Biomed Res Int. 2014;2014: 583507.
208. Tagliabue M, Ferrigno G, Horak F. Effects of Parkinson's disease on proprioceptive control of posture and reaching while standing. Neuroscience. 2009;158(4):1206–14.
209. Takakusaki K, Chiba R, Nozu T, Okumura T. Brainstem control of locomotion and muscle tone with special reference to the role of the mesopontine tegmentum and medullary reticulospinal systems. J Neural Transm (Vienna). 2016;123(7):695–729.
210. Taylor JA, Ivry RB. Cerebellar and prefrontal cortex contributions to adaptation, strategies, and reinforcement learning. Prog Brain Res. 2014;210:217–53.
211. Teasdale N, Bard C, La Rue J, Fleury M. On the cognitive penetrability of posture control. Exp Aging Res. 1993;19:1–13.
212. Teasdale N, Simoneau M. Attentional demands for postural control: the effects of aging and sensory reintegration. Gait Posture. 2001;14:203–10.
213. Termoz N, Halliday SE, Winter DA, Frank JS, Patla AE, Prince F. The control of upright stance in young, elderly and persons with Parkinson's disease. Gait Posture. 2008;27(3): 463–70.

214. Thurman DJ, Stevens JA, Rao JK. Quality Standards Subcommittee of the American Academy of Neurology. Practice parameter: assessing patients in a neurology practice for risk of falls (an evidence-based review): report of the quality standards subcommittee of the American Academy of Neurology. Neurology. 2008;70(6):473–9 Review.
215. Treleaven J. Sensorimotor disturbances in neck disorders affecting postural stability, head and eye movement control. Man Ther. 2008;13(1):2–11.
216. Vassar RL, Rose J. Motor systems and postural instability. Handb Clin Neurol. 2014;125:237–51.
217. Wing AM, Goodrich S, Virji-Babul N, Jenner JR, Clapp S. The evaluation of balance in hemiparetic stroke patients using lateral forces applied to the hip. Arch Phys Med Rehabil. 1993;74:292–9.
218. Winter DA. Sagittal plane balance and posture in human walking. IEEE Eng Med Biol Mag. 1987;6(3):8–11.
219. Winter DA, Prince FR, Frank JS, Powell CO, Zabjek KF. Unified theory regarding A/P and M/L balance in quiet stance. J Neurophysiol. 1996;75(6):2334–43.
220. Woodhull AM, Maltrud K, Mello BL. Alignment of the human body in standing. Eur J Appl Physiol Occup Physiol. 1985;54:109–15.
221. Wright WG, Gurfinkel VS, Nutt J, Horak FB, Cordo PJ. Axial hypertonicity in Parkinson's disease: direct measurements of trunk and hip torque. Exp Neurol. 2007;208(1):38–46.

RCT Design for the Assessment of Rehabilitation Treatments: The Case Study of Post-stroke Rehabilitation

Simona Ferrante, Marta Gandolla, Elisabetta Peri, Emilia Ambrosini and Alessandra Pedrocchi

1 Introduction

All of us, in our daily lives, perhaps fail to appreciate properly the extraordinary equilibrium that exists between our body and mind, which harmoniously combine to shape who we are. But as soon as we are affected by any disorder that modifies our daily life and habits, we realize just what a gift we had, and we want it back. This is why rehabilitation is so important.

Rehabilitation is the process of helping an individual to regain the highest possible level of functioning, independence and quality of life. The role of neuromotor rehabilitation, in particular, is increasingly recognized. Hence, growing importance is being attached to the evaluation of rehabilitation treatments in the panorama of the available treatment options. Thanks to ongoing technological progress, the scientific and medical communities are now able to propose a wide variety of devices, treatments and integrated solutions for tackling disease. However, for patients, the important questions before starting a specific rehabilitation treatment are always the same: Will I benefit functionally from this treatment? Is it the best treatment I can get? Will I go back to how I was before? Indeed, from a patient's point of view, improvement is not primarily a change in specific parameters, but corresponds,

S. Ferrante (✉) · M. Gandolla · E. Peri · E. Ambrosini · A. Pedrocchi
NearLab, Department of Electronic, Information and Bioengineering,
Politecnico Di Milano, Milan, Italy
e-mail: simona.ferrante@polimi.it

E. Ambrosini
Physical Medicine and Rehabilitation Unit, Scientific Institute of Lissone,
S. Maugeri Foundation, IRCCS, Lissone, Italy

G. Sandrini et al. (eds.), *Advanced Technologies for the Rehabilitation of Gait and Balance Disorders*, Biosystems & Biorobotics 19,
https://doi.org/10.1007/978-3-319-72736-3_2

rather, to improvements in functional performance, daily life activities and independence, and they want to be sure that they get the best treatment option available. It is therefore mandatory to be able to answer their questions.

The scientific community recognizes the need for classification of the level of reliability of healthcare information, in order to formulate recommendations for clinical practice. Indeed, all physicians are required to find the highest level of evidence to answer any specific clinical question. The level of evidence is strongly related to the study design, and it is usually represented by the so-called pyramid of evidence (see Fig. 1).

What the pyramid suggests is that not all evidence or information is necessarily equivalent. Systematic reviews of randomized controlled trials (RCTs) are the highest source of stable and generalizable information. They were inspired in the 1980s by Archie Cochrane, who proposed gathering information from works that, if considered singly, failed to provide full conclusions for clinical practice. Often, meta-analysis is used to statistically combine data from several studies, to increase the power and the precision of the single studies' findings. Moving down the pyramid towards the base, we find RCTs. These are widely recognized as the gold standard for drawing statistically acceptable conclusions; they are studies carried out, applying a rigorous methodology, to test the efficacy of a given treatment in a well-defined target population. Other study types, which may be found towards the base of the pyramid of clinical evidence, are accepted in the scientific community, even though the lack of clear and codified methodology often makes the results, although interesting, poorly generalizable.

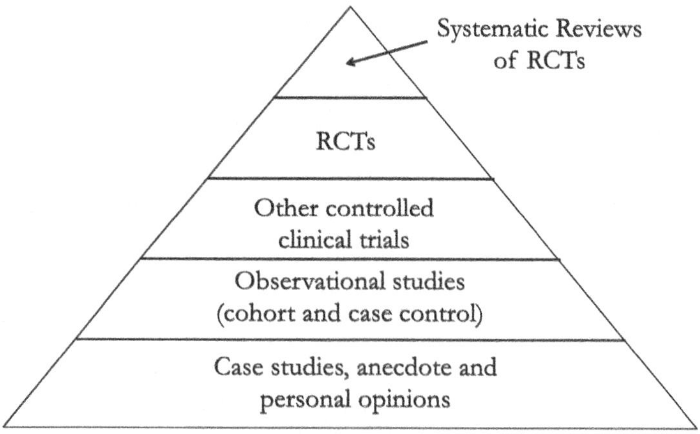

Fig. 1 Pyramid of evidence based on study design: the more systematic the observations the better the quality of the evidence

1.1 What Are RCTs?

Randomized controlled trials are studies carried out, applying a rigorous methodology, to test the efficacy of a given treatment in a well-defined target human population. The key features of an RCT are indicated by its name: the term *randomized* refers to the fact that participants are allocated to one group or another by randomization; *controlled* refers to the fact that the new treatment is given to a group of patients (called the experimental group), while another treatment, often the one currently most widely used, is given to another group of patients (called the control group). RCTs, as we know them today, are relatively recent, dating back to the time of the Second World War, with only isolated attempts made before then [12]. The precision and thoroughness of the methodology are crucially important aspects of RCTs, which, over the past 50 years, have become established as the primary and, in many instances, only acceptable source of evidence for establishing the efficacy of new treatments [12]. As stated by the Oxford Centre for Evidence-Based Medicine, Level I evidence for a given treatment efficacy is assigned if it is supported by multiple RCTs with a statistically significant number of subjects enrolled (www.cebm.net/ocebm-levels-of-evidence). Accordingly, the findings of a well-designed RCT can influence decision-making processes in healthcare, the development of international evidence-based clinical pathway guidelines, and, ultimately, the formulation of national public health policies.

With this in mind, the Consolidated Standards of Reporting Trials (CONSORT) group was created to alleviate the problems arising from inadequate reporting of RCTs (www.consort-statement.org). CONSORT published its first guidelines in 1996 [4], and these were subsequently revised in 2001 [1, 15] and again in 2010 [13]. The scientific community is currently striving to promote convergence among trials, to ensure that they are all well designed and well reported, but there still is a long way to go.

Hopewell and colleagues [9], examined the PubMed-indexed RCTs identified in the database for the years 2000 and 2006 in order to assess whether the quality of reporting improved after publication of the (CONSORT) Statement in 2001. Although they found a general improvement in the presentation of important characteristics and methodological details of RCTs, the quality of reporting was still not considered acceptable. In another study, analyzing only parallel-group design RCTs published in 2001–2010 and in 2011–2014, it was found that 88% and 94% respectively were pharmacological RCTs, meaning that non-pharmacological trials accounted for 12% and 6%; what is more, only 0% and 3% were non-pharmacological trials focusing on the use of devices, meaning that studies dealing with the use of devices had a total incidence of just 1% [18]. With advancing technology now contributing more and more to the development of rehabilitation approaches, there is clearly a need to design and perform rigorous RCTs to clarify the value of new technologies in this setting.

1.2 RCTs—The Need for Randomization

Randomization is the process of allocating study participants to the treatment(s) group(s) or the control group. It is possible that the population of interest could show certain characteristics liable to influence the selected outcome measures, and it is necessary to prevent these characteristics from being concentrated within a given treatment group, as this could result in a systematic effect between the groups that is quite distinct from any treatment effect (i.e., a confounding effect). In the long run, random allocation will equalize individual differences between groups, thus allowing, as far as possible, the treatment effect to be established without being contaminated by any potentially competing factors. In other words, the aim of random allocation is to minimize the effect of possible confounders, leading to a fair comparison between the treatment(s) under investigation and the other procedure chosen as control.

1.3 RCTs—The Need for a Control Group

The efficacy of a novel experimental treatment cannot be demonstrated merely by applying it in a group of patients, because improvements/worsening might also occur spontaneously or following other procedures. In order to demonstrate that the effects observed are attributable exclusively to the treatment under investigation, this needs to be compared with the best treatment currently available. If there is no accepted treatment available, then the control group may receive no treatment at all (which corresponds to what would happen in clinical practice in this situation), or they may receive a sham treatment known as a placebo [12]. It has to be noted that a clear set of eligibility criteria must be defined, and strictly applied, both for the experimental intervention group and for the control group, otherwise it becomes practically impossible to identify the population of patients to which the study results may subsequently be generalized.

1.4 RCTs—The Need for a Statistical Approach

In RCTs, efficacy is not evaluated on a patient-by-patient basis; the aim, rather, is to assess the efficacy of a treatment in a population as a whole. Within each group, there will be patients who perform "outstandingly" and others whose performances will correspond to the "worst" that is observed, as treatments are known to give different outcomes even in a population that is, as far as possible, homogenous.

Since the purpose of RCTs is to demonstrate the superiority (or, less often, the equivalence or non-inferiority) of a novel intervention compared to another, it is necessary to adopt a statistical approach allowing the mean behavior of the target population to be analyzed and reported. This approach requires a well-defined target population and outcome measures, which in turn determine the sample size required in order to draw conclusions, as will be detailed later in the chapter.

1.5 RCT Design

Different study designs are envisaged for RCTs (Fig. 2).

The following five designs, in particular, are commonly implemented:

- parallel-group trials: each single participant is randomized to one of the study arms (i.e., intervention or control group);
- crossover trials: each single participant is exposed to each condition in a random sequence;
- cluster trials: pre-defined homogeneous clusters of individuals (e.g., clinic 1 and clinic 2) are randomly allocated to different study arms (i.e., intervention or control group);
- factorial trials: each single participant is randomly assigned to individual interventions or a combination of interventions (e.g., participant 1 is allocated to intervention x and placebo y; participant 2 is allocated to intervention x and intervention y, participant 3 is allocated to intervention y and placebo y, etc.);
- split-body trials: for each participant, body parts (e.g., upper limbs, lower limbs, etc.) are randomized separately [9].

Among the RCTs indexed in PubMed between 2000 and 2006, 78% of reports were parallel-group trials, 16% crossover trials, and the remaining 6% were classified as "other"; specifically, this last category comprised cluster (33%), factorial (26%), and split-body (41%) trials. Among the parallel-group trials, 76% compared two groups [9]; indeed, the parallel design with two groups is by far the most used, and we therefore concentrate on this particular design in the subsequent sections.

Regardless of the chosen design, RCTs should be carried out as multicenter studies. Indeed, multicenter clinical trials, especially if the different centers are located in ethnically diverse geographical regions, have the main advantage of recruiting a more heterogeneous sample of subjects and involving different care providers. This strengthens the generalizability (external validity) of the investigation [6]. Furthermore, multicenter trials allow an ample sample size to be reached in a reasonable time.

2 Ethical Issues

The peculiarity of an RCT is that the object of investigation is the human being. This aspect differentiates it from all other types of research and makes it necessary to give careful consideration to the ethical principles that regulate the administration, in humans, of interventions with unknown effects.

In 1964, the need for universal ethical rules to govern clinical medical research led the World Medical Association to establish the Declaration of Helsinki, which incorporates ethical principles designed to regulate experiments conducted in humans. Since 1964, this document has been reviewed several times, most recently in 2013 [3]. The Declaration of Helsinki is the ethical benchmark for clinical studies and no reputable medical journal will publish studies whose designs are not based on the principles it sets forth. The main points of the Declaration are summarized below:

1. Experiments must be carried out in compliance with the principle of respect for the patient. The achievement of new knowledge can never supersede the rights of each individual.
2. A treatment that is known to be inferior should not be given to any patient in either the experimental group or the control group.
3. The privacy of the patients must be ensured and their personal information must remain confidential.
4. A patient's participation in the study is voluntary. He/she has the right to refuse to participate, and to withdraw from the study at any time. An informed written consent document, explaining the aim(s) of the study, the possible conflicts of interest, and the possible benefits and the risks entailed in the research should be read and signed by each participant before enrolment.
5. Research can be conducted only if the importance of the objectives is greater than the risks involved. A systematic analysis of the risks must be conducted before the start of the study and every effort should be made to ensure their minimization and to monitor them during the study.
6. A clear research protocol should be established. It should provide the background to the proposal, as well as indications concerning funding, affiliations of researchers, potential conflicts of interest, and compensation for subjects who might be harmed as a result of participation in the research study.

The ethics committee is the body responsible for deciding whether or not a clinical research study should be carried out. To guarantee its transparency and also that it is independent of the interests of any single category (e.g. researchers or sponsors), it is composed of individuals with different roles and areas of expertise, i.e. clinicians, pharmacists, a biostatistician, patients, and experts in medical devices, bioethics, legal and insurance issues. Ethical approval is mandatory and must be obtained before starting any study involving human subjects. Furthermore, the ethics committee has the right to monitor the progress and evolution of the study, and no amendment to the protocol may be made without its consent. At the end of the study, a report summarizing its main findings should be submitted to and evaluated by the ethics committee.

3 Bias in RCTs

Bias in clinical trials is defined as a systematic error that may induce misleading conclusions about the efficacy of one treatment over others. When designing an RCT, it is necessary to avoid all possible sources of systematic errors that could affect the treatment effect estimation. Indeed, the quality of clinical trials can be measured by evaluating the robustness of the design in this regard. However, in scientific reports, little effort is made to discuss methods for addressing sources of potential bias [10]. Typical biases in clinical trials can be classified in the following five categories [12]:

1. *Selection bias*

This type of bias can occur during the selection of the patients to be enrolled in the study. Ideally, each patient should be enrolled in the study before being randomized and allocated to a treatment group (Fig. 2). Indeed, were the medical doctor to know, in advance, the treatment group to which patients have been allocated, this could influence his/her decision to enrol a given patient.

2. *Allocation bias*

When treatment groups are not balanced in size and not similar at baseline, allocation bias is encountered [12]. The randomization procedures (Fig. 2) should be designed to balance groups at baseline with particular attention to the prognostic factors that could influence the outcome (e.g., age-matched groups).

3. *Assessment bias*

When the assessor is not blinded to treatment allocation, his/her evaluation could be influenced, leading to assessment bias (outcome measures assessment, Fig. 2). This problem is particularly important in the case of outcome measures that are characterized by low sensitivity, high subjectivity (such as patient-reported outcome measures), and low inter- and intra-rater reliability. Moreover, assessment bias can also occur when the patient is not blinded to treatment allocation, since this may lead him/her to behave differently during the assessment [12]. A recent review highlighted that trials with inadequate allocation concealment or lack of blinding tend to overestimate the intervention effect, when compared with adequately concealed trials [21]. The recent use of technologically advanced tools to flank traditional assessments based on functional scales may be helpful to reduce assessment bias. Indeed, technology provides quantitative, non-operator-dependent evaluations and promotes a consistent comparison among results of different clinical trials. Nevertheless, it often requires expensive tools that are not always available in clinical practice.

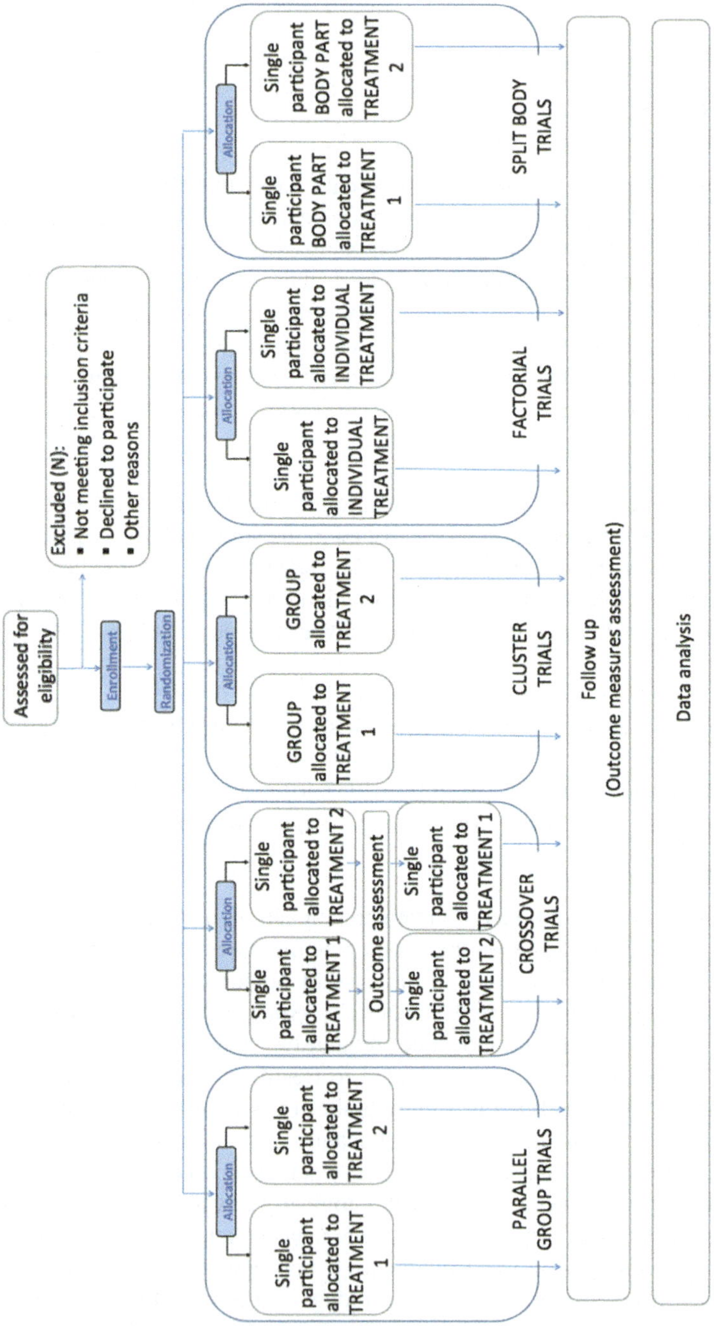

Fig. 2 Flowchart of the different RCT designs

4. *Publication bias*

The ultimate goal of any medical research is to influence clinical practice. A fundamental step, in order to share RCT findings, is to have a report of the trial published in an international scientific journal. To be published, papers undergo a peer review process, in which several experts are called upon to evaluate the quality of the clinical trial itself, and also of the report. Papers reporting positive findings are often considered more likely to be published than papers that do not show any statistically significant difference [12]. This leads to a clear bias, with the medical literature not giving equal exposure to studies with positive and negative results.

5. *Stopping bias*

To avoid a stopping bias, it is necessary to make an a priori decision on exactly when the recruitment of patients will be stopped. There are two possible choices: the first is to keep on recruiting until it is established which treatment is superior. The second is to decide beforehand the number of patients that should be recruited for the RCT. This second method is the one usually preferred, because of the bias that can potentially be induced by stopping a trial when the results obtained are considered satisfactory. Deciding the sample size in advance is not a trivial aspect. Indeed, recruiting too few patients may prevent the achievement of definitive results on the superiority of a given treatment over others. On the other hand, recruiting more patients than necessary raises an ethical issue, since the surplus patients could all be exposed directly to the superior treatment.

In response to growing evidence of bias resulting in misleading clinical trial results, several bodies have, in recent years, tried to develop guidelines to guarantee the quality of clinical trial reporting [11]. Among these, the CONSORT group defined a 25-point checklist intended to promote rigorous reporting of research and, indirectly, to prevent the publication of inadequately designed studies [14]. The checklist is intrinsically developed to minimize the risk of bias.

4 Guidelines on Designing a Parallel-Group RCT

RCTs should be adequately designed and transparently reported in order to allow critical appraisal of the validity and applicability of their results. To assess the validity of novel interventions in rehabilitation, a field in which blindness and reproducibility of the treatment are not easy to achieve, the best guidelines to follow are the CONSORT guidelines for non-pharmacological studies [19]. Below, we summarize the guidelines that should be followed in the design of a parallel-group RCT in the rehabilitation field. For each step, the example of a currently ongoing case study is provided to better clarify the point made [8].

4.1 Trial Design

The organization of an RCT starts with the formulation of a clinical question (hypothesis) that derives from the observation of patients. To demonstrate the correctness of the hypothesis a rigorous study design should be defined a priori, establishing not only the trial type (parallel group, crossover, etc.), but also the conceptual framework. In parallel-group RCTs, the conceptual framework corresponds to the hypothesis which the trial aims to demonstrate (i.e., the superiority, equivalence or non-inferiority of the novel intervention with respect to the other).

Case study. *The study proposes a novel rehabilitation program for the recovery of locomotor abilities in post-acute stroke patients. The conceptual framework is that a specific rehabilitation program (involving biofeedback cycling training, combining voluntary effort and Functional Electrical Stimulation (FES) of the leg muscles, and biofeedback balance training) is superior to standard therapy in improving walking abilities, disability, motor performance, and independence in post-acute stroke patients.*

In view of this conceptual framework, the study was designed as a parallel-group (two-group) superiority RCT.

4.2 Ethical Approval and Trial Registration

To avoid to carrying out studies whose value is undermined by methodological weaknesses, lack of transparency and/or conflicts of interest, the RCT's principal investigator prepares, as requested by an ethics committee, a series of detailed documents describing the study protocol. The RCT should be approved by this committee before the study is started.

Moreover, as already mentioned, both authors and journal editors prefer studies that give positive findings, and this leads to a publication bias, i.e. an over-representation of positive studies. One method for reducing publication bias is to register all studies undertaken in a recognized international repository. On registering the RCT, the principal investigator should declare and describe the complete methodology. Indeed, an RCT should be registered soon after securing ethical approval and before the enrolment of the first patient. Nowadays, registration is becoming mandatory for publication in the main rehabilitation journals.

Case study. *The study received the approval of the Central Ethics Committee of the rehabilitation center in which it is being carried out (Comitato Etico Centrale of the Salvatore Maugeri Foundation). The trial has been registered at clinicaltrials.gov (Identifier: NCT02439515).*

4.3 Participants' Eligibility

The profile of patients who may benefit from the intervention under investigation should be defined through clear inclusion/exclusion criteria. The more explicit these criteria are, the more the replicability of the results will be facilitated. Indeed, the aim of the trial is to obtain results that can be generalized and applied to all patients similar to those treated in the trial.

Normally the number of eligible patients is different from the number of recruited patients as a result of the need to apply the necessary ethical rules before enrolment. According to these rules, each patient should be informed in detail about the trial and should decide voluntarily whether or not to participate. Patients deciding to participate should then sign an informed consent document.

In a rehabilitation RCT it is very important to define the participants' eligibility, but also the rehabilitation centers in which the trial is performed. Indeed, the level of expertise of the care providers should be clearly stated, in order to ensure that others are equipped to reproduce the treatment correctly.

Case study: *The study participants are adult post-acute stroke patients who experienced a first stroke less than 6 months before recruitment. Other inclusion criteria were a low level of spasticity of the leg muscles (Modified Ashworth Scale score* < 2*), no limitations at the hip, knee, and ankle joints, and the ability to sit comfortably and independently for 30 min. Given that the experimental intervention includes FES, people with pacemakers and/or allergic to adhesive stimulation electrodes were excluded.*

4.4 Outcome Measures

In all rehabilitation RCTs, changes in the patients' conditions induced by the treatment(s) under investigation are assessed by collecting so-called outcome measures. These consist of internationally recognized clinical tools such as clinical scales (questionnaires or rating scales administered by the rehabilitation staff, who ask patients to perform cognitive or motor tasks) and technology-based assessment, e.g. biomechanical tests to obtain quantitative data for movements involved in the interventions, diagnostic examinations, and so forth.

When designing an RCT it is necessary to select a primary outcome measure that is strictly related to the final aim of the intervention. This measure plays a crucial role, as it is the element taken into account by the principal investigator in order to decide how large the trial ought to be. It is preferable to choose, as the primary outcome, a well-recognized measure for which it is possible to find, in the literature, the minimum clinically important difference in the population under investigation. In addition to the primary outcome, all the other measures of interest, i.e., the secondary outcome measures, should be defined a priori.

When applicable, any methods that could enhance the quality of measurements (e.g., multiple observations, training of assessors) should be defined and used.

It is also crucial to define precise time points at which all the outcome measures are collected. They should usually be collected before the beginning of the intervention, soon after the end of the intervention, and in a follow-up session, which should take place at least 6 months after the end of the intervention, thereby making it possible to evaluate changes in the medium and long term.

Case study. *The primary outcome measure was gait speed computed during a 10 m walking test performed using GAITRite® (CIR System Inc., USA), a pressure sensor system that allows measurement of spatiotemporal gait parameters. Secondary outcome measures were: other spatiotemporal gait parameters, such as cadence, stride and step length, single and double support time, swing velocity,* etc.*; clinical scales, such as the Fall Efficacy Scale, the Berg Balance Scale and the Global Perceived Effect scale; the distance covered during the 6 min walking test; lower limb EMG activations and pedal forces produced while pedaling on a sensorized cycle ergometer; and measures of postural control obtained using a sensorized balance board.*

The outcome measures were collected at baseline, soon after the end of the intervention and at 6 month follow-up.

4.5 Intervention Programs

When designing an RCT a precise definition of the interventions under investigation (both the novel one and the one used as control) should be provided. It is very important to ensure that, overall, the amount of training received by the groups is balanced.

Case study. *The experimental program consisted of 15 sessions of FES-supported volitional cycling training followed by 15 sessions of balance training. Both cycling and balance training were supported by visual biofeedback in order to maximize patients' involvement in the exercise and were performed in addition to standard therapy. The control group received standard physical therapy consisting of stretching, muscle conditioning, exercises for trunk control, standing, and walking training, and upper limb rehabilitation. Both training programs lasted 6 weeks and patients were trained for about 90 min daily. Cycling and balance training lasted about 20 min, therefore the patients in the experimental group performed only about 70 min of standard therapy. This choice ensured that the overall duration of the intervention was the same in both groups.*

4.6 Sample Size

Under the hypothesis of normal distribution of the primary outcome measure, the equation used to determine the sample size for a parallel-group RCT with two groups is the following:

$$N = \frac{2\sigma^2\left(z_\beta + z_{\frac{1}{2}\alpha}\right)^2}{\tau_M^2}$$

where τ_M is the treatment effect, i.e., the between-group difference under the hypothesis that the baseline of the two groups is similar; σ is the standard deviation of the outcome measure in the population under investigation; z_β and $z_{\frac{1}{2}\alpha}$ are the quantiles of the standard normal distribution in which β is the false positive rate, i.e., a measure of the desired power (usually set to 90% or 80%), and α is the significance level (usually set at 0.05 or 0.01). When available, τ_M is defined as the minimum clinically important difference of the outcome measure in the population under investigation.

Thus, according to this equation, the "noisier" the measurements are, i.e., the larger σ is, the larger the sample size needs to be. Also, a larger sample size is needed in order to detect a smaller difference in the means obtained in the two treatments.

Once the sample size needed in order to be able to observe a treatment effect with a given statistical power has been determined, the number should be increased to account for the possible dropout rate (normally a rate of 20% is acceptable).

Case study. *Gait speed was chosen as the primary outcome measure. Sample size was defined on the basis of ability to detect a minimal clinically important difference for gait speed, estimated as 0.16 m/s (i.e.,* $\tau_M = 0.16\,m/s$*) with a standard deviation (*σ*) of 0.22 m/s. Given that a power of 80% and a significance level of 0.05 were chosen, a sample of 60 subjects was obtained. Thus, allowing for a 20% drop-out rate, 72 patients had to be recruited.*

4.7 Randomization and Allocation Concealment

A good randomization procedure should include the generation of an unpredictable allocation sequence and the concealment of that sequence until assignment occurs [17]. Different methods have been proposed:

Simple randomization. This method requires the generation of a sequence of "A" and "B" values. Each entry in the sequence is independent of all other elements and equally likely to take both possible values. This is equivalent to the generation of a sequence in which each entry is defined by the toss of a coin. This method can result in an unbalanced number of patients per group or an unwanted imbalance between the groups at baseline.

Restricted randomization. Two main methods can be implemented: blocking randomization, which ensures that groups will be of approximately the same size, and stratification randomization, which ensures that groups will be comparable at baseline.

For blocking randomization, it is recommended to use the random permuted blocks method, based on the use of blocks of random size, because it completely avoids any selection bias. This randomization requires the choice of two even-number block sizes and it defines all the permutations of balanced values possible for each of them (e.g., if the block size is 2 there can be only two permutations, AB and BA), but if blocks of 4 and 6 elements are chosen, for example, we will have a list of 6 sequences of 4-element blocks and a list of 20 sequences of 6-element blocks (for a block of size N, the number of all possible permutations of elements is equal to $N!/((N/2)!(N/2)!)$). Then, at each iteration of the sequence generation, both the size of the block (i.e., 4 or 6) and the number of the sequence in the list (i.e., a number between 1 and 6 when 4 is extracted and a number between 1 and 20 when 6 is extracted) are randomized to create the final allocation list.

In the stratification method, the randomization can be simple or by blocks, but it is carried out separately within each of two or more subsets of participants (for example, corresponding to disease severity or study centers) in order to ensure that the patient characteristics are closely balanced within each intervention group.

In rehabilitation RCTs, it is not only the patients recruited that are randomized, but also the clinicians who will administer the intervention. Indeed, often the two interventions require different levels of clinical expertise. Therefore, the best practice to avoid biased results and improve the applicability and generalizability of the findings is to train all the possible clinicians to the same level, and then select a random sample from among them [5]. The situation is more complex, however, when the additional expertise required is not just training in the use of a novel device. Indeed, in such circumstances (e.g. surgery trials), it is impossible to recruit only clinicians who are able to perform both treatments. Recommendations for these special cases are reported in Devereaux et al. [7] and these RCTs are defined expertise-based RCTs.

Case study. *Subjects were randomized to one of two groups, one undergoing the novel rehabilitation program in addition to standard therapy (experimental group), and one undergoing standard therapy alone (control group). The randomization criteria applied were blocking randomization using blocks of random size as explained above. Given the impossibility of predicting the next value in the randomization sequence, this randomization method ensured allocation concealment.*

4.8 Blinding

Complete blindness of an RCT means that the participants, those administering the interventions, and those assessing the outcomes have to be completely unaware of the group assignment. In some studies, blindness of patients and care providers is impossible; obvious examples are trials comparing surgical with nonsurgical treatment, or different rehabilitation interventions to demonstrate the superiority of a novel device. In these cases, the minimum condition required is that the assessors be blinded to the group assignment.

A good but very difficult way of obtaining participant blindness is to compare a novel intervention with a placebo version of the same intervention. The placebo should look identical to the active treatment. One attempt to achieve this in the rehabilitation field was made by Ambrosini et al. in a study that compared an FES cycling treatment with an FES cycling placebo [2]. The patients included in the placebo group had electrodes attached correctly to their skin and underwent the same cycling sessions as the other group, but no stimulation current was delivered to their muscles. An easier and more common use of placebo concerns drug use. An example in post-stroke rehabilitation is described by Ward and colleagues (2017), who treated a chronic stroke population with motor training associated with either pharmacological modulation of neuroplasticity (atomoxetine) or placebo drugs [20].

4.9 Statistics

The method of statistical analysis should be chosen a priori during the study design phase. To analyze the treatment effect, a linear mixed model able to handle covariates (in the event of baseline imbalances) and missing values is recommended. When a significant difference between the two groups is found, it is crucial to understand whether this difference is also clinically relevant, in other words, greater than the minimum clinically important difference for the specific outcome measure in the population under investigation.

Case study. *Given the randomization method chosen (blocking randomization), the statistical analysis, performed at the end of the study, needed to take into consideration, among other things, the possibility that there was some imbalance in the baseline characteristics. For this reason, the principal investigator decided to use a linear mixed model in which, if necessary, covariates can be considered.*

5 Conclusions

This "guided tour" of the process of RCT design has highlighted the ethical and methodological principles that must be adhered to in order to demonstrate, correctly, the efficacy of a given treatment in the rehabilitation field.

Although RCTs are considered a sound basis for demonstrating treatment efficacy, they also present some limitations. First, a properly designed and conducted RCT implies quite significant costs, and therefore usually needs to be supported by a dedicated research grant. Second, many outcome measures of interest can only be verified some considerable time in the future. We may think, for example, of the long-term effects of dietary modifications on stroke prevention, or of fall prevention interventions designed for implementation in the healthy aging population—their results may not be available for decades. This makes it difficult to follow up enrolled patients effectively, and also makes the costs substantially greater than those (for personnel and resources) associated with the conducting of the trial itself. This may explain why so many RCTs encounter difficulties—failing to achieve the sample size needed in order to observe, and therefore report, the desired effect [16]. Finally, Level I evidence for a given treatment efficacy is assigned if it has been the focus of multiple RCTs (or multicenter studies). But replicating RCTs, i.e. focusing on a treatment already investigated, has two immediate implications: (i) difficulty obtaining funding, due to (ii) the lack of innovation in the study proposal.

Randomized controlled trials, even though their value is often underestimated, are the real bedrock on which to build effective conclusions on new rehabilitation treatments and can impact on clinical practice. Indeed, a well-designed RCT can influence decision-making processes in healthcare and the international evidence-based clinical pathway guidelines, and ultimately, benefit patients, who should always be placed at the heart of RCTs, and of rehabilitation research in general.

Acknowledgements This research was supported by the Italian Ministry of Healthy (grant no.: GR-2010-2312228, title "Fall prevention and locomotion recovery in post-stroke patients: a multimodal training towards a more autonomous daily life").

References

1. Altman DG, et al. The revised CONSORT statement for reporting randomized trials: explanation and elaboration. Ann Intern Med. 2001;134(8):663–94.
2. Ambrosini E, et al. Cycling induced by electrical stimulation improves motor recovery in postacute hemiparetic patients: a randomized controlled trial. Stroke; J Cereb Circ. 2011;42(4):1068–73.
3. Anon. World medical association declaration of Helsinki: ethical principles for medical research involving human subjects. JAMA. 2013;310(20):2191–4.
4. Begg C, et al. Improving the quality of reporting of randomized controlled trials. The CONSORT statement. JAMA. 1996;276(8):637–9.

5. Boutron I. Extending the CONSORT statement to randomized trials of nonpharmacologic treatment: explanation and elaboration. Ann Intern Med. 2008;148(4):295.
6. Chung KC, Song JW, WRIST Study Group. A guide to organizing a multicenter clinical trial. Plast Reconstr Surg. 2010;126(2):515–23.
7. Devereaux PJ, et al. Need for expertise based randomised controlled trials. BMJ: Br Med J. 2005;330(7482):88.
8. Ferrante S. et al. Does a multimodal biofeedback training improve motor recovery in stroke patients ? Preliminary results of a randomized control trial. 37th Annual International Conference of the IEEE Engineering in Medicine and Biology Society (*EMBC 2015*). 2005;42, p. 2011.
9. Hopewell S, et al. The quality of reports of randomised trials in 2000 and 2006: comparative study of articles indexed in PubMed. BMJ. 2010;340:c723.
10. Horton R. The rhetoric of research. BMJ (Clinical research ed.). 1995;310(6985):985–7.
11. Johansen M, Thomsen SF. Guidelines for reporting medical research: a critical appraisal. Int Sch Res Not. 2016; vol. 2016:1346026, p. 7.
12. Matthews JNS. Introduction to Randomized Controlled Clinical Trials. Second Edition, 2006.
13. Moher D, et al. CONSORT 2010 explanation and elaboration: updated guidelines for reporting parallel group randomised trials. BMJ (Clinical research ed.). 2010;340:c869.
14. Moher D, et al. CONSORT 2010 explanation and elaboration: Updated guidelines for reporting parallel group randomised trials. Int J Surg. 2012;10(1):28–55.
15. Moher D, Schulz KF, Altman DG. The CONSORT statement: revised recommendations for improving the quality of reports of parallel-group randomized trials. J Am Podiatr Med Assoc. 2001;91(8):437–42.
16. Sanson-Fisher RW, et al. Limitations of the randomized controlled trial in evaluating population-based health interventions. Am J Prev Med. 2007;33(2):155–61.
17. Schulz KF. Assessing the quality of randomization from reports of controlled trials published in obstetrics and gynecology journals. JAMA: J Am Med Assoc. 1994;272(2):125.
18. Stevely A, et al. An Investigation of the shortcomings of the CONSORT 2010 statement for the reporting of group sequential randomised controlled trials: a methodological systematic review. PLoS One. 2015;10(11):e0141104.
19. Villamar MF, et al. The reporting of blinding in physical medicine and rehabilitation randomized controlled trials: a systematic review. J Rehabil Med. 2013;45(1):6–13.
20. Ward A, et al. Safety and improvement of movement function after stroke with atomoxetine: a pilot randomized trial. Restor Neurol Neurosci. 2017;35(1):1–10.
21. Wood L, et al. Empirical evidence of bias in treatment effect estimates in controlled trials with different interventions and outcomes: meta-epidemiological study. BMJ (Clinical research ed.). 2008;336(7644):601–5.

Assessment of Balance Disorders

Marialuisa Gandolfi, Christian Geroin, Alessandro Picelli, Nicola Smania and Michelangelo Bartolo

1 Introduction

Balance is defined as "the ability to maintain the center of gravity within the body's limits of stability, under both static and dynamic conditions, including transfers" (e.g. rising from a chair) [13, 74]. According to this definition, balance is strictly related to two other axial functions, namely posture and gait. The functional goals of balance are, in fact, three-fold:

(a) maintaining a specific postural alignment (e.g. sitting, standing);
(b) facilitating voluntary movements (e.g. movement transitions between postures, gait);
(c) implementing postural reactions to recover balance after external perturbations (e.g. trips, slips, pushes).

Balance disorders (BDs) are common and debilitating in people with neurological disorders, resulting in falls, reduced mobility and loss of independence in activities of daily living [10, 15, 36]. Falls, together with other factors such as the fear of falling, are therefore a leading cause of activity restriction and social isolation from the early stages of the disease [88].

M. Gandolfi · C. Geroin · A. Picelli · N. Smania
Department of Neuroscience, Biomedicine and Movement Sciences,
Neuromotor and Cognitive Rehabilitation Research Centre (CRRNC),
University of Verona, Neurorehabilitation Unit—University Hospital AOUI Verona,
Verona, Italy

M. Bartolo (✉)
Department of Rehabilitation, Neurorehabilitation Unit — HABILITA,
Via Bologna, 1, 24040 Zingonia di Ciserano (Bergamo), Italy
e-mail: bartolomichelangelo@gmail.com

G. Sandrini et al. (eds.), *Advanced Technologies for the Rehabilitation of Gait and Balance Disorders*, Biosystems & Biorobotics 19,
https://doi.org/10.1007/978-3-319-72736-3_3

It has been reported that balance reaches an optimum in early adulthood, and subsequently deteriorates from the age of approximately 50 onwards [17, 32, 64]. Declining muscle strength, sensory functioning and speed of sensorimotor responses can be acknowledged as the primary risk factor for BDs and falls [36]. However, other risk factors include cognitive decline, especially attention and executive dysfunction, and environmental factors [2].

Adequate and timely recognition of BDs in patients with neurological disorders is crucial. First, because it allows identification of patients at risk of falling, and second because it allows balance deficits to be quantified over time in parallel with the implementation of specific rehabilitation procedures [72].

Various outcomes (e.g. tests, rating scales and questionnaires) have been reported in the literature in the context of balance evaluation in different neurological diseases (Parkinson's disease, multiple sclerosis, stroke, etc.). To date, there is no consensus on which specific tools should be preferred to assess balance, particularly in patients affected by neurological diseases [81]. Furthermore, the different etiological mechanisms involved in BDs make it very difficult to identify the best outcome measures to use. The complexity of the pathophysiology, in fact, suggests the need for a comprehensive assessment, both for diagnostic and for therapeutic purposes, and this will very often demand a multidisciplinary approach [11, 88].

As early as 2001, it was recommended, in line with the International Classification of Functioning, Disability and Health (ICF) framework, that three domains (Body Functions and Structures, Activity, and Participation) should be taken into consideration when dealing with patients with neurological disability [92]. From this perspective, balance has been classified as an "activity" and consequently, most of its outcome measures refer to this ICF domain. By contrast, few assessment protocols provide measures of body function and structure [87], and no clinical outcome measures have been developed specifically to evaluate participation.

A full review of all the outcome measures available in the literature is the beyond the scope of this chapter. Nevertheless, the overall evidence that BDs should be taken into consideration as an integral part of a comprehensive and integrated management plan in patients with neurological impairment is well established. This chapter looks at the usefulness of clinical and instrumental balance assessment in the evaluation of balance impairments in subjects with neurological disease, and their response to rehabilitation.

2 Clinical Assessment

From the perspective of BDs, the primary aim of clinical assessment is two-fold: to ascertain the presence of BDs, and to determine their underlying causes. Accordingly, clinical assessment may be divided into two main approaches: functional assessment and system assessment.

Functional assessment is designed to establish whether or not a BD exists, and (when applicable) to evaluate any changes in the disorder in response to intervention(s) [49]. In short, it allows people at risk of falling to be identified, and certain strategies then to be implemented. However, this approach does not differentiate between the reasons for BDs. System assessment, on the other hand, is helpful for determining the underlying causes of BDs, and in fact allows clinicians to implement specific interventions based on the specific pathophysiology of the disorder. In addition, a third type of assessment (quantitative) should also be undertaken in clinical practice, as will be discussed later. Quantitative assessment of postural stability is, in fact, becoming very important as a clinical tool, offering the possibility of quantifying balance disorders over time, customizing treatments and evaluating postural reactions.

2.1 Functional Assessment

Although a huge range of measurement tools has been developed in this field, there is still little agreement over which should be used in clinical practice [81]. In addition, because most of the available outcome measures lack psychometric properties and show poor clinical utility they are not readily used by clinicians and neurological physical therapists [81, 82]. Various authors agree that the ideal outcome measure should be a standardized tool able to evaluate functional and system disorders, have good psychometric properties, and, most important, be easy to use and inexpensive [31, 35, 49].

Recently, two reviews have provided clinicians with an overview of the outcome measures most commonly used to assess balance from a functional point of view in patients with neurological disease [49, 82]. These consist of two rating scales (the Berg Balance Scale [BBS] and the Tinetti Balance and Gait Assessment) [7, 8, 80], one questionnaire (the Activities-Specific Balance Confidence Scale [ABC]) [63], and three clinically-based tests, namely the Timed Up and Go [54], one-leg stance [23], and Functional Reach [21] tests.

Generally speaking, these outcome measures allow balance performance to be rated on a set of motor tasks or using a stopwatch to time how long the patient can keep his/her balance in a given posture [34]. But they have both strengths and weaknesses that should be noted. On the one hand, these outcome measures are easy to use, do not require expensive equipment, and are usually quick to administer. Furthermore, they may predict the risk of falling and the need for therapy [7]. On the other, however, their clinimetric characteristics (i.e. ceiling/floor effects, content or face validity) can vary and they may not be responsive enough to measure small changes (progression or deterioration) [12]. Finally, since the tools used in functional assessment do not make it possible to establish what type of balance problems a patient has, their capacity to indicate specific treatments is limited.

2.1.1 Rating Scales

- **The Berg Balance Scale**

The BBS is the best-known balance outcome measure able to provide a quantitative assessment of BDs [7, 8]. Originally designed to measure balance in elderly people, it has been tested in populations with different neurological diseases, such as stroke, brain injury, multiple sclerosis, Parkinson's disease, spinal cord injury, and vestibular dysfunction, as well as in orthopedic surgery patients and patients with osteoarthritis. It consists of 14 items which, by decreasing the base of support and requiring specific response strategies in static and dynamic conditions, test the ability of the patient to hold positions of increasing difficulty. Some items explore the capacity to maintain balance while sitting, standing, leaning, turning and maintaining the upright position on one leg. Others assess the ability to perform transfers between positions, reaching forward, turning around, and picking up an object from the floor.

The BBS was originally designed to be used in monitoring the clinical status of patients as well as in the evaluation of fall risk. Its administration entails observation of task performance. Each item is scored from 0 to 4: 0 denotes inability to complete the item, and 4 the ability to accomplish the task independently (total score range, 0–56; higher = better performance). Scores of less than 45 out of 56 are accepted as indicative of balance disorders in the elderly, while scores of less than 43.5 out of 56 are accepted as indicative in Parkinson's disease (www.rehabmeasures.org). This instrument refers to the ICF "Activity" domain. Its minimal clinically important difference (MCID) has not been established.

All the BBS items are situations commonly encountered in everyday life, and its administration, which does not need specialized training, requires just a few simple instruments (i.e. stopwatch, chair, step or stool). It takes from 6 to 15 min to complete, and it is free. Its psychometric properties have been extensively reported in the literature [82]. The following advantages and disadvantages of the measure might be acknowledged [60]:

Strengths	Weaknesses
Easy to use	Considerable redundancy among the items and rating structures
Free	Poor sensitivity (53% of fallers were identified)
Evaluation of static and dynamic conditions	Low sensitivity in severely affected people
No specialized training is required	Ceiling effect for active patients and/or elderly people
Minimal space and equipment requirements	No common standards for interpretation of BBS scores in relation to level of mobility and/or mobility requirements

(continued)

(continued)

Strengths	Weaknesses
Particularly suitable for use in acute stroke rehabilitation	No identification of the type of balance disorders
High inter-rater reliability (98% agreement)	No evaluation of balance during gait and/or different sensory conditions
Good specificity (96% of non-fallers were classified correctly) and high validity	No hierarchical scale

- **The Tinetti Balance and Gait test or Performance Oriented Mobility Assessment (POMA).**

This test is the oldest standardized evaluation of mobility and stability. Originally designed to measure balance (including fall risk) and gait in elderly people, it was subsequently tested in patients with amyotrophic lateral sclerosis, normal pressure hydrocephalus, Parkinson's disease and stroke. It consists of two sections, which can also be used as separate tests: balance and gait.

Balance is assessed first in the sitting position, then while arising, in standing and during turning. Additionally, it is evaluated with external perturbation and with eyes closed. The test allows evaluation of postural reactions as well as lower limb musculoskeletal constraints (e.g. muscle strength). Gait is assessed separately for the right and left foot to allow evaluation of step symmetry and step continuity. The other gait parameters evaluated are step length and clearance, path deviation, trunk stability, and stance.

A score is determined for each section, followed by a total score obtained by summing the scores of the two sections. Each item is scored on a three-point scale from 0 (highest level of impairment) to 2 (independence).

Various versions of the POMA exist, with variations existing both in the name of the test and in the means of scoring. In accordance with the original version [80], the total balance and gait scores are 16 and 12, respectively. Combining the two sections a total score of 28 indicates independence in both balance and gait activities. Scores of less than 19 are accepted as indicative of high fall risk. By contrast, scores from 9 to 24 and from 25 to 28 are taken as indicative of medium fall risk and low fall risk, respectively. The test refers to the ICF "Activity" domain.

It has been reported that the true value of this test to the healthcare team, and others, lies not only in the numerical score but also, more interestingly, in the accompanying comments. Indeed, provision is made for the addition of a list of comments for each item, reporting what deficiencies the patient exhibits and their nature. This list could help clinicians to create a differential diagnosis for each deficiency and identify further fall prevention strategies [85]. For the POMA, too, we can identify a series of advantages and disadvantages:

Strengths	Weaknesses
Easy to use	Poor specificity (only 11% of non-fallers were identified)
Free	Ceiling effect
Evaluation of static and dynamic conditions	No hierarchical scale
No specialized training is required	No clear identification of the type of balance disorders
Minimal space and equipment requirements	
Good inter-rater reliability (85% agreement)	
Good sensitivity (93% of non-fallers were identified)	
Evaluation of balance during gait and/or different sensory conditions	
Stratification of patients according to fall risk	

2.1.2 Questionnaire

- **The Activities-Specific Balance Confidence Scale (ABC)**

This is a subjective measure of confidence in performing various ambulatory activities without falling or experiencing a sense of unsteadiness (e.g. walking around the house, walking up and down stairs, picking up a slipper from the floor, getting in and out of a car). Initially tested in community-dwelling older adults, it was then tested on populations with stroke, Parkinson's disease, spinal cord injury, multiple sclerosis, vestibular disorders, unilateral transtibial amputation, traumatic brain injury, and the elderly. It is a 16-item self-report measure in which patients are required to rate their balance confidence for performing activities. The following stem is used to lead into each activity considered: "How confident are you that you will not lose your balance or become unsteady when you…". Items are rated on a rating scale that ranges from 0 (no confidence) to 100 (complete confidence). The overall score is then calculated by summing the item scores and dividing the result by the total number of items. The ABC refers to the ICF "Activity" domain. It can be self-administered or administered via interview; in the latter case, a face-to-face interview is recommended [63]. Its MCID has not been established. A cut-off score to distinguish between fallers and non-fallers has been identified in the general population as well as in specific neurological diseases. Scores lower than 67% indicate a risk of falling (people who fall 84% of the time). Instead, a cut-off score of 69% has been found to be predictive of recurrent falls based on a prospective 12-month follow-up in patients with PD (sensitivity: 93%; specificity: 69%) [48]. A cut-off score of 81.1 can provide relative certainty that patients with stroke did not have a history of multiple falls. Normative data have been provided for community-dwelling older adults and patients with stroke and Parkinson's disease (www.rehabmeasures.org). Minimal floor or ceiling effects have been reported for stroke patients. In community-dwelling older adults a score above 80% has been considered unlikely to improve after completing physical activity programs (www.rehabmeasures.org). For the ABC we can identify the points of strength and weakness listed below.

Strengths	Weaknesses
Questionnaire	Not objective
Related to activities of daily living	No evaluation of the type of BDs
Only 15 min long	Some items might not to be relevant in some populations
Good test-retest reliability (ICC: 0.7–0.92)	
Discriminates between fallers and non-fallers in Parkinson's disease	
Easy to administer and to understand	

2.1.3 Timed Test

- **Timed Up and Go test (TUG)**

The patient is asked to get up from a standard chair, walk at a comfortable and safe speed to a line 3 m away, turn at the line and walk back to the chair to sit down [62]. Individuals are permitted to use the assistive device they typically use in the community, but without the assistance of another person. Two versions have been implemented. In the TUG-Cognitive, individuals are asked to complete the test while counting backward in threes from a randomly selected number between 20 and 100. In the TUG-Manual, the patient must walk holding a cup filled with water [29, 73]. The TUG refers to the ICF "Activity" domain. Normative data have been provided for community-dwelling older adults [73]. Reported mean times taken to perform TUG, TUG-Cognitive and TUG-Manual are 8.39(± 1.36) seconds, 9.82 (± 2.39) seconds, and 11.56(± 2.11) seconds, respectively [73]. The mean values for different age groups (60–69, 70–79, 80–87 years old) differ significantly from each other. With increasing age, more time is required to perform the various tests.

Cut-off scores for elderly subjects have been estimated. Individuals completing the TUG-Cognitive in more than 15 s are classified as fallers with an overall correct prediction rate of 87% [73]. A difference of more than 4.5 s between TUG-Manual and TUG-Cognitive indicates an increased risk of falls in healthy adults [53].

In patients with Parkinson's disease, a score higher than 7.95 s may indicate a high risk of falling [37]. No ceiling effects exist, but there are floor effects with a score of 10–15 s [26, 86]. The test is easy to administer and may be useful for evaluating the effects of interventions. However, its use is limited to those who are not wheelchair bound. The TUG, too, may be considered to have various strengths and weaknesses:

Strengths	Weaknesses
Easy to use	Floor effect
Excellent inter-rater (ICC = 0.99) and test-retest (ICC = 0.99) reliability	Not possible to distinguish between balance and gait subcomponents
No specialized training is required	No clear identification of the type of balance disorders
Takes only 3 min to perform	
Evaluates dynamic conditions	
Free	
Predicts falls	
Minimal space and equipment requirements	
Correlated with the Berg Balance Scale (r = −0.72) and the Barthel Index (r = −0.51)	

2.1.4 Reaching Test

- **The Functional Reach Test (FRT)**

The FRT assesses the patient's stability by measuring the maximum distance an individual can reach forward while standing in a fixed position [91]. A modified version of the FRT has been developed for people who are unable to stand, and in this case the individual sits in a fixed position [39]. To perform the FRT, the patient has to stand close to, but not touching a wall, with the arm closer to the wall positioned at 90° of shoulder flexion with the fist closed. A ruler is mounted on the wall at shoulder height, and the subject is asked to stay with their arm outstretched. The assessor records the starting position as the position of the 3rd metacarpal head on the yardstick and then instructs the patient to "Reach as far as you can forward without taking a step". The new position of the 3rd metacarpal is then recorded, and the difference between the start and end positions, usually measured in inches or centimeters, is scored as the reach distance. Three trials are done, and the average of the last two is noted.

The modified version is performed using a leveled yardstick that has been mounted on the wall at the height of the acromion level in the patient's non-affected arm with the patient sitting on a chair. The hips, knees, and ankles are positioned at 90° of flexion, with the feet positioned flat on the floor. The initial reach is measured with the patient sitting against the back of the chair with the upper extremity flexed to 90°; the measure taken corresponds to the position of the distal end of the third metacarpal along the yardstick. The test consists of three conditions over three trials: sitting with the "unaffected" side near the wall and leaning forward, sitting with the back to the wall and leaning right, and sitting with the back to the wall and leaning left.

Patients should be instructed to lean as far as possible in each direction without rotation and without touching the wall. Once the individual leans, the position of the fifth finger along the yardstick is marked.

In people with spinal cord injury, the ulnar styloid process is used as a landmark since the tetraplegic population may not be able to make a fist. If the patient is unable to raise the affected arm, the distance covered by the acromion during leaning is recorded.

In both the FRT and the modified FRT the first trial in each direction is a practice test and should not be included in the final result. Fifteen-second rest breaks should be allowed between trials.

The FRT refers to the ICF "Activity" domain, and it is used in the following populations: community-dwelling elderly and patients with Parkinson's disease, peripheral vestibular disorders, spinal cord injury, stroke and vestibular disorders.

The MCID has not been established. Cut-off scores have been set for Parkinson's disease [6] and stroke [1]. In Parkinson's disease, different cut-offs for fall risk have been reported according to different psychometric features. A cut-off of 25.4 cm indicates fall risk with a sensitivity of 30% and specificity of 92%; a cut-off score of 30.1 increases the sensitivity to 56% and the specificity to 77%, and a score less than 31.75 cm indicates fall risk with a sensitivity of 0.86 and specificity of 0.52. In stroke patients, a cut-off score of less than 15 cm indicates fall risk. Normative data have been provided for Parkinson's disease (33.54 ± 7.36 cm), stroke with (16.8 ± 9 cm) and without arm sling (15.2 ± 8.5 cm), and vestibular disorders (31.7 ± 7.5 cm) [1, 45, 52]. This test too has its strengths and weaknesses:

Strengths	Weaknesses
Easy to use	Only one task is evaluated
Takes only 1 min to perform	No clear identification of the type of balance disorders
Good inter-rater (ICC = 0.98) and test-retest (ICC = 0.92) reliability	Not related to stabilometric limits of stability (CoP and CoM)
No specialized training is required Minimal space and equipment requirements	
Free Excellent predictive validity of subjects at risk of falls	

2.2 System Assessment

As previously discussed, a system approach should be used to determine the underlying causes of BDs [34]. As early as 1996, Lord and colleagues proposed the Physiological Balance Profile (PPA) as a reliable and valid measure of fall risk in both institutional and community settings [46]. The PPA consists of five sections (visual, proprioception, strength, reaction time, postural sway) and is therefore able to provide information on a broader array of physiological balance-related functions as well as a fall-risk score. Two versions exist: a comprehensive (long) and a screening (short) version [46]. The composite score is made up of the weighted scores of the five sections. A composite score below 0 indicates a low fall risk, a score between 0 and 1 indicates a mild risk for falling, and a score between 1 and 2 a moderate risk for falling, while scores above 2 indicate a high risk of falling.

Despite its high clinimetric properties, the PPA does not help clinicians to direct treatment [49]. By contrast, the Balance Evaluation System Test (BESTest) has been identified as the most used outcome measure for differentiating between the different types of balance deficit [33]. The BESTest consists of 36 items, grouped into six sections (biomechanical constraints, stability limits/verticality, anticipatory postural adjustment, postural responses, sensory orientation, stability in gait) and it is designed to explore all the possible systems underlying BDs. Furthermore, it is the only clinical balance test to include assessment of postural reactions to external perturbations and perception of postural verticality [33]. It also includes items from the Clinical Test of Sensory Integration for Balance [74], the BBS, and the FRT. The major limitation of BESTest is the 30 min needed to perform it. Mini-BESTest [22], developed more recently, is a short version of BESTest consisting of 14 items focusing on dynamic balance. It can be conducted in 10–15 min, and contains items belonging evenly to four of the six sections from the original BESTest. The advantages and disadvantages of BESTest are summarized below:

Strengths	Weaknesses
Determines the underlying causes of BDs	Takes a long time to perform (30 min)
Focuses treatments according to BD types	No evaluation of fall risk
Good inter-rater reliability (ICC = 0.91)	Specific equipment is required
Correlation with ABC scale ($r = 0.636$, $p < 0.01$)	
A short version is available (mini-BESTest)	

3 Instrumental Assessment

The instrumental evaluation of BDs plays an important role in rehabilitation because it helps us to understand how the postural control system works, and therefore represents an aid for the clinical diagnosis and the assessment of treatment efficacy. Moreover, the evaluation of balance can be used to identify subjects who are at risk of falling, as in the elderly population for example.

Measurement of static and dynamic balance can be obtained by means of simple tools such as clinical balance and mobility scales, and it can also be supported by instrumental tests.

Among the available instrumental measures, quantitative posturography can overcome the main drawbacks of the functional clinical balance examination, namely [88]:

(1) the variability in test performance (within/across different examiners);
(2) the subjective nature of the scoring system;
(3) its sensitivity to small changes.

The main instruments used for obtaining quantitative measurements of balance are:

(a) *force platforms*—these platforms incorporate sophisticated and expensive force transducers that make it possible to study reaction forces calculated in their three orthogonal components, x, y, and z (antero-posterior, medio-lateral, vertical directions), and the relative moments of force (Mx, My, Mz). The sway of the center of pressure (CoP) during quiet stance can be calculated from the force and moment data;
(b) *stereophotogrammetric devices*—these are used to measure whole body movements through the detection of retroreflective markers;
(c) *pedobarography walkways*—these are used to acquire spatial-temporal features of gait;
(d) *wearable inertial sensors* (WISs)—this term refers to clothing and other wearable accessories incorporating advanced electronic technologies serving to monitor functional activities (e.g. sensorized insoles to detect plantar pressures).

These tools can be used alone or variously combined with each other to assess both balance control and its modification after rehabilitation programs. More recently, movable platforms were developed and used to administer continuous and predictable perturbations, with the aim of training subjects to improve their ability to produce anticipatory postural adjustments.

3.1 Static Posturography

Static posturography is assessment of postural control obtained by characterizing displacements of the CoP while subjects maintain their stance in a relatively unperturbed state (usually quiet stance on a fixed support surface such as an instrumented platform, i.e. a *non-movable* force platform) [49, 93].

These force platforms make it possible to identify the position, on the base of support, of the instantaneous center of foot pressure during quiet stance, in tandem stance, or under more critical conditions [14, 55, 61], obtained by introducing several manipulations. In fact, the balancing task can be made more challenging:

(1) by reducing the size of the base of support;
(2) by decreasing the visual feedback (eyes closed);
(3) by decreasing the proprioceptive feedback (compliant surface);
(4) by introducing a secondary task while subjects maintain their balance.

Under the quiet stance condition, the CoP broadly reflects the position on the support base of the projection of the body's center of mass (CoM) that, in turn, partly reflects the activity of the postural muscles and the activity of the control mechanisms [16]. The movement of the CoM is what is called sway, and posturography works by measuring sway. In biomechanical terms, the CoP displacement is the controlling variable of balance, reflecting the net neuromuscular responses generated by the central nervous system to maintain control over the CoM, which is the controlled variable. For this reason, posturography approximates true sway, i.e. the movements of the CoM, on the basis of the movements of the CoP.

Overall, the results of stabilometry depend on repetition of the task, the position of the feet on the support base, and the instruction given to the subjects [41, 79, 83].

As a general consideration, the scientific literature clearly suggests that static posturography has excellent sensitivity (e.g. it is sensitive to differences in the control of balance between young, middle-aged and older subjects) [71], but poor specificity. Thus, postural sway is an excellent measure of the overall system health, but does not provide a good measure of the underlying pathophysiology since many different disorders may result in increased postural sway [19, 20, 64].

3.2 *Dynamic Posturography*

Dynamic posturography (DP) consists of assessing the subject's postural control in the presence of experimentally-induced external perturbations. These can be created using a foam cushion, or a special apparatus with a computer-controlled movable support surface that induces disequilibrium by sudden horizontal translations or rotations; alternatively, external perturbations can be applied directly to the body, for example by pushing/pulling the trunk, shoulders or pelvis, or by changing the support surface and/or visual conditions [88].

Conceptually, DP exposes the patient to different controlled visual and support surface conditions in order to quantify the failure of adaptive mechanisms to select the appropriate sensory inputs and movement response patterns.

During DP testing, the patient stands on a movable, dual force plate support surface within a movable surround (enclosure). Under the control of a computer, the force platform can either move in a horizontal plane (translate) or rotate out of the horizontal plane. It is also possible to use sensory perturbations to selectively manipulate single types of sensory input for postural control [49, 93]: horizontal translations or rotations of the support surface, movements of the visual scene,

Table 1 Sensory conditions in the SOT protocol

Eyes	Surface	Visual surround
Open	Fixed	Fixed
Closed	Fixed	
Open	Fixed	Sway referenced
Open	Sway referenced	Fixed
Closed	Sway referenced	
Open	Sway referenced	Sway referenced

galvanic vestibular stimulation or tendon vibration (to disrupt proprioception). In fact, DP is the only validated method capable of isolating the functional contributions of vestibular inputs, visual inputs, somatosensory inputs, central integrating mechanisms, and neuromuscular system outputs for postural and balance control [9].

Computerized dynamic posturography (CDP) actually provides a differential assessment of impairments through the following three sensory and motor protocols: the Sensory Organization Test (SOT), the Motor Control test (MCT) and the Adaptation Test (ADT).

The *Sensory Organization Test* is designed to identify postural control problems by assessing the patient's ability to use or to suppress different sensory information (visual, vestibular, proprioceptive). During the SOT, useful information delivered to the patient's eyes, feet and joints is effectively eliminated through calibrated "sway referencing" of the support surface and/or visual surround (Table 1). The support surface and/or visual surround tilt to directly follow the patient's anteroposterior body sway, thereby eliminating orientation information. By controlling the surface and the visual surround, while subjects' eyes are in open/closed conditions, the test may control visual and/or support surface information, also creating sensory conflict situations. The aim of the test is to isolate vestibular balance control, evoking adaptive responses of the central nervous system. Patients may express either an inability to make effective use of sensory systems, or inappropriate adaptive responses. Both situations reflect erroneous use of sensory information.

The *Motor Control Test* evaluates the patient's ability to automatically recover from unexpected external perturbations administered by means of platform translations in forward and backward directions that elicit automatic postural responses. Measurements include onset time, strength and lateral symmetry of the responses.

The *Adaptation Test* simulates daily life conditions (e.g. irregular surfaces) assessing the patient's ability to modify motor reactions and minimize sway when the support moves unpredictably in the toes-up or toes-down direction. Measurements include the magnitude of the force response required to overcome induced postural instability.

Because the measures of postural stability, as well as the motions of the support surface and visual surround, are precisely controlled and calibrated relative to the patient's height and weight, standardized graphics can be used to compare the patient's results to those of age-matched asymptomatic (normal) individuals.

Following the introduction of DP as a clinical tool in the early 1980s [59] and the development of test protocols over the subsequent years [57], this technique became regarded as the standard quantitative method for isolating and assessing the sensory and motor components of balance [9], although the high costs of the tool, the lengthy training and testing time involved, and the space needed for the equipment have, to an extent, limited its diffusion [88].

In any case, like other instrumental tools, DP should be considered a complementary component of the diagnostic process in patients with imbalance, useful for identifying the underlying sensory (vestibular, visual, somatosensory) and motor control impairments; however, by itself, DP cannot diagnose the disease or lesion site, and does not provide localizing or lateralizing information, or any information regarding the etiology. In fact, as the balance system is highly adaptive, persons with similar pathologies can present with different impairments, depending on the progression of the disease. Conversely, DP is able to provide functional information on how well an individual can use their balance and an indication of the importance of a patient's BD in their activities of daily living. Also, CDP provides a functional measure that is helpful in predicting the benefit that patients may expect to receive from therapeutic intervention with physical therapy.

3.3 Wearable Inertial Sensors

Evaluation of a patient's functional performance in daily life is essential for optimal guidance of neurological rehabilitation therapy and it can be performed using unobtrusive and ambulatory monitoring systems. Over the past decade or so, wearable technologies, clothing and accessories incorporating computer and advanced electronic technologies have been developed in order to obtain functional measurements of balance performance during activities of daily living [3–5, 40, 56, 68].

It is easy to understand the growing interest in these techniques, which make it possible to assess postural sway using built-in portable sensors, and to monitor the type, quality and quantity of the users' daily activities outside the laboratory environment.

Indeed, wearable inertial sensors [24, 25, 30, 42, 43, 58, 67, 75, 76, 89, 90] and force sensors [18, 44, 47, 78] of different kinds have been widely used to detect body sway and they work as real-time balance performance monitoring devices. WISs consisting of linear accelerometers, angular velocity sensors (gyroscopes) and magnetic sensors have been mounted on the trunk, head or lower limbs of users to capture torso, head or other body segment movements, and thus to determine any tilts in the mediolateral and anteroposterior directions [24, 25, 30, 42, 43, 58, 67, 75, 76, 89, 90]; in addition, thin-film force/pressure sensors have been placed at the plantar surface of foot to collect ground reaction force information [27, 28, 47, 65].

As mentioned, the real advantage of wearable sensors is that they allow balance monitoring to be conducted anywhere and anytime, and can therefore potentially be used as balance monitoring aids in daily life. Indeed, since they are highly transportable and need no stationary units, such as receivers or cameras, for data collection, they can easily be used outside laboratory conditions. Moreover, wearable inertial motion sensors are a good choice for human biomechanics studies as they are inexpensive devices with low power consumption.

In short, in addition to being accurate and reliable, WISs offer the following three main advantages:

(a) they are are inexpensive;
(b) they constitute a practical method for the clinical setting as well as for ecological evaluation;
(c) they allow the use of user-friendly computer interfaces with automatic analysis.

The advance of WISs has prompted the development of algorithms to automatically, objectively and quantitatively assess balance and mobility [51, 69, 70, 94, 95].

Among the actual WIS systems the *Xsens* inertial sensor was developed and has been used to investigate trunk sway with respect to gravity as well as lateral trunk postural adjustments in anticipation of step initiation. Sway parameters extracted from the planar acceleration differentiated between untreated PD and control subjects, showing smoothness of lower trunk acceleration to be the most sensitive measure of sway in early PD, apparent even before balance problems can be detected on clinical observation [50].

In conclusion, by means of WISs, it is possible to obtain an objective and systematic evaluation of the parameters involved in postural control, such as the number of oscillations and the latency of postural reactions, both in static and in dynamic conditions. What is more, these devices can be used to detect these same parameters during the performance of tests such as the TUG.

A highly satisfactory level of accuracy, usability and safety of these devices has been achieved. Maximizing the computing capacity of the micro-processer, while minimizing the size of the electronic components, appears to be the direction to follow in the future in order to optimize these devices. Wearable balance-improving devices that can be used indoors and outdoors can potentially serve as balance aids in daily life.

4 Unwitting Violation of Balance and Gait

An interesting aspect that needs to be considered when evaluating BDs in neurological patients is the clinical condition named *astasia-abasia*, a term that indicates the inability to either stand or walk in a normal way. Specifically, astasia means the inability to stand upright unassisted, while abasia means a lack of motor coordination in walking, resulting in an inconstant and unmeasurable base of gait [66]. This condition can be observed in functional neurological disorders (conversion disorders according to the DSM V) in which the bizarre gait is not related to a specific organic lesion. In these cases, a differential diagnosis with some neurological diseases (i.e. Parkinson's disease, hydrocephalus, cerebellar lesions, stroke) is necessary. The use of suggestions, distractions, and/or triggering method to differentiate between organic and psychogenic origin of the condition is useful in order to make a diagnosis. In individuals with conversion disorder, the modified gait abnormality rating scale (GARS-M) is a reliable, valid and responsive instrument that may be useful for quantifying gait abnormalities and could provide objective measures upon which to assess treatment effects [84]. Psychogenic gait can be categorized into three categories using video-recording of gait: limping of one leg, limping of two legs and truncal imbalance [38]. Recently, some authors investigated the theory that, in conversion disorders, motor symptoms are related to heightened self-monitoring and excessive cognitive control of movements [77]. They investigated patients affected by conversion disorders and matched controls maintaining static balance on a force platform under various attention conditions: (a) with eyes open; (b) with eyes closed (this condition requiring enhanced attention to proprioceptive information to regulate posture); and (c) while performing an attention-demanding cognitive task. Compared with the controls, the patients displayed a greater decrease in postural stability in the 'eyes-closed' versus 'eyes-open' condition. By contrast, cognitive distraction led to a normalization of balance. The authors concluded that attention plays an important role in postural control in conversion disorders. These findings seem to show that these patients tend to exert deliberate control of posture, which is normally an almost automatized perceptual-motor task. Attentional distraction resulted in a temporary normalization of balance; this last approach could be used to train individuals with conversion disorders to guide their attention in a more effective way.

5 Conclusions

The issue of balance assessment in neurological rehabilitation is both relevant and challenging. The concept that "not all BDs are the same" well.

The fact that BDs can be due to a wide range of causes explains the interest they attract from a wide variety of disciplines. This broad interest in the assessment of balance has led to the development of a variety of different techniques for measuring balance. It is important to bear in mind that the choice of appropriate evaluation tools depends on the patient's disease since the information collected from these tests can have different meanings. In any case, BDs should be evaluated as an integral part of a comprehensive and integrated management plan in patients with neurological impairment. To date, there is no consensus on which specific tools should be preferred in order to assess balance, especially in patients with neurological disease. However, functional and system assessment should be regarded as two sides of the same coin, both being necessary to identify the presence of BDs, and to determine the underlying causes. It is necessary to have a good understanding of the various measures and their usefulness in order to make a sensible and reasoned choice about which outcome measures to use. However, there are several aspects that still need to be addressed in the future. Namely, it would be worth assessing a possible hierarchy of rating scales, gathering information about the minimal detectable change and MCID of any given instrument, and evaluating the applicability of the various instruments across the disease spectrum. Finally, outcome measures referring to the Participation and Body Functions and Structures domains of the ICF framework still remain to be established.

It is commonly agreed that single unidimensional outcomes are unlikely to be informative on all the functional domains affected by BDs. From this perspective, it would be advisable to implement specific protocols, consisting of multiple clinical and instrumental outcomes, to assess BDs in relation to the different axial functions. Promising developments include the use of objective and automated tools. In the near future, clinicians will be able to instrument their functional and system balance assessments in order to obtain comprehensive assessment of BDs in more ecological contexts and during activities of daily living.

References

1. Acar M, Karatas GK. The effect of arm sling on balance in patients with hemiplegia. Gait Posture. 2010;32(4):641–4.
2. Ambrose AF, Cruz L, Paul G. Falls and fractures: a systematic approach to screening and prevention. Maturitas. 2015;82(1):85–93. https://doi.org/10.1016/j.maturitas.2015.06.035 Epub 2015 Jun 26.
3. Aminian K, Najafi B, Büla C, Leyvraz PF, Robert P. Spatio-temporal parameters of gait measured by an ambulatory system using miniature gyroscope. J Biomech. 2002(May);35 (5):689–99.
4. Aminian K, Robert P, Buchser EE, Rutschmann B, Hayoz D, Depairon M. Physical activity monitoring based on accelerometry: validation and comparison with video observation. Med Biol Eng Comput. 1999(May);37(3):304–08.
5. Aminian K, Trevisan C, Najafi B, Dejnabadi H, Frigo C, Pavan E, Telonio A, Cerati F, Marinoni EC, Robert P, Leyvraz PF. Evaluation of an ambulatory system for gait analysis in hip osteoarthritis and after total hip replacement. Gait Posture. 2004(Aug);20(1):102–7.
6. Behrman AL, Light KE, Flynn SM, Thigpen MT. Is the functional reach test useful for identifying falls risk among individuals with Parkinson's disease? Arch Phys Med Rehabil. 2002;83(4):538–42.
7. Berg K, Norman KE. Functional assessment of balance and gait. Clin Geriatr Med. 1996;12:705–23.
8. Berg KO, Wood-Dauphinee SL, Williams JI, Maki B. Measuring balance in the elderly: validation of an instrument. Can J Public Health. 1992;83(Suppl 2):S7–11.
9. Black FO. Clinical status of computerized dynamic posturography in neurotology. Curr Opin Otolarynogol Head Neck Surg. 2001;9:314–8.
10. Bloem BR, Marinus J, Almeida Q, Dibble L, Nieuwboer A, Post B, Ruzicka E, Goetz C, Stebbins G, Martinez-Martin P, Schrag A. Movement disorders society rating scales committee. Measurement instruments to assess posture, gait, and balance in Parkinson's disease: critique and recommendations. Mov Disord. 2016. https://doi.org/10.1002/mds.26572.
11. Bloem BR, Visser JE, Allum JH. Posturography. In: Hallet M, editor. Movement disorders—handbook of clinical neurophysiology. Elsevier; 2003. pp. 295–336.

12. Blum L, Korner-Bitensky N. Usefulness of the Berg Balance Scale in stroke rehabilitation: a systematic review. Phys Ther. 2008;88:559–66.
13. Bronstein A, Brandt T, Woolacott M. Clinical disorders of balance, posture and gait. London: Arnold; 1996.
14. Burdet C, Rougier P. Analysis of center-of-pressure data during unipedal and bipedal standing using fractional Brownian motion modeling. J Appl Biomech. 2007;23:63–9.
15. Cameron MH, Lord S. Postural control in multiple sclerosis: implications for fall prevention. Curr Neurol Neurosci Rep. 2010;10(5):407–12.
16. Caron O, Gelat T, Rougier P, Blanchi JP. A comparative analysis of the center of gravity and center of pressure trajectory path lengths in standing posture: an estimation of active stiffness. J Appl Biomech. 2000;16:234–47.
17. Chiba R, Takakusaki K, Ota J, Yozu A, Haga N. Human upright posture control models based on multisensory inputs; in fast and slow dynamics. Neurosci Res. 2016;104:96–104. https://doi.org/10.1016/j.neures.2015.12.002.
18. Crea S, Cipriani C, Donati M, Carrozza MC, Vitiello N. Providing time-discrete gait information by wearable feedback apparatus for lower-limb amputees: usability and functional validation. IEEE Trans Neural Syst Rehabil Eng. 2015;23:250–7.
19. de Haart M, Geurts AC, Huidekoper SC, Fasotti L, van Limbeek J. Recovery of standing balance in postacute stroke patients: a rehabilitation cohort study. Arch Phys Med Rehabil. 2004(Jun);85(6):886–95.
20. Dozza M, Chiari L, Chan B, Rocchi L, Horak FB, Cappello A. Influence of a portable audio-feedback device on structural properties of postural sway. J Neuroeng Rehabil. 2005 (May);31(2):13.
21. Duncan PW, Weiner DK, Chandler J, Studenski S. Functional reach: a new clinical measure of balance. J Gerontol. 1990;45:M192–7.
22. Franchignoni F, Horak F, Godi M, Nardone A, Giordano A. Using psychometric techniques to improve the Balance Evaluation Systems Test: the mini-BESTest. J Rehabil Med. 2010;42 (4):323–31.
23. Fregly AR, Smith MJ, Graybiel A. Revised normative standards of performance of men on a quantitative ataxia test battery. Acta Otolaryngol (Stockh). 1973;75:10–6.
24. Giggins OM, Sweeney KT, Caulfield B. Rehabilitation exercise assessment using inertial sensors: a cross-sectional analytical study. J Neuroeng Rehabil. 2014(Nov 27);11:158.
25. Goebel JA, Sinks BC, Parker BE Jr, Richardson NT, Olowin AB, Cholewiak RW. Effectiveness of head-mounted vibrotactile stimulation in subjects with bilateral vestibular loss: a phase 1 clinical trial. Otol Neurotol. 2009;30:210–6.
26. Herman T, Giladi N, Hausdorff JM. Properties of the 'timed up and go' test: more than meets the eye. Gerontology. 2011;57:203–10.
27. Hijmans JM, Geertzen JH, Schokker B, Postema K. Development of vibrating insoles. Int J Rehabil Res. 2007;30:343–5.
28. Hijmans JM, Geertzen J, Zijlstra W, Hof AL, Postema K. Effects of vibrating insoles on standing balance in diabetic neuropathy. J Rehabil Res Dev. 2008;45:1442–50.
29. Hofheinz M, Schusterschitz C. Dual task interference in estimating the risk of falls and measuring change: a comparative, psychometric study of four measurements. Clin Rehabil. 2010;24(9):831–42.
30. Horak FB. Clinical measurement of postural control in adults. Phys Ther. 1987;67:1881–5.
31. Horak FB. Clinical assessment of balance disorders. Gait & Posture. 1997;6:76–84.
32. Horak F, King L, Mancini M. Role of body-worn movement monitor technology for balance and gait rehabilitation. Phys Ther. 2015;95:461–70.
33. Horak FB, Macpherson JM. Postural orientation and equilibrium. In: Shepard J, Rowell L, editors. Handbook of physiology: section 12, Exercise: regulation and integration of multiple systems. New York: Oxford University Press; 1996. pp. 255–92.
34. Horak FB, Wrisley DM, Frank J. The Balance Evaluation Systems Test (BESTest) to differentiate balance deficits. Phys Ther. 2009;89:484–98.

35. Horak FB, Shupert CL, Mirka A. Components of postural dyscontrol in the elderly: a review. Neurobiol Aging 1989 (Nov, Dec);10(6):727–38.
36. Horak FB. Postural orientation and equilibrium: what do we need to know about neural control of balance to prevent falls? Age Ageing. 2006(Sep);35 Suppl 2:ii7–11.
37. Janssens J, Malfroid K, Nyffeler T, Bohlhalter S, Vanbellingen T. Application of LSVT BIG intervention to address gait, balance, bed mobility, and dexterity in people with Parkinson disease: a case series. Phys Ther 2014;94.
38. Jordbru AA, Smedstad LM, Moen VP, Martinsen EW. Identifying patterns of psychogenic gait by video-recording. J Rehabil Med. 2012;44:31–5.
39. Katz-Leurer M, Fisher I, Neeb M, Schwartz I, Carmeli E. Reliability and validity of the modified functional reach test at the sub-acute stage post-stroke. Disabil Rehabil. 2009;31 (3):243–8.
40. Keijsers NL, Horstink MW, Gielen SC. Ambulatory motor assessment in Parkinson's disease. Mov Disord. 2006(Jan);21(1):34–44.
41. Kirby RL, Price NA, MacLeod DA. The influence of foot position on standing balance. J Biomech. 1987;204:423–7.
42. Leardini A, Lullini G, Giannini S, Berti L, Ortolani M, Caravaggi P. Validation of the angular measurements of a new inertial-measurement-unit based rehabilitation system: comparison with state-of-the-art gait analysis. J Neuroeng Rehabil. 2014;11:1–7.
43. Lee BC, Kim J, Chen S, Sienko KH. Cell phone based balance trainer. J Neuroeng Rehabil. 2012;9:3–9.
44. Lee MY, Lin CF, Soon KS. Balance control enhancement using sub-sensory stimulation and visual-auditory biofeedback strategies for amputee subjects. Prosthet Orthot Int. 2007;31:342–52.
45. Lim LI, van Wegen EE, de Goede CJ, Jones D, Rochester L, Hetherington V, Nieuwboer A, Willems AM, Kwakkel G. Measuring gait and gait-related activities in Parkinson's patients own home environment: a reliability, responsiveness and feasibility study. Parkinsonism Relat Disord. 2005(Jan);11(1):19–24.
46. Lord SR, Clark RD. Simple physiological and clinical tests for the accurate prediction of falling in older people. Gerontology. 1996;42:199–203.
47. Ma CZH, Wan AHP, Wong DWC, Zheng YP, Lee WCC. A vibrotactile and plantar force measurement-based biofeedback system: paving the way towards wearable balance-improving devices. Sensors. 2015;15:31709–22.
48. Mak MK, Pang MY, Mok V. Gait difficulty, postural instability, and muscle weakness are associated with fear of falling in people with Parkinson's disease. Parkinsons Dis. 2012;2012:901721.
49. Mancini M, Horak FB. The relevance of clinical balance assessment tools to differentiate balance deficits. Eur J Phys Rehabil Med. 2010(June);46(2):239–48 (Review).
50. Mancini M, King L, Salarian A, Holmstrom L, McNames J, Horak FB. Mobility lab to assess balance and gait with synchronized body-worn sensors. J Bioeng Biomed Sci. 2011(Dec);12 Suppl 1:007.
51. Mancini M, Zampieri C, Carlson-Kuhta P, Chiari L, Horak FB. Anticipatory postural adjustments prior to step initiation are hypometric in untreated Parkinson's disease: an accelerometer-based approach. Eur J Neurol. 2009(Sep);16(9):1028–34.
52. Mann GC, Whitney SL, Redfern MS, Borello-France DF, Furman JM. Functional reach and single leg stance in patients with peripheral vestibular disorders. J Vestib Res. 1996(Sep–Oct);6(5):343–53.
53. Maranhão-Filho PA, Maranhão ET, Lima MA, Silva MM. Rethinking the neurological examination II: dynamic balance assessment. Arq Neuropsiquiatr. 2011(Dec);69(6):959–63.
54. Mathias S, Nayak US, Isaacs B. Balance in elderly patients: the "Get-up and go" test. Arch Phys Med Rehabil. 1986;67:387–9.
55. Mezzarane RA, Kohn AF. Control of upright stance over inclined surfaces. Exp Brain Res. 2007;180:377–88.

56. Moe-Nielsen R, Helbostad JL. Estimation of gait cycle characteristics by trunk accelerometry. J Biomech. 2004(Jan);37(1):121–6.
57. Monsell EM, Furman JM, Herdman SJ, Konrad HR, Shepard NT. Technology Assessment: Computerized dynamic platform posturography. Otolaryngol Head Neck Surg. 1997(Oct);117 (4):394–8.
58. Nanhoe-Mahabier W, Allum J, Pasman E, Overeem S, Bloem B. The effects of vibrotactile biofeedback training on trunk sway in parkinson's disease patients. Parkinsonism Relat Disord. 2012;18:1017–21.
59. Nashner LM, Black FO, Wall C. Adaptation to altered support and visual conditions during stance: patients with vestibular deficits. J Neurosci. 1982;5:117–24.
60. Nnodim JO, Yung RL. Balance and its clinical assessment in older adults—A review. J Geriatr Med Gerontol. 2015;1(1).
61. Piirtola M, Era P. Force platform measurements as predictors of falls among older people—a review. Gerontology. 2006;52:1–16.
62. Podsiadlo D, Richardson S. The timed "Up & Go": a test of basic functional mobility for frail elderly persons. J Am Geriatr Soc. 1991(Feb);39(2):142–8.
63. Powell LE, Myers AM. The Activities-specific Balance Confidence (ABC) Scale. J Gerontol. Series A, Biol Sci (Washington DC) 1995;50A:M28–34.
64. Prieto TE, Myklebust JB, Hoffmann RG, Lovett EG, Myklebust BM. Measures of postural steadiness: differences between healthy young and elderly adults. IEEE Trans Biomed Eng. 1996(Sep);43(9):956–66.
65. Priplata AA, Niemi JB, Harry JD, Lipsitz LA, Collins JJ. Vibrating insoles and balance control in elderly people. Lancet. 2003;362:1123–4.
66. Ropper AH, Samuels MA. Adams and Victor's principles of neurology (9th edition). New York, NY: McGraw-Hill Medical; 2009. pp. 1447–65.
67. Rossi-Izquierdo M, Ernst A, Soto-Varela A, Santos-Pérez S, Faraldo-García A, Sesar-Ignacio Á, Basta D. Vibrotactile neurofeedback balance training in patients with parkinson's disease: reducing the number of falls. Gait Posture. 2013;37:195–200.
68. Sabatini AM, Martelloni C, Scapellato S, Cavallo F. Assessment of walking features from foot inertial sensing. IEEE Trans Biomed Eng. 2005(Mar);52(3):486–94.
69. Salarian A, Zampieri C, Horak FB, Carlson-Kuhta P, Nutt JG, Aminian K. Analysing 180° turns using an inertial system reveals early signs of progression of Parkinson's disease. Conf Proc IEEE Eng Med Biol Soc. 2009;2009:224–7.
70. Salarian A, Horak FB, Zampieri C, Carlson-Kuhta P, Nutt JG, Aminian K. iTUG, a sensitive and reliable measure of mobility. IEEE Trans Neural Syst Rehabil Eng. 2010(Jun);18(3):303–10.
71. Schieppati M, Grasso M, Siliotto R, Nardone A. Effect of age, chronic diseases and parkinsonism on postural control. In: Stelmach GE, Homberg V, editors. Sensorimotor impairment in the elderly. The Netherlands: Kluver Academic Publishers; 1993. pp. 355–73.
72. Shulman LM. Understanding disability in Parkinson's disease. Mov Disord. 2010;25(Suppl. 1):S131–5.
73. Shumway-Cook A, Brauer S, Woollacott M. Predicting the probability for falls in community-dwelling older adults using the Timed Up & Go Test. Phys Ther. 2000;80 (9):896–903.
74. Shumway-Cook A, Horak FB. Assessing the influence of sensory interaction on balance: suggestion from the field. Phys Ther. 1986;66:1548–50.
75. Sienko KH, Balkwill MD, Oddsson L, Wall C. Effects of multi-directional vibrotactile feedback on vestibular-deficient postural performance during continuous multi-directional support surface perturbations. J Vestib Res. 2008;18:273–85.
76. Sienko KH, Balkwill MD, Wall C. Biofeedback improves postural control recovery from multi-axis discrete perturbations. J Neuroeng Rehabil. 2012;9.
77. Stins JF, Kemple Cl, Hagenaars MA, Beek PJ, Roelofs K. Attention and postural control in patients with conversion paresis. J Psychosom Res. 2015(Mar);78(3):249–54.

78. Sungkarat S, Fisher BE, Kovindha A. Efficacy of an insole shoe wedge and augmented pressure sensor for gait training in individuals with stroke: a randomized controlled trial. Clin Rehabil. 2011;25:360–9.
79. Tarantola J, Nardone A, Tacchini E, Schieppati M. Human stance stability improves with the repetition of the task: effect of foot position and visual condition. Neurosci Lett. 1997;228:75–8.
80. Tinetti ME. Performance-oriented assessment of mobility problems in elderly patients. J Am Geriatr Soc. 1986;34:119–26.
81. Tyson SF, Connell LA. How to measure balance in clinical practice. A systematic review of the psychometrics and clinical utility of measures of balance activity for neurological conditions. Clin Rehabil. 2009;23(9):824–40.
82. Tyson S, Watson A, Moss S, Troop H, Dean-Lofthouse G, Jorritsma S, Shannon M. Greater manchester outcome measures project. Development of a framework for the evidence-based choice of outcome measures in neurological physiotherapy. Disabil Rehabil. 2008;30(2):142–9.
83. Uimonen S, Laitakari K, Sorri M, Bloigu R, Palva A. Effect of positioning of the feet in posturography. J Vestib Res. 1992;2:349–56.
84. Vandenberg JM, George DR, O'Leary AJ, Olson LC, Strassburg KR, Hollman JH. The modified gait abnormality rating scale in patients with a conversion disorder: a reliability and responsiveness study. Gait Posture. 2015;41(1):125–9.
85. Vaught SL. Gait, balance, and fall prevention. Ochsner J. 2001;3(2):94–7.
86. Vereeck L, Wuyts F, Truijen S, Van de Heyning P. Clinical assessment of balance: normative data, and gender and age effects. Int J Audiol. 2008;47:67–75.
87. Verheyden G, Nieuwboer A, Mertin J, Preger R, Kiekens C, De Weerdt W. The Trunk Impairment Scale: a new tool to measure motor impairment of the trunk after stroke. Clin Rehabil. 2004(May);18(3):326–34.
88. Visser JE, Carpenter MG, van der Kooi JH, Bloem BR. The clinical utility of posturography. Clin Neurophysiol. 2008(Nov);119(11):2424–36.
89. Wall C, Weinberg MS. Balance prostheses for postural control. IEEE Eng Med Biol Mag. 2003;22:84–90.
90. Wall C, Wrisley DM, Statler KD. Vibrotactile tilt feedback improves dynamic gait index: a fall risk indicator in older adults. Gait Posture. 2009;30:16–21.
91. Weiner DK, Duncan PW, Chandler J, Studenski SA. Functional reach: a marker of physical frailty. J Am Geriatr Soc. 1992;40(3):203–7.
92. World Health Organization. International classification of functioning, disability and health: ICF. Geneva: WHO; 2001.
93. Yelnik A, Bonan I. Clinical tools for assessing balance disorders. Neurophysiol Clin. 2008 (Dec);38(6):439–45.
94. Zampieri C, Di Fabio RP. Improvement of gaze control after balance and eye movement training in patients with progressive supranuclear palsy: a quasi-randomized controlled trial. Arch Phys Med Rehabil. 2009(Feb);90(2):263–70.
95. Zampieri C, Salarian A, Carlson-Kuhta P, Aminian K, Nutt JG, Horak FB. The instrumented timed up and go test: potential outcome measure for disease modifying therapies in Parkinson's disease. J Neurol Neurosurg Psychiatry. 2010(Feb);81(2):171–6.

The Assessment of Gait Disorders in Neurorehabilitation

Christian Geroin, Cristina Zanga, Marialuisa Gandolfi, Nicola Smania and Caterina Pistarini

1 Introduction

Stroke survivors experience a certain degree of sensorimotor recovery. Selecting appropriate measures to assess this recovery is complex because of patient-related factors such as the heterogeneity of the stroke etiology, severity of symptoms and spontaneous recovery. Despite these heterogeneous factors, a number of approaches might help both clinicians and researchers to select appropriate outcome measures for their respective settings. The first and most important approach for selecting

C. Geroin (✉) · M. Gandolfi · N. Smania
Neuromotor and Cognitive Rehabilitation Research Center (CRRNC), Department of Neurosciences, Biomedicine and Movement Sciences, University of Verona, P.Le L.A. Scuro 10, 37134 Verona, Italy
e-mail: christian.geroin@univr.it

M. Gandolfi
e-mail: marialuisa.gandolfi@univr.it

N. Smania
e-mail: nicola.smania@univr.it

C. Zanga · C. Pistarini
Neurorehabilitation Unit, Salvatore Maugeri Foundation IRCCS, Scientific Institute of Pavia, Pavia, Italy
e-mail: cristina.zanga@fsm.it

C. Pistarini
e-mail: caterina.pistarini@fsm.it

M. Gandolfi · N. Smania
U.O.C. of Neurorehabilitation Unit, Azienda Ospedaliera Universitaria Integrata, Verona, Italy

G. Sandrini et al. (eds.), *Advanced Technologies for the Rehabilitation of Gait and Balance Disorders*, Biosystems & Biorobotics 19,
https://doi.org/10.1007/978-3-319-72736-3_4

stroke outcome measures is a framework of health and disability, such as the International Classification of Functioning, Disability and Health (ICF). The ICF provides the conceptual basis for assessing and measuring disability and health, and supports policy development in this area. Another approach is to consider an outcome measure's essential psychometric properties (reliability, validity, responsiveness, sensitivity, and minimal clinically important difference). Outcome measure selection can also be approached by considering the purpose of the measurement (discriminative, predictive or evaluative) and the nature of the study (efficacy or effectiveness) of a given intervention. It is also necessary to consider the timing of the assessment, the natural history of stroke, the severity of the disease, and the different data collection options. Finally, a distinction should also be drawn between different recovery processes (motor recovery and compensation). In this chapter, we also present a comprehensive overview of the outcome measures used to evaluate the effects of robot-assisted gait training in patients after stroke.

2 Assessment of Gait Disorders

Gait disorders and falls can commonly result in disability conditions that reduce an individual's quality of life and participation in the community [23, 24, 33]. Gait problems are common in elderly people as well as in patients affected by various pathological conditions, such as neurological, musculoskeletal, cardiovascular, respiratory and visual disorders [3].

The prevalence of gait disorders in the elderly population increases with age. Whereas gait is generally normal up to the age of 60 years, over this age, the incidence of gait problems increases [5, 32]. The most dramatic consequence of gait disorders is falling. Thirty percent of people over 65 years old have at least one fall each year. In people older than 80 years this proportion rises to 50% [35].

Recovery of walking function is one of the main objectives of neurorehabilitation. The ultimate goal of rehabilitation is to reduce the likelihood of disability, helping patients to maximize their independence and increase their interaction with the environment throughout their lifespan [31]. This is a very challenging goal that can be addressed with a tailored rehabilitation intervention that must be preceded by careful evaluation to identify the relevant problems [16].

To assess gait disorders, it is necessary to review the patient's medical history and clinical examination.

The medical history review should take into account all reports of pathological (neurological and orthopedic) conditions previously experienced by the patient which can negatively influence gait. The patient's personal data and details of past surgical and/or rehabilitation interventions (e.g. physiotherapy, occupational therapy, speech therapy, cognitive therapy) should also be clearly set out in the medical record.

The clinical examination can provide information about existing musculoskeletal and/or neurological impairments, and can allow an initial diagnosis of gait-affecting lesions. Furthermore, information on the primary pathology can also be derived from a proper evaluation of the compensatory mechanisms used by the patient to stand upright and walk [38]. This can be an observational evaluation or an assessment performed using clinical scales and instrumental measurements. The examination room must be large enough to examine patients in the sagittal and frontal planes; patients should be assessed undressed (i.e., only in their underwear), and all body segments need to be carefully inspected. They should be carefully observed while performing different activities, such as postural transfers, sitting and standing. Their complaints and wishes should be noted in their medical records. Pain, muscle weakness, sensory deficits, contractures and previous falls must also be recorded, described in both quantitative and qualitative terms. This observational evaluation is the first step in evaluating gait.

The first walking speed test should be performed at self-selected speed. Subsequently, in order to uncover any compensatory strategies adopted, the patient is asked to walk faster and more slowly. It is known that gait is composed of two main phases (% of gait), which are generally estimated during comfortable walking. The swing phase (40%) is defined as the period of time in which the reference foot is not in contact with the ground, while the stance phase (60%) corresponds to the time it is in contact with the ground. The stance phase can be further subdivided into: (i) the double stance phase (10%) during which both feet are in contact with the ground—this phase occurs at the beginning and at the end of the gait cycle, and (ii) the single limb support phase (40%) of the gait cycle, during which the opposite foot is swinging. Gait abnormalities may refer to the stance or the swing phase of the gait cycle. Stance phase dysfunctions include an abnormal base of support (equinovarus foot, claw toes, knee hyperextension) and limb or trunk instability (Trendelenburg limping). Swing phase dysfunctions can involve impaired limb advancement [3].

Clinical scales can help clinicians and researchers to quantify important aspects of walking, and have been used for this purpose in various trials. For example, clinical scales have been used to evaluate the range of motion of joints, muscle strength and spasticity, walking speed and endurance, balance, turning ability and mobility during postural transfers, kinetic and kinematic gait parameters, somatic sensation, dual task performance, and quality of life [10] (Table 1).

The use of other tools such as the Gait Assessment and Intervention Tool or videos to perform a critical appraisal is also advocated [8]. Stair climbing and descent tests can also inform about possible deficits in muscle power at the hip, knee and ankle flexors and extensors.

Table 1 List and abbreviations of scales used in the previous robot-assisted gait training clinical trials

2minWT	2-min walking test
3minWT	3-min walking test
5MWT	5-m walking test
6minWT	6-min walking test
8MWT	8-m walking test
10MWT	10-m walking test
AS	Ashworth Scale
BBS	Berg Balance Scale
BI	Barthel Index
BMI	Body Mass Index
CES-D	Center for Epidemiological Studies-depression Scale
CNS	Canadian Neurological Scale
EMS	Elderly Mobility Scale
ESS	European Stroke Scale
FAC	Functional Ambulation Category
FAI	Frenchay Activities Index
FIM	Functional Independence Measure
FM MOTOR	Fugl-Meyer Motor Subscale
FMA	Fugl-Meyer Assessment of Sensorimotor Recovery After Stroke
HR	Heart Rate
LLFDI	Late Life Function and Disability Instrument
MAS	Modified Ashworth Scale
MEFAP	Modified Emory Functional Ambulation Profile
MI	Motricity Index
MMAS	Modified Motor Assessment Scale
MMSE	Mini Mental State Examination
MOAS	Motor Assessment Scale
MRC	Medical Research council
MRS	Modified Ranking Scale
NIHSS	National Institutes of Health Stroke Scale
PROM	Passive Range of Movement
RMAS	Rivermead Motor Assessment Scale
RMI	Rivermead Mobility Index
RPE	Borg Scale of Perceived Exertion
RS	Rankin Scale
SAS	Stroke Activities Scale
SF-36	Short Form Health Survey
SPPB	Short Physical Performance Battery
SSS	Scandinavian Stroke Scale
ST	Step Test

(continued)

Table 1 (continued)

TBS	Tinetti Balance Scale
TCT	Trunk Control Test
TGS	Tinetti Gait Scale
TMS	Toulouse Motor Scale
TUG	Timed Up and Go Test

Although clinical scales are useful for quantifying gait, particularly in clinical practice, they provide subjective measurements and consequently lack accuracy and precision. These factors have a negative effect on the diagnosis, follow-up and treatment [22]. In parallel with observational and clinical assessment of gait, gait analysis has become a field of interest in neurorehabilitation because it allows quantification and objective and reliable evaluation of different gait parameters.

Gait analysis is used to quantify human motion and it is generally performed in a specialized laboratory. The aims of gait analysis are to understand the biomechanical features of human gait and to differentiate normal conditions from those defined as pathological. Other important aspects that can be studied are different biomechanical components of the body (i.e. feet, trunk, arms) and their relationship with each other during gait. Finally, gait analysis can help in drawing clinically meaningful inferences about the anatomical and biomechanical functions of the body in patients with different pathologies [20]. This is particularly important in treatment decision making (treatment planning) and in evaluating the effects of rehabilitation interventions. It is to be noted that the clinical course of gait disturbances is variable and changes over time in patients affected by neurological diseases. A better understanding of gait changes related to disease progression or treatment might help clinicians to categorize gait disorders. The classification of dysfunctional gait patterns would have important implications from the perspective of improving communication between rehabilitation experts and developing specific interventions based on patients' needs [15, 21].

The parameters used in gait analysis can be divided into five types: (i) temporal-spatial parameters; (ii) kinematic parameters; (iii) kinetic parameters; (iv) integrated biomechanics (joint moments and power); and (v) electromyography [20].

Temporal-spatial parameters are the easiest to understand and, with respect to the others, the most applicable in clinical practice. Essentially, the temporal-spatial parameters are gait speed (meters/second), stride length (meters), cadence (steps/second), step or stride width (meters), single limb support time (seconds), double limb support time (seconds), and stance time/duration [20]. Temporal-spatial parameters have often been used to quantify changes in pathological gait patterns in stroke patients after robot-assisted gait training [10, 11]. They are widely used in clinical trials, but it is important to consider that temporal-spatial parameters are a global expression of gait function and can be directly influenced by several factors (the subject's sex and age, the measurement method used, the instructions given to the subject, etc.) [20].

Kinematic parameters are used to study the movement of the body in isolation from the forces that generated the movement. They are measured as displacements of linear or angular accelerations or velocities, usually recorded using motion tracking devices and/or optical tracking cameras to derive joint angles and limb trajectories. Modern gait analysis laboratories are equipped with optical tracking cameras for either two-dimensional or three-dimensional (3D) gait analysis.

In particular, in the 3D model the cameras calibrate a defined space, and the movement of markers within that space can be tracked in all three dimensions. The markers of movement are generally placed on the skin over predefined landmarks according to existing validated models [18]; this allows measurement of a portion of the body. The markers used can be active or passive. Active markers usually transmit a signal whereas the passive ones reflect a signal from a transmitting and receiving camera. Kinematic parameters, like the temporal-spatial ones, have some limitations [20].

Kinetics is the study of the forces and moments which determine movement. Kinetic parameters include: ground reaction forces (plus the measurement of center of pressure and plantar pressure distribution), joint mechanical powers and joint moments. In general, force plates are used to measure the ground reaction force during the stance phase of gait. The ground reaction force is an overall indicator of gait performance and can distinguish abnormal curve profiles of the foot and ankle from those considered normal [20].

The center of pressure (COP) is a kinetic measure often used to study gait and postural control. It denotes the mean of the vectors of all the forces acting on the bottom of the foot during the stance phase of the gait cycle. Force plates detect and measure the COP which, in normal gait, shifts from the heel at heel strike, to the first ray at toe off. Disease or injuries can alter the location and timing of the COP [20].

Unlike the COP, which represents the average forces under the foot, plantar pressure is defined as the forces spread over the entire area of the foot that is in contact with the ground (described as the force unit per area). It is measured either with force plates or using piezo-resistive technology to produce a “map” of the pressure distribution of the plantar surface of the foot.

Kinetic and kinematic data are used to estimate the forces acting at the different joints, defined as joint moments. For instance, power (watts) is the result of the net muscle moment and the angular velocity of a segment. The net joint power offers important information about muscle contraction during the gait cycle.

Finally, electromyography measures the electrical activity flowing in the muscles. It provides insight into when a muscle is active and the degree of motor recruitment during different phases of the gait cycle.

A well-equipped movement analysis laboratory has the potential to measure and record all the above parameters. The path of movement in the three different dimensions and precise quantitative data can be collected simultaneously. Gait analysis devices are generally easy to use and non-invasive for the patient (Table 2).

Table 2 List of instrumental measures to evaluate gait and postural control

VICON system
G-sensor
GAITRite system
OPTO GAIT photoelectric cell system
Motion analysis corporation
H-GAIT system
Electromyography
Posturography

The technological devices used to study human gait fall into three different categories, namely those based on non-wearable, wearable and hybrid sensors. Systems using non-wearable sensors require a structure in which the sensors are positioned. In this case, patients walk along a marked walkway and the sensors collect all the necessary data about their gait. Systems using non-wearable sensors can be further classified, according to the method of capturing the data, into two groups: (i) those based on image processing (e.g. analog or digital cameras, laser range scanners, infrared sensors and time-of-flight cameras); and (ii) those based on the use of floor sensors (force platforms). Instead, with systems based on wearable sensors (i.e. sensors that can be positioned on the patient's body), accelerometers, gyroscopic sensors, inclinometers, magnetometers, force sensors, extensometers, goniometers and electrogoniometers, active markers and surface electromyography can all be employed [25, 34, 36].

Although the evaluation of gait disorders is a key area in the field of rehabilitation, there is no agreement on the most appropriate method of selecting outcome measures. Moreover, there is no shared consensus among researchers and clinicians about clinical scales that should be used to assess the effects of treatment, especially in the context of robot-assisted arm [29] and gait training [10].

The Italian Robotic Neurorehabilitation Research Group (IRNRG) [10] reviewed the literature on the commonly reported outcome measures in clinical trials of robot-assisted gait training in patients with stroke. They found a total of 45 outcome measures used in 27 different clinical trials. The most commonly used outcome measures were, in this order: the Functional Ambulation Category (FAC), the 10-m Walking Test, the Motricity Index, the 6-Minute Walking Test, the Rivermead Mobility Index and the Berg Balance Scale.

The FAC, first described by Holden et al. [13], differentiates six levels of walking ability on the basis of the amount of physical support required. It is a simple, cost-effective and quick instrument used to evaluate walking independence. Research indicates that the FAC score correlates with walking velocity and step length [13, 14].

The 10-m Walking Test measures the time (or number of steps) employed by a patient to cover a distance of 10 m from a standing start, when walking at their usual speed. In general, the total available distance is at least 12 m of free floor space, and parallel tapes are positioned on the floor, 10 m apart, to serve as 'start' and 'stop' lines. A stopwatch is used to measure the time taken to cover the 10 m [37].

The Motricity Index measures the patient's limb muscle strength. A sub-section of this index describes lower limb strength in three movements: ankle dorsiflexion (tibialis anterior muscle), knee extension (quadriceps muscle), and hip flexion (iliopsoas/rectus femoris muscle). The examiner monitors the movements and contraction of the respective muscles [7].

The 6-min Walking test is a quick and easy test measuring exercise endurance during walking. As its name suggests, it is used to quantify the number of meters the patient can walk in 6 min [30].

The Rivermead Mobility Index is a scale used to measure body mobility and it includes 15 mobility items: 14 relate to self-reported performances, and one (s-tanding unsupported) to direct observation. Dichotomous 'yes/no' answers are scored 1/0 and then summed; higher scores indicate better performance [6].

Finally, the Berg Balance Scale can be used to obtain a quantitative assessment of balance in older adults [4]. It consists of 14 items that require patients to hold positions or complete movement tasks of varying levels of difficulty. All items involve activities of everyday life. Scores of less than 45 out of a possible 56 are generally accepted as suggestive of balance impairment.

In conclusion, walking independence, velocity, muscle strength, endurance, mobility and balance were the main aspects of walking considered in the aforementioned clinical trials with potential implications for rehabilitation. It is interesting to note that all these outcomes come fall within the ICF's "body functions and structure" or "activity" domains. The "participation" domain, representing one of the main objectives of neurorehabilitation, has been partially neglected [10] (Fig. 1).

2.1 Selecting the Appropriate Outcome Measures

Selecting the most appropriate outcome measures and developing a standardized evaluation protocol are crucial aspects of rehabilitation. Indeed, by making it possible to select and guide the most appropriate treatment procedures, they allow clinicians and researchers to optimize patients' chances of recovery [17].

Choosing appropriate clinical measures is difficult but could be improved by considering: (i) the ICF model; (ii) essential psychometric properties; (iii) the nature of the study (effectiveness or efficacy) and (iv) the aim of the measurement; (v) the different clinical histories and (vi) recovery processes occurring in patients with stroke; and (vii) the modality of test administration and the time taken to complete the test. Once agreement is reached about the method of selecting outcome measures, the formulation of a standardized assessment protocol would enable the

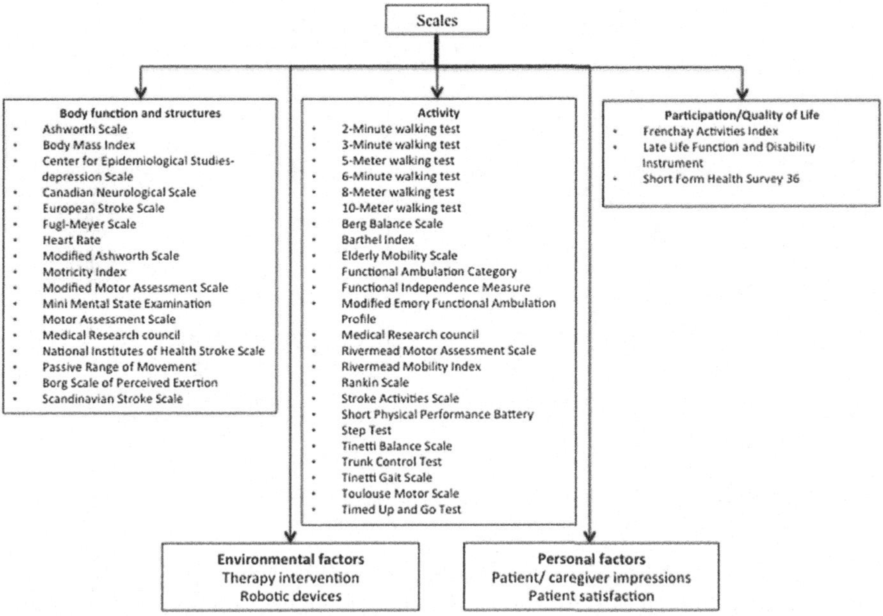

Fig. 1 The international classification of function, disability, and health framework: an example of measurement scales used in those categories

effects of different treatment procedures (e.g. robotic device end-effector versus exoskeleton) to be compared, and this could help to improve therapeutic decision making [10].

2.1.1 The International Classification of Functioning, Disability and Health

The ICF provides a scientific basis for understanding health as the interaction between an individual and his/her environment. It provides a common language for the description of health and health-related conditions, to improve communication between researchers, healthcare professionals, policy-makers, and people, including disabled people. The ICF encompasses the domains "body function and structure", "activity" and "participation", but also considers the role of "environmental factors" [39].

"Body function" refers to evaluation of the physiological and psychological function of the body, and "structure" to anatomical parts and components. Symptoms and signs such as motor weakness, sensory and proprioceptive deficits, and cognitive impairments are dysfunctions that come under the umbrella of "impairment" [28]. "Activity" is defined as a person's ability to execute a task, and a limitation in the activity domain is defined as "disability", that is, incapacity of the

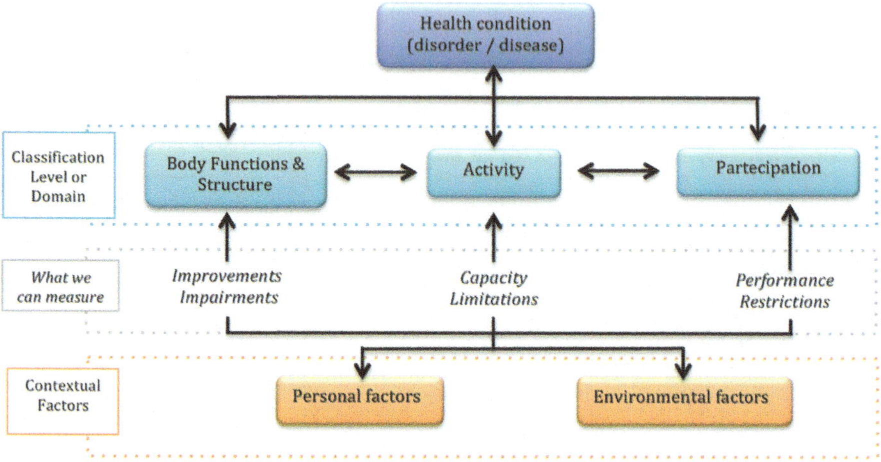

Fig. 2 The framework of the international classification of functioning, disability and health

individual to accomplish a given task [26]. Finally, "participation" is the involvement of a subject in real-life situations. If an individual has difficulty accomplishing his/her role in real-life situations, this is defined as a restriction of participation [27]. All these aspects, along with the patient's medical records, should be considered when evaluating a patient with disability caused by neurological disease [3] (Fig. 2).

2.1.2 Psychometric Properties

The analysis of psychometric properties is an important step in the selection of outcome measures. The essential psychometric properties are reliability, validity, responsiveness to change, and sensitivity, as well as the minimal clinically important difference [2].

The reliability (or reproducibility) of a score is the extent to which it is free of random error. The reliability of an instrument includes its internal consistency, and inter-rater and test-retest reliability.

The internal consistency is the degree of association between the items in a test. This can be determined by submitting a group of subjects to a test at a single time point. The data are subsequently analyzed and the internal consistency is defined according to the following reference values: ≥ 0.80 excellent; 0.70–0.79 adequate; <0.70 poor [1]. Inter-rater reliability refers to the difference between two measurements performed by two or more raters on the same group of subjects. At least 80% agreement between raters is generally required [12]. Test-retest reliability is the correlation between two measurements scored by the same individual at distinct time points. A correlation ≥ 0.75 is considered excellent, 0.4–0.74

adequate, and ≤ 0.40 poor [26]. A correlation of at least 0.90 has been suggested if the scale is used to evaluate the ongoing progress of a patient under treatment [9].

The validity of an instrument is its capacity to score what it is supposed and assumed to measure. Several types of validity exist: face, content, construct and criterion, with related subtypes (concurrent, convergent, discriminative and predictive) [26]. Criterion validity and its predictive subtype are the most important types of validity [2].

Responsiveness is the ability of an instrument to detect, over time, clinically significant changes in a patient as an effect of a treatment [26]. In the presence of evidence of a change in the measurement, the effect size can be small <0.5, moderate 0.5–0.8 or large ≥ 0.8 [26]. Evaluation of a possible "floor and ceiling" effect is also important in order to understand the limits or range of any detectable changes. The absence of a floor and ceiling effect is the best condition; the effect is considered absent when $\leq 20\%$ of patients have either the minimum (floor) or maximum (ceiling) score [26].

Sensitivity is the pertinence of an instrument in relation not only to the goals of the study but also to the ICF domains, namely body function and structure, activity and participation [2]. Finally, the minimal clinically important difference is the smallest difference in a score that is considered beneficial and worthwhile for the patient [2].

2.1.3 The Nature of the Study and the Aim of the Measurement

In the selection of outcome measures for rehabilitation interventions, it is important to distinguish between efficacy-oriented and effectiveness-oriented trials. Efficacy trials are aimed at optimizing the change so that biological changes can be detected with as few patients as possible. In this context, impairment scales might be advisable because they are most sensitive to change and have the greatest capacity to differentiate between treatment groups. By contrast, effectiveness trials aim to establish whether an intervention can have benefits in the context of ordinary clinical practice (external validity of the treatment). From this perspective, several outcomes are evaluated, including ones relevant to public health, such as comorbidity, quality of life and cost-effectiveness.

In addition to the nature of the study, measures in rehabilitation can have different aims: discriminative, predictive and evaluative. Discriminative measures are used, especially in the context of clinical trials, to separate patients into two or more homogeneous groups [2]. Predictive instruments are used to categorize patients into established measurement categories based on a gold standard. This gold standard is used to define progression of performance over time [2]. Evaluation instruments are used to measure the amount of change in single patients or patient groups over time, at different time-points such as after treatment or during follow-up [2].

2.1.4 The Discrimination of Different Clinical Histories and Recovery Processes

The choice of outcome measures should also take into consideration the phase (i.e. acute, subacute or chronic), natural history and severity of the disease. Patients may indeed present different patterns of sensorimotor recovery depending, in particular, on the disease phase and severity.

When selecting outcome measures, the distinction between motor recovery and compensation is also significant. Generally speaking, "motor recovery" means the re-acquisition of movement patterns, during the execution of a given task, that had been present before the lesion. Instead, compensation (or substitutive compensation) is the emergence, after the lesion, of new patterns of movement during the execution of a task, and it is the result of phenomena such as adaptation and/or integration of residual movement patterns. Thanks to compensation phenomena the patient is able to perform a functional task again. In the natural pattern of functional recovery, both motor recovery and compensation play fundamental roles, helping the patient to achieve a better functional outcome. It is critical for both clinicians and researchers to distinguish between these two processes, which are the basis for defining realistic and attainable goals [19].

2.1.5 Modalities of Test Administration

A further important issue in selecting outcome measures is the modality of data collection. Several can be employed: administration of instruments by trained interviewers versus self-administration, administration by a healthcare professional or other proxy, and computerized adaptive tests.

Questionnaires administered by trained interviewers are frequently used in rehabilitation; they ensure compliance and minimize errors and missing items. Self-administered questionnaires are less expensive, but they may increase the number of missing responses. From the perspective of the ICF model, impairment and activity measures can be performance-based, however participation and quality of life are often self-reported. Self-reported measures have limitations, linked for example to possible cognitive impairment and communication problems in patients with stroke.

The use of a proxy is a further interesting option. However, proxy assessors tend to assess patients as more disabled than they appear [2].

Finally, computerized adaptive testing has recently been introduced in rehabilitation and health service research. Computerized adaptive tests provide different test-item sets for each patient based on that person's estimated trait (or ability) level, and, through the administration of a small number of items, they provide precise information regarding an individual's level of functional ability [2].

3 Conclusions

The selection of appropriate outcome measures is a difficult task, and has profound implications for the choice of the most suitable treatment procedures. The identification of a shared assessment protocol, to be applied both in clinical practice and in research, is essential, but unfortunately this has not yet been achieved. The literature suggests that a common language, shared by clinicians and researchers, is important to ensure evaluation and selection of the most appropriate interventions, especially in the context of robotic rehabilitation treatment. The selection of outcome measures can be improved through the use of proposed strategies [10].

References

1. Andresen EM. Criteria for assessing the tools of disability outcomes research. Arch Phys Med Rehabil. 2000;81:S15–20.
2. Barak S, Duncan PW. Issues in selecting outcome measures to assess functional recovery after stroke. NeuroRx. 2006;3:505–24.
3. Bensoussan L, Viton JM, Barotsis N, Delarque A. Evaluation of patients with gait abnormalities in physical and rehabilitation medicine settings. J Rehabil Med. 2008;40:497–507.
4. Berg KO, Wood-Dauphinee S, Williams JL, Maki B. Measuring balance in the elderly: preliminary development of an instrument. Physiother Can. 1989;41:304–11.
5. Bloem BR, Haan J, Lagaay AM, van Beek W, Wintzen AR, Roos RA. Investigation of gait in elderly subjects over 88 years of age. J Geriatr Psychiatry Neurol. 1992;5:78–84.
6. Collen FM, Wade DT, Robb GF, Bradshaw CM. The Rivermead mobility index: a further development of the Rivermead Motor Assessment. Int Disabil Stud. 1991;13:50–4.
7. Collin C, Wade D. Assessing motor impairment after stroke: a pilot reliability study. J Neurol Neurosurg Psychiatry. 1990;53:576–9.
8. Ferrarello F, Bianchi VA, Baccini M, et al. Tools for observational gait analysis in patients with stroke: a systematic review. Phys Ther. 2013;93:1673–85.
9. Fitzpatrick R, Davey C, Buxton MJ, Jones DR. Evaluating patient-based outcome measures for use in clinical trials. Health Technol Assess 1998;2(i–iv):1–74.
10. Geroin C, Mazzoleni S, Smania N, et al., Italian Robotic Neurorehabilitation Research Group. Systematic review of outcome measures of walking training using electromechanical and robotic devices in patients with stroke. J Rehabil Med. 2013;45:987–96.
11. Geroin C, Picelli A, Munari D, Waldner A, Tomelleri C, Smania N. Combined transcranial direct current stimulation and robot-assisted gait training in patients with chronic stroke: a preliminary comparison. Clin Rehabil. 2011;25:537–48.
12. Higgins PA, Straub AJ. Understanding the error of our ways: mapping the concepts of validity and reliability. Nurs Outlook. 2006;54:23–9.
13. Holden MK, Gill KM, Magliozzi MR, Nathan J, Piehl-Baker L. Clinical gait assessment in the neurologically impaired. Reliability and meaningfulness Phys Ther. 1984;64:35–40.
14. Holden MK, Gill KM, Magliozzi MR. Gait assessment for neurologically impaired patients. Standards for outcome assessment. Phys Ther. 1986;66:1530–9.
15. Kempen JC, Doorenbosch CA, Knol DL, de Groot V, Beckerman H. Newly identified gait patterns in patients with multiple sclerosis may be related to push-off quality. Phys Ther 2016;12.
16. Küçükdeveci AA, Tennant A, Grimby G, Franchignoni F. Strategies for assessment and outcome measurement in physical and rehabilitation medicine: an educational review. J Rehabil Med. 2011;43:661–72.

17. Langhorne P, Bernhardt J, Kwakkel G. Stroke rehabilitation. Lancet. 2011;377(9778):1693–702.
18. Leardini A, Benedetti MG, Berti L, Bettinelli D, Nativo R, Giannini S. Rear-foot, mid-foot and fore-foot motion during the stance phase of gait. Gait Posture. 2007;25:453–62.
19. Levin MF, Kleim JA, Wolf SL. What do motor "recovery" and "compensation" mean in patients following stroke? Neurorehabil Neural Repair. 2009;23(4):313–9.
20. Mayich DJ, Novak A, Vena D, Daniels TR, Brodsky JW. Gait analysis in orthopedic foot and ankle surgery–topical review, part 1: principles and uses of gait analysis. Foot Ankle Int. 2014;35:80–90.
21. Mirek E, Kubica JL, Szymura J, Pasiut S, Rudzińska M, Chwała W. Assessment of gait therapy effectiveness in patients with Parkinson's disease on the basis of three-dimensional movement analysis. Front Neurol. 2016;27(7):102.
22. Muro-de-la-Herran A, Garcia-Zapirain B, Mendez-Zorrilla A. Gait analysis methods: an overview of wearable and non-wearable systems, highlighting clinical applications. Sensors (Basel) 2014;14:3362–94.
23. Pike J, Jones E, Rajagopalan K, Piercy J, Anderson P. Social and economic burden of walking and mobility problems in multiple sclerosis. BMC Neurol. 2012;12:94.
24. Pundik S, Holcomb J, McCabe J, Daly JJ. Enhanced life-role participation in response to comprehensive gait training in chronic-stroke survivors. Disabil Rehabil. 2012;34:1535–9.
25. Rowe PJ, Myles CM, Hillmann SJ, Hazlewood ME. Validation of flexible electrogoniometry as measure of joint kinematics. Physiotherapy. 2001;87:479–88.
26. Salter K, Jutai JW, Teasell R, Foley NC, Bitensky J, Bayley M. Issues for selection of outcome measures in stroke rehabilitation: ICF activity. Disabil Rehabil. 2005;27:315–40.
27. Salter K, Jutai JW, Teasell R, Foley NC, Bitensky J, Bayley M. Issues for selection of outcome measures in stroke rehabilitation: ICF Participation. Disabil Rehabil. 2005;27:507–28.
28. Salter K, Jutai JW, Teasell R, Foley NC, Bitensky J. Issues for selection of outcome measures in stroke rehabilitation: ICF body functions. Disabil Rehabil. 2005;27:191–207.
29. Sivan M, O'Connor RJ, Makower S, Levesley M, Bhakta B. Systematic review of outcome measures used in the evaluation of robot-assisted upper limb exercise in stroke. J Rehabil Med. 2011;43:181–9.
30. Steffen TM, Hacker TA, Mollinger L. Age- and gender-related test performance in community-dwelling elderly people: six-minute walk test, berg balance scale, timed up & go test, and gait speeds. Phys Ther. 2002;82:128–37.
31. Stucki G, Cieza A, Melvin J. The International Classification of Functioning, Disability and Health (ICF): a unifying model for the conceptual description of the rehabilitation strategy. J Rehabil Med. 2007;39:279–85.
32. Sudarsky L. Gait disorders: prevalence, morbidity, and etiology. Adv Neurol. 2001;87:111–7.
33. Tan D, Danoudis M, McGinley J, Morris ME. Relationships between motor aspects of gait impairments and activity limitations in people with Parkinson's disease: a systematic review. Parkinsonism Relat Disord. 2012;18:117–24.
34. Tao W, Liu T, Zheng R, Feng H. Gait analysis using wearable sensors. Sensors (Basel). 2012;12:2255–83.
35. Tinetti ME, Williams CS. Falls, injuries due to falls, and the risk of admission to a nursing home. N Engl J Med. 1997;337:1279–84.
36. Wang W, De Stefano A, Allen R. A simulation model of the surface EMG signal for analysis of muscle activity during the gait cycle. Comput Biol Med. 2006;36:601–18.
37. Watson MJ. Refining the ten-metre walking test for use with neurologically impaired people. Physiotherapy. 2002;88:386–97.
38. Whittle WM. Clinical gait analysis. Hum Mov Sci. 1996;15:369–87.
39. World Health Organization. The International Classification of Functioning, Disability and Health (ICF). Geneva: WHO; 2001. http://www.who.int/classifications/icf/en/. Accessed 23 June 2016.

Bedside Vestibular Examination

Maurizio Versino, Roberto De Icco and Silvia Colnaghi

1 Introduction

The vestibular system detects the acceleration of the head, and contributes to the detection of body position and movement in space. These vestibular signals are also used to trigger reflexes serving to stabilize gaze position (the vestibular ocular reflex —VOR) and body position (the vestibular spinal reflex) in space.

Here we report the clinical examination of VOR-related signs in dizzy patients and, more specifically, consider different kinds of acquired nystagmus, and the use of the Head Impulse Test and the Head Shaking Test.

We do not describe the positioning maneuvers used to diagnose the different kinds of benign paroxysmal positional vertigo since this, the most frequent vertigo syndrome, is a self-limiting disorder that is not underlain by a permanent lesion of the vestibular system, can be effectively treated by re-positioning maneuvers, and does not usually need supplemental rehabilitation therapy.

M. Versino · R. De Icco
Department of Brain and Behavioral Sciences, University of Pavia, Pavia, Italy

M. Versino · S. Colnaghi
Neuro-otology and Neuro-ophthamology Laboratory, C. Mondino National Neurological Institute, Pavia, Italy

S. Colnaghi
Department of Public Health, Experimental and Forensic Medicine, University of Pavia, Pavia, Italy

M. Versino (✉)
Dipartimento di Scienze del Sistema Nervoso e del Comportamento, Laboratorio Neuro-otologia e Neuro-oftalmologia Fondazione Istituto Neurologico Nazionale Mondino, IRCCS, Università di Pavia, Via Mondino 2, 27100 Pavia, Italy
e-mail: mversino@unipv.it

G. Sandrini et al. (eds.), *Advanced Technologies for the Rehabilitation of Gait and Balance Disorders*, Biosystems & Biorobotics 19,
https://doi.org/10.1007/978-3-319-72736-3_5

The topic of this chapter has also been the topic of many textbooks, to which the reader is referred for more detailed information [1–3, 7].

2 Nystagmus (Table 1)

Nystagmus [5, 6, 9–17] is an involuntary eye movement consisting of two phases in which the movement occurs in opposite directions: a slow phase followed by a quick phase, namely a saccade. Pendular nystagmus is the only form in which there is no quick phase, but rather two slow phases in opposite directions. The combination of two quick phases (back-to-back involuntary saccades) in opposite directions, with or without an interval, characterizes saccadic intrusions.

The form of nystagmus with a slow and a quick phase is called jerk nystagmus; it is described as horizontal, vertical or torsional (when the eyes rotate in the frontal plane), according to the direction of the quick phase in relation to the patient's coordinate system.

Nystagmus can be physiological, as occurring during sustained rotation or while looking at full-field image motion (optokinetic nystagmus), but it can also be a pathological sign of a vestibular and/or cerebellar dysfunction.

Nystagmus should be evaluated in all nine gaze positions and with the patient in both the sitting and supine positions. Moreover, it should be evaluated with and without fixation, because this can help in distinguishing between peripheral and central nystagmus. In the case of peripheral (but not central) nystagmus, the "central" visual-vestibular interactions can be used to dampen the nystagmus and its visual consequences. Fixation can be prevented by using Frenzel goggles, which

Table 1 Clinical features and most likely lesion sites of different kind of nystagmus

Nystagmus	Clinical features	Lesion site
Peripheral	Horizontal-torsional nystagmus, always beating toward the healthy side	Unilateral vestibular end organ/nerve/nuclei
Gaze evoked	Present only in eccentric gaze, beating in the direction of gaze	Cerebellum (flocculus)
Downbeat	Downbeating nystagmus, particularly evident in lateral gaze and downgaze	Cerebellum (floccullus)
Upbeat	Upbeating nystagmus, particularly evident in upgaze	Brainstem (paramedian medulla, pons, midbrain)
Pendular	Back-to-back slow phases leading to a circular, elliptic or diagonal eye movement	Brainstem
Periodic alternating	Spontaneous horizontal nystagmus changing beating direction after a fixed period	Cerebellum (nodulus and uvula)

consist of magnifying and retro-illuminated lenses. With another method [18], the examiner uses an ophthalmoscope to look at the head of the optic nerve of one eye, while covering or not covering the subject's other eye with his/her hand; with this method, one should bear in mind that the head of the optic nerve lies behind the center of rotation of the eyeball and all directions should be reversed, i.e. if the head of the optic nerve rotates to the right, this means that the pupil is rotating to the left. Finally, an ophthalmoscope or any other penlight can be used to flash a light on one eye, thus preventing fixation by that eye while contralateral fixation may or may not be allowed, in the latter case by covering the other eye [8].

2.1 *Peripheral Vestibular Nystagmus*

Peripheral vestibular nystagmus (PerN) is caused by a unilateral lesion affecting the vestibular end-organ and/or vestibular nerve and/or by a focal lesion within the vestibular nuclei. The most likely cause of PerN is vestibular neuritis, whose most common etiologies are infectious (viral) or vascular. From a pathophysiological perspective, PerN can be attributed to a pathological imbalance of the vestibular tonic inputs coming from the two sides.

Normally when the head is still the vestibular end organs show a tonic and balanced activity, while rotation of the head will increase the activity of one side and decrease that of the other side. For instance, rotation to the right will increase the activity of the right side and reduce the activity of the left side. This bias will trigger the VOR and drive the eyes in opposite directions, in order to maintain the stabilization of gaze in space. In the above example, a leftward movement of the eyes will compensate for the rightward rotation of the head, showing the same velocity as the head movement and without any phase shift.

In the case of left vestibular neuritis, even when the head is still the tonic activity of the two sides is unbalanced because the left input is lost and the tonic activity from the right side will prevail: this bias will trigger the VOR, causing the eyes to move to the left; however, since the head is still, the slow eye movement driven by the VOR will result in gaze displacement rather than stabilization. The slow eye movement will be quite regularly interrupted by a re-centering saccade, and this involuntary and self-perpetuating combination of slow and fast eye movement in opposite directions is a jerk nystagmus. Moreover, the retinal slip produced during the slow phase may be perceived as movement of the environment in the opposite direction, or this sensation of movement can be self-referred, namely the subject will feel a sensation of vertigo or oscillopsia (please note that during saccades we are functionally blind).

PerN is more often a horizontal-torsional nystagmus that beats toward the healthy side, and is reduced/suppressed by visual fixation. The beating direction does not change depending on the orbital position of the eye, but the amplitude and velocity of the nystagmus usually become larger as gaze is shifted toward the direction of the nystagmus.

2.2 Gaze Evoked Nystagmus

Gaze evoked nystagmus (GEN) is a nystagmus that is not detectable in the primary position of gaze, but on lateral gaze, and on upgaze and downgaze (not necessarily in all positions of gaze), and beats in the direction of gaze, i.e. changes direction depending on the gaze direction. GEN is independent of visual fixation, and may be more evident in the supine position.

The pathophysiology of GEN is an impairment of gaze-holding mechanisms: to move the eyes away from the primary position and keep them in the desired eccentric position, the ocular motor system needs to generate first a velocity signal, the pulse, to overcome the viscous forces inside the orbit, and then a position signal, the step, to overcome the elastic forces that would otherwise drive the eyes back to the primary position. The pulse, or velocity signal, is generated by the pulse generators, located in the pontine paramedian reticular formation (for horizontal saccades) and rostral interstitial nucleus of the medial longitudinal fascicles (for vertical and torsional saccades). The position signal is obtained by mathematical integration of the velocity signal, and the neural integrator is anatomically located within the medial vestibular nucleus and the nucleus prepositus hypoglossi (for horizontal saccades) or the nucleus interstitialis rostralis of the medial longitudinal fasciculus (for vertical saccades). The action of the neural integrator is reinforced by the cerebellar flocculus. Accordingly, GEN may result from a brainstem or a cerebellar lesion, but a focal brainstem lesion affecting the neural integrator only is unlikely, and GEN should suggest a floccular impairment. GEN can be associated with a downbeat nystagmus (DBN), an impairment of smooth pursuit eye movements, and an inability to suppress the VOR by visual fixation.

The combination of DBN and GEN on lateral gaze may take the form of an initially horizontal nystagmus (the GEN) that eventually becomes vertical (the DBN) with a short transitional "diagonal" phase.

Smooth pursuit eye movements are used to visually follow a moving object on a stable background, and they are driven by the velocity discrepancy between the eyes and the object. If the smooth pursuit system fails to match the velocity of the moving object, the position error between gaze and target triggers a saccade. Accordingly, on clinical examination, a smooth pursuit movement will appear abnormal when the smooth part of the movement is interrupted or completely substituted by saccades (catch-up saccades); this abnormality can equally affect all directions of movement, or it can be asymmetrical. To avoid a false-positive examination, the examiner should encourage the subject to follow the target to the very best of his/her ability, and the target should be moved through quite a large amplitude range (about 70° around primary position), and at a frequency no greater than 1 Hz, a condition in which the smooth pursuit system should not need any support from the saccade system. Please note that on clinical examination the only abnormality that can be detected is the occurrence of catch-up saccades, independently of the site of the lesion within the smooth pursuit system, and hence catch-up saccades are not pathognomonic of floccular impairment.

The VOR stabilizes gaze in space (i.e. moves the eyes in the orbit in the opposite direction to that of head movement); however, when the aim is to redirect gaze direction by moving the head, the VOR must be suppressed (i.e. the eyes must be kept still in the orbit). This suppression is provided by the cerebellar flocculus, through the visual smooth pursuit system.

VOR suppression can be tested by sitting the patient on an office chair that can be rotated.

The patient keeps his arms outstretched, with the two thumbs close to each other and in the upright position. The examiner sits in front of the patient, and rotates the chair while asking the patient to look at the examiner's nose (VOR) or at his/her own thumbs (VOR suppression).

The GEN is usually detectable as long as the subject tries to maintain the eccentric position, but can sometimes be attenuated and even disappear, and be associated with rebound nystagmus (RB) when the eyes are driven back to the primary position. The typical sequence is the following: no nystagmus in the primary position, left (or right) beating nystagmus on left (or right) gaze (GEN), followed by a right (or left) beating nystagmus when returning to the primary position (RB).

RB can be explained by the activation of a short-term adaptive mechanism. If we consider the previous example, the subject tries to keep his/her eyes on the target that is positioned to his left; because he is not able to generate a position signal for as long as it is needed, the eyes will drift (to the right) to the primary position, and the visual consequences of this retinal drift are that the target will seem to move to the left. Provided the smooth pursuit system is not greatly impaired, the subject can generate a leftward smooth pursuit signal that will be associated with, and compensate for, the time-decaying position signal, and keep the target on the fovea. On regaining the primary position, if this adaptive mechanism is not "turned off" immediately, the eyes will keep on slowly moving to the left, and a saccade, namely the RB, will be triggered to return them to the primary position. RB usually fades after a few beats of nystagmus.

The most common differential diagnosis for GEN is physiological or end-point nystagmus. It may be difficult to make the distinction on a clinical basis, but a few points can be helpful. Physiological nystagmus usually occurs in far-gaze only, is of small amplitude, and can be modulated (inhibited) by encouraging the subject to fixate the target. GEN, but not physiological nystagmus, can be associated with other cerebellar signs, in particular the following floccular signs: DBN, abnormal smooth pursuit, abnormal VOR suppression by visual fixation, RB.

2.3 Downbeat and Upbeat Nystagmus

Evidence of a vertical (downbeat or upbeat) nystagmus, but also of a pure torsional nystagmus, should always suggest a central etiology, namely a lesion in the central nervous system involving the central vestibular circuits.

Downbeat nystagmus (DBN) can be detected in all orbital positions but is usually best seen on lateral gaze; it can be positional, and can be increased by the supine position; it can be enhanced, decreased or transformed into upbeat nystagmus by convergence. DBN is not inhibited by visual fixation.

DBN is usually a consequence of a cerebellar dysfunction involving the flocculus. It can have very different underlying etiologies, but in about 30% of subjects it is idiopathic. It can be an isolated sign, but may also be associated with the other cerebellar floccular signs described elsewhere in this chapter: gaze evoked nystagmus, abnormal smooth pursuit eye movements, lack of inhibition of the VOR by visual fixation. When DBN is associated with gaze evoked nystagmus, and during lateral gaze, its direction may change, becoming more "diagonal" (directed laterally and downward).

Upbeat nystagmus (UBN) can be detected in all orbital positions but is usually best seen on upgaze; it can be positional; and it can be enhanced, decreased or transformed into downbeat nystagmus by convergence. UBN is not inhibited by visual fixation.

The sites of the lesion responsible for UBN are the paramedian medulla, pons and midbrain.

2.4 Pendular Nystagmus

In pendular nystagmus (PenN) there is no quick phase, only back-to-back slow phases in opposite directions. The direction of PenN can be purely horizontal or vertical, but it can also be a combination of both, and, depending on the relative amplitude and velocity and on the phase shift between the two, the trajectory of PenN can be diagonal, elliptical or circular. The oscillation may be conjugate, namely identical in the two eyes, but is more often slightly disconjugate, and in some cases PenN appears to be monocular. The frequency of eye oscillations ranges from 1 to 8 Hz, and may mimic saccadic oscillations. In the acquired form patients commonly complain of a disabling oscillopsia. PenN results from a combination of visual loss and brainstem demyelination, and can be seen in multiple sclerosis.

2.5 Internuclear Ophthalmoplegia

Internuclear opthalmoplegia (INO) is due to a lesion affecting the medial longitudinal fasciculus (MLF). The abducens nucleus contains some motor neurons that, through the abducens nerve, innervate the ipsilateral lateral rectus, but it also contains some interneurons that, through the MLF, reach the contralateral ocular motor neurons that innervate the contralateral medial rectus. We here refer to the motor and interneuron ensemble as the abducens nucleus complex. These anatomical connections are the basis of conjugate movement of the eyes in the horizontal plane: if you want to move your gaze to the right, you activate the right abducens neurons (both motor neurons and interneurons) that, in turn, will activate the right lateral rectus and, through the left MLF, the left medial rectus (please note that the side of the INO corresponds to the side of the ocular motor nucleus and not of the abducens nucleus). A left MLF lesion results in a left INO that, when the subject attempts to move his gaze to the right, is characterized by paresis of the adducting left eye and nystagmus of the abducting right eye. Because the neural signal, usually carried by the MLF, does not reach the neurons that innervate the left medial rectus, the adduction of the left eye will be impaired, and, depending on the severity of the lesion and on the compensatory phenomena, this impairment will range from complete paralysis (the left eye is unable to turn to the right and move further than the primary position) to more or less severe paresis (the left eye moves to the right slowly with a partial or a normal amplitude range). Since MLF lesions do not affect the right abducens nucleus, abducens nerve and lateral rectus, one would expect the movement to the right (abduction) of the right eye to be normal; actually, probably due to an increase of the neural signal generated within the abducens nucleus complex in order to increase the signal that will reach the ocular motor nerve through the dysfunctional MLF, the right eye will move more than normal and show a right beating nystagmus (Fig. 1). Overall, a left INO will appear when the subject tries to move his eyes to the right, showing up as a paresis (no or partial movement) of the adducting left eye, and with a right-beating nystagmus of the abducting right eye; since the nystagmus is not conjugate, but is detectable in the abducting eye only, it is called "dissociated nystagmus". The normal adduction of the left eye during convergence will confirm that the adduction deficit is due to an INO and not to an isolated paresis of the internal rectus. Sometimes a lesion, for instance a multiple sclerosis demyelinated plaque, can affect both MLFs and will result in bilateral INO. Finally, a lesion affecting both the abducens nuclear complex and the ipsilateral MLF will result in the one-and-half syndrome. In the case of a right MLF lesion, on the other hand, the attempt to move the eyes to the right will fail, namely there will be a gaze paresis due to the lesion of the right abducens nucleus complex (right abducens motor neurons, and right interneurons that give origin to the left MLF); the attempt to move the eyes to the left will result in an INO pattern due to the lesion of the right MLF: left beating nystagmus of the abducting left eye, impaired adduction of the right eye.

2.6 Periodic Alternating Nystagmus

Periodic alternating nystagmus (PAN) is a spontaneous horizontal nystagmus detectable in primary position that changes the beating direction after a fixed period.

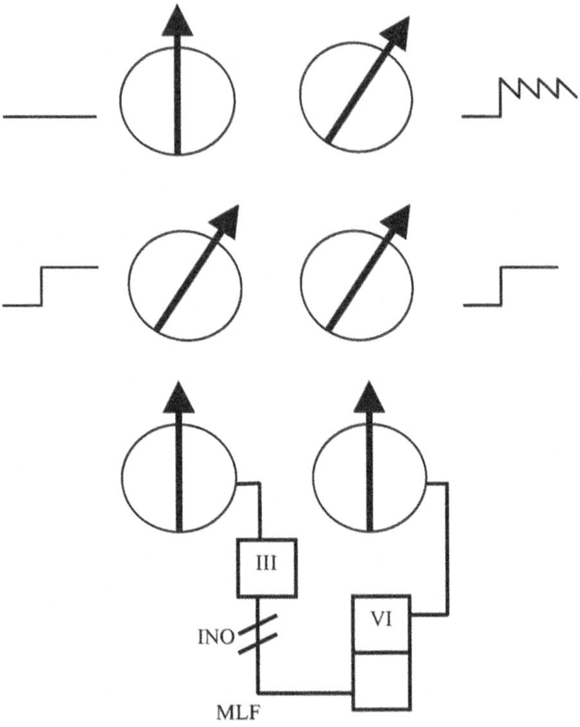

Fig. 1 Internuclear ophthalmoplegia. In the lower panel the anatomical structures involved in producing a rightward movement. In the middle panel an example of a normal rightward saccade: the movement is depicted as a "step" (time in the x-axis, position in the y-axis) near each eye. In the upper panel the same movement in the presence of INO due to lesion of the left MLF: a line, instead of a step, near the left eye means no (adducting) movement, while the saw-toothed step near the right (abducting) eye indicates right-beating nystagmus on right gaze. III: left ocular motor nucleus; VI: right abducens nucleus; INO: left internuclear opthalmoplegia due to lesion (double diagonal lines) along the left MLF

During the transition to the other direction, nystagmus may not be present or may briefly become upbeating or downbeating. In the congenital form the duration of this period is variable, while in the acquired form, it usually lasts between 90 and 120 s.

During bedside examination, PAN is not usually modified by visual fixation and can be suppressed by convergence or by head turning. In most cases, acquired PAN is secondary to a cerebellar dysfunction, in particular to a lesion involving the cerebellar nodulus and uvula.

3 Head Impulse Test

The Head Impulse Test (HIT) is a clever and simple maneuver first described by Halmagyi and Curthoys in 1988 [4]. The examiner and the subject are one in front of the other, and the subject is encouraged to relax his/her neck and to look carefully at a target, usually the examiner's nose. The examiner rotates the subject's head briskly through about 45° (2000–4000°/s), and when the head is stopped, the examiner looks at the subject's eyes. If the VOR is normal, the eyes will still be on the target and no compensatory eye movement is needed. If the VOR is hypoactive (the eyes move less than the head), a saccade in the opposite direction with respect to the head turn will bring the eyes to the target. If the VOR is hyper-active (the eyes move more than the head), a saccade in the same direction with respect to head turn will return the eyes to the target (Fig. 2).

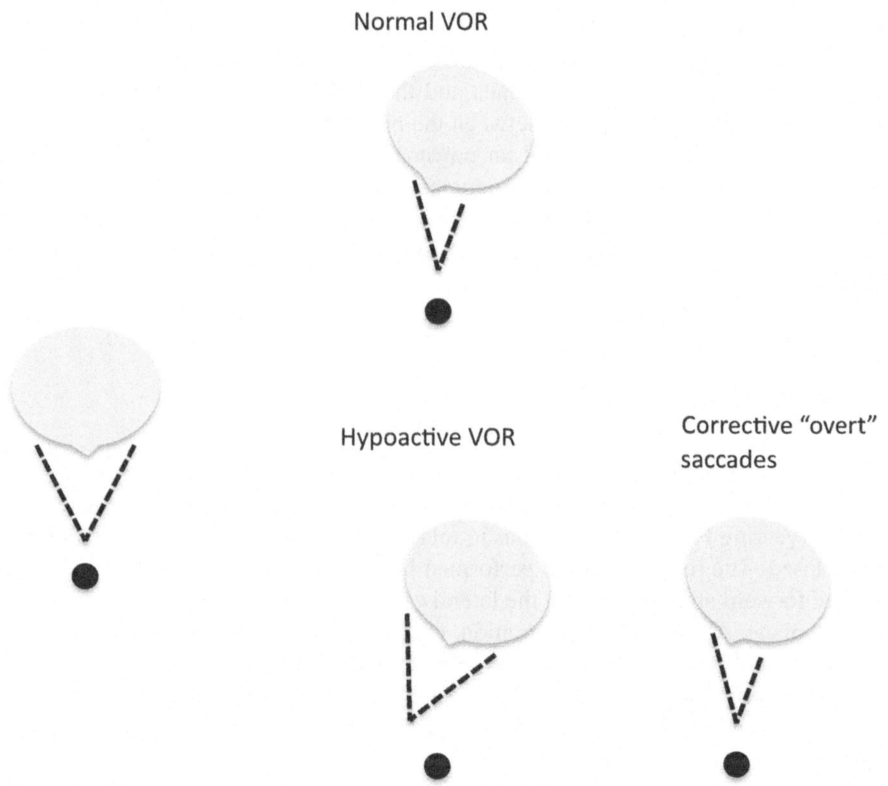

Fig. 2 Head Impulse Test. The left panel depicts a subject looking at a target. The middle panels show what happens when the subject tries to keep gaze on the target while the head is rotated to the right. If the VOR acts normally (upper middle panel), the eyes rotate to the left to compensate for the head motion, and gaze is kept on the target. If the VOR is hypoactive (lower middle panel), the movement of the eye to the left is not fully compensatory, and after the head is stopped a leftward corrective saccade is needed to foveate the target

These corrective saccades that can be seen after the head is stopped are called overt saccades, but the compensatory phenomena may also make the subject trigger covert saccades, namely corrective saccades that are already triggered during the movement of the head. Obviously, covert saccades are less easily detectable than overt ones.

A very interesting aspect of the HIT is that it evaluates the VOR by imposing very high angular acceleration, a condition in which the VOR relies almost exclusively on the activated (and not the inhibited) side. Accordingly, by rotating the head in the appropriate plane it is possible to evaluate the function of each individual canal. For instance, after asking the patient to pitch the head forward about 30°, a rotation in the horizontal plane will, respectively by rightward and leftward rotation, make it possible to evaluate the right and left lateral canal. The same holds true for vertical rotation, which allows evaluation of the vertical canals (the posterior canal of one side is functionally coupled with the anterior canal of the other side). The head is rotated by 45° with respect to the trunk and the brisk turn head turn is delivered in the vertical plane (around a bi-auricular axis). With the head turned leftward (or rightward), a vertical rotation will maximally excite the left (or right) posterior semicircular canals and the right (or left) anterior semicircular canals. Moreover, to distinguish between the posterior and the anterior semicircular canals we must bear in mind that an upward head rotation will maximally excite the posterior semicircular canals (producing a downward corrective saccade in the event of a deficit), while a downward head rotation will maximally excite the anterior semicircular canals (producing an upward corrective saccade in the event of a deficit).

4 Head Shaking Test

In the Head Shaking Test (HST) the examiner rotates the subject's head at about 2–3 Hz, for about 20 s and through an amplitude of about 60°. During the rotation the patient, wearing Frenzel goggles, has to relax his/her neck muscles and keep his/her eyes closed. The rotation can be performed both in the horizontal plane (with head pitched forward about 30° to put the lateral canals in the horizontal plane) and in the vertical plane. At the end of the rotation, the subject is asked to open his/her eyes.

The head shaking "charges" the vestibular storage mechanism, namely a central vestibular mechanism that makes the vestibular responses outlast the vestibular stimulation, and makes modulation by other sensory inputs (visual, proprioceptive) possible.

In healthy subjects, the velocity storage mechanism will be charged symmetrically, and hence the eyes will not move at the end of the rotation.

In the case of an acute unilateral vestibular loss, the velocity storage mechanism will be charged more by the healthy than by the affected side; this bias will be the same as during head rotation toward the healthy side, and hence it will trigger a jerk nystagmus toward the healthy side (at least 3 beats to be clinically significant).

In a patient with "central" vertigo, the HST may result in very different responses: no nystagmus, horizontal nystagmus, or vertical nystagmus (cross coupling). Obviously only the latter can be considered a central vestibular sign.

Glossary

DBN Downbeat Nystagmus

GEN Gaze Evoked Nystagmus

HIT Head Impulse Test

HST Head Shaking Test

INO Internuclear Ophthalmoplegia

MLF Medial Longitudinal Fasciculus

PAN Periodic Alternating Nystagmus

PenN Pendular Nystagmus

PerN Peripheral Nystagmus

RB Rebound Nystagmus

UBN Upbeat Nystagmus

VOR Vestibular Ocular Reflex

References

1. Baloh RW, Honrubia V, Kerber KA. Baloh and Honrubia's clinical neurophysiology of the vestibular system. Contemporary Neurology series. New York: Oxford University Press; 2011.
2. Brandt T. Vertigo. Its multisensory syndromes. London: Springer-Verlag; 1999.
3. Bronstein A, Lempert T. Dizziness. A practical approach to diagnosis and management. Cambridge: Cambridge University Press; 2007.
4. Halmagyi GM, Curthoys IS. A clinical sign of canal paresis. Arch Neurol. 1988;45(7):737–9.
5. Huh YE, Kim JS. Bedside evaluation of dizzy patients. J Clin Neurol. 2013;9(4):203–13. https://doi.org/10.3988/jcn.2013.9.4.203.
6. Kirchner H, Kremmyda O, Hufner K, Stephan T, Zingler V, Brandt T, Jahn K, Strupp M. Clinical, electrophysiological, and MRI findings in patients with cerebellar ataxia and a bilaterally pathological head-impulse test. Ann N Y Acad Sci. 2011;1233:127–38. https://doi.org/10.1111/j.1749-6632.2011.06175.x.
7. Leigh RJ, Zee DS. The neurology of eye movements. Contemporary Neurology series. New York: Oxford University Press; 2015.

8. Newman-Toker DE, Sharma P, Chowdhury M, Clemons TM, Zee DS, Della Santina CC. Penlight-cover test: a new bedside method to unmask nystagmus. J Neurol Neurosurg Psychiatry. 2009;80(8):900–3. https://doi.org/10.1136/jnnp.2009.174128.
9. Pierrot-Deseilligny C, Milea D. Vertical nystagmus: clinical facts and hypotheses. Brain. 2005;128(Pt 6):1237–46. https://doi.org/10.1093/brain/awh532.
10. Rett D. Gaze-evoked nystagmus: a case report and literature review. Optometry. 2007;78 (9):460–4. https://doi.org/10.1016/j.optm.2007.02.016.
11. Serra A, Leigh RJ. Diagnostic value of nystagmus: spontaneous and induced ocular oscillations. J Neurol Neurosurg Psychiatry. 2002;73(6):615–8.
12. Stahl JS, Averbuch-Heller L, Leigh RJ. Acquired nystagmus. Arch Ophthalmol. 2000;118 (4):544–9.
13. Straube A, Bronstein A, Straumann D, European Federation of Neurologic S. Nystagmus and oscillopsia. Eur J Neurol. (2012);19(1):6–14. https://doi.org/10.1111/j.1468-1331.2011.03503.x.
14. Strupp M, Hufner K, Sandmann R, Zwergal A, Dieterich M, Jahn K, Brandt T. Central oculomotor disturbances and nystagmus: a window into the brainstem and cerebellum. Dtsch Arztebl Int. 2011;108(12):197–204. https://doi.org/10.3238/arztebl.2011.0197.
15. Strupp M, Kremmyda O, Adamczyk C, Bottcher N, Muth C, Yip CW, Bremova T. Central ocular motor disorders, including gaze palsy and nystagmus. J Neurol. (2014);261(2): S542–58. https://doi.org/10.1007/s00415-014-7385-9.
16. Strupp M, Magnusson M. Acute unilateral vestibulopathy. Neurol Clin. (2015);33(3): 669–685, x. https://doi.org/10.1016/j.ncl.2015.04.012.
17. Welgampola MS, Bradshaw AP, Lechner C, Halmagyi GM. Bedside assessment of acute dizziness and vertigo. Neurol Clin. (2015);33(3):551–64, vii. https://doi.org/10.1016/j.ncl. 2015.04.001.
18. Zee DS. Ophthalmoscopy in examination of patients with vestibular disorders. Ann Neurol. 1978;3(4):373–4. https://doi.org/10.1002/ana.410030421.

Balance Rehabilitation Using Computerized Dynamic Posturographic Platforms

Isabella Springhetti and Chiara Villani

1 Introduction

Balance can be thought of as a "*complex, open, multi-functional system*":

- complex, because the system consists of several sub-systems and balance is the result of their internal interrelationship (totality, calibration);
- open, because interactions with the environment can alter the result (feedback, equifinality).

Two particular aspects of a complex, open system are important as they interfere with communication and human learning: *redundancy*, i.e. an excessive amount of converging peripheral information, and *preferentiality*, i.e. the human ability to use a preferred sensory channel (Fig. 1).

In everyday life, a normal subject has the ability to choose the information that best fits his purpose at a given time and in a given context. Preferentiality is an individual feature from the early stages of childhood development: some individuals preferentially rely on visual information, while others rely more on vestibular or proprioceptive information. Nevertheless, many everyday tasks require activation of the vestibular channel. This is particularly true when the visual cues are scarce (darkness) and/or the gait surface is unstable or uneven.

I. Springhetti (✉) · C. Villani
Neuromotor and Oncological Rehabilitation Unit,
Istituti Clinici Scientifici Maugeri, Pavia, Italy
e-mail: isabella.springhetti@icsmaugeri.it

G. Sandrini et al. (eds.), *Advanced Technologies for the Rehabilitation of Gait and Balance Disorders*, Biosystems & Biorobotics 19,
https://doi.org/10.1007/978-3-319-72736-3_6

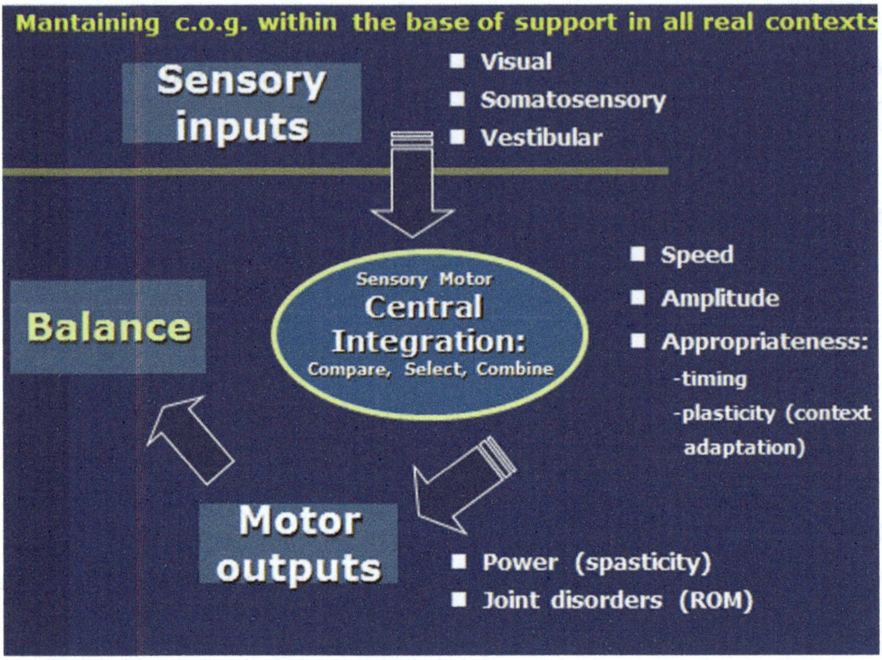

Fig. 1 Simplified framework for the balance concept. Maintaining the center of gravity within the base of support in all real contexts requires: **a** information from the periphery through different channels: visual, labyrinthine/vestibular, proprioceptive; **b** selection/integration of the central nervous system to adapt responses to changes in the environment and in the required task; **c** coordinated motor responses (amplitude, timing and spatiality) (property of the author I.S.)

The elderly may present sensory depletion, with less redundancy and more preferentiality. In other words, aging implies:

- a decrease in sensory channels;
- reduced ability to use the most appropriate channels;
- decreased central integration ability.

Furthermore, comorbidities result in impaired effector efficiency, consisting of reduced muscle trophism, loss of tendon flexibility, and skeletal deformities. Such conditions shift the center of gravity (CoG) close to the limits of stability even in a stable state.

Similarly, due to multiple sensory and/or motor deficits and constraints, the ill subject loses efficiency. This leads to a reduction in adaptive capacity [1], especially when the central nervous system is trying to select from potentially conflicting sensory information. The results of this effort are the signs and symptoms.

As an example, having to rely more on visual information, patients with peripheral vestibular lesions will suffer from vertigo whenever they see close moving images. Attempting to avoid vertigo, such patients will try to avoid relying on visual information. However, without good proprioceptive training, they will tend towards instability, with a risk of falling, especially in twilight and on uneven surfaces.

Alternatively, in the same situation, other patients might use residual vestibular information, inevitably holding their heads very stiffly, thus increasing the risk of headaches or neck pain.

Many chronic conditions have multiple causes not attributable to a single site of injury, meaning that signs and symptoms accumulate and overlap. This is why a functional model is necessary. Patients with similar pathologies may show different impairments and will respond differently to a given treatment. The best approach is multidisciplinary, impairment based and evidence based, but also takes into account pathological information [2]. To reduce the effects of impairments, patients usually use spontaneous and unconscious motor responses, related to pre-existing neurophysiological attitudes and individual clinical complexity. However, some responses are not appropriate or beneficial.

Thus, a rehabilitation specialist should consider the effectiveness of these automatic responses and the way patients implement them in response to different stimuli.

CDP analyzes how patients react to different stimuli, thus helping the rehabilitation specialist to understand and treat the imbalance.

2 The Model

2.1 The Pillars

Clinical outcome studies have demonstrated that models focusing more on impairment and functional limitations than on pathology alone produce better results and are cost effective. Taking into account an individual's interactions and the context, the model identifies three fundamental components (Fig. 2) that vary according to external and internal conditions:

1. **The subject**: according to the model, a person in an upright position acts like an inverted cone, swinging in space without losing balance. The "pivot" of the oscillations is located slightly in front of the tibiotarsal joints. The swing occurs within 8° and 4° angles anteriorly and posteriorly, thus defining the limits of stability (Fig. 3); when these limits are exceeded the subject falls.

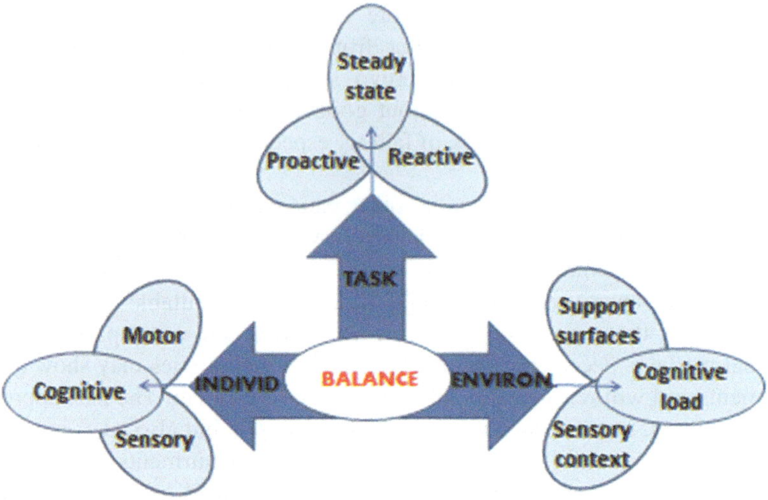

Fig. 2 Trying to translate the complexity of the balance control system into simple behavioral procedures, researchers have studied and tested several models. The one proposed by Woollacott and Shumway-Cook is extremely functional and useful. It clearly identifies the key components and interactions between subject, task and environment. (*From* Woollacott and Shumway-Cook [10], 2016 adapted with authors' permission)

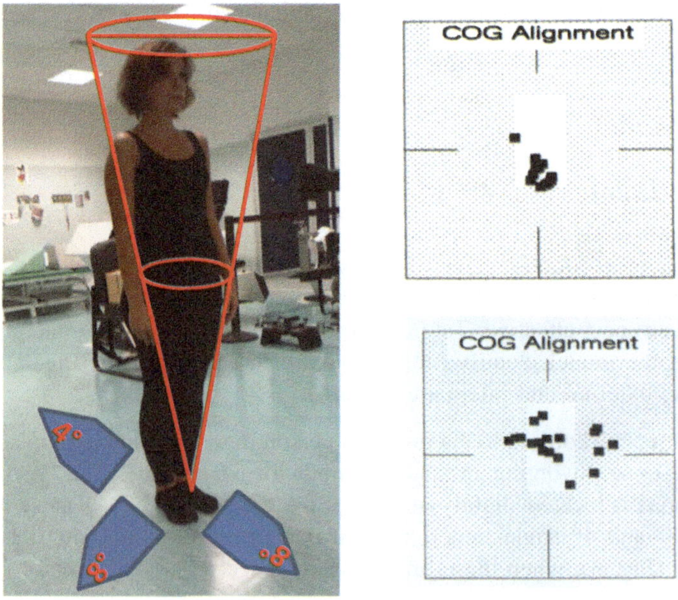

Fig. 3 During standing, the CoG of a normal subject remains within the base of support. She swings like an inverted cone within definite limits of stability: about 16° laterally, 8° anteriorly and 4.5° posteriorly. To maintain an upright position beyond these limits, the subject needs to shift the CoG or, alternatively, adopt appropriate motor strategies to keep it within the base. The amplitude of normal sway is minimal in a healthy subject, as shown in the Balance Master® sway report (top, right), but can be much wider in an impaired subject (bottom, right: cerebellar). (Property of the author)

The overall performance of humans is expressed within an interval of normality that takes into account age, sex, population categorization, etc., and reflects the sum of individual cognitive, motor and sensory features.

2. **The environment**: the context stimulates the subject to react. One sensory channel or another is stimulated depending on the characteristics of the context. For example, while standing on a cushion, the continuously changing pressure of the soft support "deceives" the proprioception of the feet. For this reason, in order to maintain an upright position, a healthy subject "prefers" to rely on vestibular information. In addition, each context brings a different cognitive load for subjects. For example, significant cognition is required of a pedestrian crossing a busy street with a bundle in his arms, while speaking on the phone.
3. **The requirements of the task**: the type of voluntary activity guides the reactions needed to complete it. Maintaining balance during any activity involves specific reactions that are appropriate to the activity. Crossing a road requires reactions different from those involved in taking a book down from a high shelf while standing on the rung of a ladder.

2.2 *Balance Conditions*

The model identifies three specific categories of balance for humans.

1. **Static Balance**: this is the ability to maintain the CoG within the support base in the absence of external perturbations while standing. Standing in an upright position is considered an unstable condition: healthy subjects minimally oscillate within their support base, but when approaching the limits of stability, a fall is prevented only by making appropriate adjustments and adopting suitable strategies.

Static equilibrium is examined with the subject in a standing position.

Locomotion at a constant pace is considered a steady state and can be investigated while walking on a treadmill at a constant speed.

A static condition can be disturbed for assessment or training purposes, recreating unexpected situations (reactive balance) or recreating voluntary actions (proactive balance).

2. **Reactive Balance**: this is the ability to recover a steady CoG *after an unexpected perturbation*, like a push or unexpected acceleration while standing on a bus.

Reactive balance is displayed by a subject whose CoG, because of external perturbations, is close to, or exceeds, the limits of stability. In these cases, the swaying motion of the ankle is insufficient to maintain the CoG within the base of support (*ankle strategy*).[1] Different strategies are progressively required in relation to the intensity of the destabilization:

1. *Hip strategy*, in which the pivot of the swing is located at the level of the subject's pelvis.
2. *Limb strategy* (upper): when destabilization is significant, this reaction results in the upper limbs being opened, as this has the effect of increasing the base of support;
3. *Step strategy*: as the final option, when an external perturbation is too powerful, the subject is forced to take a step in the same direction as the perturbation.

Reactive balance can be assessed by challenging a patient to respond to unexpected perturbations that have been recreated artificially in the gym by altering external and internal conditions. Alterations may concern:

a. the subject (e.g. eyes open vs eyes closed);
b. the environment (e.g. soft, hard or narrow surfaces); or
c. the task (e.g. holding an object).

Variations can be integrated separately, as above, or together (soft or narrow surface associated with closed eyes and holding/not holding an object), forcing the subject to make continuous sensory shifts (see below). Additional tasks with different cognitive loads can also be used (e.g. reciting poetry).

3. **Proactive Balance**: this is the ability to minimize instability during voluntary movement. It requires the use of *anticipatory reactions*, which are automated responses activated before the start of the action and aimed at achieving correct postural alignment to prevent excessive displacement of the CoG. Typically, - they occur before rising on tiptoes, lifting a suitcase, or leaning over an obstacle to reach a distant object with an upper limb, but most of voluntary activities of everyday life require this type of preparatory reactions.

Proactive balance can be assessed by challenging the patient to perform voluntary actions, in different conditions, choosing appropriate strategies. These differ in relation to:

a. the subject (e.g. eyes open vs. eyes closed);
b. the environment (e.g. soft, hard or narrow surfaces); or
c. the task (e.g. holding an object).

As above, variations in the context can be integrated, separately or together with different sensory conditions. Additional tasks at different cognitive loads (e.g. reciting poetry) can also be used.

---

[1]The reaction is initiated by the gastrocnemius tendon (due to passive anterior displacement of the body) or anterior tibialis tendon (due to passive posterior displacement) stretching. The sudden elongation makes the posterior or anterior muscle chains react, respectively.

2.3 *Sensory Interaction*

In both the reactive and the proactive state, close sensory integration is needed [3].

Proper sensory interaction is a key element in maintaining balance throughout the typical conditions of daily life. Every day, humans accomplish hundreds of voluntary actions in destabilizing contexts.

Integration at central nervous system level suppresses inaccurate and/or unreliable sensory information, supporting the most efficient channel in each case. Moreover, centralized integration provides the appropriate motor strategies in the right sequence at any given time.[2] The choice is related to the three key variables: context, task and patient.

To evaluate the efficiency of sensory interaction, one or more of the sensory channels are rendered unreliable, rather than excluded. Depending on the context and task, the subject is forced to shift from one channel to another in order to keep the CoG within the base of support. When the light is poor or the floor uneven, the visual feedback loop is too slow, it requires more than 200 ms before the subject responds. Such an interval is acceptable for changing posture during stance or during slow voluntary actions, but for preventing a fall, the vestibular channel is much more efficient.

In clinical conditions, the ability to switch channels can be tested by using altered information to mislead patients during voluntary or unexpected motions. Visual cues can be warped by specially altered lenses, or by a special helmet that acts as a dome. Proprioception is warped by using soft oscillating supports and vestibular information by bending the neck and head backwards or laterally.

3 Assessment On Computerized Posturographic Platforms: A Functional Diagnosis[3]

Clinical tests are useful and commonly used tools for investigating and quantifying different features of balance. Empirical assessment tests are detailed in the previous paragraphs. Qualitative assessment tests include, among others, the Berg Balance Scale [4], the Balance Evaluation System Test [5], and the Equiscale [6].

[2]It will be noticed that this chapter, in referring to the model, places the emphasis on the vestibular system, rather than the cerebellum, for regulating balance. This is not meant to result in the role of this important component and its related connections being overlooked. The fact that we appear to have assigned a secondary role to the cerebellum is linked to the need for simplification and a clear explanation of the functioning of the equipment. The role of the cerebellum is essential in central integration activities, especially in feed-forward loops. The reader will find more on these mechanisms elsewhere in this book.

[3]The assessment protocols performed with CDP are defined by the American Academy of Otolaryngology–Head and Neck Surgery as a gold standard in evaluation and diagnosis of vertigo/dizziness and disequilibrium of known and unknown etiologies and in medical case management.

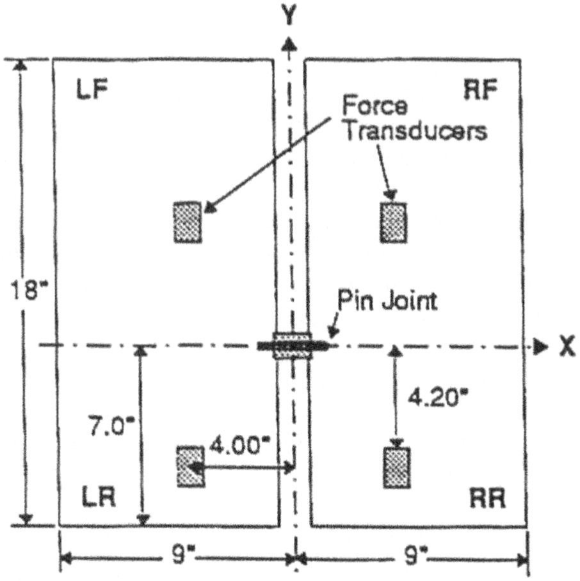

Fig. 4 The core of the instrument is the pair of force transducers (anterior F and posterior R) placed inside each plate (left and right). Transducers record forces exerted by the patient's foot. Signals are transmitted, compared and converted into numerical or graphic form by the system. (*From* Natus website, modified: http://www.natus.com/index.cfm?page=products_1&crid=484&contentid=397)

The balance domains explored by clinical tests can be better reproduced and quantified in different conditions on posturographic platforms. The references and examples of the tests reported below refer extensively to the assessment and treatment protocols performed on NeuroCom®, Equitest® and Balance Master® platforms[4] [7].

The crucial part of these equipment consists of four force transducers. They track the direction and strength of the load exerted by the patient's foot (center of pressure), thus detecting the movement of the CoG (Fig. 4). The distinctive feature of these platforms [8] is that they can be used to assess reactive balance, proactive balance and somatosensory interaction (see below). In addition, their results can be standardized for age and gender.

Specific features and properties of other types of equipment are summarized in a comparative table at the end of this chapter (Table 1).

[4]Natus Medical Incorporated-Corporate Headquarters, 6701 Koll Center Parkway Suite 120, Pleasanton, CA 94566 USA.

3.1 Reactive Balance

Reactive balance can be assessed on Equitest® platform (Fig. 5) by making a patient respond to artificially created perturbations. The footplates simulate disturbances in different planes, for example, horizontal translation and tilt.

The **Motor Control Test** (backward and forward translation) (Fig. 6) evaluates realignment between the CoG and center of force after a linear movement of the support base. The patient is required to maintain his/her balance during a series of three abrupt horizontal translations (forwards and backwards, of different amplitudes). The system assesses the ability of the patient to rapidly recover the CoG position after unexpected perturbations, by adopting the best strategy (ankle or hip) (Fig. 7). Normal subjects learn very rapidly. Depending on the type of impairment, patients' performances can be characterized by: slow responses, incorrect timing, lack of power.

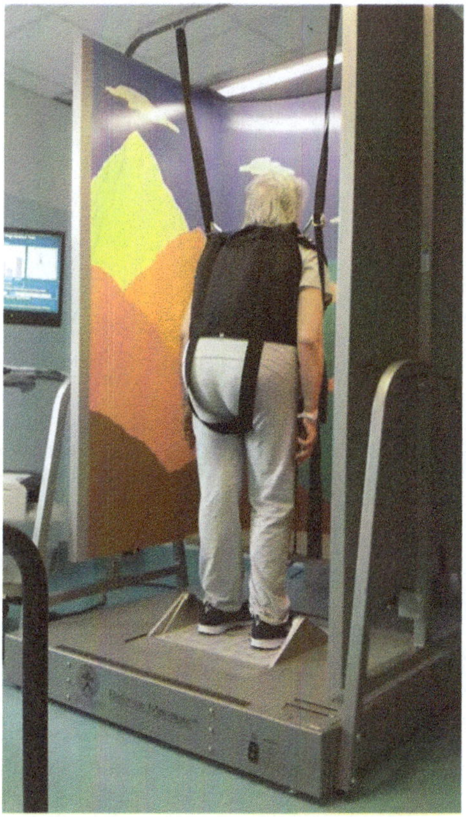

Fig. 5 Equitest® is equipped with a visual surround that alters the reliability of visual cues. The surround moves according to patient's movements: the more the patient sways, the more the surround sways. The platform also moves, by tilting or shearing in the horizontal plane. Depending on the test (see text), the platform can move concurrently with the patient or independently. Commands and feedback can be seen on the side screen and PC. (*Image* Property of the author)

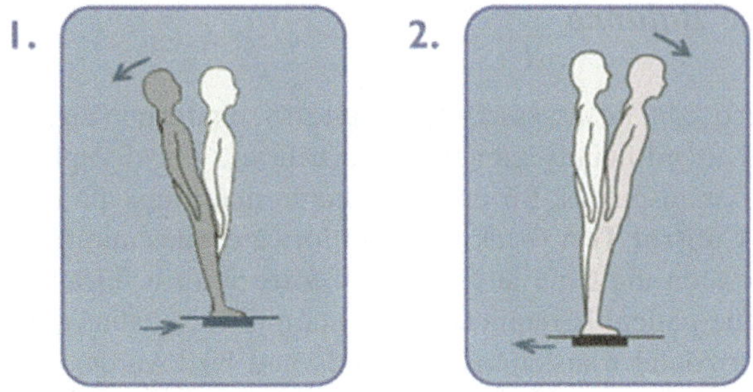

Fig. 6 Reactive Balance—Motor Control Test. The figure shows the passive motion of a subject in the early stages of a sudden translation of the platform. The consequent displacement induces a stretch reflex in the tibialis anterior muscle (left 1), and in the gastrocnemius muscle (right 2), thus starting the realignment of the CoG within the support base, operated by the anterior/posterior muscle chain. (*From* "Objective Quantification of Balance and Mobility" by NeuroCom® International Inc., Clackamas, OR 2003©)

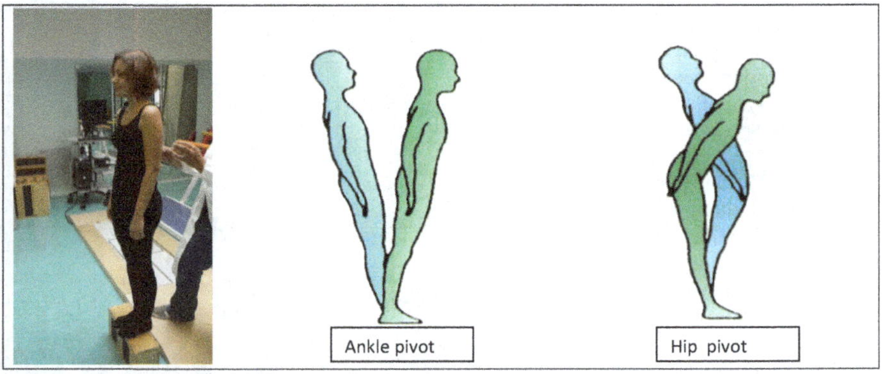

Fig. 7 The strategy adopted by the subject to regain balance depends on the magnitude of the perturbation and on the proximity to the limits of stability. Environment also influences strategies: on a narrow support (see photograph), when a major perturbation occurs, the CoG is rapidly displaced beyond the limits. In this case, a different strategy (see drawing on the right), like the hip strategy, can realign the center of force and the CoG within the support base. (*Image* Property of the author)

The system provides a graphic report of the following: symmetry in weight distribution, latency of the onset of the patient's reaction (from the start of the stimulus), and amplitude scaling (the strength of the response) for both legs during the three different translations (backwards and forwards). The gray area on each graph indicates results outside the normal range (for age and gender) (Fig. 8).

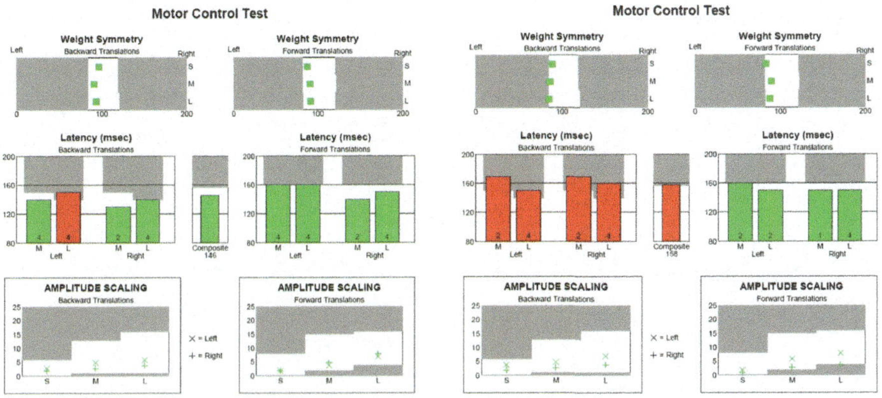

Fig. 8 The Motor Control Test report displays symmetry, latencies of backward and forward translations and the intensity of muscle strength responses. (*Image* Property of the author)

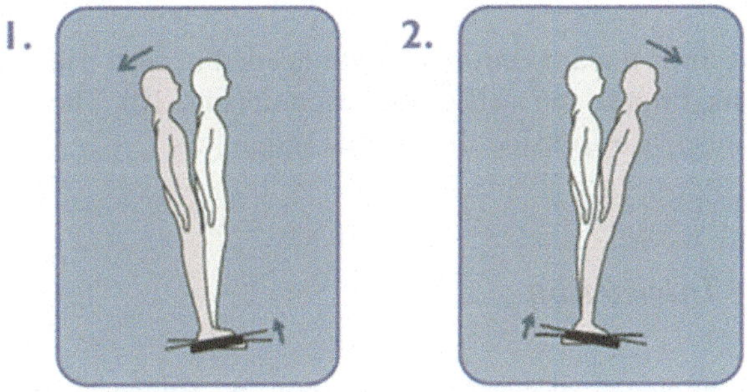

Fig. 9 Reactive Balance—Adaptation Test. The figure shows the passive motion of a subject in the early stages of a sudden rotation (tilt) of the platform. Due to the initial position of the CoG, anterior displacement occurs faster than posterior displacement; this motion induces a stretch reflex in the gastrocnemius muscle in both cases (left 1 and right 2). The test evaluates the ability of a subject to adapt to consecutive unexpected perturbations. (*From* "Objective Quantification of Balance and Mobility" by NeuroCom® International Inc., Clackamas, OR 2003©)

The **Adaptation Test** (upward and downward rotations) evaluates the time required for motor realignment of the CoG during a series of five tilting movements of the platform (Fig. 9). The patient is required to maintain balance during a series of five random upward and downward movements of the base. In this case the system assesses the ability of the patient to minimize sway when exposed to uneven surfaces, and the ability to calibrate the necessary strength. Normal subjects rapidly adapt the response pattern and, after the first unexpected perturbation, critically reduce sway and increase stability. Patients, on the other hand, can have difficulty adapting to unpredictable displacements. This may be due to ankle/hip constraints (range of movement) or muscle weakness, among other causes.

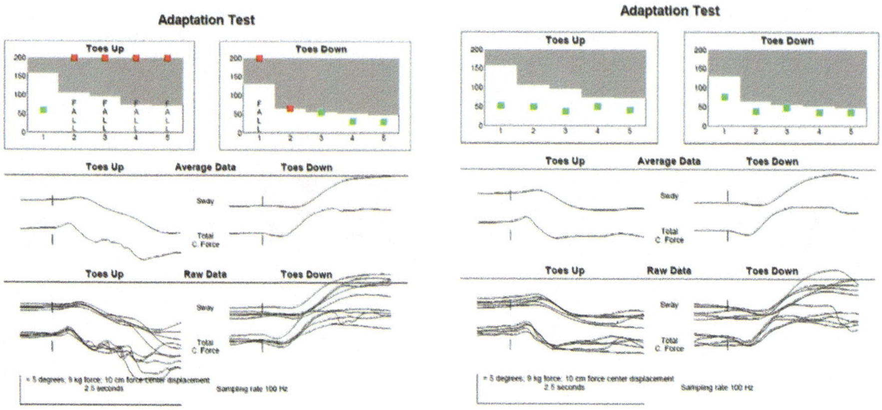

Fig. 10 Adaptation Test report. After the first disruption, the subsequent responses are faster and stronger with reduced destabilization. Comparison between before and after training shows a marked improvement in upward tilt compared with downward tilt. (*Image* Property of the author)

The system records the amount of strength needed in each trial, the amplitude of sway, and the time prior to the start of the reaction (Fig. 10). The gray area on each graph indicates responses outside the normal range.

3.2 *Sensory Interaction*

To evaluate the efficiency of sensory interaction, an Equitest® system is required (see Fig. 5). Equitest combines all the possible interactions in a single test, known as the Sensory Organization Test (SOT).

In this test, six key conditions are investigated. In two of these, the patient has to keep the CoG within the base of support, relying on only one sensory channel, the others being rendered unreliable (Fig. 11). The six conditions are the following:

1. **Standing, eyes open without external perturbations**: the patient remains standing on the platform for the duration of the test with eyes open. This is a static equilibrium condition in which the subject has all sensory systems available.
2. **Standing, eyes closed without external perturbations**: the patient remains standing on the platform for the duration of the test with eyes closed. This is a static equilibrium condition in which the subject has only two of the three sensory systems available: proprioception and the vestibular system.
3. **Standing on a fixed support, eyes open, unreliable visual information**: the patient is fed unreliable information on a screen surrounding the platform which tilts according to the patient's sway. The patient is not able to perceive the motion of the surround because it is concurrent with his/her own motion. In this

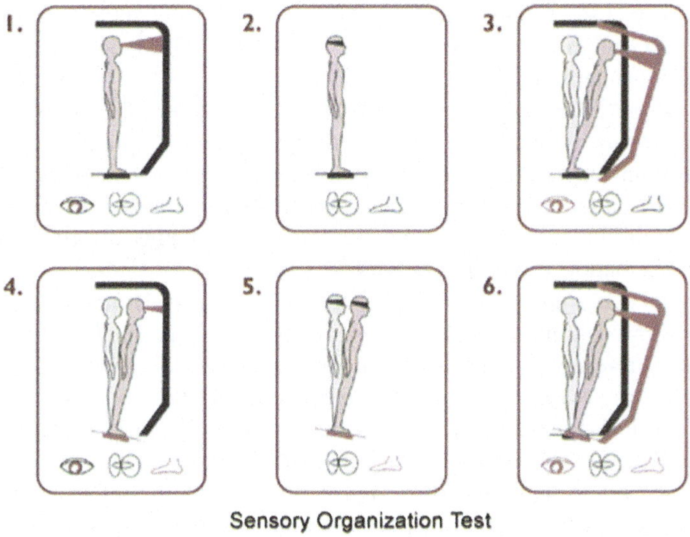

Fig. 11 The six conditions explored by the Equitest® Sensory Organization Test are illustrated above. The sensory analysis compares conditions as follows: condition 2, testing the ability of the patient to use proprioceptive information, c4 testing the ability to use the visual channel, and c5 testing the ability to use vestibular channel. Preference derives from comparison of the (3 + 6) versus (2 + 5) conditions. In 3 and 6 the visual channel is impaired, while in 2 and 5 it is excluded. In all these cases the subject must rely on channels other than the visual one; patients affected by neuropathy usually persist in using the visual channel most. (*From* "Objective Quantification of Balance and Mobility" by NeuroCom® International Inc., Clackamas, OR 2003©)

way, the patient is forced to rely only on two of the three sensory systems: proprioception and the vestibular system, because visual information is rendered unreliable by the movement of the surround.

4. **Standing, eyes open, tilting support**: the platform tilts according to the patient's spontaneous swaying. The patient is not able to perceive the platform motion because it is concurrent with his/her own motion. In this way, the patient is forced to rely only on two of the three sensory systems: vision and the vestibular system. Proprioception is rendered unreliable by the movement of the platform.
5. **Standing, eyes closed, tilting support**: the platform tilts according to the patient's spontaneous swaying. The patient is forced to rely only on the vestibular system for information. Proprioception is rendered unreliable by the movement of the platform and vision is excluded (eyes are closed).
6. **Standing, eyes open, tilting support and surround**: both platform and shield tilt according to the patient's spontaneous swaying. The patient is forced to rely only on one of the three sensory systems: the vestibular system. Proprioception and vision are rendered unreliable by the movement of the platform and surround.

The equipment analyzes the patient's movements at hip and ankle level (strategies), and their CoG alignment throughout the whole test. The report is complex and consists of four main graphs.

In the examples in Fig. 12, the *equilibrium score* shows the progress of a sensory impaired patient unable to maintain balance in the most challenging conditions (SOT conditions 4, 5 and 6, marked "Fall" on the left of the image). The comparison before and after (right image) treatment shows an improvement in keeping the CoG within the base, even in the presence of conflicting information or when only one information source is available.

The *sensory analysis* highlights how a patient uses the different sensory channels. The right column in both sensory analysis graphs displays the details of preference. "Preference" indicates the degree to which the patient relies on inaccurate or incorrect sensory channels, regardless of the availability of reliable channels, and it is determined by comparing the scores from trials' conditions 2 + 5 and 3 + 6. Patients affected by sensory disorders may be unable to make effective use of the sensory system, and show a preference for visual information when the vestibular system would be preferable, thus failing to adapt responses to the task or/ and context.

The *strategy analysis* is displaced in the central graph of both sets of images (Fig. 12). The ankle is used for minimal displacement, while the hip intervenes when the displacement is stronger. The report shows the performance strategy for each condition (symbols) and appropriateness is indicated by the relative position across the oblique strip.

The comparison of performance before and after treatment shows an increased use of all channels, and therefore that correct strategies are starting to be implemented.

A simplified test for detecting sensory interaction is also available, i.e. the modified Clinical Test of Sensory Interaction on Balance (mCTSIB) [9]. For this test a Balance Master® System is required. The main features of this instrument are illustrated in Fig. 13. Commands and feedback are provided on a screen. The whole assessment consists of a group of tests, some of which are static and some dynamic. This assessment does not include complete visual system evaluation. The patient is required to stand on firm and soft surfaces, with open and closed eyes respectively. Three trials for each of the aforesaid conditions are performed. The system provides a report showing: the mean CoG sway velocity, the CoG alignment during the trials, and a shaded area, which indicates values outside the normal range (Fig. 14). Due to the unreliability of proprioception (evaluated using foam) and the exclusion of vision (eyes closed), the most difficult trial (fourth: foam, eyes closed) forces the patient to rely only on the vestibular system. The large white area behind the fourth column, shows augmented normal ranges of sway velocity (deg/sec) indicating a remarkable variability of CoG sway in this condition.

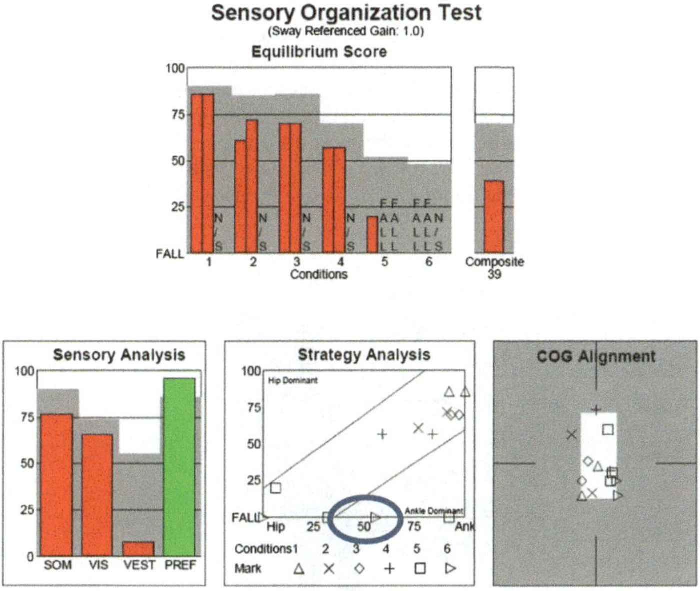
Sensory Organization Test
(Sway Referenced Gain: 1.0)
Equilibrium Score
100
75
50
25
FALL
1 2 3 4 5 6
Conditions
Composite
39
Sensory Analysis
SOM VIS VEST PREF
Strategy Analysis
Hip Dominant
Ankle Dominant
Hip 25 50 75 Ank
Conditions 1 2 3 4 5 6
Mark
COG Alignment

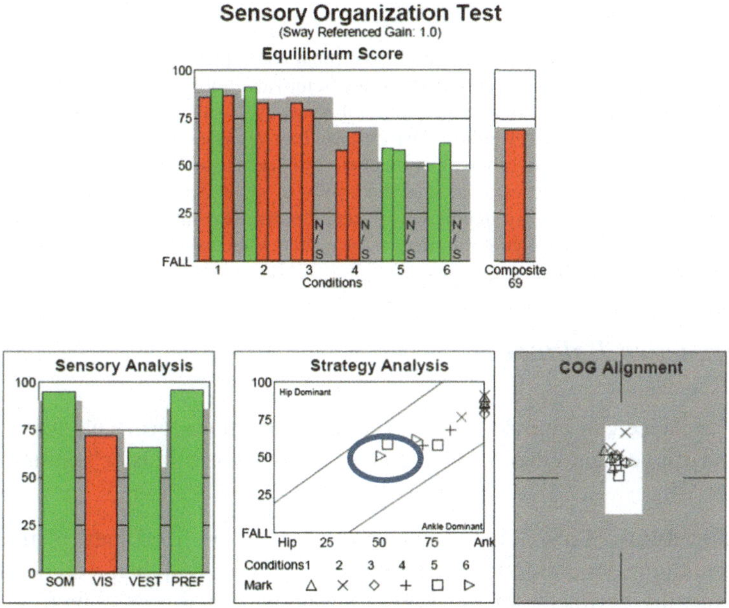
Sensory Organization Test
(Sway Referenced Gain: 1.0)
Equilibrium Score
100
75
50
25
FALL
1 2 3 4 5 6
Conditions
Composite
69
Sensory Analysis
SOM VIS VEST PREF
Strategy Analysis
Hip Dominant
Ankle Dominant
Hip 25 50 75 Ank
Conditions 1 2 3 4 5 6
Mark
COG Alignment

◀**Fig. 12** The figure shows the SOT report with the equilibrium score under each of the trials, the sensory analysis with the preference, the strategy analysis (hip or ankle), and the CoG alignment. The pre-treatment (above) and the post-treatment (below) results are shown. In the central graph there is an oblique strip with symbols in it. Symbols represent patients' performance oscillating in each trial between the hip and ankle strategies. For example, in the pre-treatment graph, the small horizontal triangle representing trial 6, the most difficult, is excessively displaced towards the ankle strategy, whereas in the post-treatment one, it is well balanced between the two strategies, lying in the center of the oblique strip. (*Image* Property of the author)

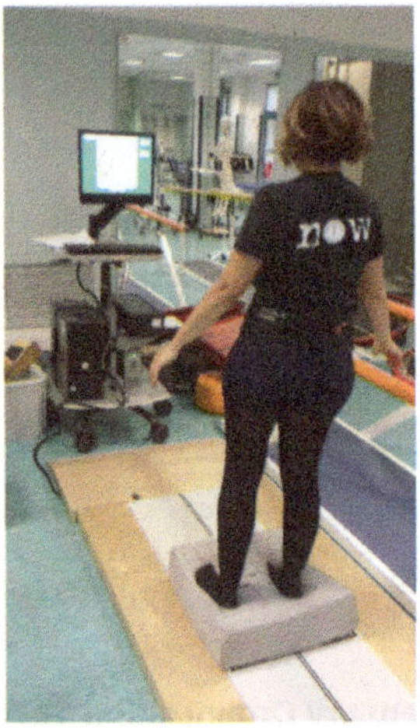

Fig. 13 Balance Master® has the same core part (dual force plate) as Equitest®, but lacks the surround and the plate motion. A set of accessories (removable tools, boxes, oscillating and fixed boards, ladders and a cushion) are provided to test the patient's behavior during different tasks and on different degrees of surface rigidity. The cushion/foot interface mimics the tilting platform movements in Equitest. Among others, this platform provides a simplified assessment of sensory interaction: the mCTSIB. The test evaluates the ability of a subject to maintain the CoG in the center of the support base over different sensory conditions. The subject's CoG movements are reproduced by a small human figure moving on the screen, concurrent with patient's movements. (*Image* Property of the author)

3.3 Proactive Balance

Proactive balance can be assessed by making a patient perform voluntary tasks on the spot. To investigate this balance condition, a Balance Master® System can be used.

Limit of Stability (LoS): This test is conducted on the fixed hard platform. The patient, standing, is required to reach a linear target first, and then a circle of targets reproducing the perimeter of the limits of stability on a screen in front of him (Fig. 15).

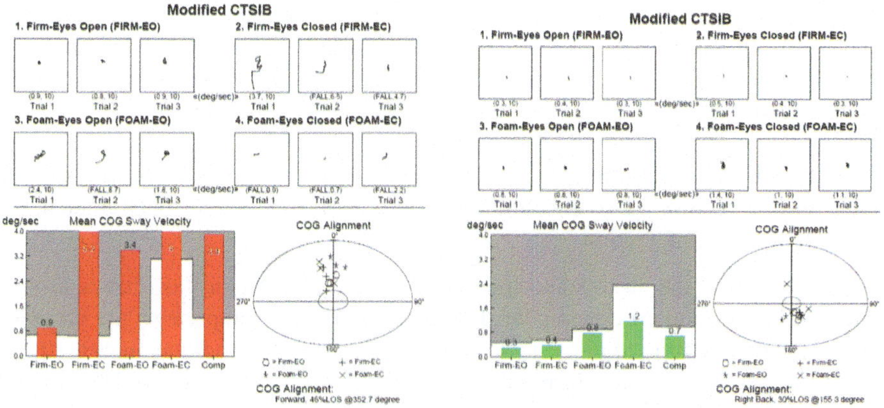

Fig. 14 The Balance Master provides a modified sensory interaction test (the modified Clinical Test of Sensory Interaction on Balance, mCTSIB, derived from the original by Horak and Shumway-Cook). The report shows the oscillation of the CoG in all trials, the CoG overall alignment, and the sway velocity (degree/sec) in all trials. (*Image* Property of the author)

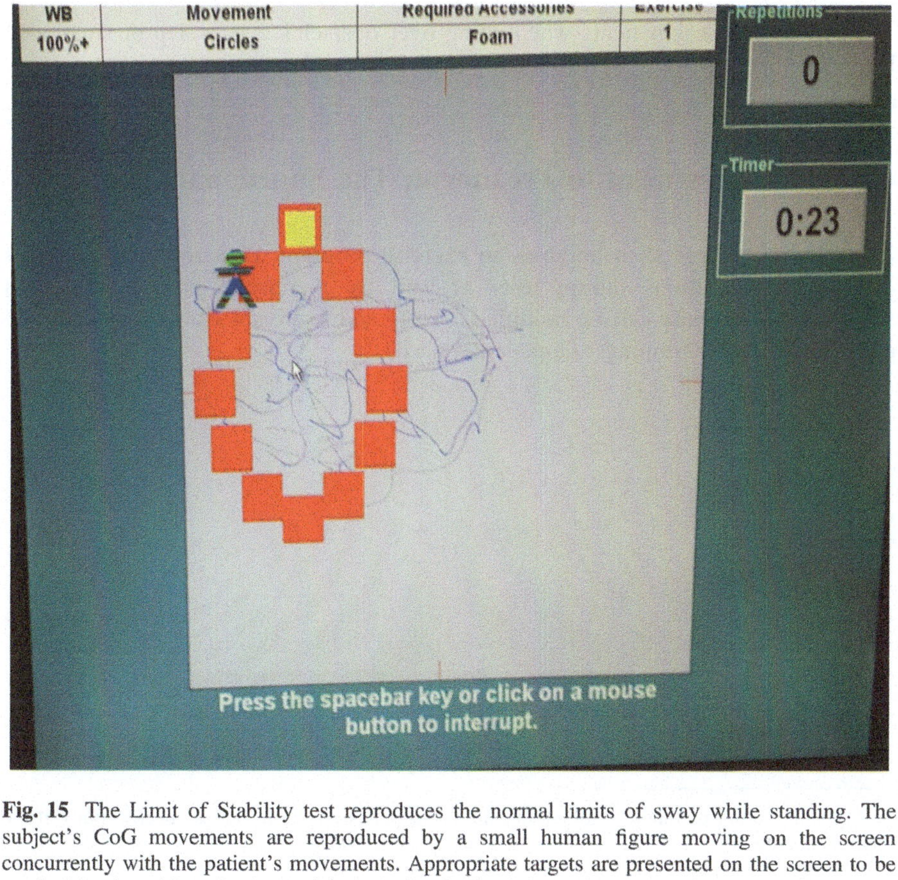

Fig. 15 The Limit of Stability test reproduces the normal limits of sway while standing. The subject's CoG movements are reproduced by a small human figure moving on the screen concurrently with the patient's movements. Appropriate targets are presented on the screen to be reached by the subject. During training, similar feedback is used to train voluntary displacements. (*Image* Property of the author)

The test evaluates the maximum distance the CoG can be displaced without loss of balance during voluntary movement. For each trial the system records: the reaction time from command to onset, the movement velocity (as CoG speed), excursion quality (endpoint and directional control), and the maximum distance covered (Fig. 16).

During the test, variations in the context (e.g. flooring type and size) and the tasks (direction, timing, swing timing) are gradually integrated, thus challenging patients' sensory interaction.

Transition tests: the sit-to-stand transition is another valuable test that is usually part of a basic standard assessment (Fig. 17). Transition components are recorded and analyzed: the time required to shift the CoG from sitting to standing, the force exerted by the lower limbs during the rising phase, the load symmetry between the two limbs, and the extent of the oscillations of the CoG during the lifting phase until stabilization (around 20 s later).

Initiation of gait can also be evaluated: a patient is required to walk three steps on a 1.5-m platform, while step length, lateral distance between steps, rate of progression and amplitude of the CoG oscillations are measured.

Other tests assess patients when going over obstacles, e.g. a step or small step ladder.

4 From Assessment to Treatment: The Functional Goal

Test results are crucial in building an exercise program. Posturography recreates challenging conditions during tests as well as exercise. Tasks, context and somatosensory inputs can be modified.[5] Tests and exercises can be selected and combined to tailor training to a patient's needs.

[5]This feature is not common to all equipment and depends on the technical specifications of the instrumentation.

Limits Of Stability

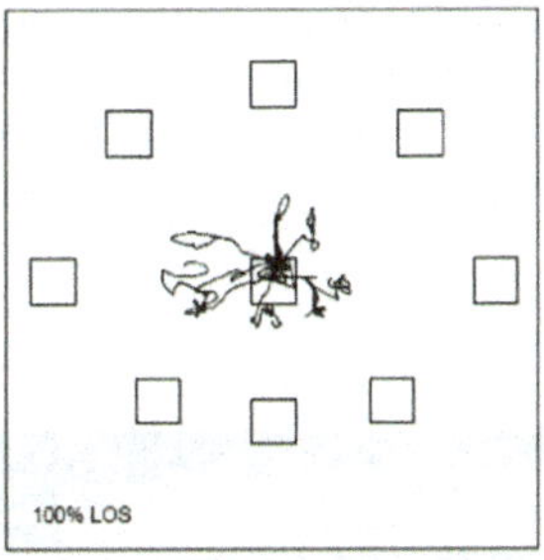

Transition	RT (sec)	MVL (deg/sec)	EPE (%)	MXE (%)	DCL (%)
1 (F)	0.94	2.8	33	43	79
2 (RF)	1.14	1.6	26	38	78
3 (R)	0.51	2.1	18	35	81
4 (RB)	0.75	2.0	26	37	69
5 (B)	0.61	2.4	29	33	49
6 (LB)	0.43	1.2	44	51	61
7 (L)	0.52	1.7	19	51	82
8 (LF)	3.41	1.3	49	49	66

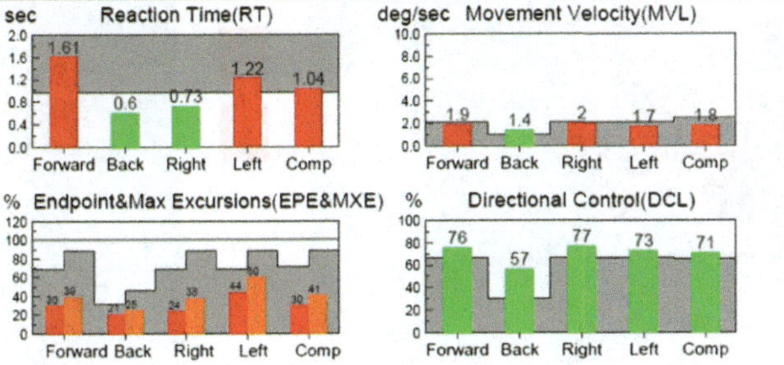

Limits Of Stability

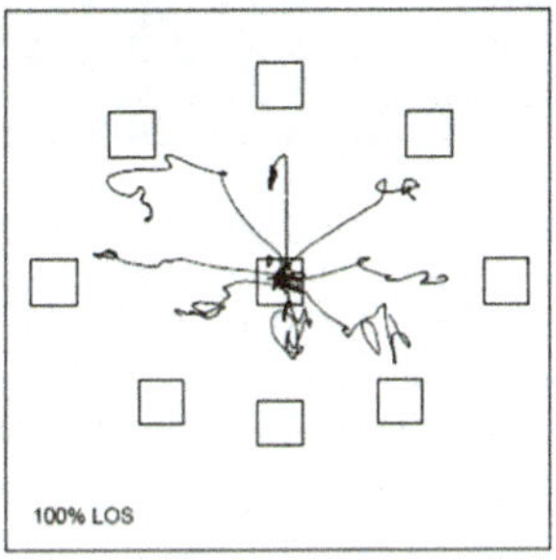

Transition	RT (sec)	MVL (deg/sec)	EPE (%)	MXE (%)	DCL (%)
1 (F)	0.93	5.6	63	63	94
2 (RF)	1.02	5.1	70	79	80
3 (R)	0.66	3.2	40	74	88
4 (RB)	1.25	1.7	49	83	61
5 (B)	0.41	1.8	28	55	45
6 (LB)	0.95	2.8	26	56	58
7 (L)	1.27	3.1	72	82	84
8 (LF)	0.75	5.3	56	92	74

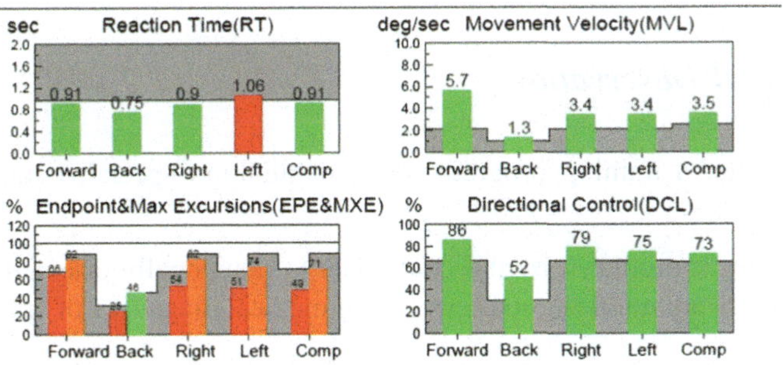

◂**Fig. 16** The LoS report shows the reaction time, the movement velocity, the endpoint excursion and the directional control of movement. Tracking the movement of her own CoG during exercise, the patient learns how to move in space without falling. As shown in the two images above, the more the patient improves, the more the times decrease, while the traces become progressively wider and smoother. (*Image* Property of the author)

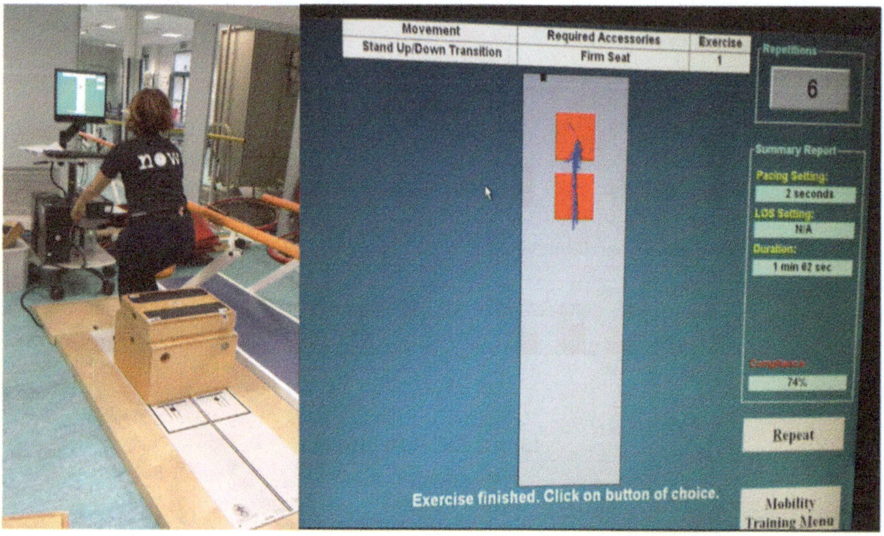

Fig. 17 Posturographic platforms are good for assessing and training proactive balance. This one is equipped with various accessories. A long platform permits gait assessment. Everyday living conditions can be recreated such as steps, stairs, obstacles, sit-to-stand transitions and others. Above left, an example of the "stand up and sit down" transition. Visual feedback guides the patient during the exercise in which CoG needs to be moved forwards and backwards during the movement. (*Image* Property of the author)

4.1 General Observations

When setting up a training program, the rehabilitation specialist must take into account that:

a. the assessment produced by the equipment is functionally oriented;
b. the platforms are not designed for making medical diagnoses of specific sites of damage;
c. the test results show the patient's failure to use sensory channels, or to adapt motor reactions—such as increased latencies in automatic responses—but do not specify the cause;

d. several dysfunctional balance patterns are common to different diseases. These patterns are well highlighted during posturography assessments, thus helping the clinician to choose the most appropriate exercises for each impairment;
e. the final choice of treatment goals is up to the physician, who knows whether the patient can effectively cope with the program.

4.2 Specific Observations

From a model perspective, training exercises can be categorized as follows:

- Mainly *reactive training* involves helping patients with their rapid automatic responses (reactive behavior), so as to address the needs of everyday life. This can be done by challenging patients with unexpected perturbations, within and up to the limits of stability (e.g. tugging on a mat on which the patient is standing).
- Mainly *proactive training* involves facilitating anticipatory reactions induced by volition and intentionality (proactive behavior) (Fig. 18). This can be achieved by introducing complexity into voluntary activities: loading the main task with additional ones (cognitive—e.g. counting—or motor—e.g. carrying an object).

The *implementation of correct strategies* is required *in reactive and in proactive* behavior. The strategy must change whenever the limit of stability is approached or exceeded. In the absence of an appropriate pattern, forcing a patient [10] to change at the right moment is another goal of treatment.

Depending on the degree of relearning, *sensory conflicts* may be introduced progressively by disturbing the visual and somatosensory channel in proactive and reactive conditions.

Exercises should be made more difficult by merging proactive and reactive aspects, by reducing timespans for exercise, and by increasing repetitions in the same session.

The patient should be provided with optimal training conditions. It is often necessary, before balance exercises, to implement a preparatory program in order to enable the best performance of the "effector" (range of motion, muscle flexibility, power and tendon elasticity). Stiffness or joint blocks, as in osteoarthritis or traumatic damage, can affect balance reactions by constraining joint strategies (ankle or hip). This aspect is investigated in the Adaptation Test for instance (see above).

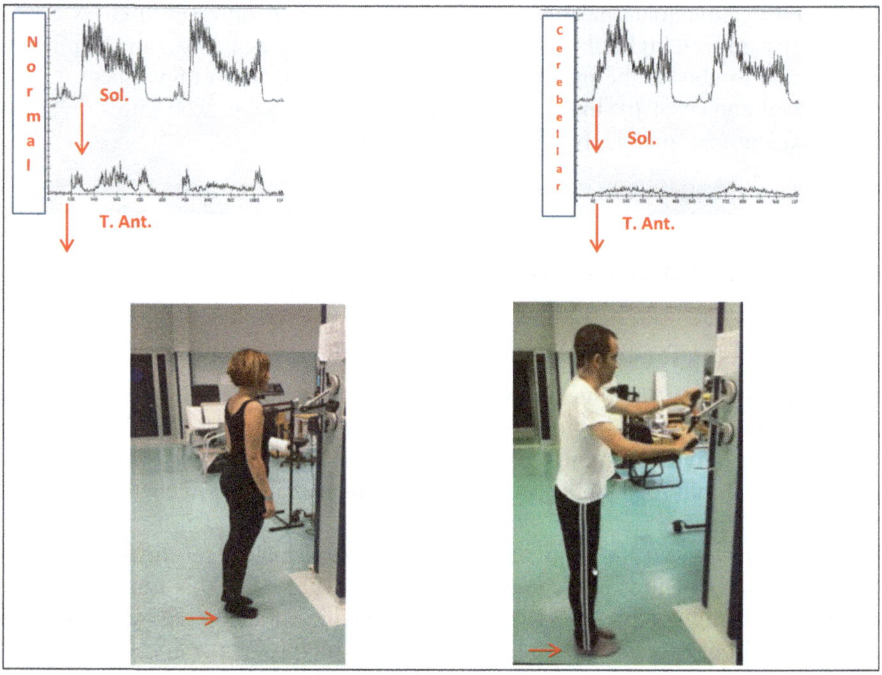

Fig. 18 Proactive behavior requires anticipatory reactions: these are activated whenever a voluntary task induces a displacement of the CoG. To maintain the CoG within a changing base of support (e.g. when rising on tiptoes), tibialis anterior muscle activation is needed prior to gastrocnemius muscle activation. The figure shows the EMG pattern of activation: in normal subjects (left) the tibialis anterior muscle starts its activation, in order to shift the CoG forward, before the subject starts to rise; in the case of a cerebellar disease, the absence of this pattern (right) results in activation of the soleus muscle alone, with an excessive posterior displacement and inability to rise on tiptoes. (*Image* Property of the author)

When possible, the joint constraint should be reduced or amended, using physical techniques and modalities. In any case, the patient should be challenged to adapt.

On the contrary, a central sensory impairment, as in multiple sclerosis, renders the vestibular pathway inefficient. Forcing patients to shift from visual to somatosensory information and reducing visual dependence are frequent treatment goals to improve sensory interaction. Patients hardly ever shift to the appropriate channel (i.e. proprioception and/or the vestibular system), even when it is partially available. In such cases, the SOT frequently reveals how much a patient relies on visual cues, even when these are unreliable.

Vision becomes less important in cases of blindness because auditory cues can partially replace visual ones in spatial exploration, nevertheless studies have demonstrated [11] that blind subjects do not have an advantage in using residual sensory channels. In truth, in the presence of neuromotor impairment, blind people behave like sighted subjects, tending to underuse vestibular information.

5 Conclusions

Many of the conditions artificially recreated by platforms are provided by clinical tests, as shown in other chapters of this book. Many exercises can also be performed by adapting the available low-tech equipment to produce challenging conditions.

The major benefits of posturographic equipment are summarized in the following points:

- The availability of reference data (for age group and gender)[6] allows comparison of the patient's performances with those of the normal population;
- Report data can be saved and stored in graphic and/or numerical form for further needs;
- The friendly interface provided by the visual and acoustic cues helps to keep the patient's attention during assessment and provides motivation during exercise;
- Objective parameters for assessment and training make reports comparable over time and across patients, particularly for variations in functional level or exercise conditions. This is useful in monitoring a patient's clinical status, in planning new training programs, and, above all, in clinical research.

[6]Equitest® equipment only.

Table 1 The table summarizes the functional characteristics of most of the existing posturographic platforms

Comparative table between static and dynamic[a] posturographic platforms												
Name/brand	Assessment	Training	Technical features				Balance					
			Safety support		Screen	Accessories	Steady	Reactive		Proactive		Sensory interaction
			Harness vest	Handrails				Vision[b]	Plate[c]	Default	Custom	
Equitest® (Natus)	✓		✓		2✓	EMG	✓	✓	✓		✓	✓
SMART Equitest® (Natus)	✓	✓	✓		2✓	EMG	✓	✓	✓	✓	✓	✓
SMART Balance Master® (Natus)	✓	✓	✓		2✓	EMG	✓	✓	✓	✓	✓	✓
Balance Master® (Natus)	✓	✓			✓	Boards, foam cushion	✓			✓	✓	
BASIC Balance Master® (Natus)	✓	✓			✓	Cushion	✓			✓	✓	
VSR™ SPORT (Natus)	✓	✓					✓			✓	✓	
VSR™ (Natus)	✓	✓				Cushion	✓			✓	✓	
Balance System™ SD (Biodex)	✓	✓		✓	✓	Vibrating feedback	✓		✓	✓		
BioSway™ (Biodex)	✓	✓			✓	Vibrating feedback	✓			✓		
Gea HD (VertigoMed)		✓		✓	✓		✓		✓	✓		
Multitest Equilibre (Framiral®)	✓	✓		✓			✓	✓	✓			

(continued)

Table 1 (continued)

Comparative table between static and dynamic[a] posturographic platforms												
Name/brand	Assessment	Training	Technical features				Balance					
			Safety support		Screen	Accessories	Steady	Reactive		Proactive		Sensory interaction
			Harness vest	Handrails				Vision[b]	Plate[c]	Default	Custom	
Prokin 212 (Woodway)	✓	✓		✓	✓		✓		✓	✓	✓	
Libra (easytech)		✓					✓			✓		
Gymplate© (Tecno Concept)	✓	✓		✓			✓		✓	✓		
Equilibrium board (Delos)	✓	✓		✓	✓	Round board	✓			✓		

The table summarizes the functional characteristics of most of the existing posturographic platforms. No selection criteria were used; after a web search, all the different pieces of equipment found were included in the comparison. These instruments currently cover most of the European market (over 90%)

[a]Dynamic platforms: grey boxes only
[b]Conditions for excluding or making unreliable visual information are provided (surrounding panel)
[c]Conditions to make somatosensory information unreliable are provided (movement of force plates)(By Alan BisioĊöproperty of the author)

References

1. Springhetti I, Tesio L. Effects of strength training on balance performance in the elderly. In: Capodaglio P, Narici MV, editors. The ageing motor system and its adaptation to training, vol. 9. Pavia: PIME; 2000. p. 91–99 ISBN 88-7963-108-X.
2. Verbrugge LM, Jette AM. The disablement process. Soc Sci Med. 1994;38:1–14 cited by Sandy LG, Gibson R in Managed care and chronic care: challenges and opportunities Manag Care Q. 1996; 4(2):5–11 (Spring).
3. Shumway-Cook A, Horak F. Assessing the influence of sensory interaction on balance. J Am. Phys Ther. 1986; 66:1584–50.
4. Berg KO, Wood-Dauphinee SL, Williams JI, Maki B. Measuring balance in the elderly: validation of an instrument. Can J Public Health. 1992;83(Suppl 2):S7–11.
5. Horak FB. The Balance Evaluation Systems Test (BESTest)—NCBI https://www.ncbi.nlm.nih.gov. PubMed Central (PMC).
6. Tesio L, Perucca L, Franchignoni FP, Battaglia MAA. short measure of balance in multiple sclerosis: validation through rasch analysis. Funct Neurol. 1997;125:255–65.
7. Management of balance and mobility disorders: Bibliography: A compilation of resources assembled by Neuro Com International Inc. Neuro Com Clackamas OR. 2003. Available at http://www.natus.com/documents/015367A_SMART-BM_EN-US_lores.pdf.
8. Monsell EM, Furman JM, Herdman SJ, Konrad HR, Shepard NT. Computerized dynamic platform posturography. Otolaryngol Head Neck Surg. 1997;117(4):394–8.
9. Shumway-Cook A, Horak FB. Assessing the influence of sensory interaction of balance. Suggestion from the field. Phys Ther. 1986;66(10):1548–50.
10. Shumway-Cook A, Woollacott M. Motor Control: Translating Research into Clinical Practice. 5th ed. Baltimore Md, Lippincott William & Wilkens; 2016.
11. Schmid M, Nardone A, De Nunzio AM, Schmid M, Schieppati M. Equilibrium during static and dynamic tasks in blind subjects: no evidence of cross-modal plasticity. Brain. 2007;130:2097–107.

The Influence of Cognitive Factors on Balance and Gait

Valentina Varalta, Cristina Fonte and Daniele Munari

1 Introduction

Gait and balance impairments are known to be omnipresent among the general elderly population, and especially among elderly people with neurological diseases (see [1] for a review).

Until recently, gait and balance were largely perceived as automated, biomechanical processes that did not require cortical control. However, extensive work has been done over the past decade to shed light on the connections between balance, gait and falls, on the one hand, and cognitive function, on the other [1–3]. The data from these studies support the notion that mobility and cognition are connected and suggest that gait is not merely an automated motor activity that utilizes minimal higher-level cognitive input. Studies on cognitive function and gait now embrace many areas of research, ranging from physiology and biomechanics to brain mapping, physics and neuropsychology.

In the present chapter we summarize the body of literature that suggests the presence of an association and relationship between cognitive function, gait and falls in the most frequent neurological diseases: stroke, Parkinson's disease (PD) and multiple sclerosis (MS).

V. Varalta (✉) · C. Fonte · D. Munari
Department of Neurosciences, Biomedicine and Movement Sciences, Neuromotor and Cognitive Rehabilitation Research Centre (CRRNC), Verona University, Verona, Italy
e-mail: valentina.varalta@univr.it

V. Varalta · C. Fonte · D. Munari
Neurorehabilitation Unit, AOUI Verona, Verona, Italy

G. Sandrini et al. (eds.), *Advanced Technologies for the Rehabilitation of Gait and Balance Disorders*, Biosystems & Biorobotics 19,
https://doi.org/10.1007/978-3-319-72736-3_7

2 The Influence of Cognitive Factors on Balance and Gait in Stroke Patients

Stroke, which is usually due to stenosis or occlusion of a blood vessel (ischemic stroke) but can also be caused by intracerebral or subarachnoid hemorrhage (hemorrhagic stroke) [4], is among the main causes of permanent adult disability in Western countries [5]. After a stroke, patients frequently experience a spectrum of motor impairments and cognitive disorders that can significantly interfere with their functions, resulting in activity and participation limitations [6]. Motor impairments after stroke typically affect one side of the body (hemiparesis, incoordination, spasticity, pain and muscle weakness) and occur in about 80% of patients [7]. These impairments often lead to gait deficits and balance disorders that in turn lead to reduced activity tolerance and an even more sedentary lifestyle [8]. They therefore result in a high level of disability in patients with stroke [9].

According to some authors, the frequency of cognitive deficits in the acute phase of stroke is over 70% [10, 11]. These deficits are present in 35.2–43.9% of patients three months after stroke and may persist for a long time in approximately 1/3 of patients [12, 13]. Typically, they include neuropsychological impairments, such as memory, visuospatial (neglect), executive, attention, perception (agnosia) and language (aphasia) deficits [14].

As indicated, motor and cognitive disorders both have a great impact on quality of life and everyday functioning of subjects with stroke. At present, neuropsychological and physical deficits are usually addressed in the rehabilitation setting as separate issues, with more attention typically paid to physical and occupational rather than cognitive therapy [6]. However, there is considerable interaction between the multiple manifestations of these patients' motor and neuropsychological impairments, and this aspect is currently poorly understood.

Specifically, stroke patients with neglect present a lateral deviation of the walking trajectory [15, 16]. This can be explained by considering gait as a consciously and actively monitored process that requires attention, and in this context, the task priority of walking is increased compared to what is observed in healthy subjects. Furthermore, it has recently been suggested that walking under usual circumstances may require attention and executive function [17], and should therefore be regarded as a not completely automated function [18]. Post-stroke subjects present abnormal gait patterns such as reduced speed, cadence and stride length [19]. On the basis of these considerations, there seems to be a need to pay greater attention to the cognitive resources required during ambulation after a stroke. When the level of processing required for two tasks exceeds the capacity of the cognitive system, we start to see interference between the tasks. In a recent study, Lee et al. showed decreases in gait ability when patients performed dual tasks. In particular, the decrease in gait velocity occurring during the manual task was more marked than that occurring during the cognitive task. This may be because the manual task interferes with ambulation, as it uses the same pathways as ambulation [20].

In the same way, it has been shown that the inability to perform dual tasks affects balance (increase in sway, asymmetrical body load distribution, and a decrease in stability limits), and may further increase the risk of falls after stroke [21]. Indeed, stroke patients may be susceptible to this risk because cortical and subcortical areas are required to implement multitasking [21].

Balance could also be affected by the presence of a visuospatial deficit (i.e. neglect). Indeed, studies have indicated a negative relationship between neglect and postural balance; in particular, patients with peripersonal neglect showed a displacement in mediolateral shift of the body's center of pressure (COP) [22].

The literature data suggest that cognitive disorders are factors that favor body imbalance. Balance deficits cause a high risk of falling in stroke patients [23], and in this case, too, cognitive deficits play an important role. Research showing that most stroke patients have difficulty maintaining stability while performing multiple tasks [24, 25] suggests that stroke survivors are more likely to fall while performing dual tasks, such as walking and talking, either simultaneously or concurrently. Thus, findings indicate that attention deficit might contribute to accident prone behavior and falling [26]. However, research on the effects of cognitive impairment on the risk of falls among community-dwelling stroke survivors is limited [27].

Executive functions are defined as a set of cognitive skills that are necessary to plan, monitor, and execute a sequence of goal-directed complex actions [28], and they seem to be a key cognitive factor in gait and balance control.

There is a growing body of studies that, on these bases, have investigated the effects of cognitive motor interference (CMI) tasks in patients with stroke [29, 30]. The changes incurred during simultaneous performance of motor and cognitive tasks are a result of CMI and they are operationalized as dual task costs by calculating the percentage change in outcome measures from the single task performance to dual task performance condition. Participants in this kind of dual task research are asked to walk or maintain their balance while performing cognitive tasks. In a recent review, dual task training in which there is CMI was found to give significant results in improving gait and balance function [8]. In particular, An et al. showed that motor and cognitive dual task gait training was more effective at improving the balance and gait abilities of chronic stroke patients than either motor dual task gait training or cognitive dual task gait training alone [31]. Accordingly, Lee et al. showed that a virtual reality physical exercise program accompanied by cognitive tasks had a positive effect on the balance and gait of stroke patients [32].

Thus, "research has emphasized the role of perception and concentration during dual task performance for posture and gait control as a paradigm of motor learning in stroke rehabilitation" [31]. It is asserted that stroke subjects need to simultaneously perform motor tasks and high cognitive functions during rehabilitation sessions, as daily living frequently requires the performance of several tasks simultaneously.

On the other hand, as previously illustrated, the presence of neglect can also affect balance and gait disorders in stroke patients. Some authors have investigated the effect of specific neglect treatment on balance skills [33, 34]. In particular, Nijboer and coworkers investigated the influence of a single session of prism adaptation on balance, and found that it may produce recalibration of disturbed representation of space as well as higher-level representations of extra-personal and internal body space in stroke subjects [33]. Furthermore, Sturt and Punt found that administration of a caloric vestibular stimulation to the contralesional ear produced an improvement in postural control [34]. These results indicate that specific treatment for a cognitive deficit (i.e. neglect) can improve balance in stroke patients.

The literature data suggest that the treatment of stroke patients should include dual task training. Furthermore, future studies should investigate the effects of specific cognitive training (e.g. attention or executive function training) on gait and balance disorders.

3 The Influence of Cognitive Factors on Balance and Gait in PD Patients

Parkinson's disease (PD) is an idiopathic neurodegenerative disorder caused by a progressive loss of dopaminergic neurons in the substantia nigra pars compacta [35, 36]. Its clinical manifestations include reduced amplitude of movement, hypokinesia, rigidity, tremor at rest and loss of balance [35]. These deficits result in abnormal gait patterns [37] that increase the risk of falls, with up to 63% of people with PD reporting more than one fall per year [38].

As well as motor impairment, about 25% of newly diagnosed, non-demented people with PD show cognitive deficits involving attention, memory, visuospatial and executive functions [39]. Specifically, PD patients show executive dysfunctions, defined as deficits in internal control of attention, set shifting, planning, inhibitory control, and conflict resolution, and impairment in dual task performance and a range of decision-making and social cognition tasks [40]. Cognitive impairments in PD are among the most consequential features of the disease, contributing to reduced quality of life [41] and increased risk of disability and mortality [42].

Previous studies support the notion that mobility and cognition are connected, perhaps because mobility shares the cortical-subcortical networks underlying cognition and balance [1, 43]. On this basis, cognitive-motor relationships have been widely explored in patients with PD.

First of all, studies have indicated that the PIGD (postural instability and gait disorders), compared with the TD (tremor dominant) subtype, is associated with cognitive impairment [44, 45] and characterized by more severe and generic motor abnormalities, specifically gait and balance disorders [45, 46].

Globally, the axial signs seem to be associated with memory, visuospatial and executive deficits [47–49]. Specifically, Varalta and coworkers found a significant correlation between executive function deficits (verbal fluency and the ability to switch attention between two tasks) and functional mobility [49]. These results are in line with those of Kelly et al. [50], who also indicated that poor global cognition, processing speed and visuospatial function are associated with more severe freezing of gait (FoG) [50]. FoG, defined as "a brief, episodic absence or marked reduction of forward progression of the feet despite the intention to walk" [51], is a gait disorder observed in half of patients with PD [52]. Since FoG is accompanied by motor and cognitive abnormalities [53], many studies have examined how these aspects interact and which factor is the most important in determining in the development of FoG [54–60]. The results indicated a clear association between presence of FoG and frontal dysfunctions ([54, 56, 58, 59), specifically FoG seemed to be strongly related to set-shifting difficulties [55, 57]. Vercruysse et al. concluded that the cognitive deficit is one of the independent determinants of FoG in people with PD [60].

Some studies have further investigated the link between cognition and motor control in PD patients, using dual task paradigms, which, as already specified, assess the ability to execute two tasks simultaneously [56, 61–63]. Usually a motor task (e.g. walking) is combined with a cognitive task (e.g. counting backwards). As previously indicated, PD patients are generally impaired in the concurrent performance of two tasks, which requires additional executive control; gait impairments, in particular, are exacerbated under dual task conditions in PD patients (for a review, see [40, 64]. Accordingly, some studies have demonstrated that patients with PD show a decrement in performance of both the cognitive task (verbal fluency, arithmetic task, counting backwards) and the motor task (gait) under dual task conditions as compared with their single task performance of either measure [61–63]. Furthermore, a significant correlation was found between functional mobility evaluated under the dual task condition (as measured by the Timed Up and Go Dual Task, TUG-COG) and cognitive impairment (as measured by the Montreal Cognitive Assessment, MoCA) [49]. These data confirm that poor cognitive ability is linked to poor functional mobility.

Functional mobility is closely linked to balance abilities. Accordingly, some studies have investigated the relationship between balance and motor/cognitive abilities in patients with PD. For example, Lee and coworkers examined the relationship between postural instability (as measured by computerized dynamic posturography) and cognitive impairment, and found a correlation between balance abilities and global cognition, visuospatial and memory functions [65]. On the other hand, some authors indicated that balance abilities are also associated with executive functions [49, 50].

In PD, gait and balance deficits often result in falls. Numerous prospective studies have investigated cognitive and motor profiles and measured the number of falls over many months in PD patients [38, 66–68]. The results obtained indicated an association between fall frequency and cognitive deficits. In particular, impaired attention and executive function seem to be significant predictors of future recurrent falls in people with PD [38, 67, 68].

The most frequent motor deficits in PD (gait and balance disorders) determine the level of disability of affected patients and contribute to their reduced quality of life. The literature data indicate a strong association between gait/balance disorders and cognitive impairments in PD.

These observations could have implications for rehabilitation in patients with PD, offering perspectives for clinical treatment protocols based on cognitive-motor relationships. In view of these considerations, some authors recently proposed rehabilitation protocols to evaluate the effects of physical training on cognitive and motor performance in patients with PD [69, 70]. In particular, Picelli and coworkers found significant improvements in cognitive performance (executive functions) and motor performance (walking) in patients who underwent a training program consisting of four weeks of treadmill training [70]. These results are in line with the study by Mirelman et al. which demonstrated improvements in motor ability (gait speed, stride length and endurance) and cognitive functions (dual task performance, attention and shifting) after six weeks of treadmill training with virtual obstacles (virtual reality) [71].

Other rehabilitation studies focusing on cognitive-motor relationships are needed to better investigate the influence of single-modality treatment (cognitive or motor training) on cognitive and motor deficits in PD patients.

4 The Influence of Cognitive Factors on Balance and Gait in MS Patients

Multiple sclerosis (MS) is a chronic neurological disease characterized by patchy inflammation, gliosis and demyelination within the central nervous system [72]. MS is the third most common cause of neurological disability in adults between 18 and 50 years of age [73].

The blockage or slowing of connections between areas of the brain and spinal cord often leads to motor, cognitive and neuropsychiatric problems [74].

Common motor symptoms in MS include muscle weakness, spasticity, ataxia and muscle spasms, increased gait variability, reduced walking speed, and impaired balance and coordination [75].

Cognitive deficits affect up to 70% of persons with MS, beginning early in the disease process [76], and worsening with disease duration and progression [77]. In particular, patients may manifest slowed information processing speed, deficits in learning and memory, and impaired perceptual skills and executive function [77, 78]. Impairment in these cognitive domains might be more pronounced in persons with progressive MS compared with relapsing-remitting MS [79]. Cognitive impairment in persons with MS is a highly disabling consequence of the disease and has been associated with many negative health outcomes and with reduced social functioning, leading to loss of independence and an increased need for assistance with activities of daily living [80].

Recently, some studies explored the relationship between cognitive factors and gait/balance impairments in people with MS.

Benedict and colleagues demonstrated that processing speed and executive functions were significant predictors of lower and upper motor function (measured by the Timed 25 Foot Walk and the Nine Hole Peg Test) in 211 MS patients with mild to moderate disability [81]. Others have reported statistically significant associations between tests of processing speed and multiple measures of walking performance [82]. Similarly, D'Orio and colleagues reported that performances on cognitive tests of IQ, processing speed and executive functioning were related to walking speed [74].

Many authors have speculated that the relationship between cognitive and motor function may be attributed, in part, to shared cerebral substrates [74, 81]. Indeed, structural imaging and post-mortem studies suggest that frontal and subcortical regions involved in cognitive processing speed and executive control are related to the spatial (e.g., step length) and temporal (e.g., double support time) aspects of gait [74, 81].

Approximately 50% of MS patients have injurious falls during the course of their illness, leading to increased disability, morbidity and even mortality [83], and these correlations may have implications for fall prevention strategies, suggesting that they should target recurrent fallers with MS. Studies investigating the relationship between falls and cognitive ability have found that processing speed and verbal memory are associated with fall frequency in MS [74, 84].

Recent evidence suggests that motor and cognitive impairments are compounded when the motor and cognitive tasks, such as walking and talking, are performed simultaneously. Changes incurred when subjects simultaneously perform motor (e.g. walking or keeping their balance) and cognitive tasks are a result of CMI.

Wajda and Sosnoff [85] reviewed studies examining CMI during walking in MS patients and found 14 investigations from 2009 to 2014 [82, 86–98]. These studies involved performance of a short walking task ($\sim$10 m) during various cognitive tasks (such as word list generation, subtraction and counting). The main finding was that the primary effect of CMI during walking in individuals with MS is a decrease in gait velocity with a percentage decline of between $\sim$6 and $\sim$27% in gait speed [85].

Other aspects found to be affected were step length [82, 86, 87, 92, 96–98], double support time as a percentage of the gait cycle [90, 92–95] and cadence [82, 92, 97, 98]. In particular, studies concluded that poorer executive functions contributed to greater decrements in walking.

Recently, rehabilitation studies, too, have explored the issue of the effect of dual tasking on gait. In particular, Peruzzi et al. [99] submitted eight people with MS to six weeks of treadmill training with virtual reality. The training introduced virtual obstacles, which required both the integration of balance strategies as well as planning, information processing and sensory integration. Gait speed and stride length showed progressive improvements throughout the single task evaluations, although these were not significant. Conversely, under the dual task condition, significant differences were observed after training, and these were further maintained at 1 month follow-up. Balance and performance-based measures also improved [99].

Like gait disorders, balance dysfunction is one of the earliest reported symptoms in MS and has been observed even in the absence of clinical disability [100].

Similarly to the studies examining CMI during walking, seven studies [91, 100–105] have examined CMI during balance tasks in MS. The majority of these investigations used COP-based measures (e.g., sway area and sway rate) generated during standing balance trials performed on a force platform. In all the studies, patients were asked to perform, during balance tasks, word list generation, counting tasks or an inhibition control task. The results, showing an increased sway velocity even in the earliest stages of the disease process [103], demonstrated an influence of CMI in balance tasks in MS. Negahban et al. [104, 105] have also observed that the COP became less regular and more complex, resulting in a decrease of variability in COP velocity, which they interpreted as delayed onset of anticipatory postural adjustments [104, 105].

Indeed, it is possible that individuals with impaired cognitive function, including decreased cognitive processing speed, are unable to select an appropriate movement correction to respond to balance perturbations. This idea is supported by data demonstrating that balance is related to cognitive processing speed in persons with MS [106] and that persons with MS have impaired postural responses to perturbations [107].

5 Conclusions

As illustrated in this chapter, the literature data suggest that there exists a strong relationship between mobility, fall risk and cognitive function in neurological patients.

These findings suggest that clinicians should also explore cognitive deficits to better understand these patients' motor deficits and risk of falling.

Furthermore, because everyday life activities usually involve both motor and cognitive resources, rehabilitation intervention in individuals with neurological disorders should be multimodal (i.e. combine cognitive tasks with motor training) in order to reduce CMI. Additionally, a multifactorial intervention may be the optimal approach to maximize efficacy, improving motor and cognitive domains.

Other rehabilitation studies are needed to better investigate the influence of single-modality (cognitive or motor) or combined (dual task) treatment on cognitive and motor disorders in neurological patients.

References

1. Segev-Jacubovski O, Herman T, Yogev-Seligmann G, Mirelman A, Giladi N, Hausdorff JM. The interplay between gait, falls and cognition: can cognitive therapy reduce fall risk? Expert Rev Neurother. 2011;11:1057–75. https://doi.org/10.1586/ern.11.69.
2. Jacobs JV, Horak FB. Cortical control of postural responses. J Neural Transm. 2007;114:1339–48. https://doi.org/10.1007/s00702-007-0657-0.

3. Yogev-Seligmann G, Hausdorff JM, Giladi N. The role of executive function and attention in gait. Mov Disord. 2008;23:329–42.
4. Cengić L, Vuletić V, Karlić M, Dikanović M, Demarin V. Motor and cognitive impairment after stroke. Acta Clin Croat. 2011;50:463–7.
5. Veerbeek JM, Kwakkel G, van Wegen EE, Ket JC, Heymans MW. Early prediction of outcome of activities of daily living after stroke: a systematic review. Stroke. 2011;42:1482–8. https://doi.org/10.1161/STROKEAHA.110.604090.
6. Chen C, Leys D, Esquenazi A. The interaction between neuropsychological and motor deficits in patients after stroke. Neurology. 2013;80:S27–34.
7. Langhorne P, Coupar F, Pollock A. Motor recovery after stroke: a systematic review. Lancet Neurol. 2009;8:741–54. https://doi.org/10.1016/S1474-4422(09)70150-4.
8. Wang XQ, Pi YL, Chen BL, Chen PJ, Liu Y, Wang R, Li X, Waddington G. Cognitive motor interference for gait and balance in stroke: a systematic review and meta-analysis. Eur J Neurol. 2015;22:555–e37. https://doi.org/10.1111/ene.12616.
9. Smania N, Picelli A, Gandolfi M, Fiaschi A, Tinazzi M. Rehabilitation of sensorimotor integration deficits in balance impairment of patients with stroke hemiparesis: a before/after pilot study. Neurol Sci. 2008;29:313–9. https://doi.org/10.1007/s10072-008-0988-0.
10. Lesniak M, Bak T, Czepiel W, Seniow J, Czlonkowska A. Frequency and prognostic value of cognitive disorders in stroke patients. Dement Geriatr Cogn Disord. 2008;26:356–63. https://doi.org/10.1159/000162262.
11. Nys G, van Zandvoort M, de Kort P, Jansen B, de Haan E, Kappelle L. Cognitive disorders in acute stroke: prevalence and clinical determinants. Cerebrovasc Dis. 2007;23:408–16.
12. Lawrence ES, Coshall C, Dundas R, Stewart J, Rudd AG, Howard R, Wolfe CD. Estimates of the prevalence of acute stroke impairments and disability in a multiethnic population. Stroke. 2001;32:1279–84.
13. Patel M, Coshall C, Rudd AG, Wolfe CD. Natural history of cognitive impairment after stroke and factors associated with its recovery. Clin Rehabil. 2003;17:158–66.
14. Jokinen H, Melkas S, Ylikoski R, Pohjasvaara T, Kaste M, Erkinjuntti T, Hietanen M. Post-stroke cognitive impairment is common even after successful clinical recovery. Eur J Neurol. 2015;22:1288–94. https://doi.org/10.1111/ene.12743.
15. Berti A, Smania N, Rabuffetti M, Ferrarin M, Spinazzola L, D'Amico A, Ongaro E, Allport A. Coding of far and near space during walking in neglect patients. Neuropsychology. 2002;16:390–9.
16. Huitema RB, Brouwer WH, Hof AL, Dekker R, Mulder T, Postema K. Walking trajectory in neglect patients. Gait Posture. 2006;23:200–5.
17. Cho KH, Lee JY, Lee KJ, Kang EK. Factors related to gait function in post-stroke patients. J Phys Ther Sci. 2014;26:1941–4. https://doi.org/10.1589/jpts.26.1941.
18. Bowen A, Wenman R, Mickelborough J, Foster J, Hill E, Tallis R. Dual-task effects of talking while walking on velocity and balance following a stroke. Age Ageing. 2001;30:319–23.
19. Chen G, Patten C, Kothari DH, Zajac FE. Gait deviations associated with post-stroke hemiparesis: improvement during treadmill walking using weight support, speed, support stiffness, and handrail hold. Gait Posture. 2005;22:57–62.
20. Lee KB, Kim JH, Lee KS. The relationship between motor recovery and gait velocity during dual tasks in patients with chronic stroke. J Phys Ther Sci. 2015;27:1173–6. https://doi.org/10.1589/jpts.27.1173.
21. Campos Sasaki A, Pinto EB, Mendel T, Sá KN, Oliveira-Filho J, D'Oliveira A Jr. Association between dual-task performance and balance during gait in community-dwelling elderly people after stroke. Healthy Aging Res. 2015;4:29. https://doi.org/10.12715/har.2015.4.29.
22. Nijboer TC, Olthoff L, Van der Stigchel S, Visser-Meily JM. Prism adaptation improves postural imbalance in neglect patients. NeuroReport. 2014;25:307–11. https://doi.org/10.1097/WNR.0000000000000088.

23. Stapleton T, Ashburn A, Stack E. A pilot study of attention deficits, balance control and falls in the subacute stage following stroke. Clin Rehabil. 2001;15:437–44.
24. Malouin F, Richards CL, Doyon J, Desrosiers J, Belleville S. Training mobility tasks after stroke with combined mental and physical practice: a feasibility study. Neurorehabil Neural Repair. 2004;18:66–75.
25. Shumway-Cook A, Brauer S, Woollacott M. Predicting the probability for falls in community-dwelling older adults using the Timed Up & Go Test. Phys Ther. 2000;80:896–903.
26. Hyndman D, Ashburn A. People with stroke living in the community: attention deficits, balance, ADL ability and falls. Disabil Rehabil. 2003;25:817–22.
27. Hwang S, Woo Y, Kim KH, Ki KI. Effects of falls experience on cognitive functions and physical activities in community-dwelling individuals with chronic stroke. Int J Rehabil Res. 2013;36:134–9. https://doi.org/10.1097/MRR.0b013e32835b667e.
28. van Iersel MB, Kessels RP, Bloem BR, Verbeek AL, Olde Rikkert MG. Executive functions are associated with gait and balance in community-living elderly people. J Gerontol A Biol Sci Med Sci. 2008;63:1344–9.
29. Her JG, Park KD, Yang YA, Ko T, Kim H, Lee J, Woo JH, Ko J. Effects of balance training with various dual-task conditions on stroke patients. J Phys Ther Sci. 2011;23:713–7.
30. Zheng J, Wang X, Xu Y, Yang Y, Shen L, Liang Z. Cognitive dual-task training improves balance function in patients with stroke. HealthMED. 2012;6:840–5.
31. An HJ, Kim JI, Kim YR, Lee KB, Kim DJ, Yoo KT, Choi JH. The effect of various dual task training methods with gait on the balance and gait of patients with chronic stroke. J Phys Ther Sci. 2014;26:1287–91. https://doi.org/10.1589/jpts.26.1287.
32. Lee IW, Kim YN, Lee DK. Effect of a virtual reality exercise program accompanied by cognitive tasks on the balance and gait of stroke patients. J Phys Ther Sci. 2015;27:2175–7. https://doi.org/10.1589/jpts.27.2175.
33. Nijboer TC, Ten Brink AF, van der Stoep N, Visser-Meily JM. Neglecting posture: differences in balance impairments between peripersonal and extrapersonal neglect. NeuroReport. 2014;25:1381–5. https://doi.org/10.1097/WNR.0000000000000277.
34. Sturt R, Punt TD. Caloric vestibular stimulation and postural control in patients with spatial neglect following stroke. Neuropsychol Rehabil. 2013;23:299–316. https://doi.org/10.1080/09602011.2012.755831.
35. Meara J, Bhowmick BK. Parkinson's disease and Parkinsonism in the elderly: introduction. In: Meara J, Koller WC, editors. Parkinson's Disease and Parkinsonism in the Elderly. Cambridge: Cambridge University Press; 2000.
36. Monchi O, Petrides M, Doyon J, Postuma RB, Worsley K, Dagher A. Neural bases of set-shifting deficits in Parkinson's disease. J Neurosci. 2004;24:702–10.
37. Picelli A, Camin M, Tinazzi M, Vangelista A, Cosentino A, Fiaschi A, Smania N. Three-dimensional motion analysis of the effects of auditory cueing on gait pattern in patients with Parkinson's disease: a preliminary investigation. Neurol Sci. 2010;31:423–30. https://doi.org/10.1007/s10072-010-0228-2.
38. Allcock LM, Rowan EN, Steen IN, Wesnes K, Kenny RA, Burn DJ. Impaired attention predicts falling in Parkinson's disease. Parkinsonism Relat Disord. 2009;15:110–5. https://doi.org/10.1016/j.parkreldis.2008.03.010.
39. Muslimovic D, Post B, Speelman JD, Schmand B. Cognitive profile of patients with newly diagnosed Parkinson disease. Neurology. 2005;65:1239–45.
40. Dirnberger G, Jahanshahi M. Executive dysfunction in Parkinson's disease: a review. J Neuropsychol. 2013;7:193–224. https://doi.org/10.1111/jnp.12028.
41. Winter Y, von Campenhausen S, Arend M, Longo K, Boetzel K, Eggert K, et al. Health-related quality of life and its determinants in Parkinson's disease: results of an Italian cohort study. Park Relat Disord. 2011;17:265–9. https://doi.org/10.1016/j.parkreldis.2011.01.003.

42. Rosenthal E, Brennan L, Xie S, Hurtig H, Milber J, Weintraub D, et al. Association between cognition and function in patients with Parkinson disease with and without dementia. Mov Disord. 2010;25:1170–6. https://doi.org/10.1002/mds.23073.
43. Stuss DT, Alexander MP. Is there a dysexecutive syndrome? Philos Trans R Soc Lond B Biol Sci. 2007;362:901–15. https://doi.org/10.1098/rstb.2007.2096.
44. Burn DJ, Rowan EN, Allan LM, Molloy S, O'Brien JT, McKeith IG. Motor sub-type and cognitive decline in Parkinson's disease, Parkinson's disease with dementia, and dementia with Lewy bodies. J Neurol Neurosurg Psychiatry. 2006;77:585–9.
45. Vervoort G, Bengevoord A, Nackaerts E, Heremans E, Vandenberghe W, Nieuwboer A. Distal motor deficit contributions to postural instability and gait disorder in Parkinson's disease. Behav Brain Res. 2015;287:1–7. https://doi.org/10.1016/j.bbr.2015.03.026.
46. Herman T, Weiss A, Brozgol M, Giladi N, Hausdorff JM. Gait and balance in Parkinson's disease subtypes: objective measures and classification considerations. J Neurol. 2014;261:2401–10. https://doi.org/10.1007/s00415-014-7513-6.
47. Domellöf ME, Elgh E, Forsgren L. The relation between cognition and motor dysfunction in drug-naive newly diagnosed patients with Parkinson's disease. Mov Disord. 2011;26:2183–9. https://doi.org/10.1002/mds.23814.
48. Poletti M, Frosini D, Pagni C, Baldacci F, Nicoletti V, Tognoni G, Lucetti C, Del Dotto P, Ceravolo R, Bonuccelli U. Mild cognitive impairment and cognitive-motor relationships in newly diagnosed drug-naive patients with Parkinson's disease. J Neurol Neurosurg Psychiatry. 2012;83:601–6. https://doi.org/10.1136/jnnp-2011-301874.
49. Varalta V, Picelli A, Fonte C, Amato S, Melotti C, Zatezalo V, Saltuari L, Smania N. Relationship between cognitive performance and motor dysfunction in patients with Parkinson's disease: a pilot cross-sectional study. Biomed Res Int. 2015;2015:365959. https://doi.org/10.1155/2015/365959.
50. Kelly VE, Johnson CO, McGough EL, Shumway-Cook A, Horak FB, Chung KA, Espay AJ, Revilla FJ, Devoto J, Wood-Siverio C, Factor SA, Cholerton B, Edwards KL, Peterson AL, Quinn JF, Montine TJ, Zabetian CP, Leverenz JB. Association of cognitive domains with postural instability/gait disturbance in Parkinson's disease. Parkinsonism Relat Disord. 2015;21:692–7. https://doi.org/10.1016/j.parkreldis.2015.04.002.
51. Nutt JG, Bloem BR, Giladi N, Hallett M, Horak FB, Nieuwboer A. Freezing of gait: moving forward on a mysterious clinical phenomenon. Lancet Neurol. 2011;10:734–44. https://doi.org/10.1016/S1474-4422(11)70143-0.
52. Giladi N, Treves TA, Simon ES, et al. Freezing of gait in patients with advanced Parkinson's disease. J Neural Transm. 2001;108:53–61.
53. Giladi N, Hausdorff JM. The role of mental function in the pathogenesis of freezing of gait in Parkinson's disease. J Neurol Sci. 2006;248:173–6.
54. Amboni M, Cozzolino A, Longo K, Picillo M, Barone P. Freezing of gait and executive functions in patients with Parkinson's disease. Mov Disord. 2008;23:395–400.
55. Naismith SL, Shine JM, Lewis SJ. The specific contributions of set-shifting to freezing of gait in Parkinson's disease. Mov Disord. 2010;25:1000–4. https://doi.org/10.1002/mds.23005.
56. Ricciardi L, Bloem BR, Snijders AH, Daniele A, Quaranta D, Bentivoglio AR, Fasano A. Freezing of gait in Parkinson's disease: the paradoxical interplay between gait and cognition. Parkinsonism Relat Disord. 2014;20:824–9. https://doi.org/10.1016/j.parkreldis.2014.04.009.
57. Stefanova E, Ječmenica Lukić M, Ziropadja L, Marković V, Stojković T, Tomić A, Dragašević Mišković N, Kostić V. Attentional set-shifting in Parkinson's disease patients with freezing of gait-acquisition and discrimination set learning deficits at the background? J Int Neuropsychol Soc. 2014;20:929–36. https://doi.org/10.1017/S1355617714000769.
58. Teramoto H, Morita A, Ninomiya S, Shiota H, Kamei S. Relation between freezing of gait and frontal function in Parkinson's disease. Parkinsonism Relat Disord. 2014;20:1046–9. https://doi.org/10.1016/j.parkreldis.2014.06.022.
59. Vandenbossche J, Deroost N, Soetens E, Spildooren J, Vercruysse S, Nieuwboer A, Kerckhofs E. Freezing of gait in Parkinson disease is associated with impaired conflict

resolution. Neurorehabil Neural Repair. 2011;25:765–73. https://doi.org/10.1177/1545968311403493.
60. Vercruysse S, Devos H, Munks L, Spildooren J, Vandenbossche J, Vandenberghe W, Nieuwboer A, Heremans E. Explaining freezing of gait in Parkinson's disease: motor and cognitive determinants. Mov Disord. 2012;27:1644–51. https://doi.org/10.1002/mds.25183.
61. Delval A, Moreau C, Bleuse S, Guehl D, Bestaven E, Guillaud E, Dujardin K, Defebvre L, Devos D. Gait and attentional performance in freezers under methylphenidate. Gait Posture. 2015;41:384–8. https://doi.org/10.1016/j.gaitpost.2014.10.022.
62. Fuller RL, Van Winkle EP, Anderson KE, Gruber-Baldini AL, Hill T, Zampieri C, Weiner WJ, Shulman LM. Dual task performance in Parkinson's disease: a sensitive predictor of impairment and disability. Parkinsonism Relat Disord. 2013;19:325–8. https://doi.org/10.1016/j.parkreldis.2012.11.011.
63. Yogev G, Giladi N, Peretz C, Springer S, Simon ES, Hausdorff JM. Dual tasking, gait rhythmicity, and Parkinson's dis- ease: which aspects of gait are attention demanding? Eur J Neurosci. 2005;22:1248–56.
64. Kelly VE, Eusterbrock AJ, Shumway-Cook A. A review of dual-task walking deficits in people with Parkinson's disease: motor and cognitive contributions, mechanisms, and clinical implications. Parkinsons Dis. 2012;2012:918719. https://doi.org/10.1155/2012/918719.
65. Lee JM, Koh SB, Chae SW, Seo WK, Kwon do Y, Kim JH, Oh K, Baik JS, Park KW. Postural instability and cognitive dysfunction in early Parkinson's disease. Can J Neurol Sci. 2012;39:473–82.
66. Camicioli R, Majumdar SR. Relationship between mild cognitive impairment and falls in older people with and without Parkinson's disease: 1-Year Prospective Cohort Study. Gait Posture. 2010;32:87–91. https://doi.org/10.1016/j.gaitpost.2010.03.013.
67. Mak MK, Wong A, Pang MY. Impaired executive function can predict recurrent falls in Parkinson's disease. Arch Phys Med Rehabil. 2014;95:2390–5. https://doi.org/10.1016/j.apmr.2014.08.006.
68. Paul SS, Sherrington C, Canning CG, Fung VS, Close JC, Lord SR. The relative contribution of physical and cognitive fall risk factors in people with Parkinson's disease: a large prospective cohort study. Neurorehabil Neural Repair. 2014;28:282–90. https://doi.org/10.1177/1545968313508470.
69. King LA, Peterson DS, Mancini M, Carlson-Kuhta P, Fling BW, Smulders K, Nutt JG, Dale M, Carter J, Winters-Stone KM, Horak FB. Do cognitive measures and brain circuitry predict outcomes of exercise in Parkinson Disease: a randomized clinical trial. BMC Neurol. 2015;15:218. https://doi.org/10.1186/s12883-015-0474-2.
70. Picelli A, Varalta V, Melotti C, Zatezalo V, Fonte C, Amato S, Saltuari L, Santamato A, Fiore P, Smania N. Effects of treadmill training on cognitive and motor features of patients with mild to moderate Parkinson's disease: a pilot, single-blind, randomized controlled trial. Funct Neurol. 2016;31:25–31.
71. Mirelman A, Maidan I, Herman T, Deutsch JE, Giladi N, Hausdorff JM. Virtual reality for gait training: can it induce motor learning to enhance complex walking and reduce fall risk in patients with Parkinson's disease? J Gerontol A Biol Sci Med Sci. 2011;66:234–40. https://doi.org/10.1093/gerona/glq201.
72. Steinman L. Multiple sclerosis: a two-stage disease. Nat Immunol. 2001;2:762–4.
73. Karni A, Kahana E, Zilber N, Abramsky O, Alter M, Karussis D. The frequency of multiple sclerosis in jewish and arab populations in greater jerusalem. Neuroepidemiology. 2003;22:82–6.
74. D'Orio VL, Foley FW, Armentano F, Picone MA, Kim S, Holtzer R. Cognitive and motor functioning in patients with multiple sclerosis: neuropsychological predictors of walking speed and falls. J Neurol Sci. 2012;316:42–6. https://doi.org/10.1016/j.jns.2012.02.003.
75. McNalley TE, Haselkorn JK. Disorders of mobility in multiple sclerosis. In: Giesser BS, editor. Primer on multiple sclerosis. New York: Oxford University Press; 2011. p. 189–96.

76. Loitfelder M, Fazekas F, Koschutnig K, Fuchs S, Petrovic K, Ropele S, Pichler A, Jehna M, Langkammer C, Schmidt R, Neuper C, Enzinger C. Brain activity changes in cognitive networks in relapsing-remitting multiple sclerosis—insights from a longitudinal FMRI study. PLoS ONE. 2014;9:e93715. https://doi.org/10.1371/journal.pone.0093715.
77. Chiaravalloti ND, DeLuca J. Cognitive impairment in multiple sclerosis. Lancet Neurol. 2008;7:1139–51. https://doi.org/10.1016/S1474-4422(08)70259-X.
78. Benedict RH, Zivadinov R. Risk factors for and management of cognitive dysfunction in multiple sclerosis. Nat Rev Neurol. 2011;7:332–42. https://doi.org/10.1038/nrneurol.2011.61.
79. Amato MP, Zipoli V, Portaccio E. Multiple sclerosis-related cognitive changes: a review of cross-sectional and longitudinal studies. J Neurol Sci. 2006;245:41–6.
80. Sandroff BM. Exercise and cognition in multiple sclerosis: The importance of acute exercise for developing better interventions. Neurosci Biobehav Rev. 2015;59:173–83. https://doi.org/10.1016/j.neubiorev.2015.10.012.
81. Benedict RH, Holtzer R, Motl RW, Foley FW, Kaur S, Hojnacki D, et al. Upper and lower extremity motor function and cognitive impairment in multiple sclerosis. J Int Neuropsychol Soc. 2011;13:1–11.
82. Motl RW, Sosnoff JJ, Dlugonski D, Pilutti LA, Klaren R, Sandroff BM. Walking and cognition, but not symptoms, correlate with dual task cost of walking in multiple sclerosis. Gait Posture. 2014;39:870–4. https://doi.org/10.1016/j.gaitpost.2013.11.023.
83. Brønnum-Hansen H, Hansen T, Koch-Henriksen N, Stenager E. Fatal accidents among Danes with multiple sclerosis. Mult Scler. 2006;12:329–32.
84. Sosnoff JJ, Balantrapu S, Pilutti LA, Sandroff BM, Morrison S, Motl RW. Cognitive processing speed is related to fall frequency in older adults with multiple sclerosis. Arch Phys Med Rehabil. 2013;94:1567–72. https://doi.org/10.1016/j.apmr.2013.02.009.
85. Wajda DA, Sosnoff JJ. Cognitive-motor interference in multiple sclerosis: a systematic review of evidence, correlates, and consequences. Biomed Res Int. 2015;2015:720856. https://doi.org/10.1155/2015/720856.
86. Allali G, Laidet M, Assal F, Armand S, Lalive PH. Walking while talking in patients with multiple sclerosis: the impact of specific cognitive loads. Neurophysiol Clin. 2014;44:87–93. https://doi.org/10.1016/j.neucli.2013.10.136.
87. Allali G, Laidet M, Assal F, Chofflon M, Armand S, Lalive PH. Dual-task assessment in natalizumab-treated multiple sclerosis patients. Eur Neurol. 2014;71:247–51. https://doi.org/10.1159/000357217.
88. Gunn H, Creanor S, Haas B, Marsden J, Freeman J. Risk factors for falls in multiple sclerosis: an observational study. Mult Scler. 2013;19:1913–22. https://doi.org/10.1177/1352458513488233.
89. Hamilton F, Rochester L, Paul L, Rafferty D, O'Leary CP, Evans JJ. Walking and talking: an investigation of cognitive-motor dual tasking in multiple sclerosis. Mult Scler. 2009;15:1215–27. https://doi.org/10.1177/1352458509106712.
90. Kalron A, Dvir Z, Achiron A. Walking while talking–difficulties incurred during the initial stages of multiple sclerosis disease process. Gait Posture. 2010;32:332–5. https://doi.org/10.1016/j.gaitpost.2010.06.002.
91. Kramer A, Dettmers C, Gruber M. Exergaming with additional postural demands improves balance and gait in patients with multiple sclerosis as much as conventional balance training and leads to high adherence to home-based balance training. Arch Phys Med Rehabil. 2014;95:1803–9. https://doi.org/10.1016/j.apmr.2014.04.020.
92. Learmonth YC, Sandroff BM, Pilutti LA, Klaren RE, Ensari I, Riskin BJ, Holtzer R, Motl RW. Cognitive motor interference during walking in multiple sclerosis using an alternate-letter alphabet task. Arch Phys Med Rehabil. 2014;95:1498–503. https://doi.org/10.1016/j.apmr.2014.03.007.
93. Nogueira LA, Dos Santos LT, Sabino PG, Alvarenga RM, Santos Thuler LC. Factors for lower walking speed in persons with multiple sclerosis. Mult Scler Int. 2013;2013:875648. https://doi.org/10.1155/2013/875648.

94. Nogueira LA, Santos LT, Sabino PG, Alvarenga RM, Thuler LC. Walking execution is not affected by divided attention in patients with multiple sclerosis with no disability, but there is a motor planning impairment. Arq Neuropsiquiatr. 2013;71:521–6. https://doi.org/10.1590/0004-282X20130080.
95. Sosnoff JJ, Boes MK, Sandroff BM, Socie MJ, Pula JH, Motl RW. Walking and thinking in persons with multiple sclerosis who vary in disability. Arch Phys Med Rehabil. 2011;92:2028–33. https://doi.org/10.1016/j.apmr.2011.07.004.
96. Sosnoff JJ, Socie MJ, Sandroff BM, Balantrapu S, Suh Y, Pula JH, Motl RW. Mobility and cognitive correlates of dual task cost of walking in persons with multiple sclerosis. Disabil Rehabil. 2014;36:205–9. https://doi.org/10.3109/09638288.2013.782361.
97. Wajda DA, Motl RW, Sosnoff JJ. Dual task cost of walking is related to fall risk in persons with multiple sclerosis. J Neurol Sci. 2013;335:160–3. https://doi.org/10.1016/j.jns.2013.09.021.
98. Wajda DA, Sandroff BM, Pula JH, Motl RW, Sosnoff JJ. Effects of walking direction and cognitive challenges on gait in persons with multiple sclerosis. Mult Scler Int. 2013;2013:859323. https://doi.org/10.1155/2013/859323.
99. Peruzzi A, Cereatti A, Della Croce U, Mirelman A. Effects of a virtual reality and treadmill training on gait of subjects with multiple sclerosis: a pilot study. Mult Scler Relat Disord. 2016;5:91–6. https://doi.org/10.1016/j.msard.2015.11.002.
100. Wajda DA, Motl RW, Sosnoff JJ. Correlates of dual task cost of standing balance in individuals with multiple sclerosis. Gait Posture. 2014;40:352–6. https://doi.org/10.1016/j.gaitpost.2014.04.209.
101. Boes MK, Sosnoff JJ, Socie MJ, Sandroff BM, Pula JH, Motl RW. Postural control in multiple sclerosis: effects of disability status and dual task. J Neurol Sci. 2012;315:44–8. https://doi.org/10.1016/j.jns.2011.12.006.
102. Jacobs JV, Kasser SL. Effects of dual tasking on the postural performance of people with and without multiple sclerosis: a pilot study. J Neurol. 2012;259:1166–76. https://doi.org/10.1007/s00415-011-6321-5.
103. Kalron A, Dvir Z, Achiron A. Effect of a cognitive task on postural control in patients with a clinically isolated syndrome suggestive of multiple sclerosis. Eur J Phys Rehabil Med. 2011;47:579–86.
104. Negahban H, Mofateh R, Arastoo AA, Mazaheri M, Yazdi MJ, Salavati M, Majdinasab N. The effects of cognitive loading on balance control in patients with multiple sclerosis. Gait Posture. 2011;34:479–84. https://doi.org/10.1016/j.gaitpost.2011.06.023.
105. Negahban H, Sanjari MA, Mofateh R, Parnianpour M. Nonlinear dynamical structure of sway path during standing in patients with multiple sclerosis and in healthy controls is affected by changes in sensory input and cognitive load. Neurosci Lett. 2013;553:126–31. https://doi.org/10.1016/j.neulet.2013.08.024.
106. Sandroff BM, Motl RW. Fitness and cognitive processing speed in persons with multiple sclerosis: a cross-sectional investigation. J Clin Exp Neuropsychol. 2012;34:1041–52. https://doi.org/10.1080/13803395.2012.715144.
107. Krishnan V, Kanekar N, Aruin AS. Anticipatory postural adjustments in individuals with multiple sclerosis. Neurosci Lett. 2012;506:256–60. https://doi.org/10.1016/j.neulet.2011.11.018.

Risk Factors and Outcome in Falls

Alessio Baricich, Marco Invernizzi and Carlo Cisari

1 The Clinical Problem

A fall is a complex event that occurs when subjects are moving of performing an action. The World Health Organization has defined a fall as "an event which results in a person coming to rest inadvertently on the ground or floor or other lower level" [1].

In the United States, falls result in 1,800,000 admissions to emergency departments and 16,000 deaths every year [2], while in the United Kingdom, about one third of elderly people fall every year, half of them recurrently.

Falls in the elderly are, indeed, common, and have a significant impact on the lives and well-being of those affected.

It has been reported that 30% of individuals aged 65 years plus have had a fall during the last 12 months, with 10% sustaining severe injuries. In addition, injuries are among the most frequent causes of death in the elderly, and up to 70% of injuries in this population are caused by falls [3].

Significant morbidity has been described in elderly fall survivors: one third required assistance in activities of daily living (ADL) for 6 months [4], while lasting disability has been found to be very common, resulting in increased dependency and/or a care home admission [5].

Moreover, falls result in increasing costs to the healthcare system, and therefore have a high economic impact; this aspect is aggravated by the growing proportion of elderly people in the population in Western countries.

A. Baricich (✉) · M. Invernizzi · C. Cisari
Physical and Rehabilitation Medicine, Department of Health Sciences, "Maggiore della Carità" University Hospital—Università del Piemonte Orientale, Viale Piazza d'armi 1, 28100 Novara, Italy
e-mail: alessio.baricich@med.uniupo.it

G. Sandrini et al. (eds.), *Advanced Technologies for the Rehabilitation of Gait and Balance Disorders*, Biosystems & Biorobotics 19,
https://doi.org/10.1007/978-3-319-72736-3_8

Several fall risk factors have been identified, e.g. sociodemographic variables, physical activity, alcohol consumption, acute and chronic health problems, dizziness, mobility and medications. These factors are amenable to assessment and are potentially modifiable though specific interventions. In detail, both physiological impairments (linked to age/lifestyle and medical conditions) and certain behaviours (linked to other factors such as habits, perception and judgement) may increase the risk of falls; moreover, environmental hazards become dangerous in inverse proportion to an individual's capacity for specific behaviours. Generally speaking, the possible contribution of each of these aspects to fall risk is highly variable, both between and within subjects.

Many neurological diseases lead to falls, as stance problems and gait disturbances are frequent symptoms in these clinical conditions.

The majority of published studies in this field focused on neurological diseases affecting elderly populations; neurological deficits are indeed considered a factor able to increase the incidence of falls in this population. However, these data were largely derived indirectly from investigations into the cause of falls that required hospital admission; instead, less is known about the relative risk of falls in patients affected by different neurological diseases.

Several studies have reported an increased risk of falls in some common neurological diseases, such as stroke, Parkinson's disease, multiple sclerosis and dementia [3, 6, 7]. However, few data concern comparative analysis of falls in different neurological conditions.

Stolze et al. [7] designed a prospective study in which all patients admitted to a neurological department were investigated for a history of falls. The aim was to assess the prevalence of falls in neurological inpatients and investigate the diseases most frequently involved. A further focus of the study was the comorbidity between falls and gait disorders in these patients. Of the 489 patients included, 165 (34%) reported one or more falls during the past year, and the prevalence of falls was nearly twice as high as that found in a community population of a similar age. About 16% of the fallers (7% of the total) had been admitted to the neurology department because of a fall; 36% of the fallers experienced a single fall, while 64% had fallen more than once. In this population, the fallers were about 8 years older than the non-fallers. In the fallers' group, falls were most frequent in patients with the following diagnoses: Parkinson's disease (62%), syncope (57%), polyneuropathy (48%), epilepsy (41%), spinal disorders (41%), motor neuron disease (33%), multiple sclerosis (31%), psychogenic disorders (29%), stroke (22%) and pain syndromes (21%). Most of the falls (53%) occurred inside the home, 14% in other buildings and 33% outside. 68% of all the fallers reported a peripheral trauma due to the fall, 9% suffered a fracture, whereas 59% sustained bruising or soft tissue damage. Fall-related peripheral traumas were most severe in patients with pain syndromes, Parkinson's disease and polyneuropathy. 5% of the fallers suffered a head trauma. Interestingly, most of the falls (55%) could be directly related to a gait disturbance; furthermore, postural disturbances were strongly correlated with falls. Both are typical findings in neurological patients. Of the drugs that may cause a fall, antidepressants, antihypertensives, diuretics and digitalis medications were identified as risk factors. In this population, the walking aid that was used by the faller at the time of admittance was deemed insufficient in 30% of the patients and, moreover, this aspect was inadequately addressed, indicating the need for optimised walking aid prescription. However, a possible limitation of this study could presumably be related to the fact that it focused on subjects who, being neurological inpatients, may be assumed to represent the most severely affected members of each diagnostic category.

In a recent prospective, case-controlled study, Homann et al. [3] compared the impact of various common neurological diseases on the risk of falls in independent community-dwelling senior citizens. They included patients aged 60 years or older, treated in a neurological outpatient clinic and, as healthy controls, subjects from the general public living in the same area. In this study, 46.5% of neurological patients, but only 16.1% healthy controls, fell at least once during the observation period (1 year). The highest proportions of fallers were found among stroke survivors (89%) and patients with Parkinson's disease (77%), dementia (60%) or epilepsy (57%). In addition, 13.2% of the neurological patients fell three or more times per year, as compared to 3.6% of the healthy subjects; neuropathies, peripheral nerve lesions and Parkinson's disease were identified as risk factors for recurrent falls. The authors also identified a series of additional risk factors, namely a higher number of neurological comorbidities, lower Barthel Index values, lower balance control, and depression, as well as older age and female gender.

As already mentioned, the majority of published studies have focused on fall risk in geriatric neurological patients. Young adults, too, can present several neurological conditions, but publications on fall risk in this population are still limited even though it is a critical issue, for several reasons: first, young adults who suffer from neurological disease can show a complex variety of physical, cognitive and emotional impairments, and, given their age, they might be subject to an increased fall risk for a longer period of time; second, young adults, being more likely to be active (working and participating in sports), may show an increased fall risk compared with older adults. In addition, the risk of fractures can be increased by the long-term use of drugs such as steroids and anti-epileptics [8, 9]. Saverino et al. [6] systematically reviewed the literature on fall risk factors in young patients affected by neurological disorders. They suggested that approximately 50% of these patients show an increased risk of falling, even though the lack of sufficient qualitative descriptions in published studies precluded comparison of different populations and the identification of characteristic patterns of falling. In addition, the studies showed contradictory results with regard to the role of physical impairments, such as muscular strength or reduced sensation, as fall predictors. However, there is strong evidence that reduced balance and gait performance is associated with fall risk, as previously reported also in older adult neurological patients and in healthy elderly people living in the community. The authors highlighted the existence of many different factors, both subject- and environment-related ones, supporting the multifactorial origin of falls. They concluded that young patients with impaired gait and balance or presenting a medium to severe level of motor disability appear to be at increased risk of falling; however, relatively independent patients with an active lifestyle could also have an increased exposure to fall risk.

2 The Pathophysiology of Falls

The pathophysiology of falls remains unclear. Even though a specific cause (gait and balance disorders) can often be identified, the event itself is probably the result of a multifactorial process. Fall prevention is definitely one of the most important topics in public health, and interest in this area has also led to an increasing interest in the neurological basis of falls.

The American Academy of Neurology identified clinical risk factors for falling, categorising them as level A (e.g. stroke, dementia and gait impairment/postural instability) and level B (e.g. Parkinson's disease, neuropathies, lower limb weakness and poor visual acuity) [10]. However, the risk of this "disease-based" approach is that it fails to take into account pathophysiological and causal mechanisms related to falls, as clearly pointed out by Fasano et al. [11] in a recent review.

Indeed, several neurological mechanisms probably underlie falls that have different clinical presentations, mechanisms that therefore do not depend on the specific disease or associated conditions.

Motor impairment

Motor impairment (muscle weakness, slowness or poor coordination) increases the risk of falling both under physiological conditions (e.g. body sway during transferring, standing or walking) and after extrinsic perturbations [11]. Perfect coordination of trunk and ankle is required in order to maintain postural stability after a perturbation. When stability is not maintained, the upper limbs have a key role in implementing rescue strategies and/or protective reactions. However, an adequate flow of information from visual, vestibular and somatosensory afferences is needed, together with the recruitment of attentive and executive resources to adapt the compensatory strategy to the external perturbation.

The motor determinants of falls can involve both the base of support and/or the center of body mass [12]. The most common disorder involving the base of support is freezing of gait (FOG), an episodic inability to generate effective stepping triggered by gait initiation, turning, spatial constraints and stress. Moreover, patients with FOG show a pathological gait pattern even in normal walking conditions; this is characterized by impairment of rhythmicity, symmetry, bilateral coordination, step scaling and dynamic postural control [13]. Patients with FOG tend to fall forward in response to due to perturbation during walking and also because of their stopped posture. FOG affects more than 50% of parkinsonian patients, and is a major cause of falling whilst walking. In addition, FOG is one of the main contributors to declining quality of life in these patients [14]. As regards disorders involving the center of body mass, postural instability is the most frequently observed. It consists of an impairment along the anteroposterior axis, typically characterized by backward body sway [15]. However, in some specific conditions in which there is conspicuous instability (e.g. ataxia, atypical parkinsonism and Huntington's disease) there can also be impairment along the mediolateral axis [16, 17]. Patients with parkinsonism could show disorders of both the base of support and the center of mass, and they show an increased fall risk in comparison with healthy elderly patients. However, mild parkinsonian signs have also been identified in elderly patients without a diagnosis of Parkinson's disease [18], a finding probably related to vascular lesions, mainly located in the frontal lobes [19].

Cognitive impairment

Postural stability and gait are automatic, subcortical motor functions. However, the strategies employed in motor reactions serving to preserve stance and stability after perturbations are under cortical control [20]. Understanding of the physiological control of stability is still limited. Postural control is generally believed to be controlled by the higher centers of the central nervous system (CNS), including the cerebral cortex. It is thought that, in response to each external perturbation, the CNS adopts the most efficient strategy in order to maintain stability, also generating protective reactions in the event of a fall. It has been reported that parkinsonian patients show a higher rate of injury after falls, also probably due to a deficit in attentive strategies that leads to an inability to generate a protective motor response with the arms [21]. Interestingly, a better prognosis was reported in elderly fallers with combined fractures of the distal radius and hip than in subjects with isolated hip fracture, highlighting the importance of the protective upper limb response [22]. In addition, attention-demanding situations are encountered in daily life, and the inability to perform a secondary task whilst walking can be a predictor of future falls [23]. There is evidence that a certain level of attention is also required in "automatic" activities such as walking. Indeed, stroke survivors and parkinsonian patients can show gait deterioration during dual-tasking, indicating impaired executive functions and attention [24, 25]. Moreover, the involvement of cognitive components in normal walking could explain the higher fall risk in patients with dementia, who are particularly vulnerable in the dual-task (talking while walking) condition [26]. As reported by Saverino et al. [6], the contribution of cognitive factors in young patients has, to date, been considered in only a limited number of studies, allowing no conclusion on their role in these subjects.

Higher-level gait disorders

Nutt et al. [27] used the term higher-level gait disorders to describe dysfunction of the highest integrative sensorimotor systems in the presence of intact basic motor and sensory functions. All these clinical conditions are characterized by a high degree of stepping variability and postural instability, related to several causes such as reduced trunk movements, poor trunk control, and impaired postural control. Affected patients show difficulties in transferring, standing and walking. Most have diffuse vascular lesions in the white matter, with impaired interactions between the basal ganglia and supplementary motor area [28, 29].

Automaticity of posture and gait control

As previously described, posture and gait are mainly automatic functions. In fact, pre-existing motor sets are generally activated to counterbalance external perturbations and to maintain the gait pattern [30, 31].

However, the association of motor impairment with decline of executive and attentive strategies could lead to dysfunction of automaticity or interlimb coordination and symmetry during gait [11].

Fear of falling

The fear of falling can develop following a fall or a near-fall episode, not necessarily with a consequent injury. It consists of a subjective, exaggerated perception of the risk of falling. Fear of falling is a risk factor for new falls [32], and it can also cause a reduction of mobility with consequences related to immobilization [33].

Other factors affecting balance and the risk of falling

Gait and balance control requires precise coordination between afferent inputs and the efferent system. The afferent system involves somatosensory, visual and vestibular inputs. Alterations in these contributions may affect balance and gait control, leading to an increased fall risk [34]. The efferent system is also important in the maintenance of balance, as it is responsible for postural reactions after a perturbation. It consists of CNS components (e.g. pyramidal tracts, basal ganglia and cerebellum) and peripheral effectors, i.e. the musculoskeletal system. Current evidence, derived from observations on fall risk in patients with conditions such as cerebellar ataxia or Parkinson's disease [35, 36], supports the role of the central efferent system in balance control.

In a very comprehensive review, Horlings et al. [34] highlighted muscle weakness as an important risk factor for falls. They also suggested that more insights into the mechanisms and patterns of muscle weakness are required in order to plan more efficacious interventions designed to increase muscle strength, improve balance and reduce falls.

3 The Outcome of Falls in Neurological Diseases

Falls are associated with many adverse health outcomes, including injury, debility and death, and the presence of neurological disease can worsen the prognosis of fallers.

As a general consideration, fractures are among the most prominent consequences of falling, and have a significant impact in terms of disability and quality of life. Some fracture risk factors are purely bone-related, e.g. bone mass, bone geometry, bone microarchitecture and bone turnover; however, fall-related factors (such as neuromuscular dysfunction, poor balance, cognitive impairment, cardiovascular instability, reduced visual acuity and use of sedative medications) can also be associated with worse fall consequences. Interestingly, Rapp et al. [37] reported an increased occurrence of femoral fractures in people with disability compared with those without disability.

As previously reported in the literature, neurological disability can lead to significant changes in the musculoskeletal system. In CNS diseases, mainly stroke and spinal cord injuries, different and specific patterns of muscle loss and muscle changes have been described, due to denervation, disuse atrophy, spasticity and myosteatosis. In fact, the pathology-related muscular modifications in neurological diseases share some pathophysiological mechanisms and characteristics with sarcopenia; however, the disability associated with these modifications is caused not only by loss of muscle mass, but also by histological modifications such as fiber switch. Therefore, these muscle tissue changes are more qualitative than quantitative [38]. Their presence could also reduce the efficacy of postural reactions and, together with muscle weakness, contribute to an increased fall risk.

In addition, bone is known to be affected in several neurological conditions, such as Parkinson's disease [39], stroke [40], spinal cord injury [41] and multiple sclerosis [42]. It could be argued that the presence of an increased fall risk together with bone loss can lead to worse fall outcomes in neurological patients, as confirmed by current evidence.

Parkinson's disease

Parkinsonian patients have a five-fold increased risk of sustaining fall-related injuries [43], and an increased risk of femoral fractures [44].

Osteoporosis and osteopenia are very common findings in patients with PD, affecting up to 91% of women and 61% of men. Reduced bone mass in parkinsonian patients seems to be caused mainly by reduced mobility through a mechanism similar to that observed in other neurological diseases. Endocrine factors (such as vitamin D deficiency), as well as nutritional and iatrogenic ones, also play an important role in bone mass depletion. Female gender, disease duration and severity (Hoehn and Yahr stages III and IV), old age and low body mass index are related to more severe osteoporosis [39]. Parkinsonian patients also potentially show longer-term complications after hip surgery and are more likely to develop pressure ulcers and be less mobile postsurgery [45]. Moreover, Fink et al. [46] confirmed that men with PD are more likely than the age-matched population to suffer a fracture, with an increased risk of mortality.

Stroke

Stroke patients have an increased fracture risk compared with the age- and sex-matched population.

Studies have reported that between 14 and 65% of people with stroke fall at least once during hospitalization. Between 37 and 73% fall during the first six months after discharge from hospital; furthermore, even at later stages of stroke recovery, the risk of falling is higher than in similarly aged subjects [47]. Periods coinciding with transitions between settings or stages (e.g. from the acute care to rehabilitation setting, and from rehabilitation to home) may be critical times. They include the early stages of rehabilitation (first week) and the first two-months after discharge from rehabilitation [47]. Fall risk in stroke has a multifactorial etiology, even though gait deficits are likely to play a major role. It has been reported that acute health problems (e.g. pneumonia, urinary tract infections) and recurrent falls can increase the risk of future falls. In addition, low levels of activity over time may result in deconditioning and increased fall risk [47].

In addition, stroke survivors who fall are at increased risk of sustaining a fracture, which is liable to have a significant impact on their clinical outcome. Ramnemark et al. [48] monitored a group of 1139 patients (630 males) admitted consecutively with acute stroke for a median of 2.9 years, reporting 154 fractures in 120 subjects, with a post stroke fracture incidence rate of 37/1000 person-years. 84% of fractures were caused by falls, and hip fracture was the most common type. Hip fracture was 2–4 times more likely in these patients than in an age-matched reference population. Subsequently, Ramnemark et al. [49] examined outcomes of hip fracture in stroke survivors, and found that survival and recovery of independent mobility after hip fracture were significantly reduced compared with what was observed in hip fracture patients who had not had a previous stroke. More recently, Kanis et al. [50] reported that post-stroke patients had a >7-fold increase in fracture risk, mainly at the hip. Fracture risk was higher in the younger age groups and during the first year after stroke.

Stroke patients are at high risk of hip fracture due to osteoporosis and falls. Stroke survivors are indeed prone to frequent falls linked to reduced strength, balance, visual problems and epilepsy [51, 52]. Forster and Young [53] found that 73% of stroke patients with mild to moderate disability had fallen in the 6 months after discharge, with falls usually occurring on the side of the paresis [54].

Multiple sclerosis

Multiple sclerosis (MS) patients show an increased risk of falls. Studies have reported that at least 50% suffer falls within prospective evaluation periods of three to six months, and that falls in these patients show a significant association with injury, fear of falling and reduced activity and social participation [55]. Various studies have identified other factors associated with falls in MS; a recently published review identified four factors showing a major association with falls in MS: the use of a mobility aid, imbalance, cognitive dysfunction, and progressive MS subtype [56]. In addition, fallers show a longer disease duration, a greater overall level of disability, a slower walking speed, and worse performances on balance tests and force platform measures with eyes open and closed [57]. Interestingly, Matsuda et al. [58] reported an association between the number of accumulated impairments and fall events. Bazelier et al. [59] reported a 1.7-fold increased risk of osteoporotic fracture and a four-fold increased risk of hip fracture in MS patients compared with population-based controls. The risk of osteoporotic fracture was significantly greater in patients with MS who had been prescribed antidepressants or hypnotics/

anxiolytics in the previous six months. The risk was also greater in patients who had been prescribed oral/intravenous glucocorticoids [60].

Spinal cord injury

The sensorimotor alterations occurring in spinal cord injury (SCI) can affect the quality and degree of ambulation, increasing the risk of falls in affected patients. Brotherton et al. [61] reported that 75% of independent ambulatory subjects with SCI sustained at least one fall in a year; of these, 18% sustained fractures and 45% reported restricted ability to function independently in the community and in productive activities. In a more recent study, Phonthee et al. [62] reported that more than one third of independent ambulatory participants with SCI experienced at least one fall during the six-month period of the study; this indicated that participants who fell had significantly poorer functional ability than those who did not fall. Having an AIS-C classification [63] and fear of falling also significantly increased the risk of falls.

4 Fall Risk Assessment

Falls are a treatable clinical syndrome. Screening is the first step in preventing future falls and the major injuries that can result from falling. Submitting a patient to a multifactorial fall assessment followed by an appropriate treatment can reduce fall risk by 30–40% [64].

Fall risk screening during clinical examination begins with collection of anamnestic data, in order to determine whether the patient has fallen during the past year. For patients who have not previously fallen, screening consists of a gait and balance assessment. It has been reported that patients who have fallen or who have a gait or balance problem showed an increased risk of future falls [65].

In this context, Gor-García-Fogeda et al. [66] analyzed the clinical and psychometric properties of observational gait assessment scales in people with neurological disorders. In their review, the authors identified the Gait Assessment and Intervention Tool (G.A.I.T.) as the most suitable scale for both clinical practice and research, as it has been shown to be valid, reliable, sensitive to change, homogeneous and comprehensive, containing a large number of items that assess most components of the gait pattern. The Rivermead Visual Gait Assessment (RVGA) has been studied in subjects with different neurological disorders, including MS. For parkinsonian patients, the Tinetti Gait Scale (TGS) showed sensitivity and the Tinetti Performance-Oriented Mobility Assessment (POMA) was predictive for falls and mortality, and also showed intra- and inter-rater reliability. Evaluation of the Tinetti POMA revealed that it showed sensitivity in subjects with normal pressure hydrocephalus, and reliability and validity in patients with Huntington's disease. In addition, the authors pointed out that further studies are needed in order to better analyze the psychometric properties of the RVGA, TGS, and G.A.I.T. in patients with neurological disorders other than stroke.

Another important aspect is the correlation between disability and fall risk. Several studies have supported the existence of this correlation, stating that the more severely affected patients are, the higher their fall risk will be [67]. However, Weerdesteyn et al. [68] observed that reducing fall frequency in stroke survivors is not necessarily good in itself, as it may be achieved by reducing physical activity, which in turn may lead to further physical decline and a reduction in postural stability and quality of life. In addition, Homann et al. [3] observed that even in patients affected by mild to moderate neurological impairments, the incidence of falling was three times higher than in healthy participants. The authors hypothesized that, in these patients, the correlation of disability with fall risk is not linear across all grades of disability, but rather corresponds to an inverse U-shaped curve. In other words, the initial propensity for an increase in falls with higher disability rises only up to a certain point; after which, as patients become more cautious and use numerous different supports, it plateaus and even decreases. The authors concluded, finally, that when patients become so disabled that they are bedridden, the risk can be presumed to approach zero, due to the lack of opportunities to fall. Similar considerations were also made by Saverino et al. [6] about young adults affected by neurological diseases. In the scientific literature, the above-described concept has previously been proposed in relation to parkinsonian patients [69], but not other neurological conditions, and further research directly comparing the risk of falling in neurological inpatients and outpatients with various degrees of disability are required to support this assumption.

In addition, as previously stated by Lee et al. [70], falls can occur in a variety of settings (e.g. home, acute-care hospital, acute rehabilitation center, skilled nursing facility). Consequently, fall risk factors, prevention strategies and also assessment tools can differ across settings. In the same review, the authors also recommended consideration of seven assessment tools, for use in conjunction with overall clinical evaluation, to assess fall risk: the Timed Up and Go Test and the Functional Gait Assessment among community-dwelling elderly; the St Thomas Risk Assessment Tool in medical inpatients <65 years old and surgical inpatients; the Hendrich fall risk model II in medical inpatients; the 10-Minute Walk Test in patients in post-stroke rehabilitation; and the Berg Balance Scale or the Step Test in patients in post-stroke rehabilitation who had fallen during their inpatient stay.

5 Conclusions

Greater attention needs to be paid to neurological diseases as a major risk factor for falls. Preventive measures should focus on reducing the risk of falling, preventing injuries, and preventing (treating) osteoporosis.

Fall risk screening assessments should be the first step, followed by a comprehensive clinical assessment to identify all potential factors. The interventions need to be interdisciplinary and may include medical treatment (medication review, optimal management of comorbidities), physiotherapy (balance, gait and mobility training), occupational therapy (function, independence, behavioral modifications), dietary support (vitamin D and calcium supplementation, general nutrition) and clinical psychology interventions to reduce anxiety and fear of falling.

References

1. World Health Organisation—Falls Fact sheet. Reviewed Sept 2016 (http://www.who.int/mediacentre/factsheets/fs344/en/).
2. Alexander BH, Rivara FP, Wolf ME. The cost and frequency of hospitalization for fall-related injuries in older adults. Am J Public Health. 1992;82(7):1020–3.
3. Homann B, Plaschg A, Grundner M, Haubenhofer A, Griedl T, Ivanic G, Hofer E, Fazekas F, Homann CN. The impact of neurological disorders on the risk for falls in the community dwelling elderly: a case-controlled study. BMJ Open. 2013;3(11):e003367.
4. Sleet DA, Moffett DB, Stevens J. CDC's research portfolio in older adult fall prevention: a review of progress, 1985–2005, and future research directions. J Saf Res. 2008;39:259–67.
5. Sattin RW, Lambert Huber DA, DeVito CA, et al. The incidence of fall injury events among the elderly in a defined population. Am J Epidemiol. 1990;131:1028–37.
6. Saverino A, Moriarty A, Playford D. The risk of falling in young adults with neurological conditions: a systematic review. Disabil Rehabil. 2014;36(12):963–77.
7. Stolze H, Klebe S, Zechlin C, Baecker C, Friege L, Deuschl G. Falls in frequent neurological diseases—prevalence, risk factors and aetiology. J Neurol. 2004;251(1):79–84.
8. Siniscalchi A, De Arro G, Michniewicz A, Gallelli L. Conventional and new antiepileptic drugs on Vitamin D and bone health: what we know to date? Curr Clin Pharmacol. 2016; 11(1):69–70.
9. Whittier X, Saag KG. Glucocorticoid-induced osteoporosis. Rheum Dis Clin North Am. 2016;42(1):177–89.
10. Thurman DJ, Stevens JA, Rao JK, Quality Standards Subcommittee of the American Academy of Neurology. Practice parameter: Assessing patients in a neurology practice for risk of falls (an evidence-based review): report of the Quality Standards Subcommittee of the American Academy of Neurology. Neurology. 2008;70(6):473–9.
11. Fasano A, Plotnik M, Bove F, Berardelli A. The neurobiology of falls. Neurol Sci. 2012; 33(6):1215–23. https://doi.org/10.1007/s10072-012-1126-6.
12. Thijs RD, Bloem BR, van Dijk JG. Falls, faints, fits and funny turns. J Neurol. 2009;256(2): 155–67.
13. Nutt JG, Bloem BR, Giladi N, Hallett M, Horak FB, Nieuwboer A. Freezing of gait: moving forward on a mysterious clinical phenomenon. Lancet Neurol. 2011;10(8):734–44.
14. Bloem BR, Hausdorff JM, Visser JE, Giladi N. Falls and freezing of gait in Parkinson's disease: a review of two inter-connected, episodic phenomena. Mov Disord. 2004;19(8): 871–84.
15. Bloem BR, Beckley DJ, van Dijk JG. Are automatic postural responses in patients with Parkinson's disease abnormal due to their stooped posture? Exp Brain Res. 1999;124(4):481–8.
16. Abdo WF, Borm GF, Munneke M, Verbeek MM, Esselink RA, Bloem BR. Ten steps to identify atypical parkinsonism. J Neurol Neurosurg Psychiatry. 2006;77(12):1367–9.
17. Stolze H, Petersen G, Raethjen J, Wenzelburger R, Deuschl G. The gait disorder of advanced essential tremor. Brain. 2001;124(Pt 11):2278–86.
18. Louis ED, Bennett DA. Mild Parkinsonian signs: an overview of an emerging concept. Mov Disord. 2007;22(12):1681–8.
19. Blahak C, Baezner H, Pantoni L, Poggesi A, Chabriat H, Erkinjuntti T, Fazekas F, Ferro JM, Langhorne P, O'Brien J, Visser MC, Wahlund LO, Waldemar G, Wallin A, Inzitari D, Hennerici MG. Deep frontal and periventricular age related white matter changes but not basal

ganglia and infratentorial hyperin- tensities are associated with falls: cross sectional results from the LADIS study. J Neurol Neurosurg Psychiatry. 2009;80(6):608–13.
20. Skoyles JR. Human balance, the evolution of bipedalism and dysequilibrium syndrome. Med Hypotheses. 2006;66(6):1060–8.
21. Bloem BR, Steijns JA, Smits-Engelsman BC. An update on falls. Curr Opin Neurol. 2003; 16(1):15–26.
22. Berner Y, Shabat S, Mann G, Stern A, Sagiv P, Nyska M. Comorbidity of distal radius (Colles' type) and hip fractures implies a better outcome in older patients. J Am Geriatr Soc. 2002;50(5):976–7.
23. Lundin-Olsson L, Nyberg L, Gustafson Y. "Stops walking when talking" as a predictor of falls in elderly people. Lancet. 1997;349(9052):617.
24. Plotnik M, Giladi N, Dagan Y, Hausdorff JM. Postural instability and fall risk in Parkinson's disease: impaired dual tasking, pacing, and bilateral coordination of gait during the "ON" medication state. Exp Brain Res. 2011;210(3–4):529–38.
25. Yang YR, Chen YC, Lee CS, Cheng SJ, Wang RY. Dual-task-related gait changes in individuals with stroke. Gait Posture. 2007;25(2):185–90.
26. Camicioli R, Howieson D, Lehman S, Kaye J. Talking while walking: the effect of a dual task in aging and Alzheimer's disease. Neurology. 1997;48(4):955–8.
27. Nutt JG, Marsden CD, Thompson PD. Human walking and higher-level gait disorders, particularly in the elderly. Neurology. 1993;43(2):268–79.
28. Chang CM, Yu YL, Ng HK, Leung SY, Fong KY. Vascular pseudoparkinsonism. Acta Neurol Scand. 1992;86(6):588–92.
29. Hennerici MG, Oster M, Cohen S, Schwartz A, Motsch L, Daffertshofer M. Are gait disturbances and white matter degeneration early indicators of vascular dementia? Dementia. 1994;5(3–4):197–202.
30. Dietz V. Do human bipeds use quadrupedal coordination? Trends Neurosci. 2002;25(9): 462–7.
31. Jacobs JV, Horak FB. Cortical control of postural responses. J Neural Transm. 2007;114(10): 1339–48.
32. Mak MK, Pang MY. Fear of falling is independently associated with recurrent falls in patients with Parkinson's disease: a 1-year prospective study. J Neurol. 2009;256(10):1689–95.
33. Brozova H, Stochl J, Roth J, Ruzicka E. Fear of falling has greater influence than other aspects of gait disorders on quality of life in patients with Parkinson's disease. Neuro Endocrinol Lett. 2009;30(4):453–7.
34. Horlings CG, van Engelen BG, Allum JH, Bloem BR. A weak balance: the contribution of muscle weakness to postural instability and falls. Nat Clin Pract Neurol. 2008;4(9):504–15.
35. Adkin AL, Bloem BR, Allum JH. Trunk sway measurements during stance and gait tasks in Parkinson's disease. Gait Posture. 2005;22(3):240–9.
36. Van de Warrenburg BP, Bakker M, Kremer BP, Bloem BR, Allum JH. Trunk sway in patients with spinocerebellar ataxia. Mov Disord. 2005;20(8):1006–13.
37. Rapp K, Becker C, Cameron ID, Klenk J, Kleiner A, Bleibler F, König HH, Büchele G. Femoral fracture rates in people with and without disability. Age Ageing. 2012;41(5):653–8.
38. Carda S, Cisari C, Invernizzi M. Sarcopenia or muscle modifications in neurologic diseases: a lexical or patophysiological difference? Eur J Phys Rehabil Med. 2013;49(1):119–30.
39. Invernizzi M, Carda S, Viscontini GS, Cisari C. Osteoporosis in Parkinson's disease. Parkinsonism Relat Disord. 2009;15(5):339–46.
40. Carda S, Cisari C, Invernizzi M, Bevilacqua M. Osteoporosis after stroke: a review of the causes and potential treatments. Cerebrovasc Dis. 2009;28(2):191–200.
41. Jiang SD, Jiang LS, Dai LY. Mechanisms of osteoporosis in spinal cord injury. Clin Endocrinol 2006;65(5):555–65.
42. Gupta S, Ahsan I, Mahfooz N, Abdelhamid N, Ramanathan M, Weinstock-Guttman B. Osteoporosis and multiple sclerosis: risk factors, pathophysiology, and therapeutic interventions. CNS Drugs 2014;28(8):731–42.

43. Hirsch MA, Toole T, Maitland CG, Rider RA. The effects of balance training and high-intensity resistance training on persons with idiopathic Parkinson's disease. Arch Phys Med Rehabil. 2003;84(8):1109–17.
44. Benzinger P, Rapp K, Maetzler W, König HH, Jaensch A, Klenk J, Büchele G. Risk for femoral fractures in Parkinson's disease patients with and without severe functional impairment. PLoS ONE. 2014;9(5):e97073.
45. Walker RW, Chaplin A, Hancock RL, Rutherford R, Gray WK. Hip fractures in people with idiopathic Parkinson's disease: incidence and outcomes. Mov Disord. 2013;28(3):334–40.
46. Fink HA, Kuskowski MA, Taylor BC, Schousboe JT, Orwoll ES, Ensrud KE, Osteoporotic Fractures in Men (MrOS) Study Group. Association of Parkinson's disease with accelerated bone loss, fractures and mortality in older men: the Osteoporotic Fractures in Men (MrOS) study. Osteoporos Int. 2008;19(9):1277–82.
47. Batchelor FA, Mackintosh SF, Said CM, Hill KD. Falls after Stroke. Int J Stroke 2012;7(6): 482–90.
48. Ramnemark A, Nyberg L, Borssén B, Olsson T, Gustafson Y. Fractures after stroke. Osteoporos Int. 1998;8(1):92–5.
49. Ramnemark A, Nilsson M, Borssén B, Gustafson Y. Stroke, a major and increasing risk factor for femoral neck fracture. Stroke. 2000;31(7):1572–7.
50. Kanis J, Oden A, Johnell O. Acute and long-term increase in fracture risk after hospitalization for stroke. Stroke. 2001;32(3):702–6.
51. Grisso JA, Kelsey JL, Strom BL, Chiu GY, Maislin G, O'Brien LA, Hoffman S, Kaplan F. Risk factors for falls as a cause of hip fracture in women. The Northeast Hip Fracture Study Group. N Engl J Med. 1991;324(19):1326–31.
52. Jørgensen L, Engstad T, Jacobsen BK. Higher incidence of falls in long-term stroke survivors than in population controls: depressive symptoms predict falls after stroke. Stroke. 2002; 33(2):542–7.
53. Forster A, Young J. Incidence and consequences of falls due to stroke: a systematic inquiry. BMJ. 1995;311(6997):83–6.
54. Chiu KY, Pun WK, Luk KD, Chow SP. A prospective study on hip fractures in patients with previous cerebrovascular accidents. Injury. 1992;23(5):297–9.
55. Nilsagård Y, Gunn H, Freeman J, Hoang P, Lord S, Mazumder R, Cameron M. Falls in people with MS—an individual data meta-analysis from studies from Australia, Sweden, United Kingdom and the United States. Mult Scler. 2015;21(1):92–100.
56. Gunn HJ, Newell P, Haas B, Marsden JF, Freeman JA. Identification of risk factors for falls in multiple sclerosis: a systematic review and meta-analysis. Phys Ther. 2013;93(4):504–13.
57. Giannì C, Prosperini L, Jonsdottir J, Cattaneo D. A systematic review of factors associated with accidental falls in people with multiple sclerosis: a meta-analytic approach. Clin Rehabil. 2014;28(7):704–16.
58. Matsuda PN, Shumway-Cook A, Ciol MA, Bombardier CH, Kartin DA. Understanding falls in multiple sclerosis: association of mobility status, concerns about falling, and accumulated impairments. Phys Ther. 2012;92(3):407–15.
59. Bazelier MT, van Staa TP, Uitdehaag BM, Cooper C, Leufkens HG, Vestergaard P, Herings RM, de Vries F. Risk of fractures in patients with multiple sclerosis: a population-based cohort study. Neurology. 2012;78(24):1967–73.
60. Bazelier MT, van Staa T, Uitdehaag BM, Cooper C, Leufkens HG, Vestergaard P, Bentzen J, de Vries F. The risk of fracture in patients with multiple sclerosis: the UK general practice research database. J Bone Miner Res. 2011;26(9):2271–9.
61. Brotherton SS, Krause JS, Nietert PJ. Falls in individuals with incomplete spinal cord injury. Spinal Cord. 2007;45(1):37–40.
62. Phonthee S, Saengsuwan J, Siritaratiwat W, Amatachaya S. Incidence and factors associated with falls in independent ambulatory individuals with spinal cord injury: a 6-month prospective study. Phys Ther. 2013;93(8):1061–72.
63. American Spinal Injury Association. International standards for neurological classification of spinal cord injury, revised 2002. Chicago: American Spinal Injury Association; 2002.

64. Chang JT, Morton SC, Rubenstein LZ, Mojica WA, Maglione M, Suttorp MJ, Roth EA, Shekelle PG. Interventions for the prevention of falls in older adults: systematic review and meta-analysis of randomised clinical trials. BMJ. 2004;328(7441):680.
65. Ganz DA, Bao Y, Shekelle PG, Rubenstein LZ. Will my patient fall? JAMA. 2007;297(1): 77–86.
66. Gor-García-Fogeda MD, Cano de la Cuerda R, Carratalá Tejada M, Alguacil-Diego IM, Molina-Rueda F. Observational gait assessments in people with neurological disorders: a systematic review. Arch Phys Med Rehabil. 2016;97(1):131–40.
67. Schmid AA, Kapoor JR, Dallas M, Bravata DM. Association between stroke severity and fall risk among stroke patients. Neuroepidemiology. 2010;34(3):158–62.
68. Weerdesteyn V, de Niet M, van Duijnhoven HJ, Geurts AC. Falls in individuals with stroke. J Rehabil Res Dev. 2008;45(8):1195–213.
69. Bloem BR, van Vugt JP, Beckley DJ. Postural instability and falls in Parkinson's disease. Adv Neurol. 2001;87:209–23.
70. Lee J, Geller AI, Strasser DC. Analytical review: focus on fall screening assessments. PM R. 2013;5(7):609–21.

Strategies to Prevent Falls

Giovanni Morone, Alessia Federici, Marco Tramontano, Roberta Annicchiarico and Antonino Salvia

1 Introduction

Falls, especially in patients with balance disorders, are a common problem in daily clinical practice and often lead to a loss of mobility and independence [1]. In the literature, between a fourth and a third of individuals aged 65 years or older reported a fall in the previous year [2, 3]. Between 10 and 15% of falls in the elderly result in serious injury, and between 5 and 10% cause a fracture [4]. Furthermore, since the elderly are the fastest growing age group in the Western population, falls are generating drastically increasing costs for public health systems. Many neurological disorders may facilitate the occurrence of falls, since balance and gait disorders are frequent symptoms in neurological patients. Moreover, in clinical experience, falls among neurological patients are frequent [5]. Despite these considerations, the prevalence, risk factors and aetiology of falls in neurological inpatients and outpatients are not well investigated.

From 2.5 to 15% of inpatients fall during hospitalisation, and from 15 to 30% of these falls result in injury (4–6% in severe injury). In rehabilitation settings, the incidence of falls ranges from 24 to 47%, with around 30% resulting in injury, and falls can lead to failure of the rehabilitation programme [6]. Falls are among the main adverse events occurring in hospitals, accounting for up to 30% of all adverse events [7, 8]. According to Wong et al. [9] the length of hospital stay and the costs of hospitalisation were increased in patients sustaining fall-related injuries, and affected patients were less likely to be discharged home [10]. Furthermore, disputes arising from injuries caused by falls are constantly on the rise, and in cases where staff negligence is ascertained in court they are associated with high and very variable costs for the hospitals involved [10]. Given the frequency and recurrence of inpatient falls, hospitals are endeavouring to identify the risk factors for this event

G. Morone (✉) · A. Federici · M. Tramontano · R. Annicchiarico · A. Salvia
IRCCS Fondazione Santa Lucia, Via Ardeatina 306, 00179 Rome, Italy
e-mail: g.morone@hsantalucia.it

G. Sandrini et al. (eds.), *Advanced Technologies for the Rehabilitation of Gait and Balance Disorders*, Biosystems & Biorobotics 19,
https://doi.org/10.1007/978-3-319-72736-3_9

and prevent its occurrence among hospitalised patients. A reduced patient fall risk in a health facility is, indeed, considered an indicator of quality of care.

2 Definition

According to Tinetti [11], a fall in the non-hospitalised geriatric population is defined as "an event which results in a person coming to rest unintentionally on the ground or lower level, not as a result of a major intrinsic event (such as a stroke) or overwhelming hazard".

3 Risk Factors

Various diagnoses (e.g. stroke, dementia, gait and balance disorders) and the use of assistive devices for walking are predictors of fall risk, as is a history of recent falls (there is strong evidence for this). Other predictors are Parkinson's disease, peripheral neuropathy, lower extremity weakness or sensory loss, and substantial loss of vision [12–14].

Community falls, as well as inpatient falls, are usually multifactorial in origin and depend on intrinsic and extrinsic factors. Intrinsic fall risk factors are specific to the patient's health status and include multiple comorbidities, the effects of certain medications such as benzodiazepine or sedative-hypnotics, impaired mental status, older age (>65 years), visual disturbances, postural hypotension, a history of unsteady gait and falls, vitamin D deficiency (alone or in combination with low creatinine clearance), and fallophobia, or a "fear of falling" [15]. Extrinsic fall risk factors include environmental obstacles that can facilitate accidental falls. For example, electrical cables, inappropriate footwear, and clutter in the patient's environment have all been found to increase fall risk in the hospitalised patient [16, 17].

4 Screening for Falls and Risk of Falling

Best practice in fall prevention and management is based on identifying risk factors for falls. Community-dwelling older people seeking medical attention because of a fall, reporting recurrent falls in the past year, or demonstrating abnormalities of gait and/or balance should be offered a multifactorial fall risk assessment. Instead, inpatients at risk of falls are those aged 65 years or older, and those aged 50–64 years who are identified by a clinician as being at higher risk of falling (for example, patients with a sensory impairment or dementia, and patients admitted to hospital with a fall, stroke, syncope, delirium or gait disturbances) [17].

When a patient suffers a fall, it is important to determine the type of fall experienced. This is crucial as it allows the most appropriate fall prevention strategies to be identified based on the patient's unique needs; it can also help caregivers to understand, in general, why falls occur, and help to ensure that staff are adequately supported in their efforts to prevent future falls. Indeed, one of the aims of a hospital or care facility is to decrease or prevent adverse outcomes in patients who are deemed at risk of falling.

Most falls can be categorised as one of four types: accidental, unanticipated physiological, anticipated physiological, or intentional [15, 16]. Accidental falls are defined as unintentional falls due to extrinsic factors: for example, the patient may trip or slip, or fall because of an environmental problem such as a spill on the floor or objects strewn in his or her path. Unanticipated physiological falls result from previously unknown intrinsic risk factors, and may therefore be associated with a patient's first syncopal episode, seizure or pathological hip fracture. An anticipated physiological fall occurs in the presence of a known intrinsic fall risk factor [15, 16].

5 Clinical and Multifactorial Assessment of Patients at Risk of Falls

In patients at risk of falling it is important to perform a multifactorial assessment. In particular, a medical examination is mandatory and must include mental status, balance and gait assessment, as well as examination of proprioception, testing of reflexes, and tests of cortical, extrapyramidal and cerebellar function [12]. It is also important to evaluate postural blood pressure, osteoporosis risk, heart rate and rhythm, and possible urinary incontinence, vitamin D deficiency and vision problems. The complexity of fall risk is such that it is also necessary to evaluate the individual's perceived functional ability and fear of falling [17]. In fact, as recently demonstrated in subacute ambulant stroke, overestimation of walking ability might lead to repeated falls [18]. It may also be useful to consider administering a standardised assessment, such as such as the Morse Falls Risk Assessment Tool [19], STRATIFY [20], and the Hendrich Falls Risk Model II [21]. However, in recent years these risk prediction tools have shown good predictive validity only in the settings in which they were validated. Other fall risk assessment tools developed to assess at-risk populations, and more useful for application in the community, are the Tinetti scores [22], the Berg Balance Test, the Elderly Fall Screening Test, the Dynamic Gait Index, and the Timed Up and Go (TUG) test [23].

Numerous clinical scores have indeed been developed, but these methods often depend on individual observation and subjective interpretation, resulting in inconsistent assessment of results with limited accuracy. Another major limitation of these standardised instruments is their low predictive value. This has been found to result in high false-positive rates, with the tools assigning high risk to large percentages of patients who did not fall [20, 24]. Another drawback is that the majority of these assessments can be performed only in a clinical environment, as their correct execution often requires supervision; this also renders them unsuitable for long-term monitoring. More recently, researchers have attempted to address some of these issues by instrumenting new or existing physical fall risk assessments with wearable motion sensors, in order to make them more objective, quicker to administer, and potentially more suitable for unsupervised use in the community [23–26]. The physical movement routines assessed can be either structured or unstructured, with several sub-options existing for each. Structured routines, for example, can be based on complex tasks that people would not normally perform in everyday life, and that may challenge an individual's strength, balance and even cognition. Examples of these include the TUG test, the Sit-to-Stand test, and the Alternate Step Test, just to name just a few. Alternatively, they may be composed of a set of simple movements that more closely resemble activities of daily living (ADL). Rispens et al. [27] in their study, showed that daily life gait characteristics are associated with fall history. However, before a conclusion can be reached on the values of these findings in fall risk prediction they need to be confirmed by others and supported by prospective data. As mentioned before, the TUG test is one of the tests most often instrumented [28]. Green et al. showed how quantitative assessment of gait and turning during the TUG test may allow more objective and sensitive determination of fall risk, improving the quality of care offered to community-dwelling elderly adults at risk of falling and allowing more timely intervention to prevent future falls. Their study aimed to show that body-worn kinematic sensors can be used to objectively quantify the TUG test and provide a comprehensive, quantitative analysis of timing, gait, and stability for each of the test's segments. Furthermore, the authors discuss how an instrumented (iTUG) tool could potentially be used in a supervised monitoring protocol, where deterioration in a subject's gait and balance would be noted as a change over time in their gyroscope-derived parameters, measured while completing the TUG test. This could form part of a continuous fall risk assessment protocol, deployed at home or in a primary care facility. Finally, several studies have verified the suitability of consumer accelerometers, like those included in recent smartphone models, for performing some clinical tests, such as the iTUG test. In the FARSEEING EU-project [29], the Android uTUG application, a stand-alone application for instrumenting the TUG test that is designed to be self-administrable at home, is the first of a series of stand-alone applications instrumenting clinical functional tests, while the uFall Android application has been developed for monitoring the user's motor activities at home. These applications take advantage of the smartphone-embedded inertial sensors and require that subjects wear the smartphone on a waist belt.

6 Multifactorial Intervention

Fall prevention protocols in acute care hospitals as well as in the community are designed to address commonly encountered fall risk factors, both extrinsic and intrinsic, and aim to minimise the occurrence of falls. The multitude of intrinsic fall risk factors in inpatients makes it difficult to isolate specific ones in this population. What is more, rehabilitation hospitals, where patients are required to do exercises that involve defying gravity, can present even more problems.

Management of fall risk may address the underlying disorder, involve adjustment of medication (minimising the use of psychoactive medications), and include an exercise programme with gait and balance training. Other interventions for fall risk reduction include management of those risk factors identified in the multifactorial assessment, specifically visual abnormalities, neurological disorders, cognitive impairment, postural hypotension, other cardiovascular abnormalities, urinary abnormalities, foot and footwear problems, and other relevant acute or chronic medical conditions, as well as prescription of and instruction in the use of assistive devices, prescription of occupational therapy, treatment of osteoporosis, management of the fear of falling, and adaptation or modification of the home environment [12, 17].

A systematic review of fall prevention interventions [30] concluded that fall prevention programmes as a group reduced the risk of falling by 11% and the monthly rate of falling by 23%. Interventions that focused on high-risk individuals (e.g., those who had previously fallen and were at increased risk of falling again) were more likely to be effective than those that targeted an unselected group of seniors. Furthermore, the most effective intervention strategies used clinical assessment combined with individualised fall risk reduction and patient follow-up. This clinical assessment consisted of gait, balance and neurological function testing, review of all medications, and development of a tailored medical management approach, and also made provision for appropriate referrals. When analysed as a group, interventions that used clinical assessment and risk reduction reduced the risk of falling by 18% and the average number of falls by 43% [30].

Multidisciplinary risk assessment and management strategies are the most effective preventive tools. In most inpatient settings, a member of the rehabilitation staff is generally the first provider to assess a patient's fall risk [31]. A recent updated Cochrane review investigating the effectiveness of interventions for fall prevention in older people in care facilities and hospitals found that vitamin D supplementation is effective in reducing the rate of falls. Furthermore, evidence on the effectiveness of exercise in subacute hospital settings was highlighted, but its effectiveness in care facilities remains uncertain. Finally, multifactorial interventions reduce falls in hospitals, but evidence on their impact on the risk of falling was inconclusive [32]. Moreover, a recent study highlighted the efficacy of multifactorial interventions (covering aspects such as post-fall review, patient education, staff education, footwear advice and toileting) with multiprofessional input [33], and also the fact that delirium avoidance programmes, reduction of sedative and hypnotic medication, patient education and sustained exercise programmes might reduce falls when implemented as single interventions [33]. Without accurate risk determination, fall prevention approaches cannot be appropriately implemented. While methods for predicting fall with injury currently remain somewhat elusive, there is a need, supported to varying degrees by the empirical literature, to develop and implement risk assessment protocols [33]. A recent Cochrane review update on interventions for preventing falls in older people living in the community found that home-based exercise programmes and home safety interventions reduce the rate of falls and the risk of falling, while multifactorial assessment and intervention programmes reduce the rate of falls but the not risk of falling. Finally, the authors pointed out that Tai Chi reduces the risk of falling [14].

7 Technology to Boost Fall Prevention

In recent years, information and communication technologies (ICT) have shown their potential to enhance the autonomy and quality of life of elderly people, by improving detection and/or prevention of falls. Furthermore, ICT solutions for fall detection and prevention could significantly reduce the costs associated with elderly care. The value and effectiveness of these solutions could be maximised through their further integration and combination, but mainly by tailoring them to specific target groups and risk factors. This tailoring could allow potential fallers to use the most appropriate devices, modalities and programmes (i.e. with optimal frequency and in the most appropriate combinations). Recent advances in the application of ICT for ageing well (and for promoting active ageing) have focused on the development and validation of technologies, tools, techniques and overall solutions for the effective management of falls. The solutions developed include the use of sensors for the timely detection of falls, pervasive applications for triggering alarms, actuators for improving the surrounding environment (e.g., lighting conditions), applications for training and improving the motor abilities of elderly end-users, as well as a rich set of applications designed to monitor and understand the status of the user with a view to identifying and applying measures that could boost fall prevention. Several solutions (mainly at component level such as fall detectors) are available as commercial products and are widely used by care service providers, housing organisations, as well as individual users at home. At the same time, more advanced integrated solutions have recently been introduced and validated as part of research projects. ICT-based fall detection and prevention solutions are usually integrated into broader fall management solutions, which combine ICT with the ever-important human care factors within appropriate processes. Despite the availability of several detection and prevention modalities, as well as the respective integrated solutions, little emphasis has so far been placed on tailoring/personalising these solutions to specific fall risk factors and target populations. Indeed, falls are associated with several risk factors, biological, economic, societal, cultural and environmental [34, 35]. In the area of biological factors, several illnesses and chronic conditions (e.g., balance/gait problems, cardiovascular diseases, vision problems, depression) are common causes of falls. At the same time, risk profiles vary according to the faller's country of origin and residence.

There is a wide range of commercially available devices for preventing fall incidents, such as bath mats, bedside rails, transfer benches, toilet seat safety and supporting devices, wall-mounted shower seats, mobility handles, raised toilet seats with arms, and so on. At the same time, research efforts have produced a wide range of wearable devices for preventing and/or detecting falls, which include systems based on accelerometers [36–39], miniaturised wearable systems [40], systems based on mobile phones [41], wrist-based systems [42], camera-based systems, systems based on movement classification, and systems involving floor pressure detection, to mention just some. Furthermore, a large number of ICT research projects (including EC co-funded projects), have striven to produce and validate more integrated solutions. For example, the FP7-CONFIDENCE project (http://fallsprevention.eu/confidence-ubiquitous-care-system-to-support-independent-living-fp7-ict) provides a ubiquitous system for detecting abnormal events (including falls), while the BIOTELEKINESY project (funded under FP7-PEOPLE-IEF-2008) provides a communication platform for the tele-monitoring and tele-management of the elderly to detect locomotion disabilities and prevent falls. Another example is the FALL-WATCH project (under FP7 "Research for SMEs", see: http://www.fallwatch-project.eu), which has developed a wearable miniaturised fall detection system for the elderly. Similarly, the FP6-IST project ENABLE has produced a wearable system supporting services to "enable" elderly people to live well, independently and at ease [43]. Various ICT innovations have been adopted to monitor falls and alert professionals or carers [44] if a fall occurs, and they include home automation systems. To date these technologies have tended to be reactive; this helps to reduce the time the faller remains lying on the ground (lying on the ground for long periods of time can cause serious health complications) and allows the person who has fallen to receive help promptly. There also exists a range of ICT systems created or adapted to be proactive in preventing falls, such as those that, to this end, provide older adults with strength and balance training opportunities, e.g. exergames, Wii-fit, Kinect [45, 46]. ICT innovations able to deliver exercise programmes in the home have the potential to reduce costs and, by providing regular feedback and motivation to older adults, increase adherence. The literature on the use of these technologies highlights, in particular, the issue of user acceptability. The numerous factors related to this aspect can be defined intrinsic—control, independence and perceived need of/requirements for safety—and extrinsic—usability, feedback gained. The technology should be chosen of the basis of the older person's preferences and customised to his/her specific needs.

References

1. Blake AJ, Morgan K, Bendall MJ, Dallosso H, Ebrahim SB, Arie TH, et al. Falls by elderly people at home: prevalence and associated factors. Age Ageing. 1988;17(365–372):2.
2. Bohannon R. Correlation of lower limb strengths and other variables with standing performance in stroke patients. Physiother Can. 1989;41(198–202):3.
3. Dunn JE, Rudberg MA, Furner SE, Cassel CK. Mortality, disability, and falls in older persons: the role of underlying disease and disability. Am J Public Health. 1992;82(395–400):4.
4. Elble RJ, Hughes L, Higgins C. The syndrome of senile gait. J Neurol. 1992;239(71–75):5.
5. Stolze H, Klebe S, Zechlin C, Baecker C, Friege L, Deuschl G. Falls in frequent neurological diseases–prevalence, risk factors and aetiology. J Neurol. 2004;25:79–84.
6. Fahn S, Elton RL. Unified's Parkinson's disease rating scale. Recent developments in Parkinson's disease. Florham Park, NJ: Macmillan Health Care Information; 1987. p. 153–63.
7. Oliver D, Connelly JB, Victor CR, Shaw FE, Whitehead A, Genc Y. Strategy to prevent falls and fractures in hospitals and care homes and effect of cognitive impairment: systematic review and meta-analyses. BMJ. 2007; 334(7584):82.
8. Hitcho EB, Krauss MJ, Birge S, Dunagan WC, Fischer I, Johnson S, Nast PA, Costantinou E, Fraser VJ. Characteristics and circumstances of falls in a hospital setting: a prospective analysis. J Gen Intern Med. 2004;19:732–9.
9. Wong CA, Recktenwald AJ, Jones ML, Waterman BM, Bollini ML, Dunagan WC. The cost of serious fall-related injuries at three midwestern hospitals. J Qual Patient Saf. 2012;37 (2):81–7.
10. Bates D, Pruess K, Souney P, Platt R. Serious falls in hospitalized patients: correlates and resource utilization. Am J Med. 1995;99:137–43.
11. Tinetti ME, Speechley M, Ginter SF. Risk factors for falls among elderly persons living in the community. N Engl J Med. 1988;319:1701–7.
12. Summary of Evidence-based Guideline for Clinicians. Assessing patients in a neurology practice for risk of falls. www.aan.org. Accessed 10 Aug 2016.
13. Guideline for the prevention of falls in older persons. American Geriatrics Society, British Geriatrics Society, and American Academy of Orthopaedic Surgeons Panel on Falls Prevention. J Am Geriatr Soc. 49(5):664–72; 2001.
14. Gillespie LD, Robertson MC, Gillespie WJ, Sherrington C, Gates S, Clemson LM, Lamb SE. Interventions for preventing falls in older people living in the community. Cochrane Database Syst Rev. (9):CD007146; 2012.
15. Currie L. Fall and injury prevention. In: Hughes R, editor. Patient safety and quality. An evidence handbook for nurses. 2008. Available at http://www.ahrq.gov/legacy/qual/nurseshdbk/.
16. Gray-Miceli D, Quigley PA. Fall prevention: assessment, diagnoses, and intervention strategies. In: Boltz M, Capezuti E, Fulmer T, Zwicker D, editors. Evidence-based geriatric nursing protocols for best practice. 4th ed. New York, NY: Springer Publishing Company; 2012. p. 268–97.
17. National Institute for Health and Care Excellence. Falls in older people: assessing risk and prevention. NICE guidelines [CG161] Published date: June 2013, ISBN: 978-1-4731-0132-6. www.nice.org.uk. Accessed 11 Aug 2016.
18. Morone G, Iosa M, Pratesi L, Paolucci S. Can overestimation of walking ability increase the risk of falls in people in the subacute stage after stroke on their return home? Gait Posture. 2014;39:965–70.
19. Morse JM, Morse RM. Calculating fall rates: methodological concerns. QRB Qual Rev Bull. 1988;14:369–71.
20. Coker E, Oliver D. Evaluation of the stratify falls prediction tool on a geriatric unit. Outcomes Manag. 2003;7(1):8–14; quiz 15-6.

21. Hendrich AL, Bender PS, Nyhuis A. Validation of the Hendrich II fall risk model: a large concurrent case/control study of hospitalized patients. Appl Nurs Res. 2003;16(1):9–21.
22. Tinetti ME. Performance-oriented assessment of mobility problems in elderly patients. J Am Geriatr Soc. 1986;34:119–26.
23. Perell KL, Nelson A, Goldman RL, et al. Fall risk assessment measures: an analytic review. J Gerontol A Biol Sci Med Sci. 2001;56:M761–6.
24. Vassallo M, Stockdale R, Sharma JC, et al. A comparative study of the use of four fall risk assessment tools on acute medical wards. J Am Geriatr Soc. 2005;53:1034–8.
25. Shany T, Redmond SJ, Marschollek M, Lovell NH. Assessing fall risk using wearable sensors: a practical discussion. A review of the practicalities and challenges associated with the use of wearable sensors for quantification of fall risk in older people. Z Gerontol Geriatr. 2012;45:694–706.
26. Zijlstra W, Aminian K. Mobility assessment in older people: new possibilities and challenges. Eur J Ageing. 2007;4:3–12.
27. Rispens SM, van Schooten KS, Pijnappels M, Daffertshofer A, Beek PJ, van Dieën JH. Identification of fall risk predictors in daily life measurements: gait characteristics' reliability and association with self-reported fall history. Neurorehabil Neural Repair. 2015;29(1):54–61.
28. Greene BR, O'Donovan A, Romero-Ortuno R, Cogan L, Scanaill CN, Kenny RA. Quantitative falls risk assessment using the timed up and go test. IEEE Trans Biomed Eng. 2010;57(12):2918–26.
29. Mellone S, Tacconi C, Schwickert L, Klenk J, Becker C, Chiari L. Smartphone-based solutions for fall detection and prevention: the FARSEEING approach. Zeitschrift für Gerontologie und Geriatrie. 2012;45(8):722–7.
30. Shekelle P, Maglione M, Chang J, Mojica W, Morton SC, Suttorp M, Roth EA, Rhodes S, Wu S, Newberry S. Evidence report and evidence-based recommendations. Zugriff am. 2003;4(2003):2010.
31. GholamHosseini H, Baig MM, Connolly MJ et al. A multifactorial falls risk prediction model for hospitalized older adults. In: 36th annual international conference of the IEEE in engineering in medicine and biology society (EMBC); 2014. p. 3484–87.
32. Cameron ID, Gillespie LD, Robertson MC, Murray GR, Hill KD, Cumming RG, Kerse N. Interventions for preventing falls in older people in care facilities and hospitals. Cochrane Database Syst Rev. 2012;12:CD005465.
33. Oliver D, Healey F, Haines TP. Preventing falls and fall-related injuries in hospitals. Clin Geriatr Med. 2010;26(4):645–92.
34. Suzhen L, Jiping L, Yijuan C. Body function and fall-related factors of the elderly in community. J Nurs Sci. 2004;19(6):5–7.
35. Prudham D, Evans J. Factors associated with falls in the elderly: a community study. Age Ageing. 1981;10:141–6.
36. Bourke A, van de Ven P, Gamble M, et al. Evaluation of waist-mounted tri-axial accelerometer based fall-detection algorithms during scripted and continuous unscripted activities. J Biomech. 2010;43(15):3051–7.
37. Li Q, Stankovic J, Hanson M, Barth A, Lach J, Zhou G. Accurate, fast fall detection using gyroscopes and accelerometer-derived posture information. In: Sixth international workshop on wearable and implantable body sensor networks. BSN 2009; 2009. p. 138–43.
38. Kangas M, Konttila A, Lindgren P, Winblad I, Jamsa T. Comparison of low-complexity fall detection algorithms for body attached accelerometers. Gait Posture. 2008;28(2):285–91.
39. Nyan N, Tay FE, Manimaran M, Seah KH. Garment-based detection of falls and activities of daily living using 3-axis MEMS accelerometer. J Phys Conf Ser. 2006;34:1059–67.
40. Chen J, Kwong K, Chang D, Luk J, Bajcsy R. Wearable sensors for reliable fall detection. In: Proceedings of 27th annual international conference of the engineering in medicine and biology society, IEEEEMBS; 2005.
41. Dai J, Bai X, Yang Z, Shen Z, Xuan D. PerFallD: a pervasive fall detection system using mobile phones. In: 8th IEEE international conference on pervasive computing and

communications workshops (PERCOM Workshops); 2010. https://doi.org/10.1109/PERCOMW.2010.5470652.
42. Degen T, Jaeckel H. Speedy: a fall detector in a wrist watch. In: Proceedings of the seventh IEEE international symposium on wearable computing; 2003. p. 184–89.
43. Hawley-Haguea H, Boultona E, Halla A, et al. Older adults' perceptions of technologies aimed at falls prevention, detection or monitoring: a systematic review. Int J Med Inform. 2014;83:416–26.
44. Brownsell S, Hawley MS. Automatic fall detectors and the fear of falling. J Telemed Telecare. 2004;10:262–6.
45. Miller CA, Hayes DM, Dye K, Johnson C, Meyers J. Using the Nintendo Wii Fit and body weight support to improve aerobic capacity, balance, gait ability, and fear of falling: two case reports. J Geriatr Phys Ther. 2012;35:95–104.
46. Williams MA, Roy LS, Jenkinson A, Stewart A. Exercising with computers in later life (EXCELL)—pilot and feasibility study of the acceptability of the Nintendo® WiiFit in community-dwelling fallers. BMC Res Notes. 2010;3:238.

Part II
Integrated Approach to Gait and Balance Rehabilitation in Neurological Diseases

Rehabilitation of Parkinson's Disease

Giovanni Abbruzzese and Elisa Pelosin

1 Introduction

Parkinson's disease (PD) is a complex neurodegenerative disorder characterized by motor and non-motor symptoms. The non-motor symptoms (involving different domains, such as sleep, mood, olfaction, autonomic regulation) may precede by many years the appearance of the classic motor features (bradykinesia/akinesia, rigidity, tremor at rest) on the basis of which the clinical diagnosis is usually made.

No curative or neuroprotective therapy is currently available and the management of PD is traditionally based on symptomatic treatment with drug therapy (levodopa being considered the "gold standard") or with neurosurgical approaches (deep brain stimulation). However, PD has a chronic progressive course and even with optimal medical or surgical management, patients still experience motor and non-motor fluctuations and a progressive loss of autonomy. In particular, the advanced stages of the disease are characterized by increasing disability, which is largely related to non-dopaminergic features [15], such as gait disorders (including freezing of gait), transfer limitations, and postural instability with falls. In addition, it should be considered that among the various presentations of the disease, the "postural instability gait disorder" subtype is characterized, from the onset, by axial involvement with a reduced levodopa responsiveness, a faster rate of cognitive decline, and a worse quality of life [40].

G. Abbruzzese (✉) · E. Pelosin
Department of Neuroscience, Rehabilitation, Ophthalmology, Genetics and Maternal Child Health, University of Genoa, Genoa, Italy
e-mail: giabbr@unige.it

G. Sandrini et al. (eds.), *Advanced Technologies for the Rehabilitation of Gait and Balance Disorders*, Biosystems & Biorobotics 19,
https://doi.org/10.1007/978-3-319-72736-3_10

For the above reasons, rehabilitation therapies are increasingly implemented as an adjuvant to pharmacological and neurosurgical treatment with the aim of maximizing functional ability and minimizing secondary complications.

2 Gait and Balance Abnormalities in PD

Gait disorders are a common manifestation among patients with PD, and according to their pattern of occurrence they can be classified as: (a) continuous, or (b) episodic [14]. Continuous (persistent) alterations in the gait pattern are more or less consistent from step to step: walking is slow and characterized by a reduced step length and step width ("shuffling gait"); furthermore, arm swing is decreased or absent, a longer double limb support phase can be observed, and patients present higher step variability with increased left/right asymmetry. These persistent gait abnormalities are usually exacerbated under dual-task conditions [31, 38]. Episodic alterations, on the other hand, are occasional, intermittent, and apparently random. They occur in an inexplicable manner, and include: (a) festination, i.e. a tendency to move forward with increasingly rapid, but ever smaller steps, associated with a forward shift of the center of gravity over the stepping feet, and (b) freezing of gait (FOG), i.e. brief, episodic absence or marked reduction of forward progression of the feet despite the intention to walk. FOG may prevent the patient from starting to walk, turning, passing through narrow spaces, and making for specific destinations.

While festination is relatively infrequent, FOG is a common and debilitating phenomenon in PD; although primarily related to progression of the disease and disease duration, it can also occur in the early stages. Although the underlying mechanisms (loss of automaticity, impaired regulation of rhythmicity, failure to release inhibition of the stepping program) are still uncertain [25], FOG is associated with an increased prevalence of falls and loss of independence [6].

Postural instability is a hallmark of PD, particularly in the more advanced stages of the disease. It reflects the interaction of complex mechanisms [37] (Table 1). Because of the need for continuous adaptation during initiation of gait, turning, negotiation of obstacles and stopping, walking poses the largest challenge to balance in PD subjects. In addition, the dual-task condition (both cognitive and motor) impairs postural stability in PD [18].

Postural instability in PD is associated with a more rapid disease progression and greater disability. Together with FOG [6], it is a major cause of falls, the incidence of which is significantly higher in patients with PD than in age-matched subjects without PD [6, 30]. Falls have a large impact (both physical and psychological) on quality of life and autonomy of patients, and are the first cause of hospitalization of PD patients.

Table 1 Mechanisms of postural instability in PD (modified from Schoneburg et al. [37])

Postural alignment	• Narrow stance	
	• Inaccurate representation of verticality	
	• Postural deformity	Camptocormia, antecollis, Pisa syndrome, scoliosis
	• Increased postural sway (in the medio-lateral direction)	
	• Impaired sensory weighting	
	• Reduced limits of stability (forward)	
Postural adjustments	• Impaired "reactive" (automatic) adjustments	Bradykinetic, multiple and smaller amplitude Lack of flexibility in strategies
	• Defective "anticipatory" postural adjustments (APA)	Reduced magnitude and prolonged latensy
Dynamic balance (walking)	• Inappropriate adaptation	Foot placement Axial control of lateral and forward stability Shifts of center of mass (CoM) from side-to-side (leg unloading) Forward movement of CoM

3 Interaction Between Cognitive Function, Gait Performance and Falls

For a long time, motor functions such as gait and balance were considered to be quasi-automatic tasks, dependent mainly on subcortical and spinal regulation. However, several neuropsychological studies demonstrated that cognitive deficits (including deficits of executive-attentional function and visuospatial abilities) are independently associated with reduced gait performances (increased gait variability and reduced gait speed) and future falls [3, 43].

Morphological and functional studies have offered additional evidence supporting the relationship between gait and cognitive resources. A nonspecific association was reported between neuroimaging findings (such as generalized brain atrophy or white matter hyperintensities) and gait and cognitive dysfunction [3]. Postural instability and a history of falls have been associated with β-amyloid deposition [23] and cholinergic dysfunction [7]. Using short-latency afferent inhibition (SAI), a transcranial magnetic stimulation technique that assesses an inhibitory circuit in the sensorimotor cortex and is regarded as a global marker of cholinergic function in the brain, Rochester et al. [35] demonstrated an association between gait dysfunction, cholinergic deficiency, and attention impairment in PD. Consistent with this idea, we recently showed a gradient of SAI reduction in PD subjects, elderly fallers and elderly non-fallers that correlated with changes in gait speed during a dual task independently of cognitive status [28]. In particular, the finding of changes in postural stability and gait ability during the performance of another demanding task (i.e. in the dual-task condition) strongly supports the idea of a common higher-order neural network (in which the cholinergic system may play a pivotal role).

In conclusion, there is robust evidence that the degree of cognitive impairment could affect the success of interventions aimed at improving gait and balance, and reducing fall risk in patients with PD. This suggests that cognitive training interventions might be successfully associated with traditional physiotherapy approaches.

4 Basic Principles of Rehabilitation in PD

Traditional approaches to rehabilitation in PD were based on empirical experience with poor knowledge of the mechanisms underlying their effects. Over the past decade, both the number and the quality of trials evaluating the efficacy of physical therapy in PD have increased substantially. A recent meta-analysis of physiotherapy interventions [41] provided evidence of a small benefit from physiotherapy over the short term (i.e. <3 months), significant only for gait speed, two- or six-minute walk test, Freezing of Gait questionnaire, the Timed Up and Go test, the Functional Reach Test, the Berg Balance Scale, and the clinician-rated Unified Parkinson's Disease Rating Scale. However, no difference between arms was found in fall rate. This review documented that physiotherapists use a wide range of approaches to treat patients with PD (without evidence of differences in treatment effect between the different types of intervention), which suggests that there is a need for consensus and large, randomized controlled trials "to demonstrate the longer-term efficacy and cost-effectiveness of *best practice* physiotherapy in PD" [41].

Experimental and clinical evidence suggests that exercise is an intervention that can help with both motor and non-motor symptoms of PD, and may be regarded as the basic element of any rehabilitation approach [42]. Brain plasticity is the ability of central nervous system cells to modify their structure and function in response to a variety of external stimuli, i.e. on the basis of experience, and exercise-induced brain plasticity can probably be considered the neural basis of the effects of rehabilitation interventions in PD [2, 29]. However, the possibility that exercise might facilitate neuroplasticity and behavior in PD depends on a number of practice variables (intensity, specificity, complexity) (Table 2).

Physical exercise and exercise-related plastic changes are the basic elements of motor learning. However, it should be pointed out that in PD the early and preferential loss of dopamine in the caudal regions of the basal ganglia (i.e. putamen) leads to diminished automatic and increased cognitive control of movements, shifting the stimulus-response "habitual" control towards a "goal-directed" control [32]. Indeed, the execution of tasks (motor or cognitive) places a greater cognitive burden on PD subjects.

Table 2 Physical exercise in Parkinson's disease: suggested features from: Abbruzzese et al. [2]

• Goal-based learning: practice of activities that will lead to improved performance (e.g. in gait/posture)
• Experience-dependent neuroplasticity, including: intensity, repetition, specificity, difficulty, and complexity of practice
• Aerobic training: vigorous and sustained activity to increase cardio-pulmonary function, oxygen consumption and blood flow to the brain
• Enhanced cognitive engagement through: feedback (verbal or proprioceptive), attentional demand (cueing or dual tasking), motivation (reward)
• Feasibility: optimal medication status, realistic objective, elimination of barriers

5 Combining the Motor and Cognitive Approach in PD Rehabilitation

Modern rehabilitation aims to bring about physiological repair of neural damage and may be seen as a "learning process" wherein old skills have to be re-acquired and new ones have to be learned through practice. This may be achieved by combining motor and cognitive training; in this context, improvements in cognitive skills may be translated into better performance of selected physical tasks or, vice versa, improvements in motor abilities may enhance cognitive performance. Indeed, a recent prospective, parallel group, single-center trial in non-demented patients with mild-to-moderate PD [9] showed that 24 months of progressive resistance exercise training improved attention and working memory.

Along these same lines, various approaches integrating cognitive and motor aspects of rehabilitation have been proposed in recent years. These include: (1) cueing training; (2) dual-task (DT) training; (3) motor imagery (MI) and action observation (AO); and (4) augmented feedback and virtual reality (VR) training (Fig. 1).

1. Cueing can be defined as the use of external stimuli, temporal or spatial, to facilitate the initiation and continuation of movement or motor activities (gait) [36]. The mechanisms underlying the effects of cueing have still not been completely elucidated, but targeted attention, self-instruction, and cueing modality and parameters are thought to play a pivotal role in its effectiveness.

In a single-blind study in 20 PD patients [19], we showed that incorporating external sensory cues into the rehabilitation protocol can extend the short-term benefit of physical therapy in moderately disabled patients with PD, possibly as a result of the learning of new motor strategies. Cueing has been found to be particularly effective in improving gait disorders [17]; the large "RESCUE" trial [24], investigating the effects of a home physiotherapy program based on rhythmic cueing, demonstrated specific positive effects on gait, freezing and balance. However, cueing therapy has some limitations since cueing seeks to trigger

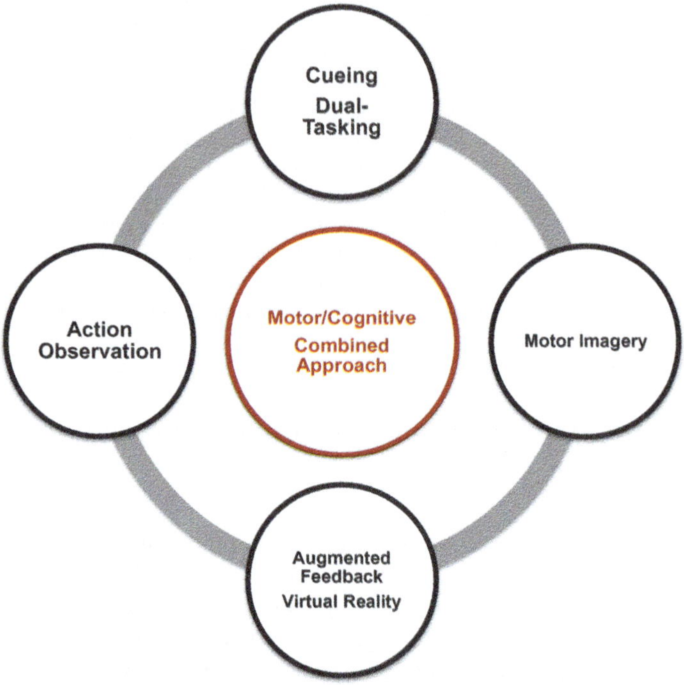

Fig. 1 Model of the integrated motor-cognitive approach to the rehabilitation of Parkinson's disease

sub-movements within a movement sequence, and does not help with the acquisition of the entire movement; therefore, cue-dependence is not the best instrument to facilitate consolidation of motor learning.

The benefits of treadmill training depend, at least in part, on a cueing mechanism since treadmill walking acts as an external pacemaker, improving gait rhythm and stability in PD [13].

2. DT training involves the simultaneous execution of two tasks with distinct goals and using different motor/cognitive task sets. DT execution ability is significantly impaired in patients with PD and the DT condition can aggravate gait disorders, leading to an increased risk of falling and reduced functional mobility. Traditionally, clinical rehabilitation guidelines for PD consider DT interventions as potentially hazardous, and indeed suggest that patients avoid performing multiple tasks simultaneously in daily life. However, this notion has recently been challenged [39], with some pilot studies demonstrating the feasibility and efficacy of DT training in PD [44]. In 15 PD patients, Fernandes et al. [12] obtained superior outcomes, in terms of static balance (mediolateral sway) and executive functions, with DT as opposed to single-task training. Rochester et al. [34] suggested that the association of cueing and the DT condition can

significantly improve the acquisition, automaticity and retention of gait performance. It has been postulated that DT gait training may enhance divided attention abilities during walking [44]. Three randomized controlled trials focusing on DT rehabilitation are currently ongoing [39].

3. MI and AO are two cognitive (mental practice) training techniques that have been proposed as promising rehabilitation tools for patients with neurological disorders [22].

MI is a cognitive process in which a subject, making use of an external (visual) or internal (kinesthetic) representation of a specific motor action, imagines that he/she is performing a movement, without actually doing it. There exists robust evidence indicating that MI could improve motor performance through the same cortical-subcortical network that is active during motor execution, thus leading to the development of neuroplasticity in the primary motor cortex [4].

Observing actions performed by others activates, in the brain, the same neural structures that are used for the actual execution of the same actions. These structures comprise the mirror neuron system (MNS). Indeed, the cerebral areas comprised in the human MNS contain specific "mirror" neurons that discharge during both the execution of goal-directed actions and the observation of other individuals performing similar actions [11].

During AO treatment, patients are requested to observe and imitate specific actions (relevant to their motor repertoire) in order to enhance the activation of the related motor areas [8]. Several studies have shown that AO treatment is effective for motor rehabilitation, for instance in patients with stroke [8].

Few clinical studies are available on the efficacy of MI and AO in PD rehabilitation (for a review, see Abbruzzese et al. [1]). We showed, that a single session of AO could reduce bradykinesia, facilitating the performance of spontaneous finger movements [27], while a rehabilitation program based on AO was able to induce an additional positive effect on recovery of walking ability in PD patients with FOG [26]. Because of their physiological background, both MI and AO can be regarded as novel and promising approaches, but their efficacy still needs to be confirmed by large, randomized controlled trials.

4. VR can be defined as interaction between a person in the real world and a virtual environment generated by a computer. The VR method has the advantage of providing rich sensory feedback (visual, auditory and haptic inputs) that can be used to train subjects, helping them to recover defective motor function through enhanced motor learning.

VR along with interactive video gaming have emerged as new treatment approaches in stroke rehabilitation settings over the past ten years [16]. More recently, VR has been proposed as a promising tool for patients with PD [10, 20], and in a few pilot studies VR-based training was shown to be feasible for gait and balance rehabilitation in PD. It should be noted that Robles-García et al. [33], in their study, found that the ability to imitate instructed motor patterns is intact in PD, which suggests that a fully-functional dopaminergic system is not essential for such imitation.

A recent multicenter, randomized controlled trial in 282 older adults, including 130 with PD [21], tested the hypothesis that an intervention combining treadmill training with a non-immersive VR component would lead to fewer falls than treadmill training alone. The results showed that the incident rate of falls was significantly lower in the treadmill training plus VR group than it had been before training, whereas the incident rate did not decrease significantly in the treadmill training alone group.

This study [21] further suggests that a rehabilitation approach targeting both cognitive and motor aspects of gait (and balance) induces a significantly beneficial outcome. It should be considered that VR systems have become much more readily available, more manageable and less expensive since commercial video gaming systems were introduced as rehabilitation tools able to provide exercises through gaming, an approach also referred to as exergaming [5].

6 Conclusions

The combined cognitive/motor approach in PD has a solid pathophysiological background, being based on re-routing of the movement through a non-automatic pathway (and therefore its removal from the sphere of automatic basal ganglia processing). Cross-sectional observations have indeed linked cognitive function (attention, working memory, executive functions) with gait disorders, postural instability and falls.

Robust evidence suggests that integrated motor and cognitive intervention is useful for enhancing gait, reducing fall risk, and improving dexterity. The optimal rehabilitation approach should target cognitive, behavioral and motor function through task-specific training and promotion of enhanced plasticity.

References

1. Abbruzzese G, Avanzino L, Marchese R, Pelosin E. Action observation and motor imagery: innovative cognitive tools in the rehabilitation of Parkinson's disease. Parkinson's Dis. 2015; 124214.
2. Abbruzzese G, Marchese R, Avanzino L, Pelosin E. Rehabilitation for Parkinson's disease: current outlook and future challenges. Parkinsonism Relat Disord. 2016;22(Suppl 1):S60–4.
3. Amboni M, Barone P, Hausdorff JM. Cognitive contributions to gait and falls: evidence and implications. Mov Disord. 2013;28:1520–33.
4. Avanzino L, Gueugneau N, Bisio A, Ruggeri P, Papaxanthis C, Bove M. Motor cortical plasticity induced by motor learning through mental practice. Front Behav Neurosci. 2015;9:105.
5. Barry G, Galna B, Rochester L. The role of exergaming in Parkinson's disease rehabilitation: a systematic review of the evidence. J Neuroeng Rehabil. 2014;11:33.

6. Bloem BR, Hausdorff JM, Visser JE, Giladi N. Falls and freezing of gait in Parkinson's disease: a review of two interconnected, episodic phenomena. Mov Disord. 2004;19:871–84.
7. Bohnen NI, Frey KA, Studenski S, Kotagal V, Koeppe RA, Scott PJ, Albin RL, Müller ML. Gait speed in Parkinson disease correlates with cholinergic degeneration. Neurol. 2013;81:1611–6.
8. Buccino G. Action observation treatment: a novel tool in neurorehabilitation. Philos Trans R Soc Lond B Biol Sci. 2014;369:20130185.
9. David FJ, Robichaud JA, Leurgans SE, Poon C, Kohrt WM, Goldman JG, Comella CL, Vaillancourt DE, Corcos DM. Exercise improves cognition in Parkinson's disease: the PRET-PD randomized, clinical trial. Mov Disord. 2015;30:1657–63.
10. dos Santos Mendes FA, Pompeu JE, Lobo AM, da Silva KG, de Paula Oliveira T, Zomignani AP, Pimentel Piemonte ME. Motor learning, retention and transfer after virtual-reality-based training in Parkinson's disease—effect of motor and cognitive demands of games: a longitudinal, controlled clinical study. Physiotherapy. 2012;98:217–23.
11. Fabbri-Destro M, Rizzolatti G. Mirror neurons and mirror systems in monkeys and humans. Physiology. 2008;23:171–9.
12. Fernandes Â, Rocha N, Santos R, Tavares JM. Effects of dual-task training on balance and executive functions in Parkinson's disease: a pilot study. Somatosens Mot Res. 2015;32:122–7.
13. Frenkel-Toledo S, Giladi N, Peretz C, Herman T, Gruendlinger L, Hausdorff JM. Treadmill walking as an external pacemaker to improve gait rhythm and stability in Parkinson's disease. Mov Disord. 2005;20:1109–14.
14. Giladi N, Horak FB, Hausdorff JM. Classification of gait disturbances: distinguishing between continuous and episodic changes. Mov Disord. 2013;28:1469–73.
15. Hely MA, Reid WG, Adena MA, Halliday GM, Morris JG. The Sydney multicenter study of Parkinson's disease: the inevitability of dementia at 20 years. Mov Disord. 2008;23:837–44.
16. Laver K, George S, Thomas S, Deutsch JE, Crotty M. Cochrane review: virtual reality for stroke rehabilitation. Eur J Phys Rehabil Med. 2012;48:523–30.
17. Lim I, van Wegen E, de Goede C, Deutekom M, Nieuwboer A, Willems A, Jones D, Rochester L, Kwakkel G. Effects of external rhythmical cueing on gait in patients with Parkinson's disease: a systematic review. Clin Rehabil. 2005;19:695–713.
18. Marchese R, Bove M, Abbruzzese G. Effect of cognitive and motor tasks on postural stability in Parkinson's disease: a posturographic study. Mov Disord. 2003;18:652–8.
19. Marchese R, Diverio M, Zucchi F, Lentino C, Abbruzzese G. The role of sensory cues in the rehabilitation of parkinsonian patients: a comparison of two physical therapy protocols. Mov Disord. 2000;15:879–83.
20. Mirelman A, Maidan I, Deutsch JE. Virtual reality and motor imagery: promising tools for assessment and therapy in Parkinson's disease. Mov Disord. 2013;28:1597–608.
21. Mirelman A, Rochester L, Maidan I, Del Din S, Alcock L, Nieuwhof F, Rikkert MO, Bloem BR, Pelosin E, Avanzino L, Abbruzzese G, Dockx K, Bekkers E, Giladi N, Nieuwboer A, Hausdorff JM. Addition of a non-immersive virtual reality component to treadmill training to reduce fall risk in older adults (V-TIME): a randomised controlled trial. Lancet. 2016;388:1170–82.
22. Mulder T. Motor imagery and action observation: cognitive tools for rehabilitation. J Neural Transm. 2007;114:1265–78.
23. Müller ML, Frey KA, Petrou M, Kotagal V, Koeppe RA, Albin RL, Bohnen NI. β-amyloid and postural instability and gait difficulty in Parkinson's disease at risk for dementia. Mov Disord. 2013;28:296–301.
24. Nieuwboer A, Kwakkel G, Rochester L, Jones D, van Wegen E, Willems AM, Chavret F, Hetherington V, Baker K, Lim I. Cueing training in the home improves gait-related mobility in Parkinson's disease: the RESCUE trial. J Neurol Neurosurg Psychiatry. 2007;78:134–40.
25. Nutt JG, Bloem BR, Giladi N, Hallett M, Horak FB, Nieuwboer A. Freezing of gait: moving forward on a mysterious clinical phenomenon. Lancet Neurol. 2000;10:734–44.

26. Pelosin E, Avanzino L, Bove M, Stramesi P, Nieuwboer A, Abbruzzese G. Action observation improves freezing of gait in patients with Parkinson's disease. Neurorehabil Neural Repair. 2010;24:746–52.
27. Pelosin E, Bove M, Ruggeri P, Avanzino L, Abbruzzese G. Reduction of bradykinesia of finger movements by a single session of action observation in Parkinson disease. Neurorehabil Neural Repair. 2013;27:552–60.
28. Pelosin E, Ogliastro C, Lagravinese G, Bonassi G, Mirelman A, Hausdorff JM, Abbruzzese G, Avanzino L. Attentional control of gait and falls: is cholinergic dysfunction a common substrate in the elderly and Parkinson's disease? Front Aging Neurosci. 2016;8:104.
29. Petzinger GM, Fisher BE, McEwen S, Beeler JA, Walsh JP, Jakowec MW. Exercise-enhanced neuroplasticity targeting motor and cognitive circuitry in Parkinson's disease. Lancet Neurol. 2013;12:716–26.
30. Pickering RM, Grimbergen YA, Rigney U, Ashburn A, Mazibrada G, Wood B, Gray P, Kerr G, Bloem BR. A meta-analysis of six prospective studies of falling in Parkinson's disease. Mov Disord. 2007;22:1892–900.
31. Plotnik M, Giladi N, Dagan Y, Hausdorff JM. Postural instability and fall risk in Parkinson's disease: impaired dual tasking, pacing, and bilateral coordination of gait during the "ON" medication state. Exp Brain Res. 2011;210:529–38.
32. Redgrave P, Rodriguez M, Smith Y, Rodriguez-Oroz MC, Lehericy S, Bergman H, Agid Y, DeLong MR, Obeso JA. Goal-directed and habitual control in the basal ganglia: implications for Parkinson's disease. Nat Rev Neurosci. 2010;11:760–72.
33. Robles-García V, Arias P, Sanmartín G, Espinosa N, Flores J, Grieve KL, Cudeiro J. Motor facilitation during real-time movement imitation in Parkinson's disease: a virtual reality study. Parkinsonism Relat Disord. 2013;19:1123–9.
34. Rochester L, Rafferty D, Dotchin C, Msuya O, Minde V, Walker RW. The effect of cueing therapy on single and dual-task gait in a drug naïve population of people with Parkinson's disease in northern Tanzania. Mov Disord. 2010;25:906–11.
35. Rochester L, Yarnall AJ, Baker MR, David RV, Lord S, Galna B, Burn DJ. Cholinergic dysfunction contributes to gait disturbance in early Parkinson's disease. Brain. 2012;135:2779–88.
36. Rubinstein TC, Giladi N, Hausdorff JM. The power of cueing to circumvent dopamine deficits: a review of physical therapy treatment of gait disturbances in Parkinson's disease. Mov Disord. 2002;17:1148–60.
37. Schoneburg B, Mancini M, Horak F, Nutt JG. Framework for understanding balance dysfunction in Parkinson's disease. Mov Disord. 2013;28:1474–82.
38. Springer S, Giladi N, Peretz C, Yogev G, Simon ES, Hausdorff JM. Dual-tasking effects on gait variability: the role of aging, falls, and executive function. Mov Disord. 2006;21:950–7.
39. Strouwen C, Molenaar EA, Münks L, Keus SH, Bloem BR, Rochester L, Nieuwboer A. Dual tasking in Parkinson's disease: should we train hazardous behavior? Expert Rev Neurother. 2015;15:1031–9.
40. Thenganatt MA, Jankovic J. Parkinson disease subtypes. JAMA Neurol. 2014;71:499–504.
41. Tomlinson CL, Patel S, Meek C, Herd CP, Clarke CE, Stowe R, Shah L, Sackley CM, Deane KH, Wheatley K, Ives N. Physiotherapy versus placebo or no intervention in Parkinson's disease. Cochrane Database Syst Rev. 2013;9: CD002817.
42. van der Kolk NM, King LA. Effects of exercise on mobility in people with Parkinson's disease. Mov Disord. 2013;28:1587–96.
43. Verghese J, Wang C, Lipton RB, Holtzer R. Motoric cognitive risk syndrome and the risk of dementia. J Gerontol Ser A Biomed Sci Med Sci. 2013;68:412–8.
44. Yogev-Seligmann G, Giladi N, Brozgol M, Hausdorff JM. A training program to improve gait while dual tasking in patients with Parkinson's disease: a pilot study. Arch Phys Med Rehabil. 2012;93:176–81.

The Treatment of Axial and Foot Dystonia

Micol Avenali, Roberto De Icco and Cristina Tassorelli

1 Introduction

Dystonia is a movement disorder that consists of sustained or intermittent muscle contractions leading to abnormal movements or sustained postures. The spectrum of dystonia is heterogeneous, as a result of the involvement of different body regions, the range of different patterns of body distribution, and the different etiologies (environmental factors, hereditary or sporadic neuronal dysfunction, neurodegenerative disease). The age at onset, body distribution, temporal pattern, and associated clinical manifestations are the main features that differentiate the various types of dystonia.

In the category of primary dystonia, cervical dystonia is the most common of the adult-onset focal axial forms. Symptoms often include pain and functional disability, and they have a devastating impact on affected individuals' daily lives.

Foot and trunk dystonia are atypical forms and they are considerably less frequent. They can be isolated or part of the phenotypical features of neurodegenerative disorders, such as Parkinson's disease (PD), atypical parkinsonism and Alzheimer's disease. The phenotype of adult-onset foot dystonia includes foot torsion usually accompanied by flexion of the forefoot and toes. Trunk dystonia, also known as Pisa syndrome, is a state of dystonic muscle contraction with a marked truncal deviation to one side; it is one of the earliest postural disorders to appear in PD patients.

M. Avenali (✉) · R. De Icco · C. Tassorelli
Neurological Rehabilitation Unit, C. Mondino National Neurological Institute,
Pavia, Italy
e-mail: avenali.micol87@gmail.com

M. Avenali · R. De Icco · C. Tassorelli
Department of Brain and Behavioral Sciences, University of Pavia, 27100 Pavia, Italy

G. Sandrini et al. (eds.), *Advanced Technologies for the Rehabilitation of Gait and Balance Disorders*, Biosystems & Biorobotics 19,
https://doi.org/10.1007/978-3-319-72736-3_11

Different mechanisms are involved in the pathogenesis of these disorders, which is yet to be completely clarified. Treatment continues to be symptomatic and the available therapies include oral medication, botulinum toxin, surgery and physical therapy. In the last few years, there has been a growing interest in the neuromodulation technique, and this applies to the field of dystonia rehabilitation, too, although literature on this issue is scant.

This chapter reviews the pathogenesis of axial and foot dystonia and the latest evidence on the treatment these conditions.

2 The Definition of Dystonia

Dystonia is a movement disorder characterized by sustained or intermittent muscle contractions causing abnormal, often repetitive, movements, postures, or both. Dystonic movements are typically patterned, usually twisting in character, and may be tremulous [1]. Dystonia is often initiated or worsened by voluntary action and associated with excessive muscle activation [2–4]. Over the years, different systems and schemes have been used for the classification of dystonia, under the influence of an increasing body of evidence. These were developed considering age at onset, body distribution, and etiology as the main differentiating factors.

In 2013, a new classification of dystonia was proposed [1], which encompasses two axes: 'clinical characteristics' and 'etiology'. The clinical characteristics are age at onset, body distribution, temporal pattern, and any associated clinical manifestations. The age at onset ranges from pediatric to adult age: infancy (birth to 2 years); childhood (3–12 years); adolescence (13–20 years); early adulthood (21–40 years), and late adulthood (40 years and older). In terms of body distribution, dystonia is described as focal (only one body region is affected), segmental (two or more contiguous body regions are affected), multifocal (two or more noncontiguous body regions are involved), generalized (the trunk and at least two other sites are involved), and hemidystonia (several body regions are involved, restricted to one side of the body). Indeed, the site and extension of the body region(s) affected are valuable considerations, which can help to guide treatment decisions. Dystonia classification also takes into account temporal definitions referring to: the modality of onset (acute or insidious), short-term variations in symptoms (diurnal, intermittent, or action induced), and long-term variations in overall severity (static or progressive). With regard to the presence of any associated clinical manifestations, dystonia is defined as "isolated" when it is the only motor feature and "combined" when it is associated with other movement disorders, such as myoclonus, parkinsonism, etc.

Regarding the etiology, the nosographic framing takes into account the existence of pathological changes or structural damage and acquired or hereditary causes. The causes of dystonia range from environmental factors to hereditary or sporadic neuronal dysfunction, neurodegenerative diseases, and pathogenic mutations in genes causing monogenic dystonia. If there is no definite etiology, dystonia can be classified as idiopathic familial or idiopathic sporadic.

3 Pathophysiology

The discovery of the first two gene mutations causing primary generalized dystonia (DYT1-TOR1A and DYT6-THAP1) prompted investigation of the molecular biology of the mutant gene products, and has facilitated studies on the pathogenesis and pathophysiology of primary dystonia. Significant progress has been made in recent years in understanding of the genetics of dystonia, and this has led to the identification of new loci and genes. New mutations have been found using whole-exome sequencing techniques, providing greater insights into the pathogenesis of the most common forms of focal dystonia [2].

Hereditary dystonia is clinically and genetically heterogeneous. The known genetic forms cover all the monogenic inheritance patterns (autosomal recessive, autosomal dominant and X-linked). In accordance with the new 2013 classification [2, 5], the different forms of hereditary dystonia are defined by their clinical features and etiology.

Dystonia was initially thought to be due to changes in somatotopically distinct regions of the internal segment of the globus pallidus. However, increasing evidence subsequently suggested a more system-wide disruption of the basal ganglia-thalamic circuitry, resulting in altered firing patterns, synchronized oscillations and broader receptive fields. Some authors suggested that changes in the cerebello-thalamo-cortical pathway may also play a role; circuit disorders underlying the development of dystonia may be related to deficiencies in cerebello-thalamo-cortical fibers. However, precisely how these abnormalities lead to the development of dystonia remains unclear [6, 7].

4 Cervical Dystonia

Cervical dystonia (CD) is the most common form of adult-onset focal dystonia [8] with a prevalence of 20-4100 cases/million and an incidence of 8–12 cases/million person-years [8]. CD is a major health problem with a devastating impact on affected individuals' daily lives [8].

The main features of CD are uncontrolled contractions of neck muscles resulting in postural deviations of the head and cervical spine. These muscle contractions can be intermittent or sustained. The main symptoms are neck pain, shoulder pain and neck rigidity [9].

4.1 Treatment

Despite the growing understanding of the disease process, treatment for dystonia remains symptomatic. The available therapies include oral medication, botulinum toxin (BoNT) and surgical procedures. For many years. symptomatic drugs of different types have been used for treating dystonia, but over the past 15–20 years, BoNT has emerged as the primary therapy [10]. As documented in randomized controlled trials, BoNT is the only treatment effective in relieving motor and non-motor symptoms of cervical dystonia in adults. Injected into dystonic muscles, it leads to reversible denervation of the neuromuscular junction by preventing the release of acetylcholine [11]. Injections should be performed under electromyography (EMG) guidance to improve precision, selecting only the muscles involved. This EMG guidance is able to ensure that the dose can be kept to the minimum and used with the longest possible dosing intervals. According to several studies that have confirmed the long-term safety and efficacy of BoNT, its benefit lasts between 12 and 16 weeks, on average, after treatment.

BoNT is available in two different types: A and B. Both have been found to be beneficial on CD severity, dystonia-related disability and pain in several double-blind, placebo-controlled trials [10]. The benefit of the treatment was indeed superior to placebo for Botox, Dysport and Myobloc, but not for Prosigne, the Chinese BoNT serotype A. In a randomized, double-blind, placebo-controlled trial, Truong et al. [12] observed a long-term effect of BoNT/A injection (Dysport, 500 units) versus placebo in 80 patients with CD. The patients were followed from baseline to 20 weeks post-injection. The authors found that Dysport was significantly more effective than the placebo at weeks 4, 9 and 12, as demonstrated by the improvements in Toronto Western Spasmodic Torticollis Rating Scale (TWSTRS) scores. Two other studies examining safety following repeated injections showed a statistically significant beneficial effect in patients who received repeated injections for up to 10 years [13, 14]. Adverse events with BoNT treatment are usually transient and mild. The main side effects, namely neck weakness, dysphagia, dry mouth, sore throat and voice changes, are seen with higher doses, and they are dose limiting. BoNT/B is used when patients become resistant to BoNT/A. Multiple studies [12, 15, 16] have shown the efficacy of BoNT/A or BoNT/B, as measured by patient self-assessment rating scales. A meta-analysis of three multi-center double-blind placebo-controlled trials showed a positive effect, reflected in a 20% improvement in the TWSTRS total score at 4 weeks after injection [17, 18]. These studies showed that BoNT/A and BoNT/B injections were safe and effective in single doses. Adverse events with BoNT/A and BoNT/B were identical, although they seemed to be more frequent with BoNT/B [18].

In the literature, articles on physical therapy interventions for the treatment of adult CD are lacking and there are no randomized controlled trials. Physiotherapy treatment for CD usually consists of EMG biofeedback training, muscle relaxation techniques, exercises to improve posture, massage, mobilization techniques, manipulation of the cervical spine, vibration, vestibular stimulation and cognitive behavioral therapy [19]. The efficacy of EMG biofeedback treatment was evaluated in five clinical trials, but only two of these were based on a sound methodology [20, 21]. EMG biofeedback training, when used as an add-on to muscle relaxation exercises, seemed effective in reducing contraction of the sternocleidomastoid muscle, and improving cervical range of motion and head alignment. In a trial conducted in a small group of patients with CD, EMG biofeedback alone seemed to reduce pain intensity, improve head-trunk alignment, and increase functional performances in activities of daily living [21]. In this study, twelve CD patients were randomly assigned to EMG biofeedback or relaxation training and graded neck exercises. The main outcome measures included physiological variables (EMG from the two sternocleidomastoid muscles, skin conductance level), behavioral parameters (angle of head deviation, range of movement of the head), self-report evaluations (depression, functional disability, perception of body schema), reports from therapists and "significant others", and independent observer video assessments. Neck muscle activity was reduced at the end of the treatment period in both groups, but the reduction was more marked in the EMG biofeedback group.

Three good quality trials have evaluated the effect of physiotherapy in combination with BoNT/A [22–24]. Tassorelli et al. [22] conducted a randomized controlled trial in 40 patients with CD to assess the efficacy of a two-week physiotherapy program combined with BoNT/A treatment and EMG biofeedback. The results showed that the addition of BONT/A treatment to a physical therapy program prolonged the duration of the therapeutic effects. In particular, there was a reduction in CD severity, as measured by the TWSTRS and the Tsui Scale (a four-item scale that evaluates amplitude and duration of sustained involuntary neck movements, shoulder elevation and head tremor in CD patients). Furthermore, the authors reported a decrease in pain symptoms and an increase in muscle functioning in the group of patients receiving BoNT/A in association with physiotherapy. It is worth noting that in the patients who had previously received the combined treatment (BoNT/A + physical therapy), a lower dose of BoNT/A was sufficient in subsequent treatments. The efficacy of BoNT/A was also confirmed by two additional studies [23, 24] which showed that associating BoNT/A with physiotherapy results in a valuable improvements in terms of neck and head posture, pain, and quality of life (as related to activities of daily life).

The sensorimotor and motor system abnormalities occurring in dystonia may be considered consequences of increased maladaptive plasticity. The sensorimotor system in these patients is abnormally sensitive to external stimuli, which may generate inappropriate and non-specific sensorimotor associations that ultimately interfere with context-specific motor actions [25]. Tools that are able to intercept and modulate the abnormal activity patterns in CD may prove effective. This is the case of non-invasive neurostimulation, delivered either as transcranial magnetic stimulation (TMS) or transcranial direct current stimulation (tDCS). Both TMS and tDCS may qualify as valid adjunctive treatments for dystonia as they offer the possibility of selectively modulating symptoms and their underlying neuropathophysiology on an individual basis. Multiple mechanisms likely contribute to the clinical effects of repetitive TMS (rTMS) and tDCS in dystonia, including normalization of cortical excitability, rebalancing of distributed neural network activity, and induction of dopamine release [26].

Studies of rTMS or tDCS in dystonia have provided abundant data on the physiology of the disorder, but quite limited evidence on the clinical effects of these techniques. Indeed, in this setting, only very few preliminary studies have been conducted on focal dystonia and they are poorly controlled. Isolated observations have suggested that abnormal excitability of network patterns may be induced by low-frequency rTMS over the primary motor cortex (M1) or dorsal premotor cortex [11, 18]. In 2007, Allam et al. [27] evaluated the effect of rTMS on the symptoms of a patient with CD who underwent five sessions of stimulation with 1200 TMS pulses delivered at a low frequency (1 Hz) over the dorsal premotor cortex. The results showed a 50% reduction in the score of the neck items on the Burke, Fahn & Marsden torsion dystonia scale. With regard to tDCS, an interesting case-control study [28] showed that both tDCS stimulation and transcranial alternating current stimulation (tACS) were capable of modulating the excitability of the cerebral cortex in a patient with idiopathic CD. In tDCS, the anode (electrode) pole showed an excitatory effect, while the cathode pole was associated with inhibitory effects on the underlying cortex. In the case of tACS, both poles showed equivalent effects on the cortex, depending on the pacing rate. The results demonstrated that tACS delivered at 15 Hz had an immediate effect in reducing dystonic symptoms, leading to a 54% reduction in the TWSTRS total score and a 75% reduction in the pain subscale. These beneficial effects persisted for at least 30 days [28]. In a recent case report, Bradnam et al. [29] evaluated the possible effect of tDCS, applied to the cerebellum and to the M1, used in combination with BoNT injections in dystonic muscles. Anodal tDCS was delivered to three different locations: the right cerebellum (5 sessions), left cerebellum (5 sessions), and combined cerebellar-M1 area (anodal DCS to the right M1, followed by anodal DCS to the left cerebellum, 10 sessions). The stimulation paradigm consisted of two 15 min blocks, separated by 5 min. BoNT/A injections followed by tDCS of the cerebellum and M1 applied over a 12 week period improved dystonia symptoms and quality of life, as shown by a 39% reduction in the TWSTRS total score, a 55% reduction in the pain sub-scale of the TWSTRS, and a significant improvement on the Cervical Dystonia Impact Profile and the Craniocervical Dystonia Questionnaire [29]. These studies provide the first evidence of a significant and long-lasting therapeutic effect of non-invasive transcranial electrical stimulation in patients with CD, and support its use as a promising new treatment option. However, more randomized controlled studies are needed in order to validate these neuromodulation methods.

5 Dystonic Foot

Adult-onset dystonia is usually confined to the upper body, especially the cranio-cervical region, and it rarely arises in the lower extremities. Indeed, primary focal foot dystonia in adults has rarely been reported. The phenotype of adult-onset lower extremity dystonia includes foot torsion, with inversion of the foot at the ankle joint, usually accompanied by flexion of the forefoot and toes. The onset of focal foot dystonia is usually subacute or insidious. Its main causes are parkinsonism, stiff-limb syndrome, trauma and stroke; it may also be of psychogenic origin [30, 31].

Pacchetti et al. [32], in 1995, described "off" painful dystonia, a type of abnormal involuntary movement usually involving the feet. This condition is induced by chronic use of levodopa, and mainly observed in the advanced stages of PD. Dopaminergic drugs, like bromocriptine, pergolide and, especially, apomorphine, may improve foot dystonia. Anticholinergics baclofen and lithium have also been used with some benefit. In their study, Pacchetti et al. used injections of BoNT/A and observed marked improvements in terms of pain and posture. More rarely, PD patients may experience dystonia during "on" periods, when dystonic posture of the foot alternates with dyskinesia. BoNT/A may also provide beneficial effects in these cases of "on dystonia" [32].

In 2005, Singer et al. described the clinical phenotype and treatment outcomes in patients with primary, adult-onset focal foot dystonia. They conducted a retrospective study of four patients diagnosed over a period of six years and followed up for five years. Primary focal foot dystonia appeared in middle age or late in life and remained restricted to the foot (indicative of a non-degenerative mechanism). Oral anti-dystonic medications were generally unsatisfactory for symptomatic relief. Similarly to what has been observed with other types of limb dystonia, BoNT injections were of substantial benefit to the patients [30].

McKeon et al. [31] characterized the clinical spectrum associated with the phenotype of lower limb dystonia. They identified 36 patients, 31 females and five males, presenting with monomelic lower limb dystonia including foot torsion [31]. Nineteen subjects were diagnosed with idiopathic dystonia and five with parkinsonisms. Dystonic foot torsion occurred with ambulation or started as task-specific and persisted during rest. In all the patients, gait was worsened to some degree by the presence of dystonia, with loss of independent ambulation. Levodopa therapy was recommended but was effective in only half of the patients. Only one in four patients obtained mild temporary benefit from the anticholinergic drug trihexyphenidyl. Three out of seven patients visibly benefited from BoNT injections into affected muscles, while pallidal deep brain simulation surgery improved deformity, pain and gait. After the failure of multiple medications and BoNT injections, orthopedic surgical interventions should be considered [31].

In 2012, Ramdhani et al. described nine patients with task-specific idiopathic focal lower extremity dystonia. The patients' main features were late age at onset, female predominance, and specific foot movement patterns: plantar flexion, inversion and involvement of the toes. Inversion of the foot was the most prevalent pattern. Specific triggers for dystonic posture were various ambulatory tasks like walking, walking down steps and running. From the pathophysiological perspective, this type of dystonia can be considered to result from both genetic and environmental factors. These patients are frequently misdiagnosed with orthopedic problems or psychogenic behavior. In these patients, too, BoNT injections are the most effective treatment [33].

6 Axial Dystonia: Pisa Syndrome

Pathological involvement of the axial muscles is often associated with PD and can lead to postural disorders and balance impairments. The pathogenesis of these disorders is not yet completely clarified, but different mechanisms are thought to be involved, such as a deficit of postural reflexes, hypertonia and rigidity, and pure dystonia. The most prevalent of the "atypical" dystonias in PD are camptocormia and lateral trunk flexion, also known as pleurothotonus or Pisa syndrome [34–36].

Pleurothotonus was first described in 1972 by Ekobm et al., who observed three patients under treatment with neuroleptics [37]. In these cases, the postural disorder regressed after suspension of the treatment. Since this original description of an association with the use of neuroleptics, several other reports have shown that Pisa syndrome may be present in PD in association with the use of antidepressants, cholinesterase inhibitors, lithium, benzodiazepines, tiapride, pergolide and pramipexole, or without any association with any specific drug [38–41].

The name Pisa syndrome derives from the characteristic posture of affected patients, which brings to mind the famous leaning Tower of Pisa (Italy). The real prevalence of the syndrome is not known, but Yassa et al. described a prevalence of 8.3% (9.3% in women and 6.4% in men) in a psychogeriatric population, while Tinazzi et al. (2015) reported a prevalence of 8.8% in a cohort of PD patients [42, 43].

Pisa syndrome is clinically characterized by:

- lateral flexion of the trunk creating a non-zero angle between the sacrum and spinous process of the 7th cervical vertebra;
- ipsilateral axial rotation of the trunk around the sagittal axis that, in the standing position, results in a higher and more anterior position of the shoulder contralateral to the side of trunk deviation;
- worsening of the postural disorder during standing, sitting and gait;
- improvement of the postural disorder in the supine position;
- limited awareness of the postural disorder on the part of the patients themselves.

The observation of dynamic variation of these patients' posture, i.e. the fact that it reverts in the supine position, clearly differentiates Pisa syndrome from scoliosis.

In the literature, different degrees of lateral trunk deviation are used for diagnosis (10° by Doherty et al., 15° by Bonanni et al.). These same authors have also proposed subdividing Pisa syndrome into mild and severe forms, on the basis of the angle amplitude: < or > 20°, respectively [44, 45]. In our experience, from the diagnostic and rehabilitation perspective, it seems more practical to consider the clinical features of the lateral trunk deviation rather than the absolute angle of deviation. A spine X-ray and quantification of the deviation angle are mandatory only when it is difficult to distinguish between Pisa syndrome and scoliosis on the basis of clinical features alone. In addition to the postural disorder, PD patients with Pisa syndrome appear to be older than PD patients without the syndrome; they also seem to show a longer and more severe disease course and a lower quality of life.

Moreover, they have a higher risk of falls, arthrosis and osteoporosis, which may expose them to orthopedic complications. Another common complaint of PD patients with Pisa syndrome is pain, in particular low back pain, which is reported by 75% of subjects [43, 46].

The relatively low prevalence of Pisa syndrome and the different possible etiologies described make its underlying pathogenesis difficult to study; central and peripheral mechanisms have both been observed [47].

6.1 Central Mechanisms

With regard to central determinants of Pisa syndrome, asymmetry in basal ganglia outflow seems to play a crucial role. Animal studies showed that an asymmetric dopaminergic signal leads to a postural disorder, with inclination of the trunk towards the side of the most impaired striatum (usually the side less affected by the akinetic symptoms of parkinsonism). Clinical observation of PD patients with Pisa syndrome confirmed this hypothesis. Tassorelli et al. described how Pisa syndrome was associated with a higher asymmetry of motor symptoms in PD, with a deviation of the trunk towards the less affected side [48].

Other data confirming these mechanisms come from reports of Pisa syndrome starting after unilateral neurosurgery involving the basal ganglia. In these cases, the side of trunk deviation was always contralateral to the side of iatrogenic damage [49–52].

Another central mechanism potentially underlying Pisa syndrome is an imbalance in the neurotransmitters involved in trunk control. Patients with the syndrome present altered levels of noradrenaline, serotonin and, above all, high levels of acetylcholine associated with a dopamine deficit. This hypothesis is corroborated by the association of Pisa syndrome with neurodegenerative disorders (Alzheimer's disease and, in particular, those characterized by dopamine deficiency such as PD and multiple system atrophy) [53, 54], and with the intake D2 receptor blockers.

Furthermore, some reports suggest close temporal relations between the clinical onset of symptoms after the assumption of typical neuroleptics and their resolution after drug discontinuation. Finally, in a few cases, a partial improvement of Pisa syndrome has been achieved with L-dopa or dopamine agonists [55].

Vitale et al. [56] found a vestibular deficit, ipsilateral to the leaning side, in all parkinsonian patients with Pisa syndrome and in four out of eleven patients without the syndrome. Interestingly, two of the latter subsequently developed Pisa syndrome, suggesting that a vestibular deficit precedes its onset and represents a subclinical marker of abnormal sensorimotor integration [56]. Another possible associated feature of PD that could explain some of the clinical characteristics of Pisa syndrome is abnormal spatial cognition, and in particular abnormal perception of postural verticality. As a consequence, patients with Pisa syndrome perceive themselves as aligned with the vertical axis when they are laterally flexed, and misaligned when passively corrected [57–59].

6.2 Peripheral Mechanisms

According to the peripheral hypothesis, the musculoskeletal system plays a primary role in the genesis of Pisa syndrome. Some authors have reported abnormal variations in fiber size, increases in internal nuclei, and increases in connective tissue. Myofibrillar disarray and similarities to protein surplus myopathies were observed in muscle biopsies of paraspinal muscles and deep neck extensor muscles of subjects with camptocormia [60]. Furthermore, necrotizing myopathy, inflammatory myopathy, and myopathy with mitochondrial abnormalities were identified in a subset of PD subjects with axial postural abnormalities, such as dropped head or bent spine [61].

Indirect evaluation of muscles involved in trunk control by means of EMG has generally failed to show neurophysiological signs of primary muscle disease; similarly, EMG recording of paraspinal muscles has not revealed denervation patterns or myopathy [48, 60, 61]. Neuroimaging techniques, such as computer tomography and magnetic resonance imaging, have shown atrophy of the paraspinal muscles in patients with Pisa syndrome, not always related to the side of trunk deviation [45, 48, 60, 61]. Taken together, these data suggest a central rather than peripheral pathogenesis of Pisa syndrome in PD. In this framework, some of the peripheral abnormalities observed (namely muscle atrophy) may represent a consequence of the chronic postural disorder. Although the peripheral musculoskeletal system does not seem to play a primary role in the genesis of the disease, EMG evaluation of the trunk muscles is important in the clinical setting to discern between different subsets of trunk dystonia and to evaluate different therapeutic approaches. For Pisa syndrome, it is important to perform an extensive EMG evaluation in both static and dynamic conditions, at least during active lateral trunk bending towards and away from the side of deviation.

Several studies have tried to classify the pattern of muscle activation, giving conflicting results. Tassorelli et al. [48] described, in the upright position, persistent tonic activity of the abdominal oblique muscle and the paraspinal thoracic muscle (T6-T7) on the bending side, whereas EMG activity was markedly reduced in muscles on the opposite side. The fact that this asymmetric tonic activation disappeared in the recumbent position confirmed it as one of the clinical features of Pisa syndrome [48]. Di Matteo et al. [60] investigated the synergies of paravertebral muscles during dynamic conditions in ten PD patients by means EMG evaluation and reported a clear dystonic pattern only in a minority of subjects. More specifically, in three subjects in static standing condition they reported tonic activation of the longissimus thoracis muscle (between T12 and L1) ipsilateral to the leaning side, and this did not recede during contralateral active lateral trunk flexion, resulting in co-activation of the left and right paravertebral muscles (dystonic pattern). The other subjects showed tonic activation of the longissimus thoracis muscle contralateral to the leaning side during the static standing condition, without co-activation of paravertebral muscles during dynamic evaluation, which thus resulted in tonic "compensatory" activation, without a pure dystonic pattern [60].

In view of these results, in 2013, an attempt was made to classify different subtypes of Pisa syndrome through more extensive EMG evaluation (paraspinal lumbar muscles, paraspinal thoracic muscles, abdominal oblique muscles, iliopsoas and rectus femoris) [61]. In particular, the following were identified:

- Pattern I: hyperactivity of lumbar paraspinal muscles ipsilateral to the trunk leaning side
  - Subtype 1: associated with hyperactivity of thoracic paraspinal muscles ipsilateral to the trunk leaning side
  - Subtype 2: associated with hyperactivity of thoracic paraspinal muscles contralateral to the trunk leaning side
- Pattern II: hyperactivity of lumbar and thoracic paraspinal muscles contralateral to the trunk leaning side, with hyperactivity of non-paraspinal muscles ipsilateral to the trunk deviation (rectus femoris, iliopsoas, abdominal oblique) [61].

Considering the physiological role played by the abovementioned muscles in trunk control in healthy subjects, it appears that in PD, pleurothotonus is subtended by dystonic activation of lumbar paraspinal muscles (Pattern I) or non-paraspinal muscles (Pattern II), and may or may not be associated with compensatory activation of muscles contralateral to the leaning side (in particular the thoracic paraspinal muscles) to limit trunk excursion [61]. It is noteworthy that the pattern of EMG evaluation may change depending on the interval since the onset of Pisa syndrome. Indeed, the dystonic features seem to represent the main underlying mechanism at onset, but may recede in the chronic stabilized phase of the syndrome, when muscular atrophy prevails. Since Pisa syndrome may be associated with other postural disorders, it may be difficult to evaluate the true severity of the lateral trunk flexion. Thus, it is advisable to monitor patients with asymmetric tone of paraspinal muscles over time with photos, videos, goniometric measures and, where possible, with kinematic analysis of movements. Moreover, it is important to assess the articular excursion of the trunk and arms, segmental strength and respiratory mechanics. The main postural alterations in Pisa syndrome can be found in the frontal plane. Physiologically the body in the frontal plane shows the following features:

- head and spine are aligned on a vertical axis;
- the line crossing the acromions and the line crossing iliac crests are horizontal and parallel to each other;
- the arms are asymmetrically aligned with the body;
- the scapulae are aligned and projected between T3 and T7.

6.3 Treatment

There are no specifically targeted studies evaluating the efficacy of drug therapy in improving Pisa syndrome, and in clinical practice the syndrome only rarely responds to antiparkinsonian drugs. Therefore, physiotherapy is considered one of the fundamental approaches to PD and to postural disorders in general, not only for attenuating the motor symptoms, but also for preserving the individual's independence in activities of daily living [62]. The rehabilitation program for Pisa syndrome mainly consists of tasks executed in front of a postural grid mirror, exercises with the Bobath balloon, and core strengthening exercises in closed kinetic chain.

Bartolo et al. [63] evaluated the effects of an ad hoc rehabilitation program on lateral trunk flexion and mobility in 22 PD patients with mild to severe lateral trunk flexion, and 22 PD patients without trunk flexion. The program consisted of 90 min daily sessions (5 days a week) for four consecutive weeks, including cardiovascular warm-up activities (10 min), stretching exercises (15 min), strengthening exercises in a functional context (15 min), over-ground gait training (20 min), balance training (15 min), and relaxation exercises (15 min). With this approach, both the upright standing position and the trunk range of motion had significantly improved at the end of the rehabilitation. Unfortunately, its effectiveness was lost after six months [63].

Another option that can be included in the rehabilitation program is injection of BoNT/A in hyperactive muscles. In a cross-over study, Bonanni et al. [45], treated nine patients with Pisa syndrome by injecting BoNT/A or placebo into the lumbar paraspinal muscles (L2–L5 levels) ipsilateral to the trunk deviation. Patients in the active group experienced a reduction in lateral trunk flexion ranging from 50% and 85.7%; moreover, in seven patients, pain associated with dystonia was reduced [45].

In 2014, Tassorelli et al. [46] designed a study to assess the efficacy of a combined therapy with rehabilitation and BoNT/A in 26 PD patients. In this series BoNT/A was injected into all hyperactive muscles (multifidus, iliopsoas, rectus abdominis, thoracic and lumbar paraspinal). The authors found that adding BoNT/A to physical rehabilitation improved lateral trunk inclination at the end of the rehabilitation period more than physical rehabilitation alone. The improvement persisted for at least three months. As previously described, pain associated with Pisa syndrome improved after BoNT/A injections and rehabilitation in all patients [46].

Pending definitive recommendations, we feel, on the basis of the data from the literature combined with our long-standing expertise, that the most rational and effective approach to the management of Pisa syndrome in PD subjects consists of optimization of the antiparkinsonian drug regimen, rapidly followed, if this proves ineffective, by BoNT injection into the hyperactive muscles, under EMG guidance, in association with physical therapy.

References

1. Albanese A, et al. Phenomenology and classification of dystonia: a consensus update. Mov Disord. 2013;28:863–73.
2. Morgante F, Klein C. Dystonia. Continuum (Minneap Minn). 2013;19:1225–41.
3. Fahn S. The varied clinical expression of dystonia. Neurol Clin. 1984;2:541–54.
4. Klein C. Movement disorders: classifications. J Inherit Metab Dis. 2005;28:425–39.
5. Balint B, Bhatia KP. Dystonia: an update on phenomenology, classification, pathogenesis and treatment. Curr Opin Neurol. 2014;27:468–76.
6. Hendrix CM, Vitek J. Toward a network model of dystonia. Ann NY Sci. 2012;46–55.
7. Skogseid IM. Dystonia—new advances in classification, genetics, pathophysiology and treatment. Acta Neurol Scand. 2014;129(Suppl. 198):13–9.
8. Defazio G, Jankovic J, Giel JL, Papapetropoulos S. Descriptive epidemiology of cervical dystonia. Tremor Other Hyperkinet Mov (N Y). 2013;4:3.
9. Snaith A, Wade D. Dystonia. Clin Evid (Online). 2014;28:2014.
10. Jankovic J. Treatment of dystonia. Lancet Neurol. 2006;5:864–72.
11. Han Y, Stevens AL, Dashtipour K, Hauser RA, Mari Z. A mixed treatment comparison to compare the efficacy and safety of botulinum toxin treatments for cervical dystonia. J Neurol. 2016.
12. Truong D, Duane DD, Jankovic J, et al. Efficacy and safety of botulinum type A toxin (Dysport) in cervical dystonia: results of the first US randomized, double-blind, placebo-controlled study. Mov Disord. 2005;20:783–91.
13. Kessler KR, Skutta M, Benecke R. Longterm treatment of cervical dystonia with botulinum toxin A: efficacy, safety, and antibody frequency. German Dystonia Study Group. J Neurol. 1999;246:265–74.
14. Haussermann P, Marczoch S, Klinger C, et al. Long-term follow-up of cervical dystonia patients treated with botulinum toxin A. Mov Disord. 2004;19:303–8.
15. Lew MF, Brashear A, Factor S. The safety and efficacy of botulinum toxin type B in the treatment of patients with cervical dystonia: summary of three controlled clinical trials. Neurology. 2000;55(12suppl 5):S29–S35.
16. Factor SA, Molho ES, Evans S, Feustel PJ. Efficacy and safety of repeated doses of botulinum toxin type B in type A resistant and responsive cervical dystonia. Mov Disord. 2005;20:1152–60.
17. Costa J, Espirito-Santo C, Borges A, et al. Botulinum toxin type B for cervical dystonia. Cochrane Database Syst Rev. 2005;(1):CD004315.
18. Delnooz CC, van de Warrenburg BP. Current and future medical treatment in primary dystonia. Ther Adv Neurol Disord. 2012;5:221–40.
19. De Pauw J, Van der Velden K, Meirte J, Van Daele U, Truijen S, Cras P, Mercelis R, De Hertogh W. The effectiveness of physiotherapy for cervical dystonia: a systematic literature review. J Neurol. 2014;261:1857–65.
20. Jahanshahi M, Sartory G, Marsden CD. EMG biofeedback treatment of torticollis: a controlled outcome study. Biofeedback Self Regul. 1991;16:413–48.
21. Smania N, Corato E, Tinazzi M, et al. The effect of two different rehabilitation treatments in cervical dystonia: preliminary results in four patients. Funct Neurol. 2003;18:219–25.
22. Tassorelli C, Mancini F, Balloni L, et al. Botulinum toxin and neuromotor rehabilitation: an integrated approach to idiopathic cervical dystonia. Mov Disord. 2006;21:2240–3.
23. El-bahrawy MN, El-tamawy MS, Shalaby NM, Abdel-alim AM. Cervical dystonia: abnormal head posture and its relation to hand function. Egypt J Neurol Psychiatry Neurosurg. 2009;46:203–8.
24. Queiroz MAR, Chien HF, Sekeff-sallem FA, Barbosa ER. Physical therapy program for cervical dystonia: a study of 20 cases. Funct Neurol. 2012;27:187–92.
25. Quartarone A, Siebner HR, Rothwell JC. Task-specific hand dystonia: can too much plasticity be bad for you? Trends Neurosci. 2006;29:192–9.

26. Wagner T, Valero-Cabre A, Pascual-Leone A. Noninvasive human brain stimulation. Annu Rev Biomed Eng. 2007;9:527–65.
27. Allam N, Brasil-Neto JP, Brandão P, Weiler F, Barros Filho Jd, Tomaz C. Relief of primary cervical dystonia symptoms by low frequency transcranial magnetic stimulation of the premotor cortex: case report. Arq Neuropsiquiatr. 2007;65:697–9.
28. Angelakis E, Liouta E, Andreadis N, Leonardos A, Ktonas P, Stavrinou LC, Miranda PC, Mekonnen A, Sakas DE. Transcranial alternating current stimulation reduces symptoms in intractable idiopathic cervical dystonia: a case study. Neurosci Lett. 2013;533:39–43.
29. Bradnam LV, Frasca J, Kimberley TJ. Direct current stimulation of primary motor cortex and cerebellum and botulinum toxin A injections in a person with cervical dystonia. Brain Stimul. 2014;7:909–11.
30. Singer C, Papapetropoulos S. Adult-onset primary focal foot dystonia. Parkinsonism Relat. Disord. 2006;12:57–60.
31. McKeon A, Matsumoto JY, Bower JH, Ahlskog JE. The spectrum of disorders presenting as adult onset focal lower extremity dystonia. Parkinsonism Relat. Disord. 2008;14:613–9.
32. Pacchetti C, Albani G, Martignoni E, Godi L, Alfonsi E, Nappi G. "Off" painful dystonia in Parkinson's disease treated with botulinum toxin. Mov Disord. 1995;10:333–6.
33. Ramdhani RA, Frucht SJ. Adult-onset idiopathic focal lower extremity dystonia: a Rare task-specific dystonia. Tremor Other Hyperkinet Mov (NY). 2013;3; pii: tre-03–142-2990-1.
34. Tolosa E, Compta Y. Dystonia in parkinson's disease. J Neurol. (2006);253(Suppl 7): VII7-I3.
35. Djaldetti R, Mosberg-Galili R, Sroka H, Merims D, Melamed E. Camptocornia (bent spine) in patients with Parkinson's disease—characterization and possible pathogenesis of an unusal phenomenon. Mov Disord. 1999;3:443–7.
36. Holler I, Dirnberger G, Pirker W, et al. Camptocormia in idiopathic Parkinson's disease: 123I beta CIT SPECT and clinical characteristics. Eur Neurol. 2003;50:118–20.
37. Ekbom, Lindholm, Ljungberg. New dystonic syndrome associated with butyrophenone therapy. Z. Neurol. 1972;202:94–103.
38. Gambarin M, Antonini A, Moretto G, et al. Pisa syndrome without neuroleptic exposure in a patient with Parkinson's disease: case report. Mov Disord. 2006;21:270–3.
39. Suzuki T, Matsuzaka H. Drug induced pisa syndrome (pleurothotonus): epidemiology and management. CNS Drugs. 2002;16:165–74.
40. Cannas A, Solla P, Floris G, et al. Reversible pisa syndrome in parkinson's disease during treatment with pergolide: a case report. Clin Neuropharm. 2005;28(5):252.
41. Kwak YT, Han IW, Baik J, Koo MS. Relation between cholinesterase inhibitor and Pisa syndrome. Lancet. 2000;355:2222.
42. Yassa R, Nastase C, Cvejic J, Laberge G. The Pisa syndrome (or pleurothotonus): prevalence in a psychogeriatric population. Biol Psychiatry. 1991;29:942–5.
43. Tinazzi M, Fasano A, Geroin C, et al. Pisa syndrome in Parkinson Disease: an observational multicenter Italian study. Neurology. 2015;85:1–11.
44. Doherty KM, Davagnanam I, Molloy S, Silveira-Moriyama L, Lees AJ. Pisa syndrome in Parkinson's disease: a mobile or fixed deformity? J Neurol Neurosurg Psychiatry. 2013;84:1400–3.
45. Bonanni L, Thomas A, Varanese S, Scorrano V, Onofrj M. Botulinum toxin treatment of lateral axial dystonia in Parkinsonism. Mov Disord. 2007;22:2097–103.
46. Tassorelli C, De Icco R, Alfonsi E, Bartolo M, Serrao M, Avenali M, De Paoli I, Conte C, Pozzi NG, Bramanti P, Nappi G, Sandrini G. Botulinum toxin type A potentiates the effect of neuromotor rehabilitation of pisa syndrome in parkinson disease: a placebo controlled study. Parkinsonism Relat Disord. 2014;20:1140–4.
47. Castrioto A, Piscicelli C, Perennou D, Krack P, Debu B. The pathogenesis of Pisa syndrome in Parkinson's disease. Mov. Dis. 2014;29:1100–7.
48. Tassorelli C, Furnari A, Buscone S, et al. Pisa syndrome in Parkinson's disease: clinical, electromyographic, and radiological characterization. Mov Disord. 2012;27:227–35.

49. Van de Warrenburg BP, Bhatia KP, Quinn NP. Pisa syndrome after unilateral pallidotomy in Parkinson's disease: an unrecognised, delayed adverse event? J Neurol Neurosurg Psychiatry. 2007;78:329.
50. Mamo H, Dondey M, Cophignon J, Pialoux P, Fontelle P, Houdart R. Transitory latero-pulsion after subthalamic and thalamic coagulations in parkinsonism patients. Rev Neurologique. 1965;112:509–20.
51. Velasco F, Velasco M, Ogarrio C, Olvera A. Neglect induced by thalamotomy in humans: a quantitative appraisal of the sensory and motor deficits. Neurosurgery. 1986;19:744–51.
52. Su PC, Tseng HM, Liou HH. Postural asymmetries following unilateral subthalomotomy for advanced Parkinson's disease. Mov Disord. 2002;17:191–4.
53. Patel S, Tariot PN, Hamill RW. Pisa syndrome without neuroleptic exposure in a patient with dementia of the Alzheimer type. J Geriatr Psychiatry Neurol. 1991;4:48–51.
54. Colosimo C. Pisa syndrome in a patient with multiple system atrophy. Mov Disord. 1998;13:607–9.
55. Villarejo A, Camacho A, Garcia-Ramos R, Moreno T, Penas M, Juntas R, et al. Cholinergic—dopaminergic imbalance in pisa syndrome. Clin Neuropharmacol. 2003;26:119–21.
56. Vitale C, Marcelli V, Furia T, et al. Vestibular impairment and adaptive postural imbalance in parkinsonian patients with lateral trunk flexion. Mov Disord. 2011;26:1458–63.
57. Yokochi F. Lateral flexion in Parkinson's disease and Pisa syndrome. J Neurol 2006;253 (Suppl 7):VII17–20.
58. Proctor F, Riklan M, Cooper IS, Teuber HL. Judgment of visual and postural vertical by parkinsonian patients. Neurology. 1964;14:287–93.
59. Bisdorff AR, Bronstein AM, Gresty M, Anastasopoulos D. Subjective postural vertical in peripheral and central vestibular disorders and Parkinson's disease. In: Taguchi KIM, Mori S, editors. Vestibular and neural front: Excerpta Medica; 1994, pp. 615–18.
60. Di Matteo A, Fasano A, Squintani G, et al. Lateral trunk flexion in Parkinson's disease: EMG features disclose two different underlying pathophysiological mechanisms. J Neurol. 2011;258:740–5.
61. Tinazzi M, Juergenson I, Squintani G, et al. Pisa syndrome in Parkinson's disease: an electrophysiological and imaging study. J Neurol. 2013;260:2138–48.
62. Tomlinson CL, Herd CP, Clarke CE, Meek C, Patel S, Stowe R, Deane KH, Shah L, Sackley CM, Wheatley K, Ives N. Physiotherapy for parkinson's disease: a comparison of techniques. Cochrane Database Syst Rev. 2014;6:CD002815.
63. Bartolo M, Serrao M, Tassorelli C, Don R, Ranavolo A, Draicchio F, et al. Four-week trunk-specific rehabilitation treatment improves lateral trunk flexion in parkinson's disease. Mov Disord. 2010;25:325–31.

Rehabilitation Approach to Stroke

Giovanni Morone, Marco Iosa and Stefano Paolucci

1 Introduction

Walking is the main determinant of independence in activities of daily living [46]. Therefore, one of the most important aims of neurorehabilitation in subjects affected by stroke should be recovery of walking and postural control during static and dynamic activities [43]. This recovery is present only in 55% of patients on discharge from a rehabilitation hospital [43]. Furthermore, even in these patients, walking ability is often not completely recovered, as they may show problems in maintaining a functional speed and balance. On average, walking speed is reduced by approximately 50% in stroke patients compared with healthy subjects [22]. But the most critical problem is the risk of falls. Falls have been reported to occur in 40–70% of stroke patients within one year of the acute event [18, 33, 51], resulting in physical complications and psychological consequences. Moreover, falls may impose a tremendous economic burden on the health care system, calling into question the efficacy of the entire rehabilitation pathway [33].

Postural balance and stability during walking have both been studied extensively in subjects after stroke, as well as in other pathologies and also in healthy elderly subjects. A recent review identified 92 different quantitative measures of gait stability obtained using different devices [19]. The most important were those related to spatiotemporal gait parameters, lower limb joint kinematics and upper body kinematics [19]. Interestingly, "upright gait stability" may be assessed in different

G. Morone (✉) · M. Iosa · S. Paolucci
Clinical Laboratory of Experimental Neurorehabilitation, IRCCS Santa Lucia Foundation, via Ardeatina 306, 00179 Rome, Italy
e-mail: g.morone@hsantalucia.it

G. Sandrini et al. (eds.), *Advanced Technologies for the Rehabilitation of Gait and Balance Disorders*, Biosystems & Biorobotics 19,
https://doi.org/10.1007/978-3-319-72736-3_12

ways. The ability to minimize oscillations during walking, in a progressive way from the lower to the upper levels of the human body, can be evaluated by keeping the head moving in a straight line at quite a constant speed [6, 21, 22]. From this perspective, it is fundamental to consider gait stability from an integrated sensorimotor perspective. Stabilization of the head during gait is crucial to allow steadying of the optic flow, thereby, through more efficient processing of vestibular system signals [4, 50], improving exploration of the environment during motor activities [47].

A pathological event can result in an abrupt loss of stability, with more severe pathologies resulting in a greater loss of upright gait stability. In recent years, many studies have suggested the use of wearable devices for assessing upright gait stability; this is done by measuring upper body accelerations [23, 24]. In patients with stroke, upper body accelerations (normalized by speed) are higher than in healthy subjects in all body axes during walking [25–28, 36]. Notably, walking speed is reduced by approximately 50% in stroke patients versus young healthy adults, while raw accelerations are not. Furthermore, trunk control is a prognostic factor for gait recovery [9, 34], and patients have been reported to show even more marked trunk asymmetries than step length and single support asymmetries [20].

Overexertion and fatigue can further impair control of gait stability in patients with stroke. One study highlighted two alternative possible strategies implemented by these patients for prolonged walking (6 min). Some subjects maintained their speed during long-lasting walking, despite a slight but progressive reduction in their upper body stability. Others applied a compensatory strategy, based on a decrease in walking speed in order to keep upper body accelerations small [28]. The former are the ones more exposed to the risk of falling.

2 Motor-Cognitive Integration

The act of walking involves many different muscles and the need to control, simultaneously, several degrees of freedom. One of the paramount discoveries related to gait is the existence of central pattern generators (CPGs), i.e. neural circuits within the spinal cord that can autonomously generate basic rhythmic locomotor patterns, even in the absence of brain connections and sensory information [16]. Evidence supporting the existence of CPGs in humans is quite compelling. However, although CPGs have been investigated in experimental models including in vitro isolated preparations, genetically engineered mice, spinal cord-transected animals, and virtual models, definitive proof is still lacking [17].

It is to be noted that supraspinal structures are involved during locomotion as well. They are responsible for initiating [29] and modifying the features of the basic gait rhythm, for stabilizing upright gait, and for coordinating movements in the environment [15]. Damage to supraspinal structures leads to specific alterations of human gait, as evident in subjects with stroke [7, 14], brain injury, cerebral palsy [26], Parkinson's disease, and cerebellar dysfunctions [31]. The cerebellum also plays a fundamental role during gait, in balance, coordination and adaptation of movements to the external environment. The cerebellum is the CNS structure where the internal models (i.e., neural representations miming significant aspects of our body, such as input/output characteristics of the sensorimotor system) are conceivably developed [53]. Internal model control has been shown to be involved in motor strategies to compensate for delays or lack of sensorimotor feedback. Some aspects of locomotion probably require internal predictive control, especially for improving dynamic stability, avoiding obstacles, or when sensory feedback is altered or compromised.

The role of superior cognitive functions during locomotion is still debated. Some authors support the idea that locomotion is a largely automated function. Indeed, people with cognitive impairment can walk without problems (e.g. Ruchinskas et al. [48]). Other authors (such as [32]) reported that a cognitive task performed during walking (i.e. dual-task condition) affected gait stability. Subjects usually show a reduced gait speed under single-task conditions, but under dual-tasking conditions subjects also showed a reduction of gait stability in the lateral-lateral direction, suggesting the need for specific integrated motor-cognitive rehabilitation to reduce the fall risk [52].

Vision plays a crucial role in gait performance, and it is probably the function that, more than any other, involves the cortical areas in exploration of the surrounding environment during walking. Aprile et al. [1] found that subjects with exotropia (an expanded visual field) showed a larger step width than subjects with esotropia (a reduced visual field), suggesting a particular neurosensory adaptation of gait to abnormal vision. These results recall the famous line "Go where I'm looking, not look where I'm going" by Berthoz in his famous book "The Brain's Sense of Movement", in which it is argued that gaze-based feed-forward control plays a role in locomotion along a desired trajectory [3].

The role of cognition may become predominant when subjects are asked to imagine a motor task before actually performing it. In recent years, rehabilitation protocols based on mental imagery have been proposed and tested with positive results. The term mental, or motor, imagery refers to the mental execution of movements, i.e. playing out the action in the mind. Although a correlation between the timing of mental imagery and the actual performance has been reported, it was recently suggested that this correlation does not mean equivalence [12]. Furthermore, it has been shown that poor awareness of the impairments, such as an underestimation of the damage caused by stroke, may affect locomotor planning and increase the risk of falling [40].

The importance attached to top-down approaches in stroke suggests that rehabilitation should incorporate cognitive-motor interventions [2]. The most popular methods are action observation therapy and mirror therapy, both acting on mirror neural systems to promote recovery [13]. More recently, new advantages seem to be offered by technology, too, such as the use of brain-computer interfaces for improving outcomes in therapy based on mental imagery [44] and the other approaches reported in the following section.

3 Technologies in Support of an Integrated Approach for Gait and Balance Recovery

In the last decade, conventional manual therapy for people affected by stroke has been enriched by the use of technological devices to improve rehabilitation outcomes [27].

The point is, why does manual therapy need technological support? Rehabilitation has been defined as the "sleeping giant" of medicine. Thus, further efforts to improve its quality care standards are required [11]. In rehabilitation, it is necessary to optimize the trade-off between the number of people treated, the intensity and duration of the treatment and the associated health care costs. This is not an easy objective to achieve, especially when considering the complexity of neurological disorders like stroke.

There is a need for deeper knowledge of the complex neural mechanisms involved, together with the development of new approaches that also take advantage of available technological support. This, in turn, will satisfy the need for more therapy performed in a more adequate and appropriate manner [23]. Recovery can indeed depend on the intensity of treatment, and on the repetition of specific skilled movements that target the motor deficits and are rewarded with performance feedback [37, 45]. In this framework, the use of technological devices may be helpful to increase intensity, repetitions, specificity and feedback during rehabilitation. In accordance with the need for an integrated top-down approach [2], recent years have seen new technologies, such as virtual reality systems, neurorobotics, muscle and neural electromagnetic stimulators, and wearable devices [27], becoming far more widespread. In this context, the 3T approach has been proposed, where the three Ts stand for: Therapy, Technology and Transnationality [41]. Neurorehabilitation should be based on evidence from the fields of neural plasticity and neuromotor physiology and constantly reviewed on the basis of updated findings in these areas of neuroscience; it should also constantly take into account the new possibilities offered by the technological development of new devices. This implies a straightforward translational approach: from neuroscience and neuroengineering to neurorehabilitation. Two clear examples of a movement towards an integrated approach to treatment are provided by constraint-induced movement therapy, which is driven by neuroscience studies [49, 54], and brain-computer interfaces, which have been developed in the field of neurotechnology and can be adapted to neurorehabilitation [44]. However, the relationship between therapy and technology is sometimes conflicting, and it can generate excessive optimism about the benefits that can be derived from the use of new technological devices for neurorehabilitation [8] or, alternatively, skepticism [10]. The challenge of integrating new technologies, recent neuroscientific findings, and conventional rehabilitation techniques should be based on scientifically collected data and rigorously tested hypotheses. On the other hand, new technological devices are often marketed before there is clear proof of their effectiveness and before clearly defined user guidelines have been developed.

4 The Need for a Multidisciplinary Team

An comprehensive, integrated approach would require the services of a health care team able, in pursuing the best restoration of functions for the single patient, to provide comprehensive assessment, treatment planning, treatment delivery, provision of equipment, and fitting of rehabilitation and adaptive devices [30]. This must therefore be a multidisciplinary team, and we would add that there is also a need for experts with interdisciplinary skills, each one highly proficient in his/her particular field, but also able to interact pro-actively with other professionals. In patients with stroke, for example, it is often fundamental to treat aphasia or unilateral spatial neglect. Improvement of these impairments may positively influence the recovery of other functional motor outcomes, such as gait and balance, and consequently improve independence in activities of daily living [35, 42]. All this, then, should be based on cooperation among members of a trans-disciplinary team that would also include speech therapists and neuropsychologists. With the addition of the technology aspect, there may also be a need for a bioengineer to maximize the exploitation of rehabilitation devices and to objectively assess the motor outcomes of patients using instrumented movement analysis.

The team should be able to tailor the right therapeutic approach to the right patient at the right time, as already suggested in relation to the use of robots in gait recovery [38, 39]. In this framework, the psychological profile of the patient can also play a fundamental role. Evidence that anxiety can limit the efficacy of robotic rehabilitation more than conventional rehabilitation [5] underlines just how closely interconnected cognitive and motor conditions are.

To quote Hippocrates, we might say that the future needs to draw a lesson from the past: "It's far more important to know what person the disease has than what disease the person has" (Hippocrates; Coo, 460 A.D.—Larissa, 377 A.D.).

References

1. Aprile I, Ferrarin M, Padua L, Di Sipio E, Simbolotti C, Petroni S, Tredici C, Dickmann A. Walking strategies in subjects with congenital or early onset strabismus. Front Hum Neurosci. 2014;8:484.
2. Belda-Lois JM, Mena-del Horno S, Bermejo-Bosch I, Moreno JC, Pons JL, Farina D, Iosa M, Molinari M, Tamburella F, Ramos A, Caria A, Solis-Escalante T, Brunner C, Rea M. Rehabilitation of gait after stroke: a review towards a top-down approach. J Neuroeng Rehabil. 2011;8:66. https://doi.org/10.1186/1743-0003-8-66.
3. Berthoz A. The Brain's Sense of Movement (translated by G.Weiss). Boston: Harvard University Press; 2000.
4. Berthoz A, Pozzo T. Head and body coordination during locomotion and complex movements. In: Swinnen S, Heuer H, Massion J, Casaer P, editors. Interlimb coordination. San Diego: Academic Press; 1994.
5. Bragoni M, Broccoli M, Iosa M, et al. Influence of psychologic features on rehabilitation outcomes in patients with subacute stroke trained with robotic-aided walking therapy. Am J Phys Med Rehabil. 2013;92(10 Suppl 2):e16–25.
6. Cappozzo A. Analysis of the linear displacement of the head and trunk during walking at different speeds. J Biomech. 1981;14:411–25.
7. Clark DJ, Ting LH, Zajac FE, Neptune RR, Kautz SA. Merging of healthy motor modules predicts reduced locomotor performance and muscle coordination complexity post-stroke. J Neurophysiol. 2010;103:844–57.
8. Datteri E. Predicting the long-term effects of human-robot interaction: a reflection on responsibility in medical robotics. Sci Eng Ethics. 2013;19(1):139–60.
9. Di Monaco M, Trucco M, Di Monaco R, Tappero R, Cavanna A. The relationship between initial trunk control or postural balance and inpatient rehabilitation outcome after stroke: a prospective comparative study. Clin. Rehabil. 2010;24:543–54.
10. Dobkin BH, Duncan PW. Should body weight-supported treadmill training and robotic-assistive steppers for locomotor training trot back to the starting gate? Neurorehabil Neural Repair. 2012;26(4):308–17.
11. Donnan GA. Rehabilitation: the sleeping giant of stroke medicine. Int J Stroke. 2013;8(1):1.
12. Fusco A, Gallotta MC, Iosa M, Morone G, Iasevoli L, Trifoglio D, Saraceni VM, Paolucci S, Baldari C, Guidetti L. The dynamic motor imagery of locomotion is task-dependent in patients with stroke. Restor Neurol Neurosci. 2016;34(2):247–56. https://doi.org/10.3233/RNN-150573.
13. Garrison KA, Winstein CJ, Aziz-Zadeh L. The mirror neuron system: a neural substrate for methods in stroke rehabilitation. Neurorehabil Neural Repair. 2010;24(5):404–12. https://doi.org/10.1177/1545968309354536.
14. Gizzi L, Feldbæk Nielsen J, Felici F, Farina D. Impulses of activation but not motor modules are preserved in the locomotion of subacute stroke patients. J Neurophysiol. 2011;106:202–10.
15. Grasso R, Ivanenko YP, Zago M, Molinari M, Scivoletto G, Castellano V, Macellari V, Lacquaniti F. Distributed plasticity of locomotor pattern generators in spinal cord injured patients. Brain. 2004;127:1019–34.
16. Grillner S. Neurobiological bases of rhythmic motor acts in vertebrates. Science. 1985;228:143–9.
17. Guertin PA. Preclinical evidence supporting the clinical development of central pattern generator-modulating therapies for chronic spinal cord-injured patients. Front Hum Neurosci. 2014;8:272.
18. Gustafson Y. Falls and injuries after stroke: time for action! Stroke. 2003;34(2):494–501.
19. Hamacher D, Singh NB, Van Dieën JH, Heller MO, Taylor WR. Kinematic measures for assessing gait stability in elderly individuals: a systematic review. J R Soc Interface. 2011;8:1682–98.

20. Hodt-Billington C, Helbostad JL, Moe-Nilssen R. Should trunk movement or footfall parameters quantify gait asymmetry in chronic stroke patients? Gait Posture. 2008;27:552–8.
21. Inman VT, Ralston HJ, Todd F. Human walking. Baltimore: Williams & Wilkins; 1981.
22. Iosa M, Fusco A, Morone G, Paolucci S. Development and decline of upright gait stability. Front Aging Neurosci. 2014; 6:14. https://doi.org/10.3389/fnagi.2014.00014.
23. Iosa M, Morone G, Cherubini A, Paolucci S. The three laws of Neurorobotics: a review on what neurorehabilitation robots should do for patients and clinicians. J Med Biol Eng. 2016;2016(36):1–11.
24. Iosa M, Picerno P, Paolucci S, Morone G. Wearable inertial sensors for human movement analysis. Expert Rev Med Devices. 2016;13(7):641–59. https://doi.org/10.1080/17434440.2016.1198694.
25. Iosa M, Fusco A, Morone G, Pratesi L, Coiro P, Venturiero V, De Angelis D, Bragoni M, Paolucci S. Assessment of upper body dynamic stability during walking in patients with subacute stroke. J Rehabil Res Dev. 2012;49:439–50.
26. Iosa M, Marro T, Paolucci S, Morelli D. Stability and harmony of gait in children with cerebral palsy. Res Dev Disabil. 2012;33(1):129–35.
27. Iosa M, Morone G, Fusco A, Bragoni M, Coiro P, Multari M, Venturiero V, De Angelis D, Pratesi L, Paolucci S. Seven capital devices for the future of stroke rehabilitation. Stroke Res. Treat. 2012;2012:187965.
28. Iosa M, Morone G, Fusco A, Pratesi L, Bragoni M, Coiro P, Multari M, Venturiero V, De Angelis D, Paolucci S. Effects of walking endurance reduction on gait stability in patients with stroke. Stroke Res Treat. 2012;2012:810415.
29. Jiang N, Gizzi L, Mrachacz-Kersting N, Dremstrup K, Farina D. A brain computer interface for single-trial detection of gait initiation from movement related cortical potentials. Clin Neurophysiol. 2014;S1388–2457(14):1–00252.
30. King JC, Nelson TR, Heye ML, Turturro TC, Titus MND. Presciptions, referals, order writing, and rehabilitation team function. In: DLisa JA and Gans BM, editors. Rehabilitation medicine: principle and practice, Third Edition. Limppincott-Raven Publishers, Philadelphia, 1998.
31. Kirtley C. Clinical gait analysis; theory and practice. Philadelphia, PA: Elsevier; 2006.
32. Lamoth CJ, van Deudekom FJ, van Campen JP, Appels BA, de Vries OJ, Pijnappels M. Gait stability and variability measures show effects of impaired cognition and dual tasking in frail people. J Neuroeng Rehabil. 2011;8:2.
33. Langhorne P, Stott DJ, Robertson L, et al. Medical complications after stroke: a multicenter study. Stroke. 2000;31(6):1223–9.
34. Masiero S, Avesani R, Armani M, Verena P, Ermani M. Predictive factors for ambulation in stroke patients in the rehabilitation setting: a multivariate analysis. Clin Neurol Neurosurg. 2007;109:763–9.
35. Matano A, Iosa M, Guariglia C, Pizzamiglio L, Paolucci S. Does outcome of neuropsychological treatment in patients with unilateral spatial neglect after stroke affect functional outcome? Eur J Phys Rehabil Med. 2015;51(6):737–43.
36. Mizuike C, Ohgi S, Morita S. Analysis of stroke patient walking dynamics using a tri-axial accelerometer. Gait Posture. 2009;30:60–4.
37. Morasso, P., Casadio, M., Giannoni, P., Masia, L., Sanguineti, V., Squeri, et al. Desirable features of a "humanoid" robot-therapist. Conference proceedings: Annual International Conference of the IEEE Engineering in Medicine and Biology Society, 2009:2418–21.
38. Morone G, Bragoni M, Iosa M, et al. Who may benefit from robotic-assisted gait training? a randomized clinical trial in patients with subacute stroke. Neurorehabil Neural Repair. 2011;25(7):636–44.
39. Morone G, Iosa M, Bragoni M, et al. Who may have durable benefit from robotic gait training? a 2-year follow-up randomized controlled trial in patients with subacute stroke. Stroke. 2012;43(4):1140–2.

40. Morone G, Iosa M, Pratesi L, Paolucci S. Can overestimation of walking ability increase the risk of falls in people in the subacute stage after stroke on their return home? Gait Posture. 2014;39(3):965–70.
41. Morone G, Paolucci S, Mattia D, Pichiorri F, Tramontano M, Iosa M. The 3Ts of the new millennium neurorehabilitation gym: therapy, technology, translationality. Expert Rev Med Devices. 2016;13(9):785–7. https://doi.org/10.1080/17434440.2016.1218275.
42. Paolucci S, Antonucci G, Pratesi L, Traballesi M, Lubich S, Grasso MG. Functional outcome in stroke inpatient rehabilitation: predicting no, low and high response patients. Cerebrovasc Dis. 1998;8(4):228–34.
43. Paolucci S, Bragoni M, Coiro P, et al. Quantification of the probability of reaching mobility independence at discharge from a rehabilitation hospital in nonwalking early ischemic stroke patients: a multivariate study. Cerebrovasc Dis. 2008;26(1):16–22.
44. Pichiorri F, Morone G, Petti M, Toppi J, Pisotta I, Molinari M, Paolucci S, Inghilleri M, Astolfi L, Cincotti F, Mattia D. Brain-computer interface boosts motor imagery practice during stroke recovery. Ann Neurol. 2015;77(5):851–65. https://doi.org/10.1002/ana.24390.
45. Pollock A, Baer G, Pomeroy V, Langhorne P. Physiotherapy treatment approaches for the recovery of postural control and lower limb function following stroke. Cochrane Database Syst Rev. 2007;(1):CD001920. Review. Update in: Cochrane Database Syst Rev. 2014;4: CD001920.
46. Preston E, Ada L, Dean CM, Stanton R, Waddington G. What is the probability of patients who are nonambulatory after stroke regaining independent walking? a systematic review. Int J Stroke. 2011;6(6):531–40.
47. Reed ES. Encountering the world: toward an ecological psychology. New York: Oxford University Press; 1996.
48. Ruchinskas RA, Singer HK, Repetz NK. Cognitive status and ambulation in geriatric rehabilitation: walking without thinking? Arch Phys Med Rehabil. 2000;81:1224–8.
49. Smania N, Gandolfi M, Paolucci S, Iosa M, Ianes P, Recchia S, Giovanzana C, Molteni F, Avesani R, Di Paolo P, Zaccala M, Agostini M, Tassorelli C, Fiaschi A, Primon D, Ceravolo MG, Farina S. Reduced-intensity modified constraint-induced movement therapy versus conventional therapy for upper extremity rehabilitation after stroke: a multicenter trial. Neurorehabil Neural Repair. 2012;26(9):1035–45. https://doi.org/10.1177/1545968312446003.
50. Spoor F, Wood B, Zonneveld F. Implications of early hominid labyrinthine morphology for evolution of human bipedal locomotion. Nature. 1994;369(6482):645–8.
51. Tilson JK, Wu SS, Cen SY, et al. Characterizing and identifying risk for falls in the leaps study: a randomized clinical trial of interventions to improve walking post-stroke. Stroke. 2012;43(2):446–52.
52. Tramontano M, Morone G, Curcio A, Temperoni G, Medici A, Morelli D, Caltagirone C, Paolucci S, Iosa M. Managing the mantainment of gait stability during dual walking task: effects of age and neurological disorders. Eur J Phys Rehabil Med. 2016.
53. Wolpert DM, Miall RC, Kawato M. Internal models in the cerebellum. Trends Cogn Sci. 1998;2:338–47.
54. Wu CY, Chang KC. Constraint-induced movement therapy translated into practice. Lancet Neurol. 2015;14(9):869–71.

Rehabilitation of Ataxias

Mariano Serrao

1 Introduction

Cerebellar disorders (which include congenital, hereditary and acquired conditions) lead to several symptoms that may vary with the cause but typically include ataxia. The term ataxia (meaning "lack of order" in ancient Greek) refers to a lack of motor coordination, although growing evidence indicates that the cerebellum also contributes to regulation of certain non-motor features such as linguistic, cognitive and affective functions. Degenerative cerebellar ataxias, which have several different causes, are a significant group of disorders with an estimated prevalence ranging from 5.2 to 18.5 per 100,000 inhabitants [2, 33]. The typical cerebellar motor syndrome includes a wide range of features such as dysmetria, asynergia or dyssynergia, a- or dysdiadochokinesia, tremor, oculomotor abnormalities, speech disturbances, hypotonia and abnormalities of posture and gait (for a review see Bodranghien et al. [3]). Gait and balance disorders are crucial features of cerebellar ataxias, having a great influence on patients' independence in daily life activities, quality of life and risk of falls [11, 28]. On these bases, and also considering the impact of these conditions in terms of economic costs and health-related quality of life [21], one of the main areas of neurorehabilitation intervention in patients with ataxia should be the treatment of gait and balance abnormalities. Over the last decade, evidence has emerged indicating that rehabilitation can improve postural and gait functions in cerebellar ataxia [15, 17, 18] and suggesting a potential role for neurorehabilitation in delaying the loss of independent walking.

M. Serrao (✉)
Department of Medical and Surgical Sciences and Biotechnologies,
Sapienza University of Rome, Corso Della Repubblica 79, 40100 Latina, Italy
e-mail: mariano.serrao@uniroma1.it

M. Serrao
Movement Analysis LAB, Rehabilitation Centre Policlinico Italia, Piazza Del Campidano 6,
00162 Rome, Italy

G. Sandrini et al. (eds.), *Advanced Technologies for the Rehabilitation of Gait and Balance Disorders*, Biosystems & Biorobotics 19,
https://doi.org/10.1007/978-3-319-72736-3_13

Gait evaluation, aimed at quantifying and typifying specific impairments of walking function in patients with neurological diseases, is crucial in order to design rehabilitation treatments tailored to individual needs. Recently, several studies have quantitatively evaluated gait and balance disorders in patients with cerebellar ataxia by means of motion analysis systems, showing differences versus healthy subjects in spatiotemporal parameters and kinematic and kinetic variables (for a review see Bodranghien et al. [3]).

The use of motion analysis systems allows a deeper characterization of walking impairment in these neurological diseases and can shed light on the nature of both the primary specific gait disorder and any compensatory mechanisms. Such deeper understanding might reasonably represent a valid pre-requisite for establishing better-targeted rehabilitation strategies.

1.1 Quantitative Evaluation of Gait and Balance in Patients with Cerebellar Ataxia

Gait ataxia has long been acknowledged and described as "clumsy, staggering movements with a wide-based gait" which resembles the gait of drunken people. While this traditional description remains useful, helping clinicians to identify cerebellar disease, modern motion analysis systems have been used to quantitatively characterize the nature and degree of the gait dysfunction. Their findings have revealed impairment of various locomotor activities, such as linear steady-state gait, turning, gait initiation and gait termination [8, 13, 14, 22, 27, 30–32, 35]. All of these motor abnormalities reflect poor limb coordination and impaired balance, which greatly restrict these patients in their daily life activities and predispose them to falls [37].

During quiet standing, the patient's body may sway back and forth and from side to side. Different mechanisms involved in postural control have been found to be impaired in patients with cerebellar ataxia. Specifically, ankle joint stretch reflexes, which are important in keeping muscle length constant and serve as a balance-related mechanism during stance, have been shown to increase [10, 25, 36]. Furthermore, patients with ataxia lose their ability to scale postural responses due to impairment of both feedback and feedforward mechanisms at several hierarchical levels of the central nervous system [1, 4, 5, 13, 14, 20].

When analyzing and detecting gait ataxia, several biomechanical abnormalities have been revealed in terms of spatiotemporal parameters, joint ROMs, joint torques, joint coordination, upper body kinematics and muscle activation patterns.

If gait speed, as an influencing factor, is controlled, the main differences in spatiotemporal and joint kinematics and kinetics between patients with ataxia and healthy controls regard the step width, step length and ankle joint kinematics [7, 22, 24]. In particular, patients with ataxia show increased step width as well as reduced step length and ankle joint excursion. All these abnormalities seem to represent balance-related compensatory mechanisms aimed at reducing dynamic imbalance, by increasing the margin of stability in the frontal plane, reducing the time in the less stable configuration (single support phase), or increasing the ankle joint strategy to control the center of mass (CoM) displacements [3].

One of the most characterizing features of gait ataxia is a marked variability of global and segmental kinematic and kinetic gait parameter values, which has been reported in almost all studies (for a review see Bodranghien et al. [3]). This feature reflects the inability of ataxic patients to maintain dynamic balance through a regular walking pattern, which leads to an increased risk of falls [28, 29].

With regard to the joint coordination deficit, abnormal intra-limb joint coupling during walking, in terms of both joint movements and interaction torques, has been reported in several studies (for a review see Bodranghien et al. [3]). In particular, increased temporal variability of intra-limb coordination has been found to relate to dynamic balance impairment and irregular foot trajectories in ataxic gait [16], while impaired inter-joint coordination leads to extremely irregular alternating joint behavior without evidence of the synchronous alternating proximal/distal joint pattern seen in healthy controls [30]. Abnormal control of the upper body leading to increase of movements and a lack of local stability of the trunk has recently been reported [7, 9], and it is an observation which suggests that upper and lower body coordination may play a pivotal role in explaining several aspect of gait ataxia.

Very recently, a detailed analysis of muscle activity patterns during locomotion in cerebellar ataxia [22, 24] showed impaired spatial and temporal profiles of EMG activity in individual muscles, as well as impaired antagonist muscle activation. In essence, ataxic patients seemed to activate both individual and paired antagonist muscles more intensely and for a longer time, possibly in an attempt to stiffen the limb and to compensate for the instability due to poor muscle coordination.

1.2 Rehabilitation of Gait and Balance in Cerebellar Ataxia

Studies on rehabilitation in cerebellar ataxia have investigated patients affected by different diseases, including degenerative ataxias, focal cerebellar lesions and multiple sclerosis. This makes it difficult to understand whether a rehabilitation treatment for a given form of ataxia can be generalized to other forms.

To date, only few studies have evaluated the efficacy of rehabilitation for improving gait and balance in patients with cerebellar degeneration, including spinocerebellar ataxia and Friedreich ataxias. Of these, only one was a randomized controlled study [26]. In general, the approaches proposed in these studies have been to seek to improve the patient's balance and independence through the use of rehabilitation techniques focusing on intensive static and dynamic balance, posture control and coordination exercises [15, 17, 18, 23, 26].

The training principles applied include progressing from simple to complex exercises, and training patients with increasingly demanding tasks (from static to dynamic balance; from slow to fast movements; and from single joint movements to complex, multi-joint coordination). In all these studies, the rehabilitation treatment was found to be effective in improving clinical scale scores (e.g. SARA, FIM, Berg Balance Scale) and gait speed and reducing the risk of falls [26, 34]. However, only in few studies were quantitative kinematic parameters used to assess the improvements induced by rehabilitation [17]. In this regard, Ilg et al. [17] found a reduction of the temporal variability in limb coordination during gait after rehabilitation treatment.

Several rehabilitation programs have been proposed for patients with degenerative ataxia. Ilg et al. [17, 18] proposed a four-week schedule of one-hour daily sessions of static and dynamic balance and coordination exercises. Miyai et al. [26] studied the effect of an intensive (11 h a week) six-week program of therapy including balance exercises, gait training, muscle strengthening and occupational therapy focusing on balance and activities of daily living.

Other rehabilitation proposals reported anecdotally include virtual reality training [19], climbing [34] and locomotion training on a treadmill with or without body weight support [6, 12, 38].

In general, the improvement in the outcome measures induced by physiotherapy has been seen to last for 6 months to 1 year after treatment [18, 19, 26]. It should be considered that in degenerative cerebellar diseases, rehabilitation treatments should be repeated over time with the aim of delaying the patient's motor decline.

References

1. Bakker M, Allum JH, Visser JE, Grüneberg C, van de Warrenburg BP, Kremer BH, Bloem BR. Postural responses to multidirectional stance perturbations in cerebellar ataxia. Exp Neurol. 2006;202:21–35.
2. Berciano J, Infante J, Mateo I, Combarros O. Hereditary ataxias and paraplegias: a clinicogenetic review. Neurologia. 2002;17:40–51.
3. Bodranghien F, Bastian A, Casali C, Hallett M, Louis ED, Manto M, Mariën P, Nowak DA, Schmahmann JD, Serrao M, Steiner KM, Strupp M, Tilikete C, Timmann D, van Dun K. Consensus paper: revisiting the symptoms and signs of cerebellar syndrome. Cerebellum. 2016;15:369–91.
4. Bruttini C, Esposti R, Bolzoni F, Vanotti A, Mariotti C, Cavallari P. Temporal disruption of upper-limb anticipatory postural adjustments in cerebellar ataxic patients. Exp Brain Res. 2015;233:197–203.
5. Bunn LM, Marsden JF, Giunti P, Day BL. Stance instability in spinocerebellar ataxia type 6. Mov Disord. 2013;28:510–6.
6. Cernak K, Stevens V, Price R, Shumway-Cook A. Locomotor training using body-weight support on a treadmill in conjunction with ongoing physical therapy in a child with severe cerebellar ataxia. Phys Ther. 2008;88:88–97.
7. Chini G, Ranavolo A, Draicchio F, Casali C, Conte C, Martino G, Leonardi L, Padua L, Coppola G, Pierelli F, Serrao M. Local stability of the trunk in patients with degenerative cerebellar ataxia during walking. Cerebellum. 2016 (in press).
8. Conte C, Serrao M, Casali C, Ranavolo A, Mari S, Draicchio F, et al. Planned gait termination in cerebellar ataxias. Cerebellum. 2012;11:896–904.

9. Conte C, Pierelli F, Casali C, Ranavolo A, Draicchio F, Martino G, Harfoush M, Padua L, Coppola G, Sandrini G, Serrao M. Upper body kinematics in patients with cerebellarataxia. Cerebellum. 2014;13(6):689–97.
10. Dichgans J, Mauritz KH. Patterns and mechanisms of postural instability in patients with cerebellar lesions. Adv Neurol. 1983;39:633–43.
11. Fonteyn EM, Schmitz-Hubsch T, Verstappen CC, Baliko L, Bloem BR, Boesch S, Bunn L, Giunti P, Globas C, Klockgether T, Melegh B, Pandolfo M, Schols L, Timmann D, van deWarrenburg BP. Prospective analysis of falls in dominant ataxias. Eur Neurol. 2013;69:53–7.
12. Freund JE, Stetts DM. Use of trunk stabilization and locomotor training in an adult with cerebellar ataxia: a single system design. Physiother Theory Pract. 2010;26:447–58.
13. Horak FB, Diener HC. Cerebellar control of postural scaling and central set in stance. J Neurophysiol. 1994;72:479–93.
14. Horak FB, Diener HC. Cerebellar control of postural scaling and central set in stance. J Neurophysiol. 1994;72:479–93.
15. Ilg W, Timmann D. Gait ataxia–specific cerebellar influences and their rehabilitation. Mov Disord. 2013;28(11):1566–75.
16. Ilg W, Golla H, Thier P, Giese MA. Specific influences of cerebellar dysfunctions on gait. Brain. 2007;130:786–98.
17. Ilg W, Synofzik M, Brotz D, Burkard S, Giese MA, Schols L. Intensive coordinative training improves motor performance in degenerative cerebellar disease. Neurology. 2009;73:1823–30.
18. Ilg W, Brotz D, Burkard S, Giese MA, Schols L, Synofzik M. Long-term effects of coordinative training in degenerative cerebellar disease. Mov Disord. 2010;25:2239–46.
19. Ilg W, Schatton C, Schicks J, Giese MA, Schols L, Synofzik M. Video game-based coordinative training improves ataxia in children with degenerative ataxia. Neurology. 2012;79:2056–60.
20. Küng UM, Horlings CG, Honegger F, Kremer HP, Bloem BR, van De Warrenburg BP, Allum JH. Postural instability in cerebellar ataxia: correlations of knee, arm and trunk movements to center of mass velocity. Neuroscience. 2009;159:390–404.
21. Lopez-Bastida J, Perestelo-Perez L, Monton-Alvarez F, Serrano-Aguilar P. Social economic costs and health-related quality of life in patients with degenerative cerebellar ataxia in Spain. Mov Disord. 2008;23(2):212–7.
22. Mari S, Serrao M, Casali C, Conte C, Ranavolo A, Padua L, Draicchio F, Iavicoli S, Monamì S, Sandrini G, Pierelli F. Turning strategies in patients with cerebellar ataxia. Exp Brain Res. 2012;222(1–2):65–75.
23. Marquer A, Barbieri G, Pérennou D. The assessment and treatment of postural disorders in cerebellar ataxia: a systematic review. Ann Phys Rehabil Med. 2014 Mar;57(2):67–78.
24. Martino G, Ivanenko YP, Serrao M, Ranavolo A, d'Avella A, Draicchio F, Conte C, Casali C, Lacquaniti F. Locomotor patterns in cerebellar ataxia. J Neurophysiol 2014;112:2810–21.
25. Mauritz KH, Dichgans J, Hufschmidt A. Quantitative analysis of stance in late cortical cerebellar atrophy of the anterior lobe and other forms of cerebellar ataxia. Brain. 1979;102:461–82.
26. Miyai I, Ito M, Hattori N, et al. Cerebellar ataxia rehabilitation trial in degenerative cerebellar diseases. Neurorehabil Neural Repair. 2012;26:515–22.
27. Morton SM, Bastian AJ. Relative contributions of balance and voluntary leg-coordination deficits to cerebellar gait ataxia. J Neurophysiol. 2003;89:1844–56.
28. Schniepp R, Wuehr M, Schlick C, Huth S, Pradhan C, Dieterich M, Brandt T, Jahn K. Increased gait variability is associated with the history of falls in patients with cerebellar ataxia. J Neurol. 2014;261:213–23.
29. Schniepp R, Schlick C, Pradhan C, Dieterich M, Brandt T, Jahn K, Wuehr M. The interrelationship between disease severity, dynamic stability, and falls in cerebellar ataxia. J Neurol. 2016;263:1409–17.

30. Serrao M, Pierelli F, Ranavolo A, Draicchio F, Conte C, Don R, Di Fabio R, LeRose M, Padua L, Sandrini G, Casali C. Gait pattern in inherited cerebellar ataxias. Cerebellum. 2012;11:194–211.
31. Serrao M, Conte C, Casali C, Ranavolo A, Mari S, Di Fabio R, et al. Sudden stopping in patients with cerebellar ataxia. Cerebellum. 2013;12:607–16.
32. Serrao M, Mari S, Conte C, Ranavolo A, Casali C, Draicchio F, et al. Strategies adopted by cerebellar ataxia patients to perform U turns. Cerebellum. 2013;12:460–8.
33. Shibata A, Oka K, Nakamura Y, Muraoka I. Prevalence and demographic correlates of meeting the physical activity recommendation among Japanese adults. J Phys Act Health. 2009;6:24–32.
34. Stephan MA, Krattinger S, Pasquier J, Bashir S, Fournier T, Ruegg DG, Diserens K. Effect of long-term climbing training on cerebellar ataxia: a case series. Rehabil Res Pract. 2011;2011:525879.
35. Timmann D, Horak FB. Prediction and set-dependent scaling of early postural responses in cerebellar patients. Brain. 1997;120(pt 2):327–37.
36. Tokuda T, Tako K, Hayashi R, Yanagisawa N. Disturbed modulation of the stretch reflex gain during standing in cerebellar ataxia. Electroencephalogr Clin Neurophysiol. 1991;81:421–6.
37. van de Warrenburg BP, Steijns JA, Munneke M, Kremer BP, Bloem BR. Falls in degenerative cerebellar ataxias. Mov Disord. 2005;20:497–500.
38. Vaz DV, Schettino RdC, Rolla de Castro TR, Teixeira VR, Cavalcanti Furtado SR, de Mello Figueiredo E. Treadmill training for ataxic patients: a single-subject experimental design. Clin Rehabil 2008;22:234–41.

An Integrated Approach to Gait and Balance Rehabilitation in Multiple Sclerosis

Maria Grazia Grasso and Luca Pace

1 Characteristics

Multiple sclerosis (MS), a chronic disease of the central nervous system (CNS), is one of the leading causes of neurological disability in young adults and it affects approximately 2.5 million people worldwide [36]. The disease is underlain by a complex, although still not fully clarified, interplay between inflammation, demyelination and neurodegeneration. The diagnosis of MS is based on the (revised) McDonald criteria [47]. From a clinical point of view, the spatial dissemination of the lesions in MS is such that the disease can manifest itself through a range of neurological symptoms. Seventy-five percent of people with MS (pwMS) present lower limb sensory-motor deficits, 66% display upper limb deficits, and 44% complain of problems in activities of daily living (ADL) [24, 54]. Lack of balance and difficulty in walking long distances are considered by healthcare professionals to be the two problems that patients report the most [20]; pwMS themselves place difficulty in walking at the top of their list of complaints, irrespective of the disease duration. Furthermore, difficulty in walking is widely known to have a negative impact on the working lives of pwMS, reducing the number of hours they work and increasing the need for changes in their work environment [31]. A number of studies based on both instrumental and clinical evaluations have shown that gait abnormalities are present in pwMS with a low degree of disability; in particular, computerized analyses have been found to detect alterations in mobility earlier than clinical examination [2, 18]. Furthermore, impaired mobility

M. G. Grasso (✉) · L. Pace
IRCCS Fondazione Santa Lucia, Rome, Italy
e-mail: mg.grasso@hsantalucia.it

G. Sandrini et al. (eds.), *Advanced Technologies for the Rehabilitation of Gait and Balance Disorders*, Biosystems & Biorobotics 19,
https://doi.org/10.1007/978-3-319-72736-3_14

can have an early impact on ADL, as assessed by means of ADL questionnaires. Balance deficits, which are highly disabling, are considered the second most common symptom overall and the most common symptom in pwMS with walking deficits [14]. Balance deficits, which occur when sensory input is disrupted and which may be the first symptom of the disease, tend to persist and to progress over time as the disease worsens. The main difficulties encountered by pwMS are in maintaining balance with a reduced base of support and in transferring their centre of mass.

2 Assessment

Here we briefly summarize the most widely used and the most specific MS scales. Kurtzke's Expanded Disability Status Scale (EDSS), with its functional systems, referring to mental, visual, brainstem, sensory, pyramidal, cerebellar and bowel and bladder functions, is the one most often used to assess the signs of the disease. The EDSS score ranges from 0, which indicates a normal neurological examination, to 10, which corresponds to death from MS [29]. Gait and balance in MS are evaluated using different scales according to the needs and interests of the referring physicians. Clinical assessment, which is the first step, includes observation of patients standing and walking and a patient interview to collect information on the quantity and quality of their gait, the state of the leg muscles, and their use of devices. Objective gait scales are scales designed and used to assess speed and endurance. Speed is assessed using the timed 25-ft walk, 10-m walk, 30-m walk, and 100-m walk tests, and endurance using the 6-min walk test (6 m WT) and two-minute walk test (2 m WT). A multicentre study that set out to identify the most reliable test to use in MS found that the timed 25-ft walk accurately describes the patient's general walking capacity, whereas an endurance measure, such as the 2 m WT, is recommended in intervention studies [17]. The Berg Balance Scale is the most widely used objective scale for assessing balance performance in MS [26]. As regards subjective scales, the validated 12-item MS walking scale [22] is considered easy to use because it is short, it helps to focus on areas of concern, it is useful for follow-up purposes, and it can be used in conjunction with objective measures. A 7-item version of the Fall Efficacy Scale–International (short FES–I) has also recently been developed and validated. This fall risk questionnaire is a patient self-report measure that assesses the risk of falls both at home and in the community, and it has proved to be valuable when time and resources are limited [13]. The Activities-specific Balance Confidence (ABC) scale is a questionnaire that investigates balance confidence during specific ADL. However, a thorough description of balance problems in pwMS demands the use of both objective and subjective balance measures [8]. Several studies have focused on 3D movement analysis. Gait analysis, in particular, may be more sensitive than timed tests, although this instrumental method is time-consuming and requires special equipment. It may, however, be used by the clinician to gather quantitative and qualitative information on functional limitations of walking and any correlations between such limitations and disability [42, 43, 53]. Furthermore, 3D gait analysis of spasticity in pwMS may help to verify the effectiveness of pharmacological and rehabilitation treatments [43].

Accelerometry is reported to be a valid approach for measuring walking limitations in ambulatory pwMS [39]. Gait and balance have more recently been assessed using the International Classification of Functioning, Disability and Health (ICF) model, which is a more functional and ecological approach. Numerous measures are available at the different levels of the ICF to assess factors affecting balance, the risk of falls and walking. When combined, these measures provide a complete assessment of the individual as well as guidance for any interventions by the healthcare team [9].

3 Rehabilitation Approaches

The rehabilitation approach needs to be individualised to each person with MS, on the basis of a comprehensive evaluation designed to ascertain both the impairment, such as weakness, spasticity or fatigue, and the broader clinical picture, including other comorbidities. After evaluating the individual's activity and participation levels, the rehabilitation programme can be planned in such a way as to optimize the patient's physical and psychological capacities. The programme is based on structured exercises of increasing difficulty with planned breaks in the course of the session, depending on the severity of the disease. There are three main physiotherapy approaches used in pwMS. The first, called the facilitation approach, incorporates the Bobath concept, proprioceptive neuromuscular facilitation and Vojta reflex locomotion, and has been combined with theoretical approaches based on motor control [34]. The second is the task-oriented therapeutic approach, which is instead a new model of motor control that focuses on the individual patient's specific disabilities, and may therefore involve, for example, constraint-induced movement therapy or a motor relearning programme. The aim of these first two approaches is to improve ADL by applying both internal (within the body) and external (environmental) stimuli to induce better movement [35]. The third approach is muscle rehabilitation, e.g. biofeedback, aerobic exercise training and resistance training, all of which have been suggested to counteract many MS symptoms [37]. Aerobic exercise training is designed to improve physical capacity; in this case, maximal oxygen uptake (VO_2max) and the mechanical power generated during the exercise are used as indicators. Resistance training programmes are instead designed to increase the impact of muscle strength, mobility, balance and performance in ADL. It involves the use of a range of machines, such as weight machines, resistance bands and aquatic training. The application of progressive resistance exercises has been shown to improve muscle strength, whereas data are lacking on other parameters, such as walking and fatigue, as well as on the effects of this approach in more severely disabled pwMS [16].

It should be noted that physical training exerts a very beneficial effect on other symptoms, as demonstrated in the Briken pilot study in which 47 pwMS with a progressive form of disease and mild-moderate disability were subdivided into four treatment groups: arm ergometry, rowing, bicycle ergometry and a waitlist control group. The 42 pwMS who completed the study displayed a significant improvement not only in aerobic fitness and walking ability but, interestingly, also in several cognitive domains, depression and fatigue [5].

Rehabilitation treatment may be designed either to improve the efficiency of a function (restorative treatment) or to help pwMS to adopt compensatory strategies (replacement treatment). These two approaches can also be combined, depending on the characteristics of the patient. Patients are advised to try to fit their difficulties into their everyday life, adapt to them, and take breaks regularly [44]. The programme needs to be revised at least every 6 months taking into account changes detected through monitoring of the disease. The prescription of assistive devices is an important point in the life of a person affected by MS. It is essential to identify both the best device for the particular patient, and the best time to prescribe it. Indeed, although the aim of assistive devices is to correct deficits and consequently improve QoL, they may negatively affect the patient's self-image. Moreover, a study conducted by the Italian MS association has shown that the devices should be prescribed by an interdisciplinary team as this significantly reduces the risk of equipment abandonment [59]. Literature on the effectiveness of ankle-foot orthoses on the walking ability of pwMS is very limited and no definitive conclusions can be drawn. However, published data suggest that more disabled pwMS tend to benefit from orthoses to a greater extent [60].

4 Evidence-Based Rehabilitation Results

Until about 15 years ago, the various approaches to MS were very conservative and cautious, the main recommendations given to patients being to take care of themselves and not get tired. Since then, however, a large body of scientific evidence has changed this stance. The first robust evidence dates back to 2005, when a Cochrane systematic review on the effectiveness of physiotherapy was published. The authors of the review concluded that physiotherapy can be effective, that no evidence exists showing that one treatment is more effective than others, and that there is no evidence of it having negative effects [49]. Another noteworthy Cochrane Database systematic review showed that although multidisciplinary rehabilitation does not change the level of impairment, it can improve activity and participation levels in PwMS [27]. A number of meta-analyses on the effectiveness of physical training were published over the following years: physical training was shown to be associated with a small but significant improvement in QoL in pwMS [38], as well as with a small but significant improvement in ambulation [52]. The effectiveness of physical training on fatigue is less conclusive, the results available being discrepant, even though exercise therapy is known to induce a positive effect on fatigue [1, 45]. No clear evidence emerged from a 2012 systematic review that investigated the effects of physiotherapy interventions on balance, considering the efficacy of specific balance exercises (motor and sensory strategies), of physical therapy based on a problem-solving approach, and of resistance and aerobic exercises. The authors concluded that physical therapy has a small but significant effect on balance in pwMS with a mild to moderate level of disability, but no effect in severely disabled people [41]. A more recent systematic review on the safety of physical therapy concluded that exercise training was not associated with an increased risk of relapse, and the risk of adverse events was not higher than in healthy populations [46]. In the light of these findings, exercise therapy may have a beneficial effect in pwMs, and may thus be recommended for rehabilitation purposes [50]. Although some deficits seem to improve following respiratory training and multidisciplinary rehabilitation, the efficacy of physical rehabilitation in non-ambulatory pwMS remains unclear [57]. However, a very recent systematic review conducted by the American Academy of Neurology (AAN) on rehabilitation treatment in MS concluded that: (1) weekly home or outpatient physical training for 8 weeks probably improves balance, disability and gait in pwMS able to walk ≥5 m, although data are insufficient to support or refute any effect on depression and anxiety; (2) 3 weeks' worth of individualised inpatient exercise followed by home exercises for 15 weeks may reduce disability in mild-moderate disease, though data are insufficient to support or refute any effect on QoL; (3) 3 weeks' worth of motor and sensory balance training may improve static and dynamic balance, and motor balance training may improve static balance. The data were found to be inadequate to support or refute the effect of this treatment on the risk of falls or on self-reported disability and handicaps [21].

As the AAN review demonstrates, there is, as yet, no conclusive evidence as to what the best treatment is, because neither studies on progressive resistance, nor those on aerobic exercises have proved the effectiveness of these approaches. However, in 2013, Canadian guidelines stated that pwMS with mild to moderate disability should perform aerobic activity of moderate intensity for 30 min twice a week, and strength training exercises for the main muscle groups twice a week [32]. Another study, in 30 pwMS, evaluated the effect of active motor rehabilitation versus passive mobilisation on the white matter microstructure by means of diffusion tensor imaging. White matter integrity in the corpus callosum and corticospinal tracts was preserved in pwMS treated with active neurorehabilitation, whereas microstructural integrity worsened in pwMS treated with passive mobilisation, thus suggesting that passive mobilisation has a detrimental effect on pwMS [3]. A review of the literature on the possible beneficial effects of exercises on disease progression concluded that any such effect is not supported by evidence yielded by clinical measures. However, some data, such as those that have previously emerged from MRI studies, patient self-reports, and immunological findings, combined with the observation that aerobic exercise (or voluntary physical activity) has the potential to modify the clinical course of the disease in experimental autoimmune encephalomyelitis (an animal model of MS), do indicate a possible effect, although the evidence is not yet conclusive [28].

5 New Approaches and Technologies

Some new approaches and technologies have been proposed in recent years, including robot-assisted training for gait and balance, which uses systems such as Lokomat®, Treadmill Training (TT) and gait training systems. The results of the few studies published to date indicate that TT, either with or without body weight support, and robot-assisted gait training (RAGT) improve the walking speed and walking distance, although it remains to be determined what kind of TT intervention is most effective [56]. From a clinical perspective, however, RAGT may represent another rehabilitation strategy for highly disabled pwMS [48, 55].

Although numerous exercise programmes designed for MS are based on hydrotherapy, the lack of studies assessing the effectiveness of this treatment on balance and gait performance alone means that no conclusions can be drawn. This technique is, however, considered useful from a clinical point of view and does not have any major side effects [10].

The efficacy of whole-body vibration was evaluated by a Cochrane review published in 2012. This review included only four MS studies whose methodological quality was deemed low [51]. Furthermore, evidence of the effectiveness of whole-body vibration on balance, gait and muscle performance is weak. Hippotherapy may also have a positive effect on balance, though this hypothesis is based on non-randomised-controlled trials alone [6]. Other techniques, such as transcutaneous electrical nerve stimulation, repetitive magnetic stimulation and electromagnetic therapy, have not been scientifically studied in RCTs, and do not appear to offer any advantages over other techniques used in rehabilitation therapy [58].

The last few years have seen increasingly widespread use of the effect of Nintendo Wii® for rehabilitation purposes in MS. Interactive visual-feedback exercises of the kind provided by Wii may improve balance disorders in MS [4].

There may also be some rationale for yoga, kickboxing, taping, pilates, vestibular rehabilitation and tai chi in MS, and some of these activities appear to yield promising results, although no conclusive evidence of their effectiveness yet exists owing to the lack of carefully planned studies [7, 11, 12, 23, 25, 40].

6 Prognostic Factors

Few studies have sought to establish what prognostic factors are predictors of a good rehabilitation outcome. In a study of 38 progressive pwMS, low motor disability upon admission, verbal intelligence and cerebellar function were found to be influential in determining rehabilitation outcome [30]. In a larger study performed in 220 progressive pwMS, the most favourable prognostic factors were a lower EDSS score, short disease duration, lack of severe cognitive deficits, and lack of severe sphincter disturbances [19]. A third, more recent, study in 212 pwMS who underwent rehabilitation for a short period of time reported that the factors able to predict beneficial results of rehabilitation were a shorter disease duration and a less marked balance impairment (in agreement with the two aforementioned papers), as well as more severe baseline impairment and activity limitation and a relapsing-remitting disease course [33].

7 Conclusions

A large body of scientific evidence indicates that rehabilitation is safe and also effective on gait and balance in pwMS with mild-moderate disability.

The potential benefits of rehabilitation in pwMS with more severe disability are not yet clear because of the lack of good quality studies. Physical activity seems to have a positive impact on other symptoms, such as fatigue, depression, cognitive deficits and QoL, although conclusive evidence is lacking. Active motor rehabilitation appears to act on the cerebral microstructure, maintaining the integrity of the white matter in the corpus callosum and corticospinal tracts; these findings suggest that rehabilitation treatment should focus, above all, on voluntary movements. Unfortunately, fewer than 20% of pwMS perform moderate to vigorous physical activity, compared with 40% of healthy controls; added to this, we know that physical activity levels decline in relapsing-remitting pwMS as the disease progresses. Few people have been able to benefit from this type of therapeutic strategy. Physical activity, chosen on the basis of individual deficits, should be encouraged in pwMS, so as to become a lifestyle choice.

Finally, well-conducted longer-term trials on rehabilitation interventions, using clinically-relevant outcome measures in patients with different types of MS and different levels of disability, are urgently needed in order to establish definitively the effectiveness of many rehabilitation interventions in this population. This is indispensable as it would improve our ability to make evidence-based decisions regarding the allocation of resources. Clearly, a key priority is to determine who benefits most from specific rehabilitation interventions. Currently, too few methodologically-rigorous studies have addressed these issues. A lack of evidence, however, does not equate with evidence against a procedure. Drawing firm conclusions from systematic reviews that summarise evidence yielded by small numbers of RCTs, possibly of poor methodological quality, is overly simplistic. Evidence-based practice acknowledges this by ensuring that clinical judgments are based on broader evidence obtained using a range of research methodologies as well as the experiences of both clinicians and patients. This is clearly reflected both in the recommendations made by national and international MS guidelines and in the opinions of people affected by MS, who regard rehabilitation as an essential component of quality healthcare [15].

References

1. Andreasen AK, Stenager E, Dalgas U. The effect of exercise therapy on fatigue in multiple sclerosis. Mult Scler. 2011;17(9):1041–54.
2. Benedetti MG, Piperno R, Simoncini L, Bonato P, Tonini A, Giannini S. Gait abnormalities in minimally impaired multiple sclerosis patients. Mult Scler. 1999;5(5):363–8.
3. Bonzano L, Tacchino A, Brichetto G, Roccatagliata L, Dessypris A, Feraco P, Lopes De Carvalho ML, Battaglia MA, Mancardi GL, Bove M. Upper limb motor rehabilitation impacts white matter microstructure in multiple sclerosis. Neuroimage. 2014;15(90):107–16.
4. Brichetto G, Spallarossa P, de Carvalho ML, Battaglia MA. The effect of Nintendo® Wii® on balance in people with multiple sclerosis: a pilot randomized control study. Mult Scler. 2013;19(9):1219–21.
5. Briken S, Gold SM, Patra S, Vettorazzi E, Harbs D, Tallner A, Ketels G, Schulz KH, Heesen C. Effects of exercise on fitness and cognition in progressive MS: a randomized, controlled pilot trial. Mult Scler. 2014;20(3):382–90.
6. Bronson C, Brewerton K, Ong J, Palanca C. Sullivan SJ Does hippotherapy improve balance in persons with multiple sclerosis: a systematic review. Eur J Phys Rehabil Med. 2010;46 (3):347–53.
7. Burschka JM, Keune PM, Oy UH, Oschmann P, Kuhn P. Mindfulness-based interventions in multiple sclerosis: beneficial effects of Tai Chi on balance, coordination, fatigue and depression. BMC Neurol. 2014;23(14):165.
8. Cameron MH, Huisinga J. Objective and subjective measures reflect different aspects of balance in multiple sclerosis. J Rehabil Res Dev. 2013;50(10):1401–10.
9. Cameron MH, Nilsagård YE. Measurement and treatment of imbalance and fall risk in multiple sclerosis using the international classification of functioning, disability and health model. Phys Med Rehabil Clin N Am. 2013;24(2):337–54.
10. Castro-Sánchez AM, Matarán-Peñarrocha GA, Lara-Palomo I, Saavedra-Hernández M, Arroyo-Morales M, Moreno-Lorenzo C. Hydrotherapy for the treatment of pain in people with multiple sclerosis: a randomized controlled trial. Evid Based Complement Alternat Med. 2012;2012:473963.
11. Costantino C, Pedrini MF, Licari O. Neuromuscular taping versus sham therapy on muscular strength and motor performance in multiple sclerosis patients. Disabil Rehabil. 2016;38 (3):277–81.
12. Cramer H, Lauche R, Azizi H, Dobos G, Langhorst J Yoga for multiple sclerosis: a systematic review and meta-analysis. PLoS One. 2014;9(11).
13. Dewan N, MacDermid JC. Fall efficacy scale-international (FES-I). J Physiother. 2014; 60(1):60.
14. Findling O, Sellner J, Meier N, Allum JH, Vibert D, Lienert C, Mattle HP. Trunk sway in mildly disabled multiple sclerosis patients with and without balance impairment. Exp Brain Res. 2011;213(4):363–70.
15. Freeman JA, Playford ED. Rehabilitation therapy in MS; a short-term, expensive, placebo. Mult Scler. 2012;18(10):1379–81.
16. Freeman J. Progressive resistance therapy is not the best way to rehabilitate deficits due to multiple sclerosis: commentary. Mult Scler. 2014;20(2):145–6.

17. Gijbels D, Dalgas U, Romberg A, de Groot V, Bethoux F, Vaney C, Gebara B, Medina CS, Maamâgi H, Rasova K, de Noordhout BM, Knuts K, Feys P. Which walking capacity tests to use in multiple sclerosis? A multicentre study providing the basis for a core set. Mult Scler. 2012;18(3):364–71.
18. Goldman MD, Marrie RA, Cohen JA. Evaluation of the six-minute walk in multiple sclerosis subjects and healthy controls. Mult Scler. 2008;14(3):383–90.
19. Grasso MG, Troisi E, Rizzi F, Morelli D, Paolucci S. Prognostic factors in multidisciplinary rehabilitation treatment in multiple sclerosis: an outcome study. Mult Scler. 2005;11(6): 719–24.
20. Hartung HP, Aktas O. Evolution of multiple sclerosis treatment: next generation therapies meet next generation efficacy criteria. Lancet Neurol. 2011;10(4):293–5.
21. Haselkorn JK, Hughes C, Rae-Grant A, Henson LJ, Bever CT, Lo AC, Brown TR, Kraft GH, Getchius T, Gronseth G, Armstrong MJ, Narayanaswami P. Summary of comprehensive systematic review: Rehabilitation in multiple sclerosis: report of the guideline development, dissemination, and implementation subcommittee of the American academy of neurology. Neurology. 2015;85(21):1896–903.
22. Hobart JC, Riazi A, Lamping DL, Fitzpatrick R, Thompson AJ. Measuring the impact of MS on walking ability: the 12-item MS walking scale (MSWS-12). Neurology. 2003;60(1):31–6.
23. Jackson K, Edginton-Bigelow K, Cooper C. Merriman H A group kickboxing program for balance, mobility, and quality of life in individuals with multiple sclerosis: a pilot study. J Neurol Phys Ther. 2012;36(3):131–7.
24. Johansson S, Ytterberg C, Claesson IM, Lindberg J, Hillert J, Andersson M et al. High concurrent presence of disability in multiple sclerosis. Associations with perceived health. J Neurol. 2007;254(6):767–73.
25. Kalron A, Rosenblum U, Frid L, Achiron A Pilates exercise training vs. physical therapy for improving walking and balance in people with multiple sclerosis: a randomized controlled trial. Clin Rehabil. 2016. pii: 02692.
26. Kanekar N, Aruin AS. The role of clinical and instrumented outcome measures in balance control of individuals with multiple sclerosis. Mult Scler Int. 2013;2013:190162.
27. Khan F, Turner-Stokes L, Ng L, Kilpatrick T. Multidisciplinary rehabilitation for adults with multiple sclerosis. Cochrane Database Syst Rev. 2007;(2).
28. Kjølhede T, Vissing K, Dalgas U. Multiple sclerosis and progressive resistance training: a systematic review. Mult Scler. 2012;18(9):1215–28.
29. Kurtzke JF. Rating neurologic impairment in multiple sclerosis: an expanded disability status scale (EDSS). Neurology. 1983;33:1444–52.
30. Langdon DW, Thompson AJ. Multiple sclerosis: a preliminary study of selected variables affecting rehabilitation outcome. Mult Scler. 1999;5(2):94–100.
31. Larocca NG. Impact of walking impairment in multiple sclerosis: perspectives of patients and care partners. Patient. 2011;4(3):189–201.
32. Latimer-Cheung AE, Martin Ginis KA, Hicks AL, Motl RW, Pilutti LA, Duggan M, Wheeler G, Persad R, Smith KM. Development of evidence-informed physical activity guidelines for adults with multiple sclerosis. Arch Phys Med Rehabil. 2013;94(9):1829–36.
33. Liberatore G, Clarelli F, Nuara A, Ungaro D, Gatti R, Rovaris M, Martinelli V, Comola M, Comi G, Rossi P, Martinelli-Boneschi F. Predictors of effectiveness of multidisciplinary rehabilitation treatment on motor dysfunction inmultiple sclerosis. Mult Scler. 2013.
34. Marcham G.A facilitation and co-ordination therapy approach to the treatment of multiple sclerosis. Aust J Physiother. 1974;20(1):23–5.
35. Mark VW, Taub E, Uswatte G, Bashir K, Cutter GR, Bryson CC, Bishop-McKay S, Bowman MH. Constraint-induced movement therapy for the lower extremities in multiple sclerosis: case series with 4-year follow-up. Arch Phys Med Rehabil. 2013;94(4):753–60.
36. Markowitz CE. Multiple sclerosis update. Am J Manag Care. 2013;19(16 Suppl):s294–300.

37. Motl RW, Arnett PA, Smith MM, Barwick FH, Ahlstrom B, Stover EJ. Worsening of symptoms is associated with lower physical activity levels in individuals with multiple sclerosis. Mult Scler. 2008;14(1):140–2.
38. Motl RW, Gosney JL. Effect of exercise training on quality of life in multiple sclerosis: a meta-analysis. Mult Scler. 2008;14(1):129–35.
39. Motl RW, Pilutti L, Sandroff BM, Dlugonski D, Sosnoff JJ, Pula JH. Accelerometry as a measure of walking behavior in multiple sclerosis. Acta Neurol Scand. 2013;127(6):384–90. https://doi.org/10.1111/ane.12036 Epub 2012 Dec 13.
40. Ozgen G, Karapolat H, Akkoc Y, Yuceyar N. Is customized vestibular rehabilitation effective in patients with multiple sclerosis? a randomized controlled trial. Eur J Phys Rehabil Med. 2016;52(4):466–78.
41. Paltamaa J, Sjögren T, Peurala SH, Heinonen A. Effects of physiotherapy interventions on balance in multiple sclerosis: a systematic review and meta-analysis of randomized controlled trials. J Rehabil Med. 2012;44(10):811–23.
42. Pau M, Coghe G, Atzeni C, Corona F, Pilloni G, Marrosu MG, Cocco E, Galli M. Novel characterization of gait impairments in people with multiple sclerosis by means of the gait profile score. J Neurol Sci. 2014;345(1–2):159–63.
43. Pau M, Coghe G, Corona F, Marrosu MG, Cocco E Effect of spasticity on kinematics of gait and muscular activation in people with multiple sclerosis. J Neurol Sci. 2015;358(1–2): 339–44 (2015.09.352).
44. Petajan JH, Gappmaier E, White AT, Spencer MK, Mino L, Hicks RW. Impact of aerobic training on fitness and quality of life in multiple sclerosis. Ann Neurol. 1996;39(4):432–41.
45. Pilutti LA, Greenlee TA, Motl RW, Nickrent MS, Petruzzello SJ. Effects of exercise training on fatigue in multiple sclerosis: a meta-analysis. Psychosom Med. 2013;75(6):575–80.
46. Pilutti LA, Platta ME, Motl RW, Latimer-Cheung AE. The safety of exercise training in multiple sclerosis: a systematic review. J Neurol Sci. 2014;343(1–2):3–7.
47. Polman CH, Reingold SC, Banwell B, Clanet M, Cohen JA, Filippi M, et al. Diagnostic criteria for multiple sclerosis: 2010 revisions to the McDonald criteria. Ann Neurol. 2011;69 (2):292–302.
48. Pompa A, Morone G, Iosa M, Pace L, Catani S, Casillo P, Clemenzi A, Troisi E, Tonini A, Paolucci S, Grasso MG. Does robot-assisted gait training improve ambulation in highly disabled multiple sclerosis people?. Mult Scler: A pilot randomized control trial; 2016.
49. Rietberg MB, Brooks D, Uitdehaag BM, Kwakkel G. Exercise therapy for multiple sclerosis. Cochrane Database Syst Rev. 2005; (1).
50. Sá MJ. Exercise therapy and multiple sclerosis: a systematic review. J Neurol. 2014;261 (9):1651–61.
51. Sitjà Rabert M, Rigau Comas D, Fort Vanmeerhaeghe A, Santoyo Medina C, Roqué i Figuls M, Romero-Rodríguez D, Bonfill Cosp Whole-body vibration training for patients with neurodegenerative disease. Cochrane Database Syst Rev. 2012;2.
52. Snook EM, Motl RW, Gliottoni RC. The effect of walking mobility on the measurement of physical activity using accelerometry in multiple sclerosis. Clin Rehabil. 2009;23(3):248–58.
53. Socie MJ MJ, Motl RW, Pula JH, Sandroff BM, Sosnoff JJ. Gait variability and disability in multiple sclerosis., Gait and Posture. 2013;38(1):51–5.
54. Spooren AI, Timmermans AA. Seelen HA Motor training programs of arm and hand in patients with MS according to different levels of the ICF: a systematic review. BMC Neurol. 2012;2(12):49.
55. Straudi S, Fanciullacci C, Martinuzzi C, Pavarelli C, Rossi B, Chisari C, Basaglia N. The effects of robot-assisted gait training in progressive multiple sclerosis: A randomized controlled trial. Mult Scler. 2015.
56. Swinnen E, Beckwée D, Pinte D, Meeusen R, Baeyens JP. Kerckhofs E treadmill training in multiple sclerosis: can body weight support or robot assistance provide added value? A systematic review. Mult Scler Int. 2012;2012:240274.
57. Toomey E, Coote SB. Physical rehabilitation interventions in nonambulatory people with multiple sclerosis: systematic review. Int J Rehabil Res. 2012;35(4):281–91.

58. Tyler ME, Kaczmarek KA, Rust KL, Subbotin AM. Skinner KL1, Danilov YP. Non-invasive neuromodulation to improve gait in chronic multiple sclerosis: a randomized double blind controlled pilot trial. J Neuroeng Rehabil. 2014;1(11):79.
59. Verza R, Carvalho ML, Battaglia MA, Uccelli MM. An interdisciplinary approach to evaluating the need for assistive technology reduces equipment abandonment. Mult Scler. 2006;12(1):88–93.
60. Wening J, Ford J, Jouett LD. Orthotics and FES for maintenance of walking in patients with MS. Dis Mon. 2013;59(8):284–9.

Balance and Walking Training in Ataxic Neuropathies

Philippe Thoumie, Maeva Ferrari, Samy Bendaya, Michèle Mane and Besma Missaoui

1 Introduction

Neuropathies are characterized by a sensorimotor deficit of the extremities, especially the lower limbs. According to the clinical signs, they can be divided into motor, sensory or trophic forms. With regard to the sensory forms, the main disorders are subjective and objective sensory disorders without motor impairment. Ataxic neuropathies are severe deep sensory disorders that, in turn, cause balance and walking disorders, with a reduction of distal sensitivity on tuning fork testing and greater imbalance with eyes closed (Romberg sign).

2 Consequences of Proprioceptive Disorders on Balance Function

Proprioception of the lower limbs plays an important role in static and dynamic balance. As early as the middle of the 19th century, Romberg showed the main signs of so-called locomotor ataxia. Through experimental studies of manipulation of sensory inputs, the consequences of damage to proprioceptive pathways soon became well understood.

The main characteristic of proprioception loss at the lower limbs is visual dependence, which the Romberg sign clearly shows. Loss of balance with eyes closed (under the shower for example) or difficulty walking in the dark are the first symptoms that patients complain of.

P. Thoumie (✉) · M. Ferrari · S. Bendaya · M. Mane · B. Missaoui
Service de Rééducation Neuro-Orthopédique, APHP Hôpital Rothschild,
5 Rue Santerre 75012, Paris, France
e-mail: philippe.thoumie@rth.aphp.fr

G. Sandrini et al. (eds.), *Advanced Technologies for the Rehabilitation of Gait and Balance Disorders*, Biosystems & Biorobotics 19,
https://doi.org/10.1007/978-3-319-72736-3_15

In dynamic conditions, e.g. while walking, balance is also impaired but much less so than in static conditions [1] because there is less use of proprioceptive afferents during movement than during balance moments [2]. Therefore, some ataxic patients can walk without a cane but need to lean when they pause. Patients thus keep their dynamic balance while walking, which nonetheless remains ataxic (loss of controlled leaning on the heel on the ground and increase of the base of support, both of which improve under visual control).

3 Presentation of Ataxic Neuropathies

Ataxic neuropathies can be linked to various disorders [3]:

- Ganglionopathies or sensory neuropathies (dysimmune, medication-related, mainly linked to platinum compounds, or hereditary).
- Demyelinating polyneuropathies, dysimmune or associated with IgM monoclonal gammopathies (anti-MAG neuropathies) and chronic idiopathic polyradiculoneuropathy with predominantly sensory disorders or, rarely, exclusively with sensory disorders.
- Axonal neuropathy with infectious, toxic, metabolic or degenerative etiology.

These different diseases are all characterized by peripheral nerve impairment involving large sensory fibers. Their differences lie in their etiologies and in certain possible specific treatments aimed at controlling their evolution.

Pharmacological treatment of some of these diseases has improved recently [4] and specific evaluation scales have been developed (some of which are presented later).

In sequential treatments, as well as treatments using immunoglobulins, we have to adapt patient care to the frequency of the treatment. This aspect also influences the evaluation of our patient care as consideration should be given to the impact of the treatment on neurological disease and, in particular, on fatigue that may be related to the underlying disease. We carry out our evaluation tests mostly during the « on » phase; the goal is to define our objectives based on the symptoms not reacting to the basic treatment and to avoid attributing positive pharmacological results to physiotherapy.

4 Clinical Trials of Rehabilitation: Summary of Results

Physiotherapy has long been considered for neuropathies as well for other chronic nervous system diseases. The authors of a Cochrane review [5], evaluating this aspect, found only one trial that fully met their inclusion criteria, and also included an additional two trials that assessed outcomes less than eight weeks after randomization. The three studies included 82 patients. Physiotherapy for neuropathies includes muscle strengthening [6, 7], balance work [8] and endurance work [9] with differences in terms of duration (3 to 24 weeks) and type of reeducation training (muscular strength training or balance rehabilitation).

Despite the low overall number of patients involved in these studies, it seems that exercise and muscle strengthening do not worsen neurological injuries and that they have a short-term positive effect not only on criteria such as muscle strength, balance and endurance, but also on the quality of life of these patients: Ruhland and Shields [7] showed increases on the SF-36 subscales physical activity (+25 points), social integration (+8 points) and emotional factors (+11 points). This shows that rehabilitation in neuropathy can have a positive impact. However, the programs offered so far focused on one aspect of rehabilitation without taking into account the nature of the impairment; therefore, patients presenting very different clinical aspects were evaluated together (i.e. those with more motor deficiency or mainly sensory disorders). Other studies carried out in different clinical situations show that the degree of sensory disorders is directly linked to the risk of falling in neuropathy in the elderly [10], with a relative risk factor of 17 for falls and 13 for instability, and consequences on muscle strength deficit, which in turn has an impact on walking speed in other diseases such as multiple sclerosis [11].

Two recent experimental studies also showed that vibration stimulation on the soles of the feet increases the stability of elderly patients or patients suffering from neuropathy [12, 13].

5 Clinical Evaluation of Ataxic Neuropathies

Neurological examination allows the diagnosis of ataxic neuropathies when deep sensory disorders are more prominent than other sensory and motor disorders.

Several scales have been considered, especially for inflammatory chronic polyradiculoneuropathies (these are among the most common ataxic neuropathies) in order to create a quantitative evaluation of the various corresponding deficiencies and impairments.

5.1 Motricity Index

This is based on clinical evaluation of muscles according to the classical scale (0–5) of the Medical Research Council, validated in Guillain-Barré syndrome [14] on key muscles such as the anterior tibialis muscle. This muscle rating derives from the scale considered for the Charcot Marie Tooth neuropathy (hereditary neuropathy) [15].

0 = normal
1 = motor disorders of anterior tibialis muscle (4 + to 4−) walking on heels and toes
2 = motor disorder of anterior tibialis muscle less or equal to 3 (heel −, tip+)
3 = anterior tibialis muscle less than 3 and disorder of triceps surae (heel −, tip −)
4 = anterior tibialis muscle less to 3 and proximal disorder (gluteus medius, psoas)

5.2 *Sensibility Test*

Merkies et al. proposed an evaluation, based on application of pin-prick and turning fork testing, and the Weber test, to the upper and lower limbs to obtain a score between 0 and 20 [16].

Score	Pin prick uppers limbs	Pin prick lowers limbs	Tuning fork upper limbs	Tuning fork lowers limbs	Weber index
Normal = 0	Index DIP +	Hallus IP +	Index DIP +	Hallus IP +	<5 mm
1	Index DIP −	Hallus IP −	Index DIP −	Hallus IP −	5–9 mm
2	Ulnar Styloid −	Medial malleolus −	Ulnar styloid −	Medial malleolus −	10–14 mm
3	Epicondylitis −	Patella −	Epicondylitis −	Patella −	15–19 mm
4	Acromio Clavicular −	Anterior superior iliac spine −	Acromio clavicular −	Anterior superior iliac spine −	20 mm and +

5.3 *ODSS (Overall Disability Sum Score)*

This is a mixed scale (0–12 points), including a scale of impairment of the upper limbs (0–5 points) and lower limbs (0–7 points), deriving from a functional evaluation [17] and validated for chronic inflammatory neuropathy.

5.4 Evaluation of Walking and Balance Disorders

This evaluation takes place through a series of clinical tests and validated instruments. These are generic tests usually used for balance or walking disorders in neurological pathologies or in the elderly.

- Clinical examination using the Berg Balance scale (BBS) [18], the timed Get-up and Go test (TUG), the functional Reach Test (FRT) [19].
- Instrumental analysis of balance on a force platform, both with eyes open, eyes closed and on foam.
- Instrumental analysis of walking using the Locomètre®.
- Analysis of muscle strength of the knee extensors and flexors during isokinetic contraction.

We also evaluate walking on stairs and falls, and look for avoidance behaviours which are positive if they help the patient adapt to the evolution of the disease but detrimental if they lead to social isolation or falling phobia.

6 Day Hospital Rehabilitation Protocol

The program carried out at the Rothschild Hospital aims to provide proprioceptive stimulation based on vibratory stimulation of soles of the feet, balance work with decrease of visual afferents, and rehabilitation for muscle deconditioning.

Three sessions, lasting 3 h, take place every week for 4 weeks; each session includes:

Sensory training (20 min)

Exercises to be carried out seated, aiming at increasing basic sensitivity: alternation of hot and cold baths, vibratory stimulation above the perception threshold of the soles of both feet with Vibralgic® (Fig. 1).

Exercises to be carried out seated or lying down, with the aim of improving dexterity: pressure exercises, handling and picking up objects, writing.

Exercises to be carried out standing, such as walking with eyes closed on different surfaces and different volumes.

Range of motion improvement

Non-specific and specific mobilizations depending on the joints being evaluated, possibly after immersion of the feet in a basin.

Analytical muscular strengthening (20 min)

Strengthening of the muscles found to be weaker on testing. Exercises are split up, alternated in time and type, mainly isotonic, and performed at 60% of maximum

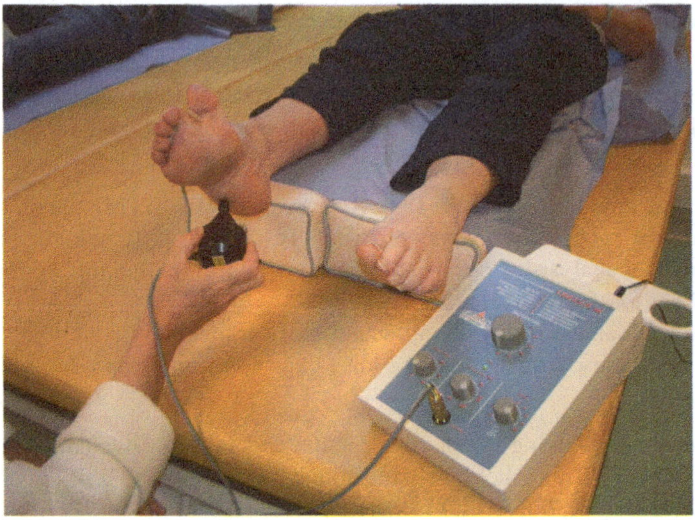

Fig. 1 Vibratory stimulation, above the perception threshold of the soles of both feet, with Vibralgic®

resistance, with two series of 10 repetitions during the day, according to the pain and fatigability of the patient.

Balance training (30 min)

This includes static and dynamic balance training.

Static balance: the therapist can choose from the following: exercises to be carried out with eyes open, eyes closed, with shoes on or bare footed, with head movements, on a stable surface, on a steady surface and then an unsteady surface. The exercises progress from the least to the most difficult and are adapted to the patients: work on seated balance: first steady surface and feet, and then unsteady; Klein ball with exercises for the upper limbs; standing up, on all fours then upright on two knees and kneeling on one knee; work on standing position introducing an unsteady surface (Fig. 2) then double task involving upper limbs; work on standing on one foot:

Dynamic balance: different walking exercises, from the least to the most difficult, should be considered in order to stimulate simultaneously:

- **Proprioceptive compensation**: on irregular surface, on an inclined plane, walking backwards and with little light;
- **Visual compensation**: walking sideways, partial vision and walking over obstacles (Fig. 3).

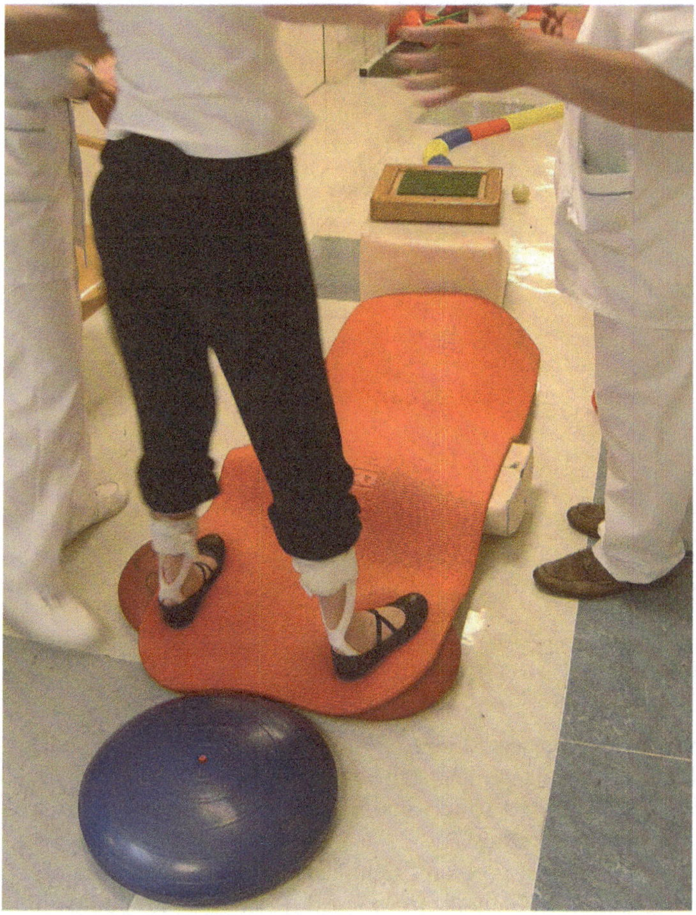

Fig. 2 Standing position on an unsteady surface

Two other programs may be associated with this balance training program:

- Manual rehabilitation of grip: this is done with occupational therapists, according to the initial evaluation (on a scale of 400 points). The approach is similar to that for lower limbs but will not be explained here.
- Endurance training for improvement of aerobic capacities (20–30 min). This is done on ergometric bicycles with maximum resistance or treadmills, at 60% of the theoretical heart rate.

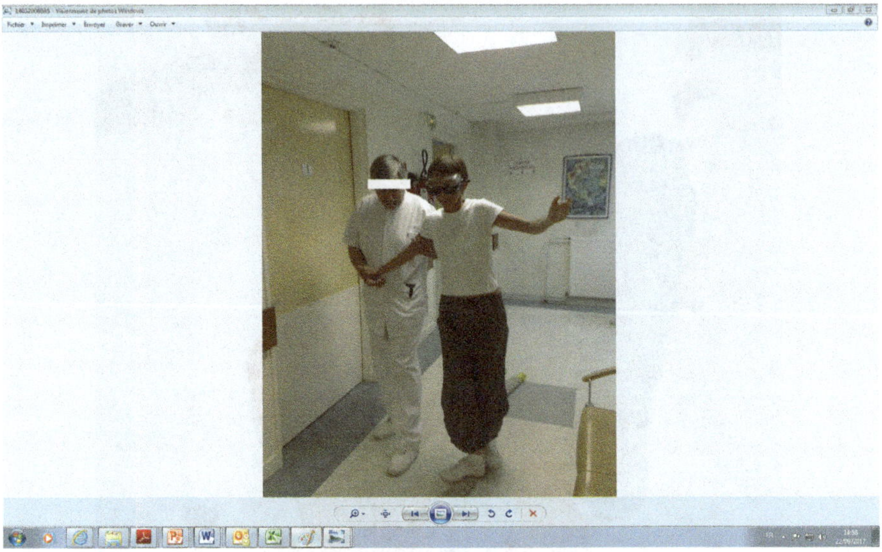

Fig. 3 Visual compensation training: walking sideways, partial vision and walking over obstacles

7 Summary of Our Experience

Our experience was presented in a recent paper [20]. The main goal of our study was to characterize balance and gait impairment in thirty patients with proprioceptive ataxia and to assess the value of a rehabilitation program through a preliminary non-controlled study.

Following the training program, significant improvements were observed on all clinical balance tests. Gains corresponded to 4.7 ± 4.8 points on the BBS, 5.6 ± 5 cm on the FRT, and -2.2 ± 2.4 s on the TUG. After training, patients unable to stand eyes with closed numbered 11/30 (vs 15/30 before) and patients unable to stand with eyes open on a foam surface numbered 8/30 (vs 12/30 before), but these changes were not significant. A significant correlation was observed between the pallesthetic score and instability assessed with sway area on a firm surface with eyes open at the final evaluation.

Limited changes on instrumental tests were observed after training: a trend to reduction of sway area was observed during a balance test on a force platform in eyes open condition and an increased cadence was observed at different velocities corresponding to an only slightly but significantly higher speed during spontaneous gait.

The confounding effects of age and neuropathy-related impairment were assessed using correlation studies. No correlation was found between age and pallesthetic score but a significant and negative correlation was observed between age and FRT values. A positive effect of training was observed on the BBS, without change when considering age as a covariate.

The conclusion of this study is that all patients with sensory ataxia, including the oldest, can benefit from rehabilitation aimed at improving their dynamic balance. Nevertheless, improvement in static conditions was not observed in our instrumental evaluations and patients with high degrees of sensory loss remained at greater risk of visual dependence despite rehabilitation.

8 Conclusion

Ataxic neuropathies are associated with severe balance impairment affecting static balance and gait. These changes can be improved by following a training program aimed at compensating for a variable part of the sensory impairment.

This training program is composed of a multisensory approach using compensation with tactile sensory and visual control.

In our experience, dynamic balance appears to be more improved than static balance at the end of such a training program. The long-term effects depend on the origin of the neuropathy and whether patients have the opportunity to continue with regular exercises.

References

1. Nardone A, Grasso M, Schieppati M. Balance control in peripheral neuropathy: are patients equally unstable under static and dynamic conditions? Gait Posture. 2006;23:364–73.
2. Capaday C, Stein RB. Amplitude modulation of the soleus H-reflex in the human during walking and standing. J Neurosci. 1986;6:1308–13.
3. Kuntzer T, Antoine JC, Steck AJ. Clinical features and pathophysiological basis of sensory neuronopathies (ganglionopathies). Muscle Nerve. 2004;30:255–68.
4. Leger JM. A review of the medical management of chronic inflammatory demyelinating polyradiculoneuropathy. Expert Opin Pharmacother. 2005;6:569–82.
5. White CM, Pritchard J, Turner-Stokes L. Exercise for people with peripheral neuropathy. Cochrane Database Syst Rev 2004;CD003904.
6. Lindeman E, Leffers P, Spaans F, Drukker J, Reulen J, Kerckhoffs M, et al. Strength training in patients with myotonic dystrophy and hereditary motor and sensory neuropathy: a randomized clinical trial. Arch Phys Med Rehabil. 1995;76:612–20.
7. Ruhland JL, Shields RK. The effects of a home exercise program on impairment and health-related quality of life in persons with chronic peripheral neuropathies. Phys Ther. 1997;77:1026–39.
8. Richardson JK, Sandman D, Vela S. A focused exercise regimen improves clinical measures of balance in patients with peripheral neuropathy. Arch Phys Med Rehabil. 2001;82:205–9.
9. Pitetti KH, Barrett PJ, Abbas D. Endurance exercise training in Guillain-Barre syndrome. Arch Phys Med Rehabil. 1993;74:761–5.
10. Richardson JK, Hurvitz EA. Peripheral neuropathy: a true risk factor for falls. J Gerontol A Biol Sci Med Sci. 1995;50:M211–5.
11. Thoumie P, Mevellec E. Relation between walking speed and muscle strength is affected by somatosensory loss in multiple sclerosis. J Neurol Neurosurg Psychiatry. 2002;73:313–5.

12. Priplata AA, Patritti BL, Niemi JB, Hughes R, Gravelle DC, Lipsitz LA, et al. Noise-enhanced balance control in patients with diabetes and patients with stroke. Ann Neurol. 2006;59:4–12.
13. Priplata AA, Niemi JB, Harry JD, Lipsitz LA, Collins JJ. Vibrating insoles and balance control in elderly people. Lancet. 2003;362:1123–4.
14. Kleyweg RP, van der Meche FG, Schmitz PI. Interobserver agreement in the assessment of muscle strength and functional abilities in Guillain-Barre syndrome. Muscle Nerve. 1991;14:1103–9.
15. Shy ME, Blake J, Krajewski K, Fuerst DR, Laura M, Hahn AF, et al. Reliability and validity of the CMT neuropathy score as a measure of disability. Neurology. 2005;64:1209–14.
16. Merkies IS, Schmitz PI, van der Meche FG, van Doorn PA. Psychometric evaluation of a new sensory scale in immune-mediated polyneuropathies. Inflammatory Neuropathy Cause and Treatment (INCAT) Group. Neurology. 2000;54:943–9.
17. Merkies IS, Schmitz PI, van der Meche FG, Samijn JP, van Doorn PA. Clinimetric evaluation of a new overall disability scale in immune mediated polyneuropathies. J Neurol Neurosurg Psychiatry. 2002;72:596–601.
18. Berg KO, Wood-Dauphinee SL, Williams JI, Maki B. Measuring balance in the elderly: validation of an instrument. Can J Public Health. 1992;83(Suppl 2):S7–11.
19. Duncan PW, Weiner DK, Chandler J, Studenski S. Functional reach: a new clinical measure of balance. J Gerontol. 1990;45:M192–7.
20. Missaoui B, Thoumie P. Balance training in ataxic neuropathies. Effects on balance and gait parameters. Gait Posture. 2013;38(3):471–6.

Approach to Gait and Balance Rehabilitation in Spinal Cord Injury

Federica Tamburella, Marcella Masciullo, Marco Molinari and Giorgio Scivoletto

1 Introduction

In 1700 BC, the Edwin Smith Papyrus, an ancient Egyptian medical text, described spinal cord injury (SCI) as an "ailment not to be treated." [1] SCI can actually be defined as a lesion that occurs in any portion of the spinal cord and results in complete or incomplete impairment of motor, sensory and autonomic functions below the level of the injury [1]. The aetiology of SCI may be traumatic (TSCI) or non-traumatic (NTSCI).

The estimated global incidence of SCI is 40 to 80 new cases per million population per year, based on quality country-level incidence studies of SCI of all causes. This means that every year, between 250,000 and 500,000 people become spinal cord injured [2]. The proportion made up of TSCI cases varies widely, and appears to differ across regions. Historically, up to 90% of SCI is of traumatic origin, but data from the most recent epidemiological studies indicate a trend towards an increase in the incidence of NTSCI. The NTSCI population is generally older and affected by progressive diseases; this population has more costly care needs, but for shorter periods of time [2].

F. Tamburella · M. Masciullo · M. Molinari · G. Scivoletto (✉)
Spinal Cord Unit, IRCCS Fondazione S. Lucia, via Ardeatina 306, 00179 Rome, Italy
e-mail: g.scivoletto@hsantalucia.it

F. Tamburella · G. Scivoletto
Spinal Rehabilitation Laboratory, IRCCS Fondazione S. Lucia, via Ardeatina 306, 00179 Rome, Italy

M. Masciullo · M. Molinari
Laboratory of Robotic Neurorehabilitation, IRCCS Fondazione S. Lucia, via Ardeatina 306, 00179 Rome, Italy

G. Sandrini et al. (eds.), *Advanced Technologies for the Rehabilitation of Gait and Balance Disorders*, Biosystems & Biorobotics 19,
https://doi.org/10.1007/978-3-319-72736-3_16

Improvements in SCI recognition, evaluation and pre-hospital management, as well as in trauma care services, general clinical care and rehabilitation services, have resulted in a longer life expectancy for people with SCI in high-income countries, together with a decreased risk of mortality from secondary conditions [2].

People with TSCI go through three consecutive clinical phases after sustaining the lesion: acute, sub-acute and chronic. In the acute phase, immediately after the lesion, they need to be stabilised. In the sub-acute phase, when they are rehabilitation hospital inpatients, major cognitive and physical rehabilitation interventions are implemented with the aim of maximising their functional outcome and independence. Once in the chronic phase, when they are no longer being treated intensively in hospital, patients undergo less intensive rehabilitation interventions as outpatients. Indeed, it is now generally recognised that SCI patients, in particular those with complete or near-complete lesions, can develop severe and often life-threatening complications even in the chronic phase. For instance, muscle wasting, osteopenia or osteoporosis, hormone dysregulation, and cardiovascular problems are among the problems typically encountered in chronic SCI. For this reason, these patients require continuous rehabilitation training.

In affected subjects the overall goal of rehabilitation interventions is to help them regain a level of independence compatible with a good quality of life. Quality of life can be scored in different ways: from the patient's perspective, restoration of bladder and bowel function is the principal goal for subjects with paraplegia, while subjects with tetraplegia consider recovery of upper limb function to be a priority [3].

Recovery of locomotor ability is also a high priority for SCI subjects, independently of their disease severity, time since injury, and age at the time of injury [3], and is thus becoming the target of several SCI rehabilitation approaches. In fact, walking recovery is one of the main goals after SCI, and even though it is almost never attainable in subjects with complete lesions, it is a realistic objective for those with incomplete lesions, among whom recovery of walking has been rated at first place among rehabilitation objectives [4].

2 Cortical and Spinal Neuroplasticity

The main aims of rehabilitation in an individual with SCI are to compensate for the functional loss and to make use of those parts of the sensory-motor system that are still intact [5]. In general, SCI is followed by cortical re-organisation, and there is evidence that the sensory-motor cortex may play a role in the recovery of function in SCI subjects [6]. This re-organisation may be attributed to the exploitation of both pre-existing and new neural circuits [7]. Re-activation of parts of the sensory-motor system that are still intact [8] can be optimised during rehabilitation by using task-specific sensory cues and by favouring the recruitment of both spinal circuitries and spared supra-spinal connections.

Neuroplasticity after SCI occurs not only at cortical level but also at other anatomical and physiological levels of the central nervous system, such as the spinal cord and brainstem [9], and it consists, for example, of changes in synaptic formations and synaptic strength, axonal sprouting and changes in intracellular properties [10, 11].

Indeed, as described in several animal studies, neuronal circuits for locomotion in the spinal cord have the capacity to 'learn' through training independently of their connection to the brain [12]. The mechanisms underlying this training-induced plasticity that leads to improved recovery of locomotion include, among others, adaptation of neurotransmitter systems within the spinal cord (glycinergic and GABAergic systems) and enhanced collateral sprouting [13]. On the basis of findings in animal studies, methods for training functional movements (e.g. stepping) have been successfully developed for individuals with incomplete SCI [14, 15].

Spinal neuronal circuits below the level of the lesion can be activated by an appropriate afferent input, leading to training effects [16]. By contrast, the movement disorders typically observed after SCI, e.g., spastic movement disorders, are due to defective utilisation of afferent inputs in combination with secondary compensatory mechanisms [17]. Rehabilitation interventions after SCI should therefore focus on exploiting the plasticity of neuronal circuits, i.e., at supraspinal and/or spinal level, rather than focusing on improving isolated clinical signs, such as muscle tone or reflex excitability.

3 Activity-Dependent Plasticity-Based Gait Rehabilitation and Its Physiological Prerequisites

Gait rehabilitation strategies are currently based on the above-mentioned evidence demonstrating that the adult mammalian cortex and spinal cord have a remarkable capacity for activity-dependent plasticity when exposed to walking training. In people who retain some control of their leg muscles, treadmill training with body weight support, performed according to the rules of spinal locomotion, may result in an improvement of locomotion, as reflected in greater speed, strength, coordination and endurance, and reduced need for assistive devices.

The success of the training depends on the presence of various physiological prerequisites necessary to evoke a pattern of muscle activation similar to that found in individuals without injury of the nervous system, as this is the basic requirement for facilitating meaningful plasticity [16].

In accordance with the rules of spinal locomotion, body un-loading and re-loading are considered crucially important for inducing training effects on the neurological locomotor centres, because the afferent input from receptors signalling contact forces during the stance phase (corresponding to the initiation of newborn stepping by foot sole contact) is essential for activation of the spinal neuronal circuits underlying locomotion.

The most important sensory input for locomotion comes from stretch- and load-sensitive mechanoreceptors located in the muscles and skin. Furthermore, in humans, skin receptors on the dorsal foot play a role during the swing phase of walking over obstacles [18].

Load information for proprioceptive input comes from leg extensor muscles, and is transmitted as Ib afferent signals from Golgi tendon organs, and probably also from mechanoreceptors in the sole of the foot [19–21]. This information is thought to be integrated into polysynaptic spinal reflex pathways that adapt the autonomous locomotor pattern to the actual ground condition. Furthermore, it is assumed that Ib afferent input from leg extensors during the stance phase inhibits flexor activity.

Afferent input from load receptors is a crucial factor, necessary to trigger a locomotor EMG pattern in individuals with SCI [20, 21]. This affirmation is based on the observation that without loading of the sole of the foot during the stance phase no meaningful leg muscle activation occurs in individuals with complete SCI during supported stepping. The role of this specific afferent input is to generate and shape the locomotor pattern, to control phase transitions, and to reinforce ongoing activity.

In addition, as observed in studies in cats [22], hip extension movements, i.e. hip joint-related afferent input (more than knee or ankle joint excursions), are essential for the initiation of the swing phase and the generation of a locomotor EMG pattern in people with incomplete SCI [23]. In addition to load receptor information, a hip joint-related afferent input was shown to be required for the generation of a locomotor pattern, as has also been shown to be the case for stepping in human infants [23].

In accordance with animal models, in motor complete paraplegic subjects, the execution of assisted stepping movements within a driven gait orthosis and with restricted movements of the hips (blocked knees) induces a normal pattern of leg electromyographic activity, thus highlighting the significance of hip joint receptors in the generation of locomotor activity [24]. These assisted stepping movements, restricted to imposed ankle joint movements, were followed by no, or only focal reflex responses in the stretched muscles [24].

4 Implicit and Explicit Learning

During treadmill training and conventional gait training, both explicit and implicit clues can be used to improve the recovery of patients. An example of explicit input is visual feedback. Augmented visual feedback is an approach commonly used to help patients with incomplete SCI detect stepping errors. For example, clinicians usually place visual cues on the floor to help patients to see the difference between expected and actual stride lengths [25]. According to the visual goal, patients modify their motor plan to minimise errors. This requires the engagement of a cognitive process (i.e., the patient makes a conscious decision to take a longer step), and it is regarded as an example of explicit learning. On the other hand, the use of a resistance applied to the leg during the swing phase can be regarded as an implicit input.

While swing resistance and augmented visual feedback may induce different motor learning processes, they may modulate stride/step length through similar pathways, including: (a) modification of motor commands for stepping at supraspinal level; (b) enhancement of neural descending drive in the residual spinal pathways. Specifically, error signals detected by the visual and proprioceptive channels can induce motor adaptation, causing recalibration of motor commands for stepping so as to minimise the difference between the actual and expected stride/step length [26]. The neural descending drive appears to increase when an individual moves against resistance [27]. Providing augmented visual feedback during gait training can enhance active involvement and thus increase descending drive and motor outputs [28]. These considerations lead us to postulate that, in patients with incomplete SCI, providing swing resistance and augmented feedback together (multisensory feedback) may enhance gait training outcomes compared to providing either type of feedback alone (unisensory feedback). Specifically, multisensory feedback may further augment neural descending drive in the residual spinal pathways. Also, error-driven learning may be more effective (i.e., effects may last longer) when different learning pathways (implicit and explicit) are engaged simultaneously. However, the literature on the effect, on motor training outcomes, of combining implicit and explicit learning is contradictory. While some investigators reported beneficial effects of explicit information on implicit motor learning [29], others reported detrimental [30, 31] or modest effects [32, 33]. These contradictory findings may result from a combination of factors such as task differences, the type, timing and salience of the explicit information, and the characteristics of participants [34].

5 Other Approaches: Balance Training and Sensory Enhancement

Functional gait training is classically considered the most effective approach for promoting recovery of gait function [9], however, in addition to task-specific training, ad hoc protocols aimed at improving impaired functions involved in gait control might also help to boost recovery. Below we examine the effects of isolated balance training and enhancement of somatosensory inputs in reducing spasticity and improving both balance and gait functions.

Lower extremity muscle strength has commonly been considered the main factor affecting walking function in individuals with SCI [35]. Therefore, the aim of most rehabilitation approaches has been to reinforce the lower extremities. However, as recently reported by our group, many factors besides muscle strength influence the recovery of walking function [36]. In particular, we demonstrated that balance and spasticity, as well as weight, are key factors affecting walking performance in SCI subjects [36].

Good balance allowed patients to walk with fewer aids and also enabled them to record lower times (i.e. to walk faster) on a timed test and to walk longer distances [36]. Recently, other authors claimed similar findings in a randomised clinical trial where balance was used together with walking speed and other outcome measures [37].

Furthermore, lack of postural control is regarded as one of the main reasons underlying the fear of falling observed among people with SCI during rehabilitation programmes aimed at improving their ability to walk and stand [38, 39]. The incidence of falls in people with SCI is 75%, which is higher than that reported for healthy subjects aged 65 and older (35%) [39], and also higher than the rates reported for subjects with neurological disease resulting in peripheral neuropathy (50%) or with Parkinson's disease (38–62%) [40]. In addition, in SCI subjects, the incidence of fractures due to accidental falls has been reported to be 18%, which is 5–6% greater than the incidence in healthy older adults.

Various groups have addressed the issue of balance, suggesting it to be important in determining gait performance after SCI [36, 37, 40]. Accordingly, several authors have examined the efficacy of re-education of balance function in SCI patients through task-specific oriented training [41], focusing on sitting [41–44] and standing balance recovery [45, 46]. However, only a single study addressed the efficacy of task-specific balance training based on visual biofeedback (vBFB) in supporting walking functions in chronic motor incomplete SCI patients [47]. The results indicated that vBFB training improves balance and gait in these subjects. Furthermore, inclusion of vBFB training in a rehabilitation protocol resulted in greater gait improvements than were obtained with conventional gait rehabilitation alone, and these improvements were maintained at follow-up examinations.

With regard to the enhancement of sensory inputs, SCI is followed by cortical re-organisation which, as already mentioned above, consists of re-organisation of pre-existing neural circuits and the formation of new ones. Additionally, recovery of function can also be related to re-activation of parts of the sensory-motor system that are still intact [48]. It has been suggested that these neuroplasticity phenomena might be improved, and supraspinal centres activated, by exteroceptive afferents [49]. In line with this hypothesis, it was recently proposed [50] that disrupted plantar pressure sensation during standing resulted in balance deficits, implying that cutaneous afferents might contribute not only to the control of locomotion, but also to posture. It is generally assumed that the sensory information projecting to the spinal cord and brain serves to correct errors during movement execution, i.e., provides corrective feedback in response to sensory input from a wide range of tissues and environments that change in a predictable way. One approach for re-activating the sensory-nervous system is to use rehabilitation strategies that include somatic sensory afferents and activate functional movements [51]. In recent years, increasing cutaneous stimuli through neuromuscular kinesiotaping (KT) has been proposed as a means of enhancing somatosensory inputs [52]. In healthy humans, KT seems to decrease the H-reflex amplitude, thus influencing (inhibiting) muscle tone through proprioceptive feedback [53, 54]. KT has been used in neurological pathologies [55–57] including stroke and multiple sclerosis, and in various orthopaedic disorders [53, 54], and has generally been found to improve muscle tone, range of motion, balance parameters, and pain symptoms. On the basis of evidence that major gait impairments in incomplete SCI are caused by ankle spasticity and decreased balance [36], both of which are positively affected by KT [53–57] we recently performed a study to examine the effect of KT in chronic SCI subjects [58]. We demonstrated that short-term application of KT reduces lower limb spasticity and pain. Furthermore, KT application resulted in balance and gait improvement, while not influencing other neurological deficits such as strength.

References

1. Silva NA, Sousa N, Reis RL, Salgado AJ. From basics to clinical: a comprehensive review on spinal cord injury. Prog Neurobiol. 2014;114:25–57.
2. World Health Organization, International Spinal Cord Society. 2013. International Perspectives on Spinal Cord Injury. In: Bickenbach J. editor. 2013.
3. Hubli M, Dietz V. The physiological basis of neurorehabilitation–locomotor training after spinal cord injury. J Neuroeng Rehabil. 2013;10:5.
4. Ditunno PL, Patrick M, Stineman M, Morganti B, Townson AF, Ditunno JF. Cross-cultural differences in preference for recovery of mobility among spinal cord injury rehabilitation professionals. Spinal Cord. 2006;44:567–75.
5. De Biase ME, Politti F, Palomari ET, Barros-Filho TE, De Camargo OP. Increased EMG response following electromyographic biofeedback treatment of rectus femoris muscle after spinal cord injury. Physiotherapy. 2011;97:175–9.
6. Green JB, Sora E, Bialy Y, Ricamato A, Thatcher RW. Cortical motor reorganization after paraplegia: an EEG study. Neurology. 1999;53:736–43.
7. Raineteau O, Schwab ME. Plasticity of motor systems after incomplete spinal cord injury. Nat Rev Neurosci. 2001;2:263–73.
8. van Tuijl JH, Janssen-Potten YJ, Seelen HA. Evaluation of upper extremity motor function tests in tetraplegics. Spinal Cord. 2002;40:51–64.
9. Dietz V, Fouad K. Restoration of sensorimotor functions after spinal cord injury. Brain. 2014;137:654–67.
10. Boulenguez P, Liabeuf S, Bos R, et al. Down-regulation of the potassium-chloride cotransporter KCC2 contributes to spasticity after spinal cord injury. Nat Med. 2010;16:302–7.
11. Murray KC, Nakae A, Stephens MJ, et al. Recovery of motoneuron and locomotor function after spinal cord injury depends on constitutive activity in 5-HT2C receptors. Nat Med. 2010;16:694–700.
12. Courtine G, Song B, Roy RR, Zhong H, Herrmann JE, Ao Y, Qi J, Edgerton VR, Sofroniew MV. Recovery of supraspinal control of stepping via indirect propriospinal relay connections after spinal cord injury. Nat Med. 2008;14:69–74.
13. Fouad K, Tetzlaff W. Rehabilitative training and plasticity following spinal cord injury. Exp Neurol. 2012;235:91–9.
14. Dietz V, Colombo G, Jensen L, Baumgartner L. Locomotor capacity of spinal cord in paraplegic patients. Ann Neurol. 1995;37:574–82.

15. Harkema SJ, Hillyer J, Schmidt-Read M, Ardolino E, Sisto SA, Behrman AL. Locomotor training: as a treatment of spinal cord injury and in the progression of neurologic rehabilitation. Arch Phys Med Rehabil. 2012;93:1588–97.
16. Rossignol S, Dubuc R, Gossard JP. Dynamic sensorimotor interactions in locomotion. Physiol Rev. 2006;86:89–154.
17. Dietz V, Sinkjaer T. Spastic movement disorder: impaired reflex function and altered muscle mechanics. Lancet Neurol. 2007;6:725–33.
18. Schillings AM, van Wezel BM, Mulder T, Duysens J. Muscular responses and movement strategies during stumbling over obstacles. J Neurophysiol. 2000;83:2093–102.
19. Bastiaanse CM, Duysens J, Dietz V. Modulation of cutaneous reflexes by load receptor input during human walking. Exp Brain Res. 2000;135:189–98.
20. Harkema SJ, Hurley SL, Patel UK, Requejo PS, Dobkin BH, Edgerton VR. Human lumbosacral spinal cord interprets loading during stepping. J Neurophysiol. 1997;77:797–811.
21. Dietz V. Neuronal plasticity after a human spinal cord injury: positive and negative effects. Exp Neurol. 2012;235:110–5.
22. Pearson KG. Role of sensory feedback in the control of stance duration in walking cats. Brain Res Rev. 2008;57:222–7.
23. Dietz V. Do human bipeds use quadrupedal coordination? Trends Neurosci. 2002;25:462–7.
24. Dietz V, Muller R, Colombo G. Locomotor activity in spinal man: significance of afferent input from joint and load receptors. Brain. 2002;125(12):2626–34.
25. Amatachaya S, Keawsutthi M, Amatachaya P, Manimmanakorn N. Effects of external cues on gait performance in independent ambulatory incomplete spinal cord injury patients. Spinal Cord. 2009;47(9):668–73.
26. Bastian AJ. Understanding sensorimotor adaptation and learning for rehabilitation. Curr Opin Neurol. 2008;21(6):628–33.
27. Aagaard P, Simonsen EB, Andersen JL, Magnusson P, Dyhre-Poulsen P. Neural adaptation to resistance training: changes in evoked V-wave and H-reflex responses. J Appl Physiol. 2002;92(6):2309–18.
28. Banz R, Bolliger M, Colombo G, Dietz V, Lünenburger L. Computerized visual feedback: an adjunct to robotic-assisted gait training. Phys Ther. 2008;88(10):1135–45.
29. Boyd LA, Winstein CJ. Implicit motor-sequence learning in humans following unilateral stroke: the impact of practice and explicit knowledge. Neurosci Lett. 2001;298(1):65–9.
30. Green TD, Flowers JH. Implicit versus explicit learning processes in a probabilistic, continuous fine-motor catching task. J Mot Behav. 1991;23(4):293–300.
31. Malone LA, Bastian AJ. Thinking about walking: effects of conscious correction versus distraction on locomotor adaptation. J Neurophysiol. 2010;103(4):1954–62.
32. Reber PJ, Squire LR. Encapsulation of implicit and explicit memory in sequence learning. J Cogn Neurosci. 1998;10(2):248–63.
33. Shea CH, Wulf G, Whitacre CA, Park JH. Surfing the implicit wave. Q J Exp Psychol A. 2001;54(3):841–62.
34. Boyd LA, Winstein CJ. Providing explicit information disrupts implicit motor learning after basal ganglia stroke. Learn Mem. 2004;11(4):388–96.
35. Burns SP, Golding DG, Rolle WA Jr, Graziani V, Ditunno JF Jr. Recovery of ambulation in motor-incomplete tetraplegia. Arch Phys Med Rehabil. 1997;78:1169–72.
36. Scivoletto G, Romanelli A, Mariotti A, et al. Clinical factors that affect walking level and performance in chronic spinal cord lesion patients. Spine. 2008;33:259–64.
37. Ditunno JF Jr, Barbeau H, Dobkin BH, et al. Validity of the walking scale for spinal cord injury and other domains of function in a multicenter clinical trial. Neurorehabil Neural Repair. 2007;21:539–50.
38. Arazpour M, Bani MA, Hutchins SW, Curran S, Javanshir MA. The influence of ankle joint mobility when using an orthosis on stability in patients with spinal cord injury: a pilot study. Spinal Cord. 2013;51:750–4.

39. Kannus P, Niemi S, Palvanen M, Parkkari J. Continuously increasing number and incidence of fall-induced, fracture-associated, spinal cord injuries in elderly persons. Arch Intern Med. 2000;160:2145–9.
40. Brotherton SS, Krause JS, Nietert PJ. Falls in individuals with incomplete spinal cord injury. Spinal Cord. 2007;45:37–40.
41. Alexeeva N, Sames C, Jacobs PL, et al. Comparison of training methods to improve walking in persons with chronic spinal cord injury: a randomized clinical trial. J Spinal Cord Med. 2011;34:362–79.
42. Boswell-Ruys CL, Harvey LA, Barker JJ, Ben M, Middleton JW, Lord SR. Training unsupported sitting in people with chronic spinal cord injuries: a randomized controlled trial. Spinal Cord. 2010;48:138–43.
43. Betker AL, Desai A, Nett C, Kapadia N, Szturm T. Game-based exercises for dynamic short-sitting balance rehabilitation of people with chronic spinal cord and traumatic brain injuries. Phys Ther. 2007;87:1389–98.
44. Bjerkefors A, Carpenter MG, Thorstensson A. Dynamic trunk stability is improved in paraplegics following kayak ergometer training. Scand J Med Sci Sports. 2007;17:672–9.
45. Sayenko DG, Alekhina MI, Masani K et al. Positive effect of balance training with visual feedback on standing balance abilities in people with incomplete spinal cord injury. Spinal Cord. 2010;48(12):886–93.
46. Harkema SJ, Ferreira CK, van den Brand RJ, Krassioukov AV. Improvements in orthostatic instability with stand locomotor training in individuals with spinal cord injury. J Neurotrauma. 2008;25:1467–75.
47. Tamburella F, Scivoletto G, Molinari M. Balance training improves static stability and gait in chronic incomplete spinal cord injury subjects: a pilot study. Eur J Phys Rehabil Med. 2013;49(3):353–64.
48. Lam T, Eng JJ, Wolfe DL, Hsieh JT, Whittaker M. A systematic review of the efficacy of gait rehabilitation strategies for spinal cord injury. Top Spinal Cord Inj Rehabil. 2007;13:32–57.
49. Delwaide PJ, Crenna P. Cutaneous nerve stimulation and motoneuronal excitability. II: evidence for non-segmental influences. J Neurol Neurosurg Psychiatry. 1984;47:190–6.
50. Nakazawa K, Miyoshi T, Sekiguchi H, Nozaki D, Akai M, Yano H. Effects of loading and unloading of lower limb joints on the soleus H-reflex in standing humans. Clin Neurophysiol. 2004;115:1296–304.
51. Lynskey JV, Belanger A, Jung R. Activity-dependent plasticity in spinal cord injury. J Rehabil Res Dev. 2008;45:229–40.
52. Halseth T. The effects of kinesio^{TM} taping on proprioception at the ankle. J Sports Sci Med. 2004;3:1–7.
53. Alexander CM, Stynes S, Thomas A, Lewis J, Harrison PJ. Does tape facilitate or inhibit the lower fibres of trapezius? Manual Ther. 2003;8:37–41.
54. Lin JJ, Hung CJ, Yang PL. The effects of scapular taping on electromyographic muscle activity and proprioception feedback in healthy shoulders. J Orthop Res. 2011;29:53–7.
55. Cortesi M, Cattaneo D, Jonsdottir J. Effect of kinesio taping on standing balance in subjects with multiple sclerosis: a pilot study\m{1}. NeuroRehabilitation. 2011;28:365–72.
56. Kilbreath SL, Perkins S, Crosbie J, McConnell J. Gluteal taping improves hip extension during stance phase of walking following stroke. Aust J Physiotherapy. 2006;52:53–6.
57. Karadag-Saygi E, Cubukcu-Aydoseli K, Kablan N, Ofluoglu D. The role of kinesiotaping combined with botulinum toxin to reduce plantar flexors spasticity after stroke. Top Stroke Rehabil. 2010;17:318–22.
58. Tamburella F, Scivoletto G, Molinari M. Somatosensory inputs by application of KinesioTaping: effects on spasticity, balance, and gait in chronic spinal cord injury. Front. Hum Neurosci. 2014;30(8):367.

Part III
New Technologies for the Evaluation and Rehabilitation of Gait and Balance Disorders

Advanced Methods for Gait Analysis Data Processing

Manuela Galli and Mariano Serrao

1 Introduction

Gait analysis (GA), or the computerized multifactorial (3D kinematics, kinetics and electromyography) evaluation of walking, is becoming increasingly widespread in clinical settings. GA is a means of evaluating walking ability for the purposes of arriving at an exhaustive diagnosis, of better characterizing the functional limitations of a patient with a certain pathology, and of evaluating the efficacy of rehabilitation treatments. Nowadays, there is growing recognition of the importance of measuring and analyzing gait variability, and GA is becoming increasingly accepted and used in rehabilitation and in clinical research. In the current era of evidenced-based medicine, continuous development of quality, which includes the careful measurement and recording of results, contributes to more efficient application of diagnostic procedures and interventions and to a reduction of expenditure on unnecessary procedures. In this context, GA is a fundamental tool for characterizing gait patterns in quantitative terms.

M. Galli
Department of Electronics, Information and Bioengineering,
Politecnico di Milano, Milan, Italy

M. Serrao (✉)
Department of Medical and Surgical Sciences and Biotechnologies,
Sapienza University of Rome, Rome, Italy
e-mail: mariano.serrao@uniroma1.it

G. Sandrini et al. (eds.), *Advanced Technologies for the Rehabilitation of Gait and Balance Disorders*, Biosystems & Biorobotics 19,
https://doi.org/10.1007/978-3-319-72736-3_17

2 Gait Analysis Data Acquisitions: Gait Analysis Lab Equipment

The clinical GA output is the result of integration of different data (spatiotemporal parameters, kinematics, kinetics and electromyography).

The instrumentation used in a Movement Analysis Lab (MAL) must meet a series of technical requirements, namely it must offer:

- three-dimensionality (3D);
- non-invasiveness;
- the capacity to provide quantitative information with high precision;
- the capacity to execute an integrated multifactorial analysis, i.e. to acquire, contemporaneously, data on kinematics, dynamics and muscular activation during movement, together with video-recording data;
- ease of use;
- cost-effectiveness.

The instruments typically found in a "traditional" MAL are shown below (Fig. 1).

- Sterophotogrammetry systems: these are systems able to provide three-dimensional coordinates of markers positioned on the subject's body on specific landmarks (Fig. 2a). The markers, composed of reflective material, are illuminated at regular intervals by each camera, thanks to an infrared source, while the reflex is captured by the camera coaxial with the light source. The

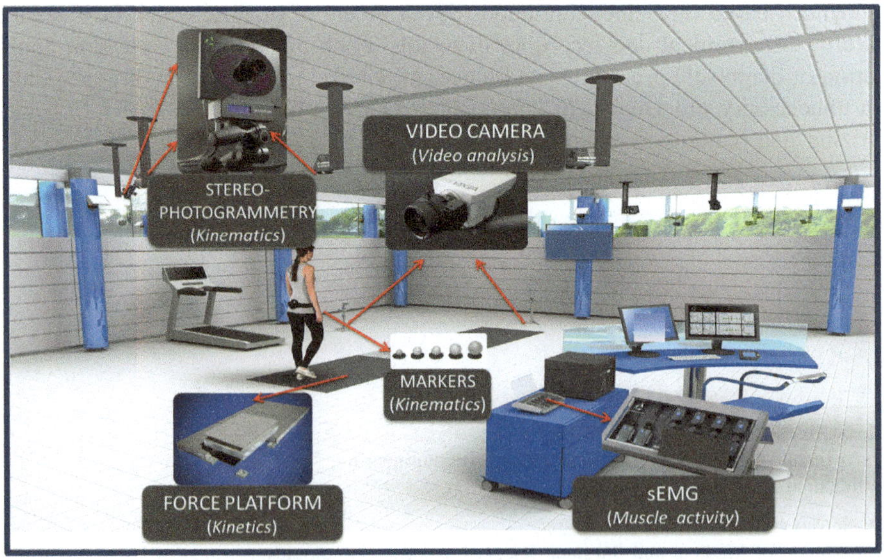

Fig. 1 Typical equipment of a Gait Analysis Lab

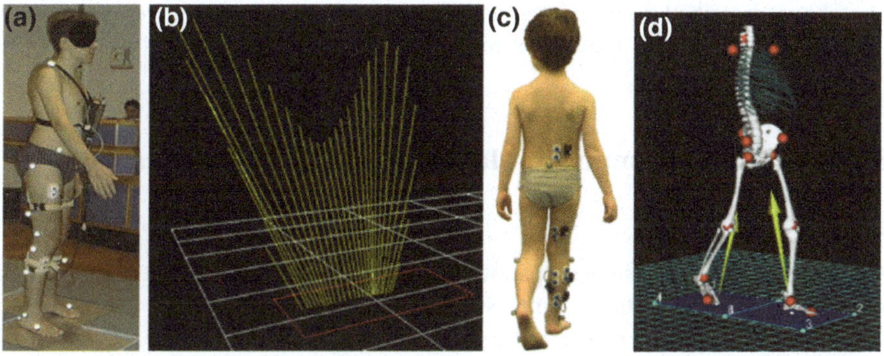

Fig. 2 **a** Positioning of markers on the subject's body in accordance with Davis' protocol [23], **b** the vectogram generated during foot contact on the force platform during walking,**c** Markers' placement, **d** 3D reconstruction of body and ground reaction forces

system is totally non-invasive. This simply functioning instrumentation—for a more detailed description see Ferrigno et al. [30]—allows dedicated software to calculate (from the three-dimensional coordinates (XYZ) of markers placed on specific body parts according to international protocols) the internal joint positions and trajectories, velocities, accelerations and angles (flexion-extension angles, ab-adduction angles and extra-internal rotation angles) of the principal joints involved in walking (pelvis, hip, knee, ankle). In this way, it is easy to measure the kinematics of movement of the body segment on which the markers are placed. The markers are usually taped to the subject's body, and do not cause any pain or discomfort.

- Force platforms: a force platform is used to record the contact forces exchanged with the ground when the foot is in contact with its surface (Fig. 2b). From the measurement of the system of forces exchanged with the ground, together with the acquisition of the kinematics by the optoelectronic system, it is possible to calculate, by means of an inverse dynamic approach, the torques and powers at the main joints [23].
- Electromyography: this system (surface electromyography, sEMG, Fig. 1) is able, by means of surface electrodes, to acquire electrical signals generated by muscular contraction. These last-generation systems are based on wireless technology, and use light miniaturized probes for recording and transmission. Thanks to the lack of wires and the lightness of the probes, patients can quickly be prepared for the examination, without altering their motor patterns (Fig. 2c).
- Video recording systems: by making video recordings of patients, we are able to observe their movements and analyze them in a qualitative way. Video recording analysis is important to support the GA data interpretation: it is far easier to understand a graph depicting the kinematics of a joint if this can be compared with the patient's actual movements.

The above described equipment is used in an integrated way to give a 3D multi-factorial measure of the movement to be evaluated.

3 GA Output, Summary Measures and Their Clinical Applications

A GA report usually shows spatiotemporal parameters (like cadence, walking velocity, stride time, stance time, swing time, step length, stride length, etc.), kinematic variables (flexion-extension, ab-adduction internal-external rotation of the pelvis, hip, knee and ankle joints), internal moments and joint powers on the sagittal plane, by means of specific graphic organization of the data. Several studies in the literature refer to the use of GA graph analysis for specific pathologies, such as cerebral palsy (CP) in children; numerous courses are organized to provide instruction in the administration of GA trials, in how to read and clinically interpret GA data, and in how to apply these data for rehabilitation purposes. Several scientific publications have demonstrated that the use of GA has radically changed the treatment of children with CP [24, 25, 33, 47] for the following reasons:

- Before treatment, GA allows better evaluation of the motor disorder and better identification of the rehabilitation/therapeutic pathway to be followed in the single patient;
- After treatment, GA makes it possible to measure the efficacy of the treatment, and to assess whether a new intervention or modification of the therapeutic strategy is needed. The availability, before treatment, of quantitative information on the efficacy of one treatment with respect to another equates with greater knowledge and a greater likelihood of a successful treatment.

Given the importance of GA in clinical settings, what is clearly needed is the ability to produce a report able to highlight a subject's gait pattern deviation and summarize his/her specific gait pattern. GA variables are numerous (spatiotemporal parameters, 3D kinematics, kinetics, EMG signals, etc.) and if we also consider that, in each patient, the data from several reports (each corresponding to a different trial) must be analyzed in order to verify their consistency, then it is clear that reading and evaluating a GA trial is a very time-consuming process. In an attempt to address these issues, the traditional approach was based on the identification of certain specific parameters, starting from basographic, kinematic and kinetic data, like spatiotemporal parameters (velocity, step length, step width, etc.), joint angle values at specific instants of the gait cycle (hip range of motion, value of knee angle in midstance, value of ankle angle at initial contact, etc.), and peaks in moment and power graphs (maximum value of ankle moment and ankle power in terminal stance, etc.). This approach to report analysis has some limitations, namely:

- the identification of the parameters to be considered is subjective (some investigators will choose to highlight a specific joint angle at a specific instant, but this is a matter of preference);
- the choice of parameters to be considered is pathology dependent (as some variables are good for identifying a typical gait pattern related to a specific movement disorder, but not for identifying patterns associated with other disorders).

New methods for GA data processing have been proposed and, in particular, some summary measures have been developed in order to provide simple measures of gait function, making it possible to quantify and represent in a single number, or a few numbers, the deviation of a patient' gait pattern from normality [11, 13, 17, 19, 21, 27, 35, 45, 51, 60, 65–68, 74]. In particular, these indices have been shown to be useful for objectifying clinical impressions, quantifying the degree of the deviation of gait from normal, stratifying the severity of the pathology, documenting changes in gait over time, and evaluating the effects of rehabilitation interventions. The literature has proposed several summary measures that can be computed starting from GA trial data, and that have clinical applications. Most parameters (Normalcy Index, Gait Deviation Index, Gait Profile Score, Movement Deviation Profile) were computed starting from kinematic GA data; some attempts have also been made to propose summary measures related partially (Hip Flexor Index) or totally (GDI-Kinetics) to kinetic data. Table 1 lists the most widely used summary measures capable of providing a GA evaluation result that may feasibly be used in clinical practice.

3.1 Normalcy Index (NI) or Gillette Gait Index (GGI)

The Normalcy Index (NI) or Gillette Gait Index (GGI) [59] represents the first attempt to define a single parameter able to describe the quality of the gait pattern in a global sense. It is a measure of the extent to which a patient's gait differs from the mean gait pattern for healthy individuals computed from 16 univariate gait parameters that were considered, by the developers of the instrument, significant for capturing the important features of the gait pattern. The NI is computed using standard multivariate statistical techniques (principal component analysis) applied to 16 3D GA variables, specifically three spatiotemporal parameters (percentage of stance phase, normalized velocity and cadence) and 13 kinematic parameters (mean pelvic tilt, range of pelvic tilt, mean pelvic rotation, minimum hip flexion, range of hip flexion, peak abduction in swing, mean hip rotation in stance, knee flexion at initial contact, time of peak knee flexion, range of knee flexion, peak of dorsiflexion in stance, peak of dorsiflexion in swing, and mean foot progression angle). The sum of the square of these 16 independent variables is interpreted as the deviation of the

Table 1 Main summary measures proposed in the literature

Name of the index	Authors	Considerations about the index	Fields of application
Indices based on kinematic data			
Normalcy Index (NI) or Gillette Gait Index (GGI)	Schutte et al. [59]	1. The selected parameters are pathology dependent 2. Dependent on reference dataset 3. Too synthetic 4. No kinetics	Cerebral palsy (mainly)
Gait Deviation Index (GDI)	Schwartz and Rozumalski [61]	1. Dependent on reference dataset 2. Too synthetic 3. No kinetics	Cerebral palsy, Batten disease, muscular dystrophy, Parkinson's disease, lower limb amputees, etc.
Gait Profile Score (GPS) and Movement Analysis Profile (MAP)	Baker et al. [4]	1. Possibility to highlight each joint deviation (gait variable score) 2. No kinetics 3. Independent of large reference dataset	Cerebral palsy, multiple sclerosis, Helers-Danlos syndrome hereditary spastic paraparesis Parkinson's disease Down's syndrome
Movement Deviation Profile (MDP)	Barton et al. [9]	1. Independent r of large reference dataset 2. It provides more detail than a single number, like the GPS	Cerebral palsy (mainly)
Index based on kinetic data			
GDI-Kinetic	Rozumalski and Schwartz [56]		Cerebral palsy, rheumatoid arthritis

subject's gait from normal. Using this statistical method, it is possible to measure and represent, as a single number, the deviation of a pathological gait pattern from a normal average profile. The NI has a mean value of 15.7, with high values reflecting more abnormal gait patterns. It has been the most widely cited and validated summary measure. In particular, its use has been widely validated in CP and idiopathic toe walker populations. It has been shown to be effective when used to evaluate the range of pathology present in specific diagnoses, to compare a subject's gait to that of others with the same diagnosis, to track a subject's gait pathology over time, and to examine the effectiveness of an intervention [26, 59, 69, 73].

3.2 *Gait Deviation Index (GDI)*

The Gait Deviation Index (GDI) was developed [61] in order to address the limitations of the NI. It uses data from across the gait cycle for the nine joint angles (the pelvis and hip in three planes, the knee and ankle in the sagittal plane and foot progression) and is generally regarded as most clinically significant index in GA. From a large dataset of people who had been evaluated with GA, 15 gait features were extracted from the GA kinematics using the singular value decomposition. Applied to a control group, these gait features define an averaged, non-pathological gait. The root mean square distance of the 15 gait features between a subject exhibiting gait pathology and the control group is computed. As the resulting measure was not normally distributed, its logarithm was taken and scaled such that the mean value for the healthy population was 100; 10 points below 100 corresponds to one standard deviation away from the healthy group mean [4, 61]. The GDI was moderately correlated with the NI ($r2 = 0.56$), suggesting that these two parameters are both measures of the same underlying construct, although a large spread at any given level indicates that they measure different aspects of the gait pathology [61].

The GDI was found to be normally distributed across people with different Functional Assessment Questionnaire (FAQ) scores, and mean values for the different levels were similar increments apart. The validity of the GDI was first assessed in healthy subjects and in individuals with CP, and in both children [18, 46, 48, 50, 61] and adults [2]. The GDI in adults demonstrated similar results in terms of distributional properties to those reported in studies conducted in healthy children and children with CP [61]. The GDI has now been applied successfully not only in CP, but also in patients with different pathological conditions, such as Batten disease [34], muscular dystrophy [62], lower limb amputees [29, 39], Parkinson's disease [63], hip osteoarthritis [55], rheumatoid arthritis [14, 28], slipped capital femoral epiphysis [15] and lumbar spinal stenosis [38].

Compared with the NI, the GDI has several advantages. The fact that it uses the entire variability in kinematic variables across the gait cycle, rather than a small number of discrete parameters specific for children with CP, removes much of the subjectivity in the choice of parameters. In addition, the GDI values seem to be much less sensitive to differences in the reference data, in contrast with the NI which requires a reasonably large number of people in the reference dataset and also gives values that can vary significantly according to the selected reference datasets [49]. The GDI proceeds naturally from the analysis of gait features, and it provides considerable data compression and a framework for other analytical techniques, such as cluster analysis for gait classification [61]. In addition, it was shown in a previous study that uncertainty on the GGI increases when the GGI value increases with the pathology [3]. This could be related to the fact that the GGI increases indefinitely with the pathology, and this, in turn, participates in the increase of the uncertainty; instead, variation of the GDI remains confined within a finite interval from 0 to 100.

It is also important to note that calculation of the GDI, based on the whole gait cycle, for each curve, could limit the propagation of errors, unlike the GGI which uses punctual parameters in specific instants of the gait cycle [48].

3.3 Gait Profile Score (GPS) and Movement Analysis Profile (MAP)

More recently, the Gait Profile Score (GPS) was proposed as the direct root mean square distance between an individual's data and the mean normal data computed across the gait cycle for the same nine joint angles of one side. Thus, it represents a simpler interpretation of the distance measures underlying the GDI: the GPS results in a modified measure that can be calculated independently of the feature analysis. In addition, to a global measure of the overall gait quality, i.e. the GPS, it can be deconstructed to provide the Gait Variable Score (GVS) for nine kinematic variables (the pelvis and hip in three planes, the knee and ankle on the sagittal plane and the foot progression) [4]. The GPS is generally presented with the GVSs in a bar chart, generating the Movement Analysis Profile (MAP). The MAP describes the magnitude of deviation of the nine individual variables averaged over the gait cycle, providing insight into which variables contribute to the increase in GPS.

The GPS is normally distributed for the control population (mean 5.3°). In patient data, the distribution categorized either by the Gross Motor Function Classification System (GMFCS) (for CP) or the Functional Activities Questionnaire (FAQ) (all patients) is not normal, but its log transform is Baker et al. [4]. The GPS was validated against established index measures of gait abnormality and general measures of mobility in children with CP [4]. The authors [5] proposed a rationale for defining a minimal clinically important difference for the GPS, which was found to be 1.68.

Strong positive correlations were found between the GPS and MAP component scores, and clinicians' ratings of kinematic gait deviation [12], thus providing evidence that these indices have criterion-related validity relative to clinician judgments. The authors proposed that the GPS, particularly the MAP, might be useful in clinical practice and education as an adjunct to the traditional presentation of complex kinematic data. It could also be useful as a measure of both the group and individual outcomes following an intervention or over time. Thus, the availability of MAP and GVS components together with GPS represents an advantage of this summary measure over the other measures [12].

The GPS has strong face validity because it is based on the root mean square distance between gait data for an individual child and the averaged data from children with no gait pathology. Analysis of the intra-session variability suggests that it is also a reliable measure, and the findings of a moderate correlation with the NI and a strong relationship between the GPS and the GDI are based on essentially similar measures of distance. The GPS shows a very strong nonlinear correlation with the GDI (r = 0.995) and analysis showed a close mathematical relationship between the GPS and the unscaled GDI. The GDI and GPS are in fact different ways of scaling the same underlying construct and therefore there is little point in using both these outcome measures [4]. However, there is debate over the use of the GDI and GPS in clinical practice and research. At present, there are pros and cons for both indices and choosing one over the other is often based on personal preference. The choice between the two parameters depends primarily on whether a scaled or unscaled score is preferred and whether reference to the MAP enhances the interpretation of the results [6]. Recently, Rasmussen et al. (2015) investigated the intra-rater reliability and agreement of GDI and GPS (with its GVSs) in a group of children with CP. They found that GDI and GPS demonstrated excellent reliability and acceptable agreement, demonstrating that they can both be used in research and clinical practice. However, the large variability observed for some of the GVSs means that cautious consideration is warranted when selecting outcome measures. However, the same authors pointed out that the size of the sample of children considered in their research (n = 18) might be considered relatively low, and this may have influenced the results; in addition, the relatively narrow inclusion criteria for their study might have limited its results in terms of reliability and external validity.

The literature contains several research studies conducted using the GPS, and not only in CP. The outcomes of orthopedic surgery in children [31, 32, 57, 58, 70–72] and adults [54] with CP and the effects, on gait, of ankle foot orthoses [37] have been assessed using the GPS. The suitability of the GPS and of other gait summary measures (NI and GDI) for use in lower limb amputees [39], in young hemiplegics [22] and in Parkinson's disease [63] has also been assessed. Kark et al. [39] found that the GPS, like the NI, detected significant differences between the levels of amputation on the intact side, whereas the GDI did not. The differences in the results between the GDI and the GPS could be a result of the calculation methods used. The GDI is calculated against a matrix of data from able-bodied subjects, whereas the GPS is calculated against a single column of data from able-bodied subjects. The method of calculation may have resulted in greater variability of the GDI, and may have been responsible for its failure to detect significant differences between levels of amputation on the intact side. In addition, the MAP was shown to be useful for the elucidation of the underlying causes of gait pathology, which could not be achieved using the other overall gait summary measures [39]. Another element that might justify these different results between the GPS and GDI may be the fact that the GPS is defined as a raw score, whereas the GDI is transformed and scaled. Danino et al. [22] used the GPS, NI and GDI to evaluate the use of functional electrical stimulation neuroprostheses as a method for improving gait in hemiplegic patients.

They found that the GPS and GDI provided similar results, however decomposition of the GPS into the nine MAP scores was found to be a helpful tool for evaluating gait studies, as it highlighted the main components responsible for the overall change displayed in their study. Conversely, the GGI showed no significant improvement, although the trend was positive. This result can be attributed to the fact that this index has been found to have some shortcomings, including the arbitrary and unbalanced nature of the 16 parameters that comprise it, as well as difficulties in its implementation [22, 61]. Speciali et al. [63] assessed the effects of subthalamic deep brain stimulation and levodopa on gait in people with Parkinson's disease using the GPS and the GDI, and found them to show similar treatment effects, as did the GVS for hip and knee flexion/extension. These authors' overall conclusion was that GDI, GPS and GVS results reflect the known responses to medication and stimulation of people with PD. This strongly suggests that these measures are valid for use in people with this condition and further suggests a general validity of their use in populations other than that for whom they was designed, namely, children with CP.

The GPS has also been applied in other pathologies, such as multiple sclerosis [20, 52, 53], Helers-Danlos syndrome, [16], hereditary spastic paraparesis [1], Parkinson's disease [64] and Down's syndrome [36], and appears to be a suitable measure for representing gait deviations from physiological patterns in these pathological states.

With respect to the other summary measures, the GPS has some advantages. Previous indices derived from the conventional gait model could not easily be extended to data derived from different gait models or to different activities (running, stair climbing, etc.); by contrast, the GPS is independent of the feature analysis and can be calculated directly from the data of an individual and the averaged data of people with no gait pathology. Another potential advantage of the GPS is its deconstruction, or MAP. The MAP provides useful insights into which variables contribute to an elevated GPS. A lack of strong correlations of individual GVSs with the GPS and with each other suggests that there is considerably more information contained within the MAP than in the GPS alone. In addition, because the score is derived from the control database alone, this score (unlike the GDI and NI, which are based on the outputs of the conventional gait model) makes it easier to compute equivalent scores for different gait models.

One of the limits of the GPS is that, like the GDI, no spatiotemporal parameters and kinetics were included in its computation. With regard to the spatiotemporal parameters, it is important to stress that, because gait speed is not correlated with the GPS [4], it is recommended that self-selected speed be reported in addition to the GPS in clinical studies. However, in a first attempt to compute the GVS for kinetics, Firth et al. [32] considered ankle dorsi-plantar flexion moment and ankle power.

3.4 Movement Deviation Profile (MDP)

As an alternative to conventional analysis of complex data, artificial neural networks, specifically the self-organizing map (SOM) described by Kohonen [43, 44], have been used to detect deviation from normality in a wide range of applications. The use of the SOM's quantization error to quantify the deviation of gait from normality has been described by Barton et al. [8] and was illustrated with examples from patients with CP. Barton et al. [7] also used the power of self-organizing artificial neural networks or the SOM in order to visualize complex gait patterns in the form of single curves. The SOM operates by converging gait data to stem patterns, which are arranged on a relational map in the context of the total data space presented to the SOM during training. This method enables the identification of existing gait patterns and opens up the possibility of defining new gait patterns, which are otherwise difficult to identify in multi-dimensional data space. This method provides repeatable dimensionality reduction with a resolution that can be controlled by careful selection of the input data. The multi-dimensional ranking of subjects is possible both cross-sectionally and longitudinally. This method was used to identify differences in lower extremity coordination between different types of foot orthoses and to assess gait quality in a group of patients with various gait problems [8].

In a more recent paper, a refined procedure, which generates the Movement Deviation Profile (MDP) from information provided by the SOM, was proposed [9]. The MDP was validated by comparing it to the GDI, FAQ scores, and clinical diagnoses of patients from a large dataset. In particular, the MDP represents a single curve showing the deviation of an individual's movement from normality. Joint angles, recorded from typically developing children over one gait cycle, were used to train a SOM, which then generated MDP curves for patients with gait problems. The mean MDP over the gait cycle showed a high correlation with the GDI, a statistically significant difference between groups of patients with a range of functional levels (Gillette FAQ Walking Scale 7–10) and a trend of increasing values for patients with CP through hemiplegia I–IV, diplegia, triplegia and quadriplegia. The small difference between the MDP and GDI can be explained by the SOM's method of operation—it compares biomechanical patterns to the nearest abstract reference pattern—, and by its flexibility in compensating for temporal shifts in movement data. Contrary to the GDI, and similarly to the GPS, the MDP does not depend on a condensed representation of a large database containing control and patient data. In addition, while simple averaging of the MDP can provide a single score, the MDP is similar to the GPS in that it can provide more detail than a single number expressing deviation from normality in the same units as the data used (degrees). The MDP could be considered an alternative method of processing complex biomechanical data, potentially supporting clinical interpretation. The ability of the MDP versus the GDI to detect gait changes was evaluated in a child with CP [10]. The GDI showed a symmetric response on the two opposite sides of normality but the neural network-based MDP gave an asymmetric response, thereby faithfully reflecting the unequal biomechanical consequences of joint angle changes. In conclusion, the MDP can detect altered gait even if the changes are missed by the GDI, and the authors suggested that to complement the advantages of the GDI, additional use of other gait indices (e.g. MDP) is recommended.

While many synthetic indices for summarizing patterns of gait kinematics have been proposed in the literature, only one developed for evaluating gait kinetics has been proposed, namely the GDI-Kinetic.

3.5 GDI-Kinetic

The GDI-Kinetic, which is an index based on kinetic variables, was developed [56] using essentially the same method used to develop the GDI. The method extracted 20 gait features from the raw gait kinetic data using the singular value decomposition. Linear combinations of the 20 gait features produced a 91% faithful reconstruction of the data. Concurrent and face validity for the GDI-Kinetic are presented through comparisons with the GDI, Gillette FAQ Walking Scale, and topographic classifications used in the diagnosis of CP. The GDI-Kinetic and GDI are linearly related, but are not strongly correlated, indicating that for any given level of GDI-Kinetic, there can be a wide variety of kinematic patterns, and vice versa; this suggests that each index measures a different aspect of gait pathology. As with the GDI, the GDI-Kinetic scalewith FAQ level is suitable for distinguishing different levels of functional limitation. The GDI-Kinetic also scales with respect to clinical involvement based on topographic CP classification in hemiplegia types I–IV, diplegia, triplegia and quadriplegia. Interestingly, in hemiplegia, the unaffected limb exhibits lower GDI-Kinetic scores than the affected side, indicating that compensations in the unaffected limb result in greater deviations from normal gait than those observed in the affected limb [56]. The GDI-Kinetic can complement the GDI, allowing a more comprehensive measure of gait pathology that includes not only kinematics but also kinetics. However, to the best of our knowledge, only few applications of this index are reported in the literature. Brostrom et al. [14] used GDI and GDI-Kinetic to quantify the impact of treatment with anti-tumor necrosis factor-alpha inhibitors on gait dynamics in patients with rheumatoid arthritis; they showed that GDI and GDI-Kinetic scores appeared to be useful outcome measures for quantifying changes in gait deviations after this intervention. Kiernan et al. [40, 41] used the GPS and GDI-Kinetic to investigate the clinical agreement of different regression equations based on pelvic anatomy routinely used to estimate the hip joint center during gait analysis. In another study, the effect of using different anthropometric sets on predicted sagittal plane moments during normal and diplegic CP gait was investigated using GDI-Kinetic [42].

4 Example of a Gait Analysis Report

Figure 3 shows a sample page of a report of a GA performed using last-generation software. It includes two of the summary measures previously described (GPS, with its GVSs, and GDI).

The report gives the GPS and GDI values for the right limb (first column) and left limb (second column) of a child with CP (spastic right hemiplegia), as well as the normal value ranges.

The GPS results show that the right limb is characterized by higher values than the left limb (14.5° vs. 10.8°), thereby confirming, in a summary way, that the right

Gait Profile Score	RIGHT LIMB	LEFT LIMB	NORMAL VALUES
Gait Profile Score (deg):	14.5 ± 0	10.8 ± 0	<7

Gait Variable Scores	RIGHT LIMB	LEFT LIMB
Pelvis Obliquity (deg):	4.2 ± 0	3.8 ± 0
Pelvis Tilt (deg):	1.9 ± 0	2.1 ± 0
Pelvis Rotation (deg):	6.8 ± 0	4.6 ± 0
Hip Ab-Adduction (deg):	6.1 ± 0	8.9 ± 0
Hip Flex-Extension (deg):	9.6 ± 0	7.4 ± 0
Hip Rotation (deg):	38.1 ± 0	23.6 ± 0
Knee Flex-Extension (deg):	19.8 ± 0	11.4 ± 0
Ankle Dorsi-Plantarflex (deg):	10.1 ± 0	6.4 ± 0
Foot Progression (deg):	7.2 ± 0	12.3 ± 0

Gait Deviation Index	RIGHT LIMB	LEFT LIMB	NORMAL VALUES
Gait Deviation Index:	63.93 ± 0	88.82 ± 0	>100

Fig. 3 A sample page of a GA report using two synthetic indices (GPS and GDI). The report concerns a child with spastic right hemiplegia

limb is the more compromised. Through analysis of the GVSs, on the other hand, it is possible to identify the main alterations responsible for the worse right limb GPS. In particular, it can clearly be seen that hip flexion-extension, hip rotation, knee flexion-extension and ankle dorsi-plantarflexion show higher values for the right side with respect to the left; these results make it possible to identify the main joints involved in the gait alteration.

This great opportunity to identify the more compromised joints is lost if we instead consider the GDI. The GDI confirms that the right limb is the more compromised (63.93 vs. 88.82) but analysis of this index does not allow us to pinpoint which joint angle values are impaired.

5 Conclusions

In this chapter we have provided an overview of the summary measures most widely used in order to express the deviation of an individual's gait pattern from normal walking. On the basis of the literature found on this topic, the clinical applications of these measures and our own personal experience, we conclude that summary measures could represent a useful tool, mainly in clinical settings, for objectifying clinical impressions, quantifying the degree of deviation of gait from normal, stratifying the severity of pathology, documenting changes in gait over time, and evaluating interventions. However, it is common opinion that they should always be used in conjunction with all of the other specific information contained in a GA report, i.e. spatiotemporal parameters, kinematics, kinetics and EMG data.

References

1. Adair B, Rodda J, McGinley JL, et al. Kinematic gait deficits at the trunk and pelvis: characteristic features in children with hereditary spastic paraplegia. Dev Med Child Neurol. 2016;58:829–35.
2. Andersson C, Mattsson E. Adults with cerebral palsy: a survey describing problems, needs, and resources, with special emphasis on locomotion. Dev Med Child Neurol. 2001;43:76–82.
3. Assi A, Ghanem I, Lavaste F, et al. Gait analysis in children and uncertainty assessment for Davis protocol and gillette gait index. Gait Posture. 2009;30:22–6.
4. Baker R, McGinley JL, Schwartz MH, et al. The gait profile score and movement analysis profile. Gait Posture. 2009;30:265–9.
5. Baker R, McGinley JL, Schwartz M, et al. The minimal clinically important difference for the gait profile score. Gait Posture. 2012;35:612–5.
6. Baker R. Measuring walking: a handbook of clinical gait analysis. London: Mac Keith Press; 2013.
7. Barton G, Lees A, Lisboa P, et al. Visualisation of gait data with Kohonen self-organising neural maps. Gait Posture. 2006;24:46–53.
8. Barton G, Lisboa P, Lees A, et al. Gait quality assessment using self-organising artificial neural networks. Gait Posture. 2007;25:374–9.
9. Barton GJ, Hawken MB, Scott MA, et al. Movement deviation profile: a measure of distance from normality using a self-organizing neural network. Hum Mov Sci. 2012;31:284–94.
10. Barton GJ, Hawken MB, Holmes G, et al. A gait index may underestimate changes of gait: a comparison of the movement deviation profile and the gait deviation index. Comput Methods Biomech Biomed Eng. 2015;18:57–63.
11. Begg RK, Wytch R, Major RE. Instrumentation used in clinical gait studies: a review. J Med Eng Technol. 1989;13(6):290–5.
12. Beynon S, McGinley JL, Dobson F, et al. Correlations of the gait profile score and the movement analysis profile relative to clinical judgments. Gait Posture. 2010;32:129–32.
13. Brehm MA, Harlaar J, Schwartz M. Effect of ankle-foot orthoses on walking efficiency and gait in children with cerebral palsy. J Rehabil Med. 2008;40:529–34.
14. Broström EW, Esbjörnsson AC, von Heideken J, et al. Change in gait deviation index after anti-tumour necrosis factor-α treatment in individuals with rheumatoid arthritis: a pilot study. Scand J Rheumatol. 2013;42:356–61.
15. Caskey PM, McMulkin ML, Gordon AB, et al. Gait outcomes of patients with severe slipped capital femoral epiphysis after treatment by flexion-rotation osteotomy. J Pediatr Orthop. 2014;34:668–73.
16. Celletti C, Galli M, Cimolin V, et al. Use of the gait profile score for the evaluation of patients with joint hypermobility syndrome/Ehlers-Danlos syndrome hypermobility type. Res Dev Disabil. 2013;34:4280–5.
17. Choi SJ, Chung CY, Lee KM, et al. Validity of gait parameters for hip flexor contracture in patients with cerebral palsy. J Neuroeng Rehabil. 2011;8:4.
18. Cimolin V, Galli M, Vimercati SL, et al. Use of the gait deviation index for the assessment of gastrocnemius fascia lengthening in children with Cerebral Palsy. Res Dev Disabil. 2011;32:377–81.
19. Cimolin V, Galli M. Summary measures for clinical gait analysis: a literature review. Gait Posture. 2014;39:1005–10.

20. Coghe G, Pau M, Corona F, et al. Walking improvements with nabiximols in patients with multiple sclerosis. J Neurol. 2015;262:2472–7.
21. Cretual A, Bervet K, Ballaz L. Gillette gait index in adults. Gait Posture. 2010;32:307–10.
22. Danino B, Khamis S, Hemo Y, et al. The efficacy of neuroprosthesis in young hemiplegic patients, measured by three different gait indices: early results. J Child Orthop. 2013;7:537–42.
23. Davis RB, Ounpuu S, Tyburski D, Gage JR. A gait analysis data collection and reduction technique. Hum Mov Sci. 1991;10:575–87.
24. Davids JR. Quantitative gait analysis in the treatment of children with cerebral palsy. J Pediatr Orthop. 2006;26(4):557–9.
25. De Luca PA. Cerebral Palsy. In: Drennan JC, editor. The child's foot and ankle. New York: Raven Press; 1992. p. 279–304.
26. Domagalska M, Szopa A, Syczewska M, et al. The relationship between clinical measurements and gait analysis data in children with cerebral palsy. Gait Posture. 2013;38:1038–43.
27. Dreher T, Vegvari D, Wolf SI, et al. Development of knee function after hamstring lengthening as a part of multilevel surgery in children with spastic diplegia: a long-term outcome study. J Bone Joint Surg Am. 2012;18:121–30.
28. Esbjörnsson AC, Rozumalski A, Iversen MD, et al. Quantifying gait deviations in individuals with rheumatoid arthritis using the gait deviation index. Scand J Rheumatol. 2014;43:124–31.
29. Eshraghi A, Abu Osman NA, Karimi M, et al. Gait biomechanics of individuals with transtibial amputation: effect of suspension system. PLoS ONE. 2014;9:e96988.
30. Ferrigno G, Pedotti A. Elite: a digital dedicated hardware system for movement analysis via real-time TV signal processing. IEEE Trans Biomed Eng. 1985;32:943–50.
31. Ferreira LA, Cimolin V, Costici PF, et al. Effects of gastrocnemius fascia lengthening on gait pattern in children with cerebral palsy using the gait profile score. Res Dev Disabil. 2014;35:1137–43.
32. Firth GB, Passmore E, Sangeux M, et al. Multilevel surgery for equinus gait in children with spastic diplegic cerebral palsy: medium-term follow-up with gait analysis. J Bone Joint Surg Am. 2013;95:931–8.
33. Gage JR. (2004). The treatment of gait problems in cerebral palsy. In: Gage JR. editor. London: Cambridge University Press.
34. Galli M, Cimolin V, De Pandis MF, et al. Use of the gait deviation index for the evaluation of patients with Parkinson's disease. J Mot Behav. 2012;44:161–7.
35. Galli M, Ferrario D, Patti P, et al. The use of 3d motion analysis in a patient with an atypical juvenile neuronal ceroid lipofuscinoses phenotype with CLN1 mutation and deficient PPT activity. J Dev Phys Disabil. 2012;24(2):155–65.
36. Galli M, Cimolin V, Rigoldi C, et al. Use of the Gait Profile Score for the quantification of gait pattern in Down syndrome. J Dev Phys Disabil. 2015;27:609–15.
37. Galli M, Cimolin V, Rigoldi C, et al. Quantitative evaluation of the effects of ankle foot orthosis on gait in children with cerebral palsy using the Gait profile score and gait variable scores. J Dev Phys Disabil. 2016;28:367–79.
38. Garbelotti SA Jr, Lucareli PR, Ramalho A Jr, et al. An investigation of the value of tridimensional kinematic analysis in functional diagnosis of lumbar spinal stenosis. Gait Posture. 2014;40:150–3.
39. Kark L, Vickers D, McIntosh A, et al. Use of gait summary measures with lower limb amputees. Gait Posture. 2012;35:238–43.
40. Kiernan D, Malone A, O'Brien T, et al. The clinical impact of hip joint centre regression equation error on kinematics and kinetics during paediatric gait. Gait Posture. 2015;41:175–9.
41. Kiernan D, Hosking J, O'Brien T. Is adult gait less susceptible than paediatric gait to hip joint centre regression equation error? Gait Posture. 2016;45:133–6.
42. Kiernan D, Walsh M, O'Sullivan R, et al. The influence of estimated body segment parameters on predicted joint kinetics during diplegic cerebral palsy gait. J Biomech. 2014;47:284–8.

43. Kohonen T. Self-organisation and associative memory. Berlin: Springer; 1988.
44. Kohonen T. Self-organizing maps. Berlin: Springer; 2001.
45. Lee KM, Chung CY, Kwon DG, et al. Reliability of physical examination in the measurement of hip flexion contracture and correlation with gait parameters in cerebral palsy. J Bone Joint Surg Am. 2011;93:150–8.
46. Lee SY, Kwon SS, Chung CY, et al. Rectus femoris transfer in cerebral palsy patients with stiff knee gait. Gait Posture. 2014;40:76–81.
47. Lee EH, Goh JC, Bose K. Value of gait analysis in the assessment of surgery in cerebral palsy. Arch Phys Med Rehabil. 1992;73(7):642–6.
48. Massaad A, Assi A, Skalli W, et al. Repeatability and validation of gait deviation index in children: typically developing and cerebral palsy. Gait Posture. 2014;39:354–8.
49. McMulkin ML, MacWilliams BA. Intersite variations of the Gillette Gait Index. Gait Posture. 2008;28:483–7.
50. McMulkin ML, Gordon AB, Caskey PM, et al. Outcomes of orthopaedic surgery with and without an external femoral derotational osteotomy in children with cerebral palsy. J Pediatr Orthop. 2016;36:382–6.
51. Novacheck TF, Trost J, Schwartz MH. Intramuscular psoas lengthening improves dynamic hip function in children with cerebral palsy. J Pediatr Orthop. 2002;22:158–64.
52. Pau M, Coghe G, Atzeni C, et al. Novel characterization of gait impairments in people with multiple sclerosis by means of the gait profile score. J Neurol Sci. 2014;345:159–63.
53. Pau M, Coghe G, Corona F, et al. Effect of spasticity on kinematics of gait and muscular activation in people with multiple sclerosis. J Neurol Sci. 2015;358:339–44.
54. Putz C, Döderlein L, Mertens EM, et al. Multilevel surgery in adults with cerebral palsy. Bone Joint J (2016);98-B:282–8.
55. Rosenlund S, Holsgaard-Larsen A, Overgaard S, et al. The gait deviation index is associated with hip muscle strength and patient-reported outcome in patients with severe hip osteoarthritis-a cross-sectional study. PLoS ONE. 2016;11:e0153177.
56. Rozumalski A, Schwartz MH. The GDI-Kinetic: a new index for quantifying kinetic deviations from normal gait. Gait Posture. 2011;33:730–2.
57. Rutz E, Baker R, Tirosh O, et al. Tibialis anterior tendon shortening in combination with Achilles tendon lengthening in spastic equinus in cerebral palsy. Gait Posture. 2011;33:152–7.
58. Rutz E, Donath S, Tirosh O, et al. Explaining the variability improvements in gait quality as a result of single event multi-level surgery in cerebral palsy. Gait Posture. 2013;38:455–60.
59. Schutte LM, Narayanan U, Stout JL, et al. An index for quantifying deviations from normal gait. Gait Posture. 2000;11:25–31.
60. Schwartz MH, Novacheck TF, Trost J. A tool for quantifying hip flexor function during gait. Gait Posture. 2000;12:122–7.
61. Schwartz MH, Rozumalski A. The gait deviation index: a new comprehensive index of gait pathology. Gait Posture. 2008;28:351–7.
62. Sienko Thomas S, Buckon CE, Nicorici A, et al. Classification of the gait patterns of boys with Duchenne muscular dystrophy and their relationship to function. J Child Neurol. 2010;25:1103–9.
63. Speciali DS, Oliveira EM, Cardoso JR, et al. Gait profile score and movement analysis profile in patients with Parkinson's disease during concurrent cognitive load. Braz J Phys Ther. 2014;18:315–22.
64. Speciali DS, Corrêa JC, Luna NM, et al. Validation of GDI, GPS and GVS for use in Parkinson's disease through evaluation of effects of subthalamic deep brain stimulation and levodopa. Gait Posture. 2014;39:1142–5.
65. Syczewska M, Dembowska-Bagińska B, Perek-Polnik M, et al. Gait pathology assessed with gillette gait index in patients after CNS tumour treatment. Gait Posture. 2010;32:358–62.
66. Sutherland DH. The evolution of clinical gait analysis part I: kinesiological EMG. Gait Posture. 2001;14(1):61–70.

67. Sutherland DH. The evolution of clinical gait analysis. Part II kinematics. Gait Posture. 2002;16(2):159–79.
68. Sutherland DH. The evolution of clinical gait analysis part III—kinetics and energy assessment. Gait Posture. 2005;21(4):447–61.
69. Szopa A, Domagalska-Szopa M, Czamara A. Gait pattern differences in children with unilateral cerebral palsy. Res Dev Disabil. 2014;35:2261–6.
70. Terjesen T, Lofterød B, Skaaret I. Gait improvement surgery in ambulatory children with diplegic cerebral palsy. Acta Orthop. 2015;86:511–7.
71. Thomason P, Baker R, Dodd K, et al. Single-event multilevel surgery in children with spastic diplegia: a pilot randomized controlled trial. J Bone Joint Surg Am. 2011;93:451–60.
72. Tinney A, Thomason P, Sangeux M, et al. The transverse Vulpius gastrocsoleus recession for equinus gait in children with cerebral palsy. Bone Joint J. (2015);97-B:564–71.
73. Trost JP, Schwartz MH, Krach LE, et al. Comprehensive short-term outcome assessment of selective dorsal rhizotomy. Dev Med Child Neurol. 2008;50:765–71.
74. Westhoff B, Martiny F, Reith A, et al. Computerized gait analysis in Legg-Calvé-Perthes disease–analysis of the sagittal plane. Gait Posture. 2012;35:541–6.

Exoskeletons for Over-Ground Gait Training in Spinal Cord Injury

Marco Molinari, Marcella Masciullo, Federica Tamburella, Nevio Luigi Tagliamonte, Iolanda Pisotta and José L. Pons

1 Introduction

Both in Europe and beyond, spinal cord injury (SCI) is becoming an increasingly major public health problem. The consequences of sustaining a SCI can be devastating and affect many aspects of a patient's life.

According to recent estimates, the incidence rate of SCI in Europe is around 6/million population/year; furthermore, every year, worldwide, between 250,000 and 500,000 people suffer a SCI. The number of people living with SCI is increasing year by year, reflecting the increased frequency of spinal lesions, but also the improvements in the life expectancy of subjects affected by SCI. However, although knowledge in this field is advancing all the time, there exist no interventions able to promote regeneration of spinal cord nerve pathways. In many cases, the aim of rehabilitation interventions is to help patients achieve greater autonomy in daily life, through the use of a wheelchair, which is currently the main tool capable of helping SCI patients to regain a degree of mobility and independence, even though in some cases the pursuit of greater independence can be impeded by obstacles, both physical and psychological [53].

M. Molinari (✉) · F. Tamburella · N. L. Tagliamonte · I. Pisotta
Neuro-Robot Rehabilitation Lab, Fondazione Santa Lucia IRCCS, Rome, Italy
e-mail: m.molinari@hsantalucia.it

M. Masciullo · F. Tamburella · N. L. Tagliamonte
Spinal Rehabilitation Lab, Fondazione Santa Lucia IRCCS, Rome, Italy

J. L. Pons
Neural Rehabilitation Group, Cajal Institute, Spanish National Research Council (CSIC), Madrid, Spain

G. Sandrini et al. (eds.), *Advanced Technologies for the Rehabilitation of Gait and Balance Disorders*, Biosystems & Biorobotics 19,
https://doi.org/10.1007/978-3-319-72736-3_18

Therefore, recovery of locomotor ability continues to be the top priority for SCI patients, irrespective of the severity of their conditions, the time that has elapsed since the injury, and their age when they sustained it [34]; it has indeed become the target of several SCI rehabilitation approaches.

Robotic gait assistance allows increased training duration, reproducible gait patterns, and close monitoring of the patient's progress during the treatment [33, 49]. Both the manual method, in which physical therapists manipulate the individual's lower limbs manually to reproduce a correct gait pattern [32], and the robotic gait method have led to improved patient outcomes, but there is not yet enough statistical evidence to affirm, definitively, the advantages of robotic training [62].

Robotic devices for gait training have undergone considerable technological development in recent years.

The first devices developed for gait rehabilitation were stationary robotic devices combining body weight support platforms and lower-limb active orthoses (e.g. Lokomat) [8].

With regard to these static solutions, wearable exoskeletons (WRs) present a number of advantages for rehabilitation, for example they enhance mobility, allow the patient to be trained in a range of different tasks, and get the patient more actively involved. In particular, the over-ground walking systems are robotic devices that help patients to practice gait, postural and balance exercises in a safe, controlled manner, and allow them to control their own movements, rather than moving only according to predetermined movement patterns.

However, all currently existing lower-limb WRs have been developed mainly to provide assistance: they are pre-programmed to help patients rehearse a certain gait pattern, and the repetition of these "imposed" gait kinematics through a number of cycles is expected to lead to improved motor function.

Substantial advances have been made in terms of the safety and portability of these exoskeletons, and also the skills they train and the enhancement of the effort required to use them [37, 63]. Unfortunately, however, while exoskeleton technology continues to advance, likely leading to psychological as well as physical benefits of legged mobility, the anticipated benefits across multiple physiological systems remain largely unproven. Moreover, these systems require considerable resources, due to their complex design, aspects of which include the type of actuators chosen to drive the robot, the base of support, which must be compact enough to allow indoor manoeuvrability, and the need for a well-designed mechanism to support the patients' body.

2 Learning in the Damaged Spinal Cord

Currently applied gait rehabilitation strategies are also based on evidence that the adult mammalian cortex and spinal cord have a remarkable capacity for activity-dependent plasticity when a subject undergoes gait training (e.g. on a treadmill).

Neural plasticity, a rather broadly used term, refers to a mechanism of reorganization of neuronal circuits that is activated during motor learning, for example, or after a neurotrauma at either cortical or spinal level [11]. Therefore, strategies for recovering gait ability are based on intensive training programmes designed to stimulate the central pattern generator (CPG) [13, 41]. Also, intensive training has other benefits, improving muscle tone and coordination of muscle groups. Neural plasticity, improved muscle tone and coordination, and changes in functional strategies to achieve walking (i.e. strategies not related to neurological changes) are the main elements that can contribute to improved locomotion [59]. In view of these considerations, a new rehabilitation intervention, based on the hypothesis that CPGs can be reactivated by rhythmic proprioceptive stimulation and body weight support gait training (BWST), was developed. Several nonrandomized trials reported that in motor-incomplete SCI patients, BWST produces some form of functional walking, with significant improvements in home and/or community walking [2–4, 14, 16, 22, 60].

By contrast, in motor-complete SCI patients, unsupported walking is seldom, if ever, recovered [19], even after BWST [29, 42]. In fact, even though individuals with a clinically complete SCI can, after BWST, generate 3–10 consecutive steps without assistance under optimal conditions in terms of limb loading, treadmill speed, and kinematics, they do not reach functional ambulation [29, 42].

A recent randomized trial [21] in which BWST plus over-ground practice was compared with over-ground practice alone, the two approaches were associated with an equal likelihood of functional over-ground walking in incomplete SCI patients admitted for rehabilitation. If gait can be recovered through rhythmic stimulation, robotic devices that can sustain rhythmic leg movements according to the rules of spinal locomotion may be of value. In fact, mechanical assistive devices have been developed and used clinically, being reported to be at least as effective as treadmill and conventional training.

More recently the idea that injured pathways have the capacity recover and uninjured ones to increase their activity has been supported by increasing experimental evidence of axonal sprouting, unmasking of relatively ineffective functional connections, and modification of synaptic strength—observations that provide neurobiological bases for the concept of spinal cord neuroplasticity [50]. However, if the recovery of gait is subtended by circuits other than those responsible for normal walking, this may be reflected in the characteristics of the recovered gait.

Robotic intervention in neuromotor rehabilitation is intended to promote the motor learning that is crucial for recovery. The efficacy of human-robot interactions in promoting learning depends on the sequence of actions either imposed on or self-selected by the patient. In the main, the strategies applied are intended to promote effort and self-initiated movements, and they are thought to: (a) allow a margin of error around a target path without providing assistance, (b) trigger assistance in relation to the amount of exerted force or velocity, (c) enable a compliance at the level of the joint, and (d) detrend the robotic assistance by means of what has been proposed as a forgetting factor [7, 43] comparable to the human controller. The use of robotics for training of specific motor tasks has recently become more prevalent, and we here report that using an "assist-as-needed" approach to step training after a severe SCI carries a high probability of resulting in successful rehabilitation. The "assist-as-needed" paradigm allows variability in the step trajectory within specific boundaries, with the robotic arms constraining the deviations in a manner mimicking that observed under normal, intact conditions. Another apparently critical feature of robotic devices or step training is their ability to integrate normal hip and leg motion, as occurs during normal stepping. Robotic devices of this kind have the potential to aid therapists in the clinical setting and to enhance the ability of SCI patients to regain their maximum possible level of locomotor activity.

3 The Sensory System as a Critical Source of Control After a Severe Spinal Cord Injury

It is generally assumed that the sensory information projecting to the spinal cord and brain serves to correct errors in movement, i.e., provides corrective feedback in response to the activation of sensory receptors. In cases of incomplete SCI, however, there appear to occur extensive adaptations in the interaction of multiple supraspinal centers having access, directly or indirectly, to the more restricted descending systems remaining to the spinal circuitry.

For example, a dramatic level of plasticity can occur after severe, but incomplete, SCIs in humans, and result in recovery of reasonably successful locomotion [20, 21].

The most relevant sensory input for locomotion comes from stretch- and load-sensitive mechanoreceptors located in the muscles and skin. Furthermore, skin receptors on the dorsal foot play a role during the swing phase of walking over obstacles in humans [48].

Proprioceptive input from leg extensor muscles, in the form of Ib afferent signals from Golgi tendon organs, and probably also from mechanoreceptors in the sole of the foot, provides load information [5]. This information is thought to be integrated into polysynaptic spinal reflex pathways that adapt the autonomous locomotor pattern to the actual ground condition. Furthermore, it is assumed that Ib afferent input from leg extensors during the stance phase inhibits leg flexor activity.

Afferent input from load receptors is a crucial factor that is needed to trigger a locomotor EMG pattern in individuals with SCI [18, 30]. This statement is based on the observation that unless the sole of the foot is loaded during the stance phase, no meaningful leg muscle activation occurs in individuals with complete SCI during supported stepping. The role of this specific afferent input is to generate and shape the locomotor pattern, to control phase transitions, and to reinforce ongoing activity.

In addition, in accordance with observations in cats [48], hip extension movements, i.e. hip-joint-related afferent input (minus inputs relative to knee or ankle joint excursions), are essential for the initiation of the swing phase and the generation of a locomotor EMG pattern in people with incomplete SCI [17]. Besides load receptor information, a hip joint-related afferent input was shown to be required for the generation of a locomotor pattern, and this was also shown to be the case for the generation of stepping in human infants [17].

In accordance with animal models, in motor-complete paraplegic subjects, assisted stepping movements within a driven gait orthosis and with restricted movements of the hips (blocked knees) induce a patterned leg EMG activity, highlighting the significance of hip joint receptors in the generation of locomotor activity [15].

4 Exoskeletons to Support Human Walking

Exoskeletons incorporate lightweight, wearable electrically-powered joints that mimic their (impaired) biological counterparts, and thus extend the patient's functional body. Exoskeletons, based on innovative medical technology, acquire the wearer's motion intentions, and they are designed to: (i) assist the wearer's locomotion; (ii) enhance the strength of the wearer's joints; and (iii) achieve a high level of performance in rehabilitation [8].

Several complex lower limb exoskeletons are commercially available, and others are in the prototype stage [6, 10, 23, 37, 46, 51, 54, 56, 57, 63]. These clinically applicable, assistive devices offer renewed hope to immobile individuals [45], and also the possibility, at least in principle, of partial recovery or functional substitution of the damaged body part.

Given the complex nature of locomotor control, compensatory strategies, and neuronal network plasticity, there is still a lack of knowledge on the effect of robotic gait assistance on locomotor function and its recovery in injured humans. It has been established that the synergistic nature of muscle coordination is maintained in healthy subjects during robotic gait training at various walking speeds and with different levels of assistance [44]. Four motor modules were sufficient to represent the variety of behavioural goals demanded during robotic guidance, with similar relationships between muscle patterns and biomechanical parameters across subjects, confirming that the low-dimensional and impulsive control of human walking is maintained using robotic force guidance.

A key feature of robots that support over-ground gait is that they enable individuals to practice, in the rehabilitation setting, the types of activity they will need to be proficient in before returning home and into the community. Indeed, the chance to practice walking over ground, standing up and sitting down, and other functional tasks is important, as all these tasks are critical components of functional independence, yet they are often difficult for patients with significant levels of impairment to practice safely; and it is not only the patient that is at risk of injury, but also the therapist. The integration of robotic technologies into neurorehabilitation can play a critical role in the safe and effective delivery of gait training.

Numerous wearable robots or powered exoskeletons for legged mobility are currently under development, undergoing clinical trials in human subjects, or already available on the market. Exoskeletons for the lower extremities have joints that match the patient's lower limb joints and motors that drive movements of these joints to assist leg movements. These "mechanical suits" can help people with SCIs to stand up and walk away from their wheelchairs. These robots were designed around the function and shape of the human body, and the wearer is able to control the robotic limbs; this may improve his ability to walk, run and jump, and can also enable him to lift objects he would not normally be able to lift.

Here we differentiate between:

- exoskeletons for human strength augmentation, and
- exoskeletons for rehabilitation purposes.

(i) *Exoskeletons for human strength augmentation*

The idea of using technology to replace limb function lost as a result of trauma or disease is not a prerogative of the modern era: archaeological data show that hip replacements were constructed even in ancient Greek and Roman times [31]. Over the centuries the approach did not change much, and it is only in the modern era that developments in the field of computer science have ushered in an approach based on greater interaction between technological apparatuses and human beings. Considering the complexity of the interrelationships between patient and orthosis, and of efforts to restore the complete loop, including incoming movement-related sensory information [31], the road is anything but simple and has indeed proven more difficult, complex and above all slower than initially envisaged.

SARCOS (USA) was the first exoskeleton, developed for military use. It was funded by DARPA in 2000. It implements rotary hydraulic actuators at the hip and knee and a linear hydraulic actuator at the ankle, and uses elastic joints (to reduce the required joint torques) in combination with variable dampers at the knee. The drawback is that the exoskeleton increased the metabolic energy consumption of subjects wearing it. Moreover, the elastic joints are symmetrical, i.e. they have a similar torque-angle relationship for flexion and extension and are mono articular.

BLEEX (USA), the Berkeley Lower Extremity Exoskeleton (BLEEX), consists of a metal frame that holds a backpack and two exoskeletal legs. Actuation is performed at the hip, knee and ankle joint in the sagittal plane; the remaining degrees of freedom movements of the hip and ankle can be achieved passively. Force sensors are attached under the soles of both feet. It is designed for autonomous operation by a small fuel engine that supplies the onboard computer and the hydraulics with power [64]. The principle of the control scheme is to minimize the interaction forces between the human and the machine [36]. There are no algorithms implemented to control postural stability in the event of unexpected forces acting on the operator.

MIT quasi-passive leg exoskeleton (USA). This, too, is based on the working principle of using elastic joints (to reduce the required joint torques) in combination with variable dampers at the knee. This exoskeleton also has the drawback of increasing the metabolic energy consumption of subjects wearing it. Moreover, the elastic joints are symmetrical, i.e. they have a similar torque-angle relationship for flexion and extension and are mono articular.

The NTU Exoskeleton (Singapore) [39, 40] developed at the Nanyang Technological University features two actuated legs that hold a payload frame, and the operator (patient) stands on the footplates of the exoskeleton. The idea of the control scheme is that the exoskeleton footplate follows the trajectory of the operator's foot during the swing phase of each leg. This allows the operator to provide information about the desired velocity and stride length. The exoskeleton utilizes the ZMP (zero moment point) concept to ensure that balance is maintained during motion.

Power Assisting Suit (Japan). Researchers at the Kanagawa Institute of Technology have developed an exoskeleton for assisting nursing personnel when handling patients. The suit weighs 30 kg. It supports the operator (patient) at the elbows, waist and knees with pneumatic actuators. The controller structure calculates the joint torques required to maintain a statically stable position by computing the inverse of a rigid body model that takes into account the current joint angles and masses of the components of the exoskeleton and the weight of the patient. The patient is weighed beforehand [61].

ReWalk (Israel) developed by Argo Medical Technologies. Upper body motions are analyzed and used to trigger and maintain walking (gait) patterns and other modes of operation (such as stair climbing and shifting from sitting to standing), leaving the hands free for self-support and/or other functions. This approach relies on the use of crutches by the wearer.

Indego® (USA) consists of a hip segment, a right and left thigh segment, and a right and left shank segment. Although the exoskeleton does not explicitly contain a foot segment or ankle joint, it is designed to be used in conjunction with a set of standard ankle-foot orthoses. In addition, the Indego® does not have any exposed cables or anything heavy to carry on the back and does not require a backpack. According to the Indego® website (Indego. Nashville, TN; 2014 Available from: http://indego.com/indego/en/home), the device is quick and easy to put on, take off and adjust with just one hand, without assistance. The average walking speed is 0. 22 m/s (0.8 km/h). The Indego® has six modes (sit-to-stand transitions, standing, stand-to-walk transitions, walking, walk-to stand transitions, and stand-to-sit transitions), weighs 12.3 kg, and the battery allows up to 4 h of use (Indego, Nashville, TN; 2014 Available from: http://indego.com/indego/en/home, last accessed 25 Jul 2014). A recent study [24] compared the usefulness of in-lab training with Indego® versus knee-ankle-foot orthoses (non-powered), between parallel bars, considering distance, time and speed: Indego® was found to be much more effective.

(ii) *Exoskeletons for rehabilitation purposes*

The **Powered Lower Limb Orthosis** (USA) developed at the University of Michigan is designed for rehabilitation of patients with neurological injuries. Investigations focus on consequences for the patient (immediate and long term), changes in movement behaviour, and whether certain simple control modes can, in practice, be handled by patients. The orthosis is powered at the knee and ankle joint by artificial pneumatic muscles with movement limited to the sagittal plane.

The air supply and the controller are not mounted on the exoskeleton. Since it is mainly designed as a rehabilitation device for use in a clinical environment, this is not a major restriction. A detailed description of the design and construction can be found in Ferris et al. [25]. The different modes of operation can be found in Sawicki et al. [52]. Experiments showed that after a couple of minutes healthy volunteers could adapt their muscle activations properly, resulting in a close-to-normal kinematic gait pattern.

TUPLEE (Germany) [26, 27] is an exoskeleton for the lower extremities, developed at Technische Universität Berlin (TUB). It uses electrical signals from the muscles as the main means of information transportation between the human operator and the exoskeleton. It is designed to support the movement of a subject at the knee joint (in activities like walking, climbing stairs, sit-to-stand movements) by contributing extra torque through an electrical actuator.

These electrical (EMG) signals are picked up from the skin overlying selected muscles and reflect the activation of the observed muscle. They are evaluated using a sophisticated but simplified biomechanical model of the human body in order to derive the operator's desired action. A support action is computed in accordance with the desired action and is executed by the exoskeleton. The biomechanical model contains parameters that reflect properties of the human operator and his or her current body state. A calibration algorithm for these parameters has also been developed which relies exclusively on sensors mounted on the exoskeleton.

EKSO (Eksobionics Ltd, Richmond, CA, USA) is a wearable lower extremity robotic exoskeleton with two legs connected to a torso structure containing the computer and batteries. The torso is aligned with the user's lower back, and the exoskeleton legs are fastened to the user's legs by hook-and-loop fastener straps that align the user's lower back and joints with those of the device. Two additional straps are tightened over the user's shoulders to help support the torso structure. The device has powered (bilaterally) hip and knee joints in the sagittal plane and other movement directions are restricted. The ankle joints of the exoskeleton allow passive (spring) movement limited to the sagittal plane.

Currently, Ekso has four walk modes: in the first two walk modes, either a physical therapist or the user actuates sit-to-stand transitions and steps with a button push; whereas in the other two walk modes, gait intent detection, to command the exoskeleton, is accomplished by detecting the forward and lateral movement of the user's hips (to accomplish weight shift), or by the user's weight shift and initiation of forward leg movement. Ekso requires walking aids, and crutches are provided to ensure the stability and safety of the user; the bottoms of the crutches are fitted with force sensors to ensure firm placement on the ground and at least partial weight bearing. No step will be triggered unless both crutches are firmly on the ground. Additionally, the controller uses a hierarchical finite-state machine to transition between the different movements without forcing the user into unsafe positions [55].

The Hybrid Assistive Leg (HAL) (Japan) was developed in cooperation between the Japanese University of Tsukuba and the company Cyberdyne Systems. The project focuses on supporting elderly and gait-disordered people. Different control strategies have been developed with the primary interface being EMG signals from the operator's muscles. Early prototypes consisted of a system with four actuated joints (DC motors) at the hip and knee of both legs, with passive joints at the ankles. The latest development (HAL 5) also includes actuated shoulder and elbow joints. The controller relies on estimated torques based on the EMG measurements which are used as the target values of the control algorithm [35]. In a single case experimental A-B (pre-post) design study, Aach et al. [1] tested the HAL in 8 chronic SCI patients. The results obtained revealed a highly significant improvement in over-ground walking abilities evaluated by the 10MWT, the 6MWT, and the TUG test, and a partial reduction of physical assistance and walking aids in the WISCI II score.

Kinesis (Technaid, Madrid, Spain) is a lower limb rehabilitation robot designed for providing hybrid gait training to patients with incomplete SCI. The target population is patients with a prognosis for functional recovery of walking, i.e. patients who can walk short distances but depend on a wheelchair for community ambulation, and usually conserve some hip flexor function. Kinesis is a knee-ankle-foot exoskeleton, equipped with an active actuator at the knee, and a passive elastic actuator at the ankle for plantar and dorsal flexion; it is equipped with force-sensitive resistors to detect foot-ground contact, potentiometers to monitor joint angular position, and an embedded strain gauge-based Wheatstone bridge to measure user-robot interaction torques [12]. As a hybrid-therapy system, Kinesis can provide functional electrical stimulation (FES) to the knee extensor (rectus femoris and vastus lateralis) and flexor (semitendinosus and biceps femoris) muscles through surface electrodes. Its controller comprises four main components: (1) a robotic or joint controller, (2) a FES controller, (3) a muscle fatigue estimator, and (4) a finite-state machine.

There is some evidence that FES-assisted walking can enable walking or enhance walking speed in incomplete or complete SCI. Also, regular use of FES in gait training or activities of daily living can lead to improvement in walking even when the stimulator is not in use [38]. However, FES also raises challenges, such as rapid fatigue in muscles and poor control of joint trajectories [58], and these preclude its widespread use for gait compensation. The addition of FES to an exoskeleton system can allow exploitation of the muscle power generation, reducing the power demand of the exoskeleton and allowing the use of less powerful joint actuators, leading to a less heavy and power-demanding system. Also, the combination of FES and exoskeleton technologies can allow longer use of the neuromuscular electrical stimulation, and therefore increase the benefits derived from FES-induced gait: muscle strength and cardio-respiratory fitness [9, 28, 38, 47].

5 Conclusions

Overall, existing exoskeletons at best allow subjects to walk on regular ground, and in all cases, support is needed for balance. Anecdotal reports indicate that paraplegic subjects may use an exoskeleton to participate in a marathon. The first symbolic kick-off in the 2014 World Cup in Brazil was made by a young paraplegic man equipped with a Brain Computer Interface-controlled exoskeleton. Nevertheless, the use of exoskeletons among people with SCIs is still extremely limited and almost exclusively confined to supervised environments. To become more widely used, exoskeletons have to overcome many of their present limitations. The critical aspects needing to be addressed in the near future include reducing their bulkiness, and increasing patient autonomy in their use, as well as other aspects such as velocity, adaptability to all terrains, balance, and portability. It seems that technological advances will allow these issues to be overcome within the foreseeable future.

On the other hand, a challenge with no clear solutions in the foreseeable future is that of developing physiological symbiotic control mechanisms. The currently available exoskeletons allow very little interaction with the user. In general stepping is produced in a stereotyped way through a binary command coming either from a hand-controlled tool or from weight shifting. No on-line control of either balance or velocity is implemented, and the subject is more or less passively transported by the machine. The development of human-machine interaction modules capable of collecting biological signals to drive exoskeleton movement is the real challenge. In this regard, balance control might represent an area worth exploring. An exoskeleton not requiring crutches or other tools would free the wearer's hands, and allow him to cope with obstacles and irregularities in the terrain. Furthermore, a balance shared control module will represent an extremely important step for the development of gait shared control modules.

To achieve better acceptance in clinical rehabilitation, exoskeletons need to show a greater capacity to adapt to rehabilitation needs, allowing interactions with rehab professionals, thereby allowing customable evaluation and training sessions. The development of closed-loop real-time control mechanisms, based on biological signals and capable of adapting exoskeleton performances to the ever-changing needs of patients, currently appears to be the right direction to follow for future developments in this field.

To rise from their wheelchair and walk, at will, in all environments and at a reasonable speed is the dream of all subjects with paraplegia. This once unimaginable goal now seems within reach, but many obstacles still have to be overcome before exoskeletons can allow paraplegics to stand easily, balance effortlessly and walk at the same pace as anyone else—or maybe even run along a beach! Biologically inspired shared control mechanisms that would include mastering of balance, pace and obstacles may represent the answer to these high expectancies of persons with damage of the spinal cord.

References

1. Aach M, Cruciger O, Sczesny-Kaiser M, et al. Voluntary driven exoskeleton as a new tool for rehabilitation in chronic spinal cord injury: a pilot study. Spine J. 2014;14:2847–53.
2. Barbeau H, Fung J. The role of rehabilitation in the recovery of walking in the neurological population. Curr Opin Neurol. 2001;14:735–40.
3. Barbeau H, Ladouceur M, Norman KE, et al. Walking after spinal cord injury: evaluation, treatment and functional recovery. Arch Phys Med Rehabil. 1999;80:225–35.
4. Barbeau H, McCrea DA, O'Donovan MJ, et al. Tapping into spinal circuits to restore motor function. Brain Res Rev. 1999;30:27–51.
5. Bastiaanse CM, Duysens J, Dietz V. Modulation of cutaneous reflexes by load receptor input during human walking. Exp Brain Res. 2000;135:189–98.
6. Belforte G, Gastaldi L, Sorli M. Pneumatic active gait orthosis. Mechatronics. 2001;11:301–23.
7. Belda-Lois J-M, Mena-del Horno S, Bermejo-Bosch I, et al. Rehabilitation of gait after stroke: a review towards a top-down approach. J Neuroeng Rehabil. 2011;8:66.
8. Chen G, Chan CK, Guo Z, et al. A review of lower extremity assistive robotic exoskeletons in rehabilitation therapy. Crit Rev Biomed Eng. 2013;41:343–63.
9. Creasey GH, Ho CH, RJ, et al. Clinical applications of electrical stimulation after spinal cord injury. J Spinal Cord Med. 2004;27:365–75.
10. Cruciger O, Tegenthoff M, Schwenkreis P, et al. Locomotion training using voluntary driven exoskeleton (HAL) in acute incomplete SCI. Neurology. 2014;83:474.
11. Curt A, Hedel HV, Klaus D, Dietz V, Group ESS. Recovery from a spinal cord injury: significance of compensation, neural plasticity, and repair. J Neurotrauma. 2008;25:677–85.
12. del-Ama A, Koutsou A, Moreno J. Review of hybrid exoskeletons to restore gait following spinal cord injury. J Rehabil Res Dev. 2012;49(4):497–514.
13. Dietz V. Spinal cord pattern generators for locomotion. Clin Neurophysiol. 2003;114:1379–89.
14. Dietz V, Colombo G, Jensen L, et al. Locomotor capacity of spinal cord in paraplegic patients. Ann Neurol. 1995;37:574–82.
15. Dietz V, Colombo G. Effects of body immersion on postural adjustments to voluntary arm movements in humans: role of load receptor input. J Physiol. 1996;497:849–56.
16. Dietz V, Wirz M, Curt A, et al. Locomotor pattern in paraplegic patients: training effects and recovery of spinal cord function. Spinal Cord. 1998;36:380–90.
17. Dietz V. Do human bipeds use quadrupedal coordination? Trends Neurosci. 2002;25:462–7.
18. Dietz V. Neuronal plasticity after a human spinal cord injury: positive and negative effects. Exp Neurol. 2012;235:110–5.
19. Ditunno JF, Graziani V, Tessler A. Neurological assessment in spinal cord injury. Adv Neurol. 1997;72:325–33.
20. Ditunno JF Jr, Barbeau H, Dobkin BH, et al. Validity of the walking scale for spinal cord injury and other domains of function in a multicenter clinical trial. Neurorehabil Neural Repair. 2007;21:539–50.
21. Dobkin B, Apple D, Barbeau H, et al. Weight-supported treadmill vs. over-ground training for walking after acute incomplete SCI. Neurology. 2006;66:484–93.
22. Dobkin B, Harkema S, Requejo P, et al. Modulation of locomotor-like EMG activity in subjects with complete and incomplete spinal cord injury. J Neurol Rehabil. 1995;9:183–90.
23. Esquenazi A, Talaty M, Packel A, Saulino M. The ReWalk powered exoskeleton to restore ambulatory function to individuals with thoracic-level motor-complete spinal cord injury. Am J Phys Med Rehabil. 2012;91:911–21.
24. Farris R, Quintero H, Murray S, et al. A preliminary assessment of legged mobility provided by a lower limb exoskeleton for persons with paraplegia. IEEE Trans Neural Syst Rehabil Eng. 2014;22:482–90.

25. Ferris DP, Czerniecki JM, Hannaford B. An ankle-foot orthosis powered by artificial pneumatic muscles. J Appl Biomech. 2005;21:189–97.
26. Fleischer C. Controlling exoskeletons with EMG signals and a biomechanical body model. Dissertation, TU Berlin; 2007.
27. Fleischer C, Hommel G. Calibration of an EMG-based body model with six muscles to control a leg exoskeleton. In: Proceedings of the 2007 IEEE International Conference on Robotics and Automation (ICRA07). 2007, p. 2514–2519.
28. Graupe DH, Cerrel-Bazo H Kern, et al. Walking performance, medical outcomes and patient training in FES of innervated muscles for ambulation by thoracic-level complete paraplegics. Neurol Res. 2008;30:123–30.
29. Harkema S, Dobkin BH, Edgerton VR. Pattern generators in locomotion: implications for recovery of walking after spinal cord injury. Top Spinal Cord Injury Rehabil. 2000;6:82–96.
30. Harkema SJ, Hurley SL, Patel UK, et al. Human lumbosacral spinal cord interprets loading during stepping. J Neurophysiol. 1997;77:797–811.
31. Hernigou P. Ambroise pare IV: the early history of artificial limbs (from robotic to prostheses). Int Orthop. 2013;37:1195–7.
32. Hesse S, Werner C, Paul T, et al. Influence of walking speed on lower limb muscle activity and energy consumption during treadmill walking of hemiparetic patients. Arch Phys Med Rehabil. 2001;82:1547–50.
33. Hidler J, Sainburg R. Role of robotics in neurorehabilitation. Top Spinal Cord Inj Rehabil. 2011;17:42–9.
34. Hubli M, Dietz V. The physiological basis of neurorehabilitation–locomotor training after spinal cord injury. J Neuroeng Rehabil. 2013;10:5.
35. Kawamoto H, Kanbe S, Sankai Y. Power assist method for HAL3 estimating operator's intention based on motion information. In: Proceedings of the 2003 IEEE International Workshop on Robot and Human Interactive Communication. 2003, p. 67–72.
36. Kazerooni H. Exoskeletons for human power augmentation. Intelligent Robots and Systems, 2005 (IROS). In: Proceedings of the 2005 IEEE/RSJ International Conference. 2005;3459–64.
37. Kolakowsky-Hayner SA. Safety and feasibility of using the EksoTM bionic exoskeleton to aid ambulation after spinal cord injury. J Spine 2013;S4:1–8.
38. Lam T, Wolfe D, Eng J, Domingo A. Lower limb rehabilitation following spinal cord injury. In: Eng JJ, Teasell RW, Miller WC, Wolfe DL, Townson AF, Hsieh JTC, Connolly SJ, Mehta S, Sakakibara BM, editors. Spinal Cord Injury Rehabilitation Evidence. 2010;1–47.
39. Liu X, Low KH. Development and preliminary study of the NTU lower extremity exoskeleton. Cybernetics and Intelligent Systems, IEEE Conference on 2004 (vol. 2, p. 1099–106).
40. Liu X, Low KH, Yu HY. Development of a lower extremity exoskeleton for human performance enhancement. Intelligent Robots and Systems, 2004 (IROS). Proceedings of the 2004 IEEE/RSJ International Conference on, 2004 (vol. 4, p. 3889–94).
41. MacKay-Lyons M. Central pattern generation of locomotion: a review of the evidence. Phys Ther. 2002;82:69–83.
42. Maegele M, Muller S, Wernig A, et al. Recruitment of spinal motor pools during voluntary movements versus stepping after human spinal cord injury. J Neurotrauma. 2002;19:1217–29.
43. Marchal-Crespo L, Reinkensmeyer DJ. Review of control strategies for robotic movement training after neurologic injury. J Neuroeng Rehabil. 2009;6:20.
44. Moreno JC, Barroso F, Farina D, et al. Effects of robotic guidance on the coordination of locomotion. J NeuroEng Rehabil. 2013;10:79.
45. Moreno JC, Del Ama AJ, de Los Reyes-Guzman A, et al. Neurorobotic and hybrid management of lower limb motor disorders: a review. Med Biol Eng Comput 2011;49:1119–1130.
46. Neuhaus PD, Noorden JH, Craig TJ, et al. Design and evaluation of mina: a robotic orthosis for paraplegics. IEEE Int Conf Rehabil Robot. 2011;2011:5975468.

47. Nightingale EJ, Raymond J, Middleton JW, et al. Benefits of FES gait in a spinal cord injured population. Spinal Cord. 2007;45:646–57.
48. Pearson KG. Role of sensory feedback in the control of stance duration in walking cats. Brain Res Rev. 2008;57:222–7.
49. Pons JL. Wearable Robots. Chicester, UK: Wiley; 2008.
50. Rainetau O, Schwab ME. Plasticity of motor systems after incomplete spinal cord injury. Nat Rev Neurosci. 2001;2:263–73.
51. Sanz-Merodio D, Cestari M, ArevaloJ C, et al. A lower-limb exoskeleton for gait assistance in quadriplegia. EEE international conference on robotics and biomimetics: ROBIO. 2012;2012:107511–4.
52. Sawicki GS, Gordon KE, Ferris DP. Powered lower limb orthoses: applications in motor adaptation and rehabilitation. In: Rehabilitation Robotics, 2005 (ICORR). 9th International Conference on 2005, p. 206–11.
53. Simpson LA, Eng JJ, Hsieh JTC, et al. The Health and life priorities of individuals with spinal cord injury: a systematic review. J Neurotrauma. 2012;29:1548–55.
54. Stein J, Bishop L, Stein DJ, et al. Gait training with a robotic leg brace after stroke: a randomized controlled pilot study. Am J Phys Med Rehabil. 2014;93:987–94.
55. Strausser KA, Kazerooni H. The development and testing of a human machine interface for a mobile medical exoskeleton. In: IEEE/RSJ International Conference on Intelligent Robots and Systems (IROS), 2011. Piscataway, NJ: IEEE.
56. Strausser KA, Swift TA, Zoss AB et al. Prototype medical exoskeleton for paraplegic mobility: first experimental results. In: ASME 2010 dynamic systems and control conference: DSCC, 2010.
57. Sylos-Labini F, La Scaleia V, d'Avella A, et al. EMG patterns during assisted walking in the exoskeleton. Front Human Neurosci. 2014;8:423.
58. Thrasher TA, Popovic MR. Functional electrical stimulation of walking: function, exercise and rehabilitation. Ann Readapt Med Phys. 2008;51:452–60.
59. Van Hedel H, Dietz V. Rehabilitation of locomotion after spinal cord injury. Restor Neurol Neurosci. 2010;28:123–34.
60. Wernig A, Muller S, Nanassy A, et al. Laufband therapy based on "rules of spinal locomotion" is effective in spinal cord injured persons. Eur J Neurosci. 1995;7:823–9.
61. Yamamoto K, Ishii M, Noborisaka H et al. Stand alone wearable power assisting suit-sensing and control systems. Robot and Human Interactive Communication, 2004. ROMAN 2004. 13th IEEE International Workshop on 2004, p. 661–6.
62. Yang JF, Musselman KE. Training to achieve over ground walking after spinal cord injury: a review of who, what, when, and how. J Spinal Cord Med. 2012;35:293–304.
63. Zeilig G, Weingarden H, Zwecker M, et al. Safety and tolerance of the ReWalk exoskeleton suit for ambulation by people with complete spinal cord injury: a pilot study. J Spin Cord Med. 2012;35:96–101.
64. Zoss A, Kazerooni H, Chu A. On the mechanical design of the Berkeley Lower Extremity Exoskeleton (BLEEX). Intelligent Robots and Systems, 2005 (IROS). Proceedings of the 2005 IEEE/RSJ International Conference on 2005, p. 3465–72.

The End-Effector Device for Gait Rehabilitation

Nicola Smania, Christian Geroin, Nicola Valè and Marialuisa Gandolfi

1 Introduction

Today's concepts of motor learning address the demand for adequate therapy solutions with a task-specific approach. Since the 1990s, robot-assisted gait training (RAGT) has become a promising approach, alongside conventional rehabilitation, for treating gait disturbances in patients with neurological disease. RAGT devices enable the patient to practice an intensive, repetitive and assisted gait-like movement and have been found to improve mobility and independence in activities of daily living [31]. On the basis of their driving principles, robotic devices for gait rehabilitation can be divided into two categories: exoskeleton and end-effector

N. Smania (✉)
Neurorehabilitation Unit, Department of Neurological, Biomedical and Movement Sciences, Hospital Trust of Verona, Neuromotor and Cognitive Rehabilitation Research Centre (CRRNC), University of Verona, P.le L.a. Scuro 10, 37134 Verona, Italy
e-mail: nicola.smania@univr.it

C. Geroin · N. Valè · M. Gandolfi
Department of Neurosciences, Biomedicine and Movement Sciences, Neuromotor and Cognitive Rehabilitation Research Centre (CRRNC), University of Verona, Verona, Italy
e-mail: christian.geroin@univr.it

N. Valè
e-mail: nicola.vale22@gmail.com

M. Gandolfi
e-mail: marialuisa.gandolfi@univr.it

N. Smania · M. Gandolfi
U.O.C. of Neurorehabilitation, A.O.U.I. Verona, Verona, Italy

G. Sandrini et al. (eds.), *Advanced Technologies for the Rehabilitation of Gait and Balance Disorders*, Biosystems & Biorobotics 19,
https://doi.org/10.1007/978-3-319-72736-3_19

robots [20]. The former, extensively described elsewhere in this book, consist of treadmill-centered technology combined with an exoskeleton and a body weight support system. The latter represent an alternative approach in which footplates are used to guide the feet and thereby reproduce the gait trajectory.

A full review of the neural correlates of walking control is beyond the scope of this chapter. Nevertheless, the overall evidence that locomotion control relies on the integrity of spinal central pattern generators, along with feedback and feed-forward mechanisms of movement control supports the use of robotic gait training technology in patients with neurological impairment [33].

There is plenty of literature indicating that repetitive gait-like movements promote gait recovery. Interestingly, however, the training effects of end-effector-type systems may extend beyond this, enhancing not only gait but also balance recovery [11].

In this chapter, we briefly review (1) the types of end-effector devices employed in clinical trials; (2) the scientific evidence on the effects of end-effector robot-assisted training in patients with neurological impairment, and (3) the potential mechanisms involved in robot-induced gait recovery.

2 Existing End-Effector Robotic Gait Training Devices

A number of devices have been used in the gait rehabilitation of patients with neurological impairments. Some of them are commercially available products, while others have been built and applied only in the laboratory setting. With regard to the commercially available devices, four end-effector robotic gait training systems have been investigated in the literature: the Gait Trainer (GT1), the G-EO System, the Gait Master and the LokoHelp (LH).

The GT1 (Reha-Stim, Berlin) is the first electromechanical device developed for the rehabilitation of gait in patients with stroke [13]. In accordance with its tenet "learning to walk by walking", the GT1 focuses on improving the patient's ability to walk through the repetitive training of lost movements. The GT1 enables wheelchair-bound subjects to practice a gait-like movement with minimal assistance and with a reduced number of constraints, acting at different lower limb levels. The training can be intensified or lightened thanks to a body weight support system and by adapting the pace to the individual patient's ability. Compared with traditional treadmill therapy, the GT1 demands significantly less effort on the part of the attending staff, while increasing the amount of gait rehabilitation provided.

The GT1 follows the end-effector principle. The patient stands on two movable footplates, whose movements are controlled by a planetary gear system. The footplates are motor driven and control 1 degree of freedom (DOF) of the foot in the sagittal plane. The stance and swing phases of the gait cycle are simulated in an assisted gait-like movement. The patient's horizontal and vertical trunk movements are also assisted according to the gait phase. Spatiotemporal gait parameters (i.e. step length, gait speed) can be set individually taking into account the patient's impairments and, over time, improvements. Accordingly, the body weight support system allows the patient to be trained in different assistance conditions according to his/her neurological impairment. During therapy, the integrated servo drive automation supports the patient's own effort, ensuring that the rotation speed is kept constant. Note that the patient's knees are not fixed. The physiotherapist, if necessary, can assist the patient's movement through physical manual contact to correct certain deficits of mobility that need to be compensated for e.g. exaggerated knee flexion, knee hyperextension, lack of full knee extension. Furthermore, a knee support system has been developed to make the knee perform a natural gait pattern and to stabilize the patient's gait. Training can also be combined with functional electrical stimulation (FES) to stimulate the activity of lower limb muscles during the task-specific exercise.

Two main advantages can be acknowledged. First, the GT1 is easy to use. Before the therapy session, the patient puts on the harness system, which is customizable to his/her physical characteristics. The patient is positioned using the built-in swivel device, the feet being secured on the base plates and the wire mounts attached to compensate for lateral movement of the body. Second, several diseases such as cerebral palsy [34], multiple sclerosis [11], stroke [12] and Parkinson's disease [27, 28] may benefit from the therapeutic possibilities of the GT1, and the system can also be used in patients with joint replacements. Possible limitations of the GT1 are the incomplete unloading of the lower limb in the swing phase of gait, and the impossibility of training other aspects related to patients' mobility, such as climbing up and down stairs. These drawbacks have been partially overcome by the HapticWalker [32], which is the first end-effector device to enable harness-secured patients to perform repetitive practice of climbing up and down stairs. The system comprises two 3-DOF robot modules that allow each foot to move in the sagittal plane. Foot movement along the horizontal and vertical base axes is performed by linear direct drive motors, which run independently on a common rail, but are connected via a slider-crank system. The HapticWalker comprises a translatory and rotatory footplate workspace that ensures permanent foot attachment along arbitrary walking trajectories during all phases of gait. The HapticWalker footplate dynamics were designed to simulate walking speeds of up to 5 km/h with a maximum acceleration of 3.5 g and 120 steps/min [31]. The foot module contains a 6-DOF force/torque sensor and the footplate. Note that the dimensions of this device and the high voltage required during natural gait of healthy subjects have limited its clinical utility.

The G-EO System (Reha Technologies, Swiss) [15] may be considered the latest innovation in the field of electromechanical end-effector devices. It offers the unique feature of realistically simulating walking and climbing stairs. It can be operated effortlessly by a single physiotherapist. The graphic user interface shows the actual trajectory so that the physiotherapist can control and correct it, if needed. Spatiotemporal parameters (e.g. step length, step height, terminal stance, and initial contact) can be modified, as can inclination angles of the feet and the vertical and lateral excursions of the center of mass. The footplates each have 3 DOFs, allowing control of the length and height of the steps and the footplate angles. The binding opens and the machine stops immediately in the event of incorrect trajectory settings. Two further DOFs control the lateral displacement of the hip and of the body weight support system.

Two therapy modes are mastered: the active mode and the active-assistive mode. The former allows the patient to self-initiate the gait simulation by overcoming a pre-selected resistance (threshold). This mode is thought to increase the level of active participation during the therapy session. The latter, instead, senses the patient's efforts to overcome the pre-selected resistance threshold and then augments the patient's effort during the initiation of his/her gait movement. The adaptive control is applied only to two of the 3 DOFs intended to control the legs, while the other 2 DOFs controlling the center of mass (body weight support system and the lateral displacement of the hip) are not activated [36].

As mentioned, the G-EO System offers the unique feature of simulated up-and-down stair climbing. This is generated by motion capture data and calculated based on Blondel's Rule for an 18 cm step. This feature offers the possibility of a creating complete rehabilitation pathway leading to full recovery of mobility. The short setup time and the easy accessibility of the device, even for patients in wheelchairs (thanks to the rear platform), are the main features contributing to its clinical utility. Finally, the G-EO System can be flexibly deployed for the treatment of several diseases (e.g. stroke, multiple sclerosis, Parkinson's disease).

The other two commercially available mechanical gait devices are the LokoHelp (LokoHelp Group, Germany) and the GaitMaster4. The former is an electromechanical gait device designed to be placed on a treadmill [9]. The patient is secured with a harness that supports his/her body weight. Each lower leg is placed in an orthosis, which keeps the ankle joint at a 90° angle. The LokoHelp device is then fixed onto the belt of the motor-driven treadmill and transmits the treadmill movement to levers positioned on the two sides of the device. The orthoses are then attached to these lateral levers. Simulation of gait is obtained thanks to the path followed by the levers, which imitate the stance and swing phases in a sequentially accurate manner. Ropes attached to the side and front bars control the movements of the center of mass. Gait speed can be set individually from 0 to 2.5 km/h, while step length is fixed at 400 mm. Physical assistance can be provided according to the patient's needs (e.g. to control knee or hip extension in the stance phase).

The GaitMaster4 (Department of Intelligent Interaction Technologies of the Graduate School of Systems and Information Engineering, University of Tsukuba) consists of two slider cranks and two ball-screw actuators, serving to move the footpads back and forth, and up and down respectively [40]. Gait movement is thus carried out by footpads passively moving the patient's feet back and forth, and up and down. As a result, a patient can perform repetitive hip extension exercises. A computer controls gait trajectories and speed, which can be set according to the patient's condition. No body weight support system is provided. Indeed, during training, the physical therapist has to assist the patient's body and lower limb movements, and support the trunk if needed.

In summary, these end-effector devices share similar pros and cons. Movements are not constrained to only one anatomical plane (i.e. the sagittal plane), thus increasing the patient's influence on the walking trajectory and allowing meaningful balance training. The patient is not largely guided through the movements, as is the case with exoskeleton devices. As a result, the patient is able to produce movements more volitionally, and be more involved in the gait training. The absence of an exoskeleton structure does not allow support of the knee joint. This condition might be challenging for some patients, who may require assistance from the therapist and support from orthoses. By contrast, for other patients, it could be a means of improving control strategies, offering more scope for patient influence on the walking trajectory.

3 Clinical Outcomes of End-Effector Robotic Gait Training Devices

A systematic review of studies involving electromechanical and end-effector robot-assisted gait training clinical trials (RAGTCTs) was performed. First, a search of MEDLINE, EMBASE, CINALH, PubMed, PsychINFO and Scopus databases was carried out to identify relevant studies. The keywords used were: Stroke, Traumatic Brain Injury, Cerebral Palsy, Parkinson's Disease, Spinal Cord Injury, Multiple Sclerosis, Lower limb, Rehabilitation, Gait training and Physiotherapy.

Inclusion criteria were: studies published from January 2001 until June 2016; studies involving subjects affected by neurological disorders such as stroke, traumatic brain injury, cerebral palsy, Parkinson's disease, spinal cord injury, and multiple sclerosis; RAGTCTs involving end-effector devices. Exclusion criteria were: studies involving only healthy subjects, use of robotic orthosis devices, and articles published in a language other than English.

The table lists the main RAGTCTs dealing with end-effector devices, giving key information: device name, study design, type and stage of neurological disease, number of subjects enrolled, treatment procedures and main findings.

3.1 Results

A total of 20 articles published from 2001 to 2016 (involving 904 individuals) fulfilled the inclusion criteria for the review. A total of four different end-effector devices were evaluated in terms of clinical efficacy using different study designs: 13 randomized controlled clinical trials, three crossover clinical trials, and four clinical trials (three feasibility studies and one prospective observational study). Several neurological conditions were explored: stroke (16 studies), spinal cord injury (2 studies), traumatic brain injury (2 studies), Parkinson's disease (2 studies), multiple sclerosis (1 study) and cerebral palsy (1 study).

These studies explored the effects of end-effector devices in the acute, subacute and chronic phases of disease and at different stages of evolution. The treatment duration ranged from 20 to 50 min, and was performed 3–6 times per week for 3–8 weeks. The net time of application of the different devices ranged from 15–20 to 30 min (Table 1).

The incorporation of virtual reality (VR) and brain-machine interfaces (BMIs) during training can enhance the patient's experience. VR is a further modality that can be used to augment gait improvements. It provides the patient with positive bio-signals linked to gait performance, such as forces/torques at lower limb joints, thereby motivating conscious control of movements [18]. Useful signals about movement errors, and immediate feedback on motor performance can also be provided. The VR modality, combined with RAGT, can enhance improvement more than robot therapy alone [21]. People with stroke can show, at ankle level, motor control improvements in terms of power and force after training with VR [22].

BMIs associated with robotic devices for paralyzed and severely impaired stroke patients have been investigated in several studies [38]. This approach bridges the gap that exists between missing movements (due to a brain lesion), the intention to move in the central nervous system, and the actual movement of a robotic device (or orthosis) [4]. Most of the existing studies focused on upper limb recovery, but emerging evidence points to the value of this approach for gait and balance rehabilitation, too [6].

Chung and collaborators evaluated the effects of brain-computer interface (BCI)-based FES on balance and gait function in patients with stroke [2]. Ten patients were randomly assigned to an experimental BCI-FES group (n = 5) or a FES group (n = 5). The experimental group underwent ankle dorsiflexion training with FES and BCI for 30 min daily for 5 consecutive days, while FES group received dorsiflexion ankle training combined with electrical stimulation only for the same duration of time. The results indicate that BCI-based FES training is a useful exercise for balance and gait function. Indeed, after training, the BCI-FES group showed significant differences in Timed Up and Go test score, cadence and step length on the affected side. The FES group showed no significant differences after the intervention. Although there were no significant differences between the two groups after the intervention, the combined therapy may be seen as a promising approach for post-stroke recovery of gait function.

To date, limited attention has been paid to the potential role of robotic devices in measuring particular gait performances. By measuring several dimensions of interest, such as spasticity, reflexes, the level of voluntary control, as well as functional movements, they allow monitoring of motor recovery and of the patient's improvements [19], and are therefore of particular interest from the rehabilitation perspective.

Table 1 Summary of end-effector studies for gait rehabilitation in neurological diseases

Authors	Device	Study design	Disease	Phase of disease	Number of subjects	Training times (–Total treatment net time; –ET; –CT)	Main results
Chua et al. [1]	GT	RCT	Stroke	Subacute	106	– Total of 45 min; 6 times/week; 8 weeks – GT (20 min) + stance or gait training (15 min) + cycling (10 min) – Stance/gait training (35 min) + cycling (10 min)	No difference was found between GT and CT in FAC, Barthel index, gait speed and endurance, or stroke impact scale
Picelli et al. [28]	GT	RCT	PD	H&Y = 3	66	– Total of 30 min; 3 times/week; 4 weeks – GT (30 min) – Balance training (30 min)	No difference was found between GT and CT in BBS, activities-specific balance confidence scale; TUG; UPDRS
Gandolfi et al. [11]	GT	RCT	MS	EDSS = 1.5–6.5	22	– Total of 50 min; 2 times/week; 6 weeks – GT (30 min) + passive joint mobilization and stretching (10 min) – Sensory integration balance training (50 min)	No difference was found between GT and CT in walking speed and BBS, activities-specific balance confidence scale, sensory organization balance test, stabilometric assessment, fatigue severity scale, cadence, step length, single and double support time, multiple sclerosis quality of life-54. SIBT was more effective than GT on sensory organization balance test, compliant surface-dome condition at follow-up (1 month)
Picelli et al. [27]	GT	RCT	PD	H&Y = 2.5–3	41	– Total of 40 min; 3 times/week; 4 weeks – GT (30 min) – Active joint mobilization (10 min) + gait training (PNF) (30 min)	GT was more effective than CT on 10-m walking speed, 6 MWT, stride length and ratio between single, double support duration, Parkinson's fatigue scale, UPDRS post-treatment and at follow-up (1 month)
Conesa et al. [3]	GT	Observational report	Stroke	Subacute	69	– Total of 4.5 h; 5 times/week; 4 weeks – GT (20–40 min) + multidisciplinary treatment (4 h/day)	GT was effective in improving FAC, 10 MWT, and Tinetti gait and balance scales. Non statistically significant differences were found between GT and CT

(continued)

Table 1 (continued)

Authors	Device	Study design	Disease	Phase of disease	Number of subjects	Training times (–Total treatment net time; –ET; –CT)	Main results
						– Gait training (1 h) + multidisciplinary treatment (4 h/day)	
Tanaka et al. [35]	GM4	Pilot crossover study	Stroke	Chronic	12	– Total of 20 min; 4–6 weeks (total of 12 sessions) – GM4 (20 min) – No training	GM phase was more effective than no training phase in improving maximum gait speed but no statistically significant difference was found in TUG between phases
Hesse et al. [14]	G-EO	Clinical trial	Stroke	Subacute	30	– Total of 60 min; 5 times/week; 4 weeks – G-EO (15–20 min) + gait and stair climbing training (30 min) – Gait training + stair climbing training (60 min)	G-EO was more effective than CT in improving FAC 0–5; gait velocity, RMI and lower limb MI. At follow-up (3 months) only differences in FAC and MI persisted

ET Experimental treatment; *CT* control treatment; *GT* gait trainer; *GM4* GaitMaster4; *RCT* randomized controlled trial; *PD* Parkinson's disease; *MS* multiple sclerosis; *H&Y* Hoehn and Yahr scale score; *PNF* proprioceptive neuromuscular facilitation; *EDSS* expanded disability status scale score; *FAC* functional ambulation category; *BBS* Berg Balance Scale; *TUG* Timed Up and Go test; *UPDRS* unified Parkinson's disease rating scale; *SIBT* sensory integration balance training; *6 MWT* 6 min walking test; *10 MWT* 10 min walking test; *RMI* rivermead mobility index; *MI* motricity index

Authors	Device	Study design	Disease	Phase of disease	Number of subjects	Training times (–Total treatment net time; –ET; –CT)	Main results
Smania et al. [34]	GT	RCT	CP	GMFC II to IV	18	– Total of 40 min; 5 times/week; 2 weeks – GT (30 min) + passive joint mobilization and stretching (10 min) – Passive joint mobilization and stretching (10 min) + strengthening exercises (15 min) + balance and gait exercises (15 min)	GT more effective than CT on 10 MWT; 6 MWT, hip kinematics, gait speed, and step length at the end of the treatment and at follow-up (1 month). No difference was found in WeeFIM score within and between groups

(continued)

Table 1 (continued)

Authors	Device	Study design	Disease	Phase of disease	Number of subjects	Training times (–Total treatment net time; –ET; –CT)	Main results
Geroin et al. [12]	GT	Pilot RCT	Stroke	Chronic	30	– Total of 50 min; 5 times/week; 2 weeks – GT with TDCS (20 min) + joint mobilization and strengthening exercises (30 min) – GT with STDCS (20 min) + joint mobilization and strengthening exercises (30 min) – Overground walking (20 min) + joint mobilization and strengthening exercises (30 min)	GT with/without TDCS was more effective than overground walking in improving 6 MWT and 10 MWT, kinematic gait parameters, FAC, RMI, MI-leg subscore. Improvements were maintained at follow-up (1 month). No difference was found between GT with and without TDCS groups
Morone et al. [23]	GT	RCT	Stroke	Subacute	48	– Total of 2.5 h; 5 times/week; 4 weeks – GT (20 min) + conventional physiotherapy (2 h) – Gait training (40 min) + conventional physiotherapy (2 h) Patients were divided in low MI group and high MI group. Both groups were divided between ET and CT	GT was more effective than CT in improving FAC at the end of the treatment and RMI, trunk control test, BI, Rankin scale, and 6MWT at discharge. All differences were found only in low MI groups
Freivogel et al. [10]	LH	RCr	Stroke/ TBI/ SCI	Subacute-chronic	16	– Total of 30 min; 3–5 times/week; 6 weeks – LH (30 min) – Gait training with treadmill (30 min)	No difference was found between groups in FAC, gait velocity, MI, RMI

(continued)

Table 1 (continued)

Authors	Device	Study design	Disease	Phase of disease	Number of subjects	Training times (–Total treatment net time; –ET; –CT)	Main results
Peurala et al. [25]	GT	RCT	Stroke	Acute	56	– Total of 75 min; 5 times/week; 3 weeks – GT (20 min) + conventional physiotherapy (55 min) – Walking overground (20 min) + conventional physiotherapy (55 min) – Conventional physiotherapy (55 min)	GT and walking overground were better than CT in improving FAC at the end of the treatment and at follow-up (6 months)
Ng et al. [24]	GT	Pilot RCT	Stroke	Subacute	54	– Total of 2.5 h; 5 times/week; 4 weeks – GT with FES (20 min) + conventional physiotherapy (40 min) + multidisciplinary treatment (1.5 h) – GT without FES (20 min) +conventional physiotherapy (40 min) + multidisciplinary treatment (1.5 h) – Gait training overground (20 min) + conventional physiotherapy (40 min) + multidisciplinary treatment (1.5 h)	GT with/without FES was more effective than CT in improving Elderly Mobility Scale, and gait speed at the end of the treatment. Only GT with FES was more effective than CT in improving FAC. At follow-up (6 months) the GT with/without FES groups scored better than CT in all outcomes
Freivogel et al. [9]	LH	Feasibility	SCI/ TBI/ Stroke	Subacute-chronic	6	– Total of 30 min; 20 times over 6 weeks – LH (30 min) + conventional physiotherapy	LH was effective in improving FAC, MI, BBS and RMI

(continued)

Table 1 (continued)

Authors	Device	Study design	Disease	Phase of disease	Number of subjects	Training times (–Total treatment net time; –ET; –CT)	Main results
Pohl et al. [29]	GT	RCT	Stroke	Subacute	155	– Total of 45 min; 5 times/week; 4 weeks – GT (20 min) + gait training (25 min) + group physiotherapy – Gait training (45 min) + group physiotherapy	After treatment, significantly more patients in GT group had a BI > 75 (no difference at 6 months) and were able to walk independently. GT was better than CT in improving walking velocity, walking endurance, RMI and motor power of the paretic lower limb at the end of the treatment
Dias et al. [5]	GT	RCT	Stroke	Chronic	40	– Total of 40 min; 5 times/week; 5 weeks – GT (20 min) + joint mobilization and strengthening exercises (20 min) – Physiotherapy—Bobath method (20 min) + joint mobilization and strengthening exercises (20 min)	GT was effective in improving MI-lower limb, Toulouse Motor Scale, BBS, RMI, 10 MWT and 6 MWT. Only patients in GT showed functional gain at follow-up (3 months)
Tong et al. [37]	GT	RCT	Stroke	Subacute	46	– Total of 2.5 h; 5 times/week; 4 weeks – GT with FES (20 min) + conventional physiotherapy (40 min) + multidisciplinary treatment (1.5 h) – GT without FES (20 min) + conventional physiotherapy	GT with/without FES was more effective than CT in improving 5-m walking speed test, MI, elderly mobility scale and FAC. No difference was found between GT with/without FES groups

ET Experimental treatment; *CT* control treatment; *GT* gait trainer; *LH* LokoHelp; *RCT* randomized controlled trial; *RCr* randomized crossover study; *CP* cerebral palsy; *TBI* traumatic brain injury; *SCI* spinal cord injury; *GMFC* gross motor function classification system; *TDCS* transcranial direct current stimulation; *STDCS* sham transcranial direct current stimulation; *MI* motricity index; *FES* functional electrical stimulation; *10 MWT* 10 min walking test; *6MWT* 6 min walking test; *WeeFIM* functional independence measure for children; *FAC* functional ambulation category; *RMI* rivermead mobility index; *BI* Barthel index; *BBS* Berg balance scale

(continued)

Table 1 (continued)

Authors	Device	Study design	Disease	Phase of disease	Number of subjects	Training times (–Total treatment net time; –ET; –CT)	Main results
						(40 min) + multidisciplinary treatment (1.5 h) – Gait training (20 min) + conventional physiotherapy (40 min) + multidisciplinary treatment (1.5 h)	
Peurala et al. [26]	GT	RCT	Stroke	Chronic	45	– Total of 75 min; 5 times/week; 3 weeks – GT with FES (20 min) + conventional physiotherapy (55 min) – GT without FES (20 min) + conventional physiotherapy (55 min) – Walking overground (20 min) + conventional physiotherapy (55 min)	No difference was found between GT with/without FES and CT in improving 10 MWT 6 MWT, MMAS, dynamic balance test time and test trip. CT was better in reducing ankle spasticity. GT with FES was better in improving ankle dorsiflexion force. GT without FES was better in improving hip flexion force. MMAS score decreased in all groups at follow-up
Werner et al. [39]	GT	RCr	Stroke	Subacute	30	– Total of 15–20 min; 5 times/week; 2 weeks – GT (15–20 min for 2 weeks) – Gait training using treadmill (15–20 min for 2 weeks)	GT was better than CT in improving gait ability. No difference between groups was found in gait velocity, RMI and MMAS. No difference between groups was found at follow-up (6 months)
Hesse et al. [17]	GT	Feasibility	Stroke	Subacute-chronic	14	– 65 min; 5 times/week; 4 weeks – GT (20 min) + conventional physiotherapy (45 min)	GT was effective in improving gait velocity, cadence, and stride length. Electromyography showed a more physiological pattern at the end of treatment

ET Experimental treatment; *CT* control treatment; *GT* gait trainer; *RCT* randomized controlled trial; *RCr* randomized crossover study; *FES* functional electrical stimulation; *BI* Barthel index; *MI* motricity index; *BBS* Berg balance scale; *RMI* rivermead mobility index; *10 MWT* 10 min walking test; *6 MWT* 6 min walking test; *MMAS* modified motor assessment scale

4 How Might End-Effector Robotic Gait Training Devices Exert Their Effects?

In the last decade, several end-effector robotic devices for gait rehabilitation have been tested for feasibility, efficacy and effectiveness, giving promising results [20]. Most of the existing studies were performed using the GT1 or the G-EO System. These studies involved patients with stroke in either the sub-acute or chronic phase [12]. Only two studies were conducted in patients with Parkinson's disease [27, 28], one study in children with cerebral palsy [34], and one study in patients with multiple sclerosis [11]. Only two studies, involving patients affected by different diseases (stroke, traumatic brain injury and spinal cord injury), have been performed using the LokoHelp [9, 10]. Some therapeutic benefits of end-effector gait training in stroke patients have been reported. In general, improvements in several domains have been highlighted. Beneficial training effects on walking independence, endurance, functional walking ability and gait speed were reported [5, 12, 14, 17, 23–25, 29, 37, 39]. It must, however, be noted that GT1 training failed to induce significant improvements over conventional training alone in two studies [1, 3] that involved patients with stroke in the sub-acute phase.

In clinical practice there is a lack of consensus on which type of device (end-effector/exoskeleton), timing (acute/subacute/chronic phase), training modalities (passive/active/assisted), and training protocols (duration, frequency, doses) should be preferred [33]. These decisions can only be based on the intrinsic characteristics of the devices, because, to date, no evidence is available about what type of device (end-effector or exoskeleton) should be chosen on the basis of patients' clinical characteristics and rehabilitation aims [33].

Balance might be better improved with an end-effector device because fewer movement constraints are applied during the exercise, meaning that it simulates the effects of a sensory integration balance training program [11]. Notwithstanding the added value of end-effector devices in improving postural control, there has still been no direct comparison aimed at investigating their superiority over exoskeleton devices in improving balance and gait [20].

It could be argued that less physical assistance and more freedom during the exercises might work as sensory augmentations for sensorimotor integration processes (weighting and reweighting of sensory information). These sensory augmentations might be further enriched with sensory manipulations using sub-sensory mechanical noise or vibration applied to the sole, haptic learning (without vision) and FES cycling to strengthen the activity of leg muscles during walking. Finally, amplification of the patient's movement errors [8], in order to induce postural adaptations and unexpected perturbation during the swing phase of walking, might be useful [8].

With regard to the way in which end-effector robotic gait training devices work, it is not entirely clear why these devices might positively influence gait [20].

Robotics represents an additional instrument for the physiotherapist and should be applied in conjunction with a conventional training modality.

These technological devices do not make physiotherapists redundant; rather, by making it possible to better tailor individual treatments, they support physiotherapists involved in administering intensive training [16].

Physiotherapy aimed at restoring walking can be now offered more intensively with the same manpower and for a wider audience, since the number of repetitions of gait movement that can be achieved with a robotic device (and hence the intensity of the treatment) is probably unattainable with conventional treatments like treadmill training. Moreover, robotic devices can improve strength, cardiovascular performance and other domains associated with exercise.

From the ongoing debate on motor learning and its related effects on neuroplasticity, it appears that many of its aspects might have a strong impact on almost all of the elements of gait recovery in patients with neurological impairment. First, the level of active participation and motivation plays a crucial role. Assistance offered by a robot can help a patient to reach a movement target, even when he/she is not able, alone, to achieve the necessary range of motion. The robot also plays a coaching role, adjusting, step by step, the progression towards an optimal motor performance. Also, the assistive mode allows many thousands of repetitive movements to be performed. Evidence suggests that robot assistance during training might increase motivation, allowing activities, and also levels of performance, that could not be achieved without its help [30].

Second, the modality of therapy heavily influences the level of participation and motor learning processes. Increasing the difficulty and inducing error augmentation in order to obtain motor adjustments in a given task might represent a considerable learning stimulus. Indeed, both strategies can render the training more challenging and promote "errorless" motor learning phenomena. Although there is a lack of direct comparative evidence to suggest the superiority of one method over another, the hypothesis that error amplification leads to an increased rate of motor skill acquisition has been emphasized in the literature [7]. From this perspective, patient-robot interaction can also provide feedback for sensorimotor-type rehabilitation training [38], allowing task-specific balance training [5, 11, 28]. The reduced number of constraints, the higher degrees of freedom, especially for pelvic movements, and the possibility of setting different levels of difficulty (i.e. walking, climbing up and down stairs) add up to an ideal environment for promoting motor learning processes [11].

Finally, repetitive task practice might enhance neural plasticity phenomena. The potential role of rehabilitation in promoting recovery of function through neuroplasticity processes has been demonstrated in people with stroke (Takeuchi et al. 2013). The particular function of robot-mediated therapy in inducing neuroplasticity has been described in healthy subjects [38]. By contrast, it has not been entirely established in patients affected by neurological diseases [38]. Future studies should be performed to further investigate this field of research.

5 Conclusions

The literature suggests that end-effector devices can improve gait and balance performance in patients with neurological disorders. Despite the lack of common and shared treatment protocols, 20 min of gait training is generally considered to be the shortest time potentially able to produce changes in gait and balance performance.

To speed up progress in this field of research, clinical randomized controlled trials on larger samples of patients are needed. These trials should be designed with the aim of improving knowledge of robot-mediated learning mechanisms and, in particular, of robotic assistance, robotic perturbation, VR, and the interfacing of the brain with robotic devices, and also their combined effects. In addition, software designed to enhance sensory augmentations and sensorimotor integration processes (i.e. using vision manipulations) should be implemented.

References

1. Chua J, Culpan J, Menon E. Efficacy of an electromechanical gait trainer poststroke in Singapore: a randomized controlled trial. Arch Phys Med Rehabil. 2016;97(5):683–90.
2. Chung E, Kim JH, Park DS, Lee BH. Effects of brain-computer interface-base functional electrical stimulation on brain activation in stroke patients: a pilot randomized controlled trial. J Phys Ther Sci. 2015;27(3):559–62.
3. Conesa L, Costa Ú, Morales E, et al. An observational report of intensive robotic and manual gait training in sub-acute stroke. J Neuroeng Rehabil. 2012;9:13.
4. Daly JJ, Wolpaw JR. Brain-computer interfaces in neurological rehabilitation. Lancet Neurol. 2008;7(11):1032–43.
5. Dias D, Laíns J, Pereira A, et al. Can we improve gait skills in chronic hemiplegics? A randomised control trial with gait trainer. Eura Medicophys. 2007;43(4):499–504.
6. Dobkin BH. Brain-computer interface technology as a tool to augment plasticity and outcomes for neurological rehabilitation. J Physiol. 2007;579(3):637–42.
7. Domingo A, Ferris D. The effects of error augmentation on learning to walk on a narrow balance beam. Exp Brain Res. 2010;206(4):359–70.
8. Emken JL, Reinkensmeyer DJ. Robot-enhanced motor learning: accelerating internal model formation during locomotion by transient dynamic amplification. IEEE Trans Neural Syst Rehabil Eng. 2005;13(1):33–9.
9. Freivogel S, Mehrholz J, Husak-Sotomayor T, Schmalohr D. Gait training with the newly developed 'LokoHelp'-system is feasible for non-ambulatory patients after stroke, spinal cord and brain injury. A feasibility study. Brain Inj. 2008;22(7–8):625–32.
10. Freivogel S, Schmalohr D, Mehrholz J. Improved walking ability and reduced therapeutic stress with an electromechanical gait device. J Rehabil Med. 2009;41(9):734–9.
11. Gandolfi M, Geroin C, Picelli A, et al. Robot-assisted vs. sensory integration training in treating gait and balance dysfunctions in patients with multiple sclerosis: a randomized controlled trial. Front Hum Neurosci. 2014;22(8):318.
12. Geroin C, Picelli A, Munari D, Waldner A, Tomelleri C, Smania N. Combined transcranial direct current stimulation and robot-assisted gait training in patients with chronic stroke: a preliminary comparison. Clin Rehabil. 2011;25:537–48.

13. Hesse S, Sarkodie-Gyan T, Uhlenbrock D. Development of an advanced mechanised gait trainer, controlling movement of the centre of mass, for restoring gait in non-ambulant subjects. Biomed Tech. 1999;44:194–201.
14. Hesse S, Tomelleri C, Bardeleben A, Werner C, Waldner A. Robot-assisted practice of gait and stair climbing in nonambulatory stroke patients. J Rehabil Res Dev. 2012;49(4):613–22.
15. Hesse S, Waldner A, Tomelleri C. Innovative gait robot for the repetitive practice of floor walking and stair climbing up and down in stroke patients. J Neuroeng Rehabil. 2010;28 (7):30.
16. Hesse S, Werner C. Connecting research to the needs of patients and clinicians. Brain Res Bull. 2009;78(1):26–34.
17. Hesse S, Werner C, Uhlenbrock D, von Frankenberg S, Bardeleben A, Brandl-Hesse B. An electromechanical gait trainer for restoration of gait in hemiparetic stroke patients: preliminary results. Neurorehabil Neural Repair. 2001;15(1):39–50.
18. Koenig A, Omlin X, Bergmann J, et al. Controlling patient participation during robot-assisted gait training. J Neuroeng Rehabil. 2011;23(8):14.
19. Krebs HI, Volpe BT, Aisen ML, Hogan N. Increasing productivity and quality of care: robot-aided neuro-rehabilitation. J Rehabil Res Dev. 2000;37(6):639–52.
20. Mehrholz J, Pohl M. Electromechanical-assisted gait training after stroke: a systematic review comparing end-effector and exoskeleton devices. J Rehabil Med. 2012;44:193–9.
21. Mirelman A, Bonato P, Deutsch JE. Effects of training with a robot-virtual reality system compared with a robot alone on the gait of individuals after stroke. Stroke. 2009;40(1): 169–74.
22. Mirelman A, Patritti BL, Bonato P, Deutsch JE. Effects of virtual reality training on gait biomechanics of individuals post-stroke. Gait Posture. 2010;31(4):433–7.
23. Morone G, Bragoni M, Iosa M, et al. Who may benefit from robotic-assisted gait training? A randomized clinical trial in patients with subacute stroke. Neurorehabil Neural Repair. 2011;25(7):636–44.
24. Ng MF, Tong RK, Li LS. A pilot study of randomized clinical controlled trial of gait training in subacute stroke patients with partial body-weight support electromechanical gait trainer and functional electrical stimulation: six-month follow-up. Stroke. 2008;39(1):154–60.
25. Peurala SH, Airaksinen O, Huuskonen P, et al. Effects of intensive therapy using gait trainer or floor walking exercises early after stroke. J Rehabil Med. 2009;41(3):166–73.
26. Peurala SH, Tarkka IM, Pitkänen K, Sivenius J. The effectiveness of body weight-supported gait training and floor walking in patients with chronic stroke. Arch Phys Med Rehabil. 2005;86(8):1557–64.
27. Picelli A, Melotti C, Origano F. Robot-assisted gait training in patients with Parkinson disease: a randomized controlled trial. Neurorehabil Neural Repair. 2012;26:353–61.
28. Picelli A, Melotti C, Origano F, et al. Robot-assisted gait training is not superior to balance training for improving postural instability in patients with mild to moderate Parkinson's disease: a single-blind randomized controlled trial. Clin Rehabil. 2015;29:339–47.
29. Pohl M, Werner C, Holzgraefe M, et al. Repetitive locomotor training and physiotherapy improve walking and basic activities of daily living after stroke: a single-blind, randomized multicentre trial (DEutsche GAngtrainerStudie, DEGAS). Clin Rehabil. 2007;21(1):17–27.
30. Reinkensmeyer DJ, Patton JL. Can robots help the learning of skilled actions? Exerc Sport Sci Rev. 2009;37(1):43–51.
31. Sale P, Franceschini M, Waldner A, Hesse S. Use of the robot assisted gait therapy in rehabilitation of patients with stroke and spinal cord injury. Eur J Phys Rehabil Med. 2012;48:111–21.
32. Schmidt H, Werner C, Bernhardt R, Hesse S, Krüger J. Gait rehabilitation machines based on programmable footplates. J Neuroeng Rehabil. 2007;9(4):2.
33. Schwartz I, Meiner Z. Robotic-assisted gait training in neurological patients: who may benefit? Ann Biomed Eng. 2015;43:1260–9.
34. Smania N, Bonetti P, Gandolfi M, et al. Improved gait after repetitive locomotor training in children with cerebral palsy. Am J Phys Med Rehabil. 2011;90:137–49.

35. Tanaka N, Saitou H, Takao T, et al. Effects of gait rehabilitation with a footpad-type locomotion interface in patients with chronic post-stroke hemiparesis: a pilot study. Clin Rehabil. 2012;26(8):686–95.
36. Tomelleri C, Waldner A, Werner C, Hesse S. Adaptive locomotor training on an end-effector gait robot: evaluation of the ground reaction forces in different training conditions. IEEE Int Conf Rehabil Robot. 2011;2011:5975492.
37. Tong RK, Ng MF, Li LS. Effectiveness of gait training using an electromechanical gait trainer, with and without functional electric stimulation, in subacute stroke: a randomized controlled trial. Arch Phys Med Rehabil. 2006;87(10):1298–304.
38. Turner DL, Ramos-Murguialday A, Birbaumer N, Hoffmann U, Luft A. Neurophysiology of robot-mediated training and therapy: a perspective for future use in clinical populations. Front Neurol. 2013;13(4):184.
39. Werner C, Von Frankenberg S, Treig T, Konrad M, Hesse S. Treadmill training with partial body weight support and an electromechanical gait trainer for restoration of gait in subacute stroke patients: a randomized crossover study. Stroke. 2002;33(12):2895–901.
40. Yano H, Masuda T, Nakajima Y, et al. Development of a gait rehabilitation system with a spherical immersive projection display. J Robotics Mechatronics. 2008;12:836–45.

Early Verticalization in Patients in a Vegetative or Minimally Conscious State

Giuseppe Frazzitta, Ilaria Zivi, Roberto Valsecchi and Leopold Saltuari

1 Background

Brain injuries acquired as a result of trauma, brain hypoxia, cerebrovascular diseases, tumors, infections and toxic substances can affect consciousness in the acute phase. In severe cases, complete recovery from a comatose state may not be achieved, leaving the patient in a vegetative state (VS) or a minimally conscious state (MCS) [1].

The prevalence of disorders of consciousness (DOC) in the population is around 0.2–6 1/100,000. Although advances in acute medical care mean that nowadays more and more people with DOC survive, standard rehabilitation approaches continue to present limitations, with the result that we are also seeing an increase in the number of people surviving these injuries with residual disabilities.

G. Frazzitta (✉) · I. Zivi
Department of Brain Injury and Parkinson's Disease Rehabilitation, Ospedale "Moriggia-Pelascini", via Pelascini, 22015 Gravedona ed Uniti (CO), Italy
e-mail: frazzittag62@gmail.com

I. Zivi
e-mail: ilaria.zivi@gmail.com

R. Valsecchi
Department of Intensive Care, Ospedale "Moriggia-Pelascini", via Pelascini, 22015 Gravedona ed Uniti (CO), Italy
e-mail: valsecchi.dott@gmail.com

L. Saltuari
Research Unit for Neurorehabilitation South Tyrol, Landeskrankenhaus Hochzirl-Natters, Hochzirl 1, 6170 Zirl, Austria
e-mail: leopold.saltuari@tirol-kliniken.at

G. Sandrini et al. (eds.), *Advanced Technologies for the Rehabilitation of Gait and Balance Disorders*, Biosystems & Biorobotics 19,
https://doi.org/10.1007/978-3-319-72736-3_20

Considering the high clinical and social impact of this situation, the main goal of current rehabilitation science should be to find new treatment strategies capable of reducing the effects of the main injury, preventing secondary and tertiary complications and exploiting the brain's plastic potential in order to promote functional recovery.

2 Management of Patients

With a view to improve the management of primary and secondary mechanisms of brain damage, international guidelines recommend hospitalizing brain injured patients in neurological intensive care units and suggest an integrated approach in which both the acute care and the rehabilitation treatment are carried out in conjunction, under a single interdisciplinary team [2–4].

Indeed, the possibility of starting rehabilitation in the acute setting helps to improve patient outcome: mobilization has been shown to reduce ventilator dependence and the risk of complications (e.g. infections, pressure ulcers, osteoporosis) and to improve circulation, arousal and functional communication, thus limiting physical deconditioning and allowing shorter intensive care unit (ICU) stays [5, 6].

Nonetheless, there is currently no widely approved rehabilitation protocol for patients affected by acquired brain injury and the appropriate timing of intensive out-of-bed mobilization is still a matter of debate.

3 Passive Verticalization as Part of the Rehabilitation Program

One of the first and most important aims of rehabilitation in acquired brain injuries is the restoration of the orthostatic position. Indeed, orthostatism, by activating the proprioceptive, tactile and vestibular pathways, is thought to provide strong sensory stimulation in comatose patients, and leads to increased cortical activation [7–9].

In the rehabilitation of unconscious patients, this condition is achieved through passive verticalization sessions involving the use of tilt tables, which allow the patient to be moved gradually from a 0° to a maximum 90° position, and are reported to induce an improvement of the level of consciousness.

In this context, Elliott and Walker, using the Wessex Head Injury Matrix, assessed the behavior of 12 VS and MCS patients while lying in bed and during a 20-minute period of standing, achieved with the aid of a standard tilt table. They reported consistent improvements in the highest ranked behavior and in the total number of behaviors in the standing position [7].

Riberholt et al. studied the effects of verticalization with a normal tilt table in 16 patients with VS/MCS within the first 3 months of injury. The authors observed an increased level of arousal (time with eyes open) in the upright compared with the supine position [8].

With the same purpose, Toccolini et al. treated 23 mechanically ventilated patients with daily sessions of gradual verticalization with a standard tilt table, performed in the ICU. The patients showed significant improvements in Glasgow Coma Scale (GCS) and Richmond Agitation Sedation Scale scores during tilt between the beginning and the end of treatment [9].

In addition to sensory stimulation, a lowering of intracranial pressure could be another mechanism contributing to the neurological improvement after head-up tilt. Indeed, postural changes are known to redistribute the cerebrospinal fluid within the craniospinal space and to modify the venous outflow (thus the cerebral blood volume) through the valveless jugular veins [10]. However, head elevation in trauma patients was reported to be dangerous if not balanced by activation of the cerebral autoregulation mechanisms, because of a marked decrease in mean arterial pressure with consequent reduction in cerebral perfusion pressure. On the other hand, a study performed with transcranial Doppler in patients with cerebral vasospasm after subarachnoid hemorrhage did not show any significant change in cerebral blood flow after gradual head-of-bed elevation to 45° [11].

Unfortunately, the use of the standard tilt table, mostly in severely brain injured patients, often provokes vasovagal syncope symptoms, thus limiting or delaying this type of treatment [12].

4 A Novel Approach: "Stepping Verticalization"

Bearing in mind the collateral effects of verticalization of patients, Luther et al., in 2008, studied the effects of a new device, composed of a tilt table and an integrated robotic stepping device (Erigo®, Hocoma, Switzerland) [12]. This device is equipped with a harness to fasten the patient's upper body to the table and straps to secure the feet to two footplates and the distal thighs to the stepping device (Fig. 1). Leg stepping movements are therefore passively obtained via the rhythmic alternating pushing up of the feet. An inner computer controls all the modifiable parameters, basically stepping frequency and slope variations (possible from 0° to 90°).

Patients affected by VS or MCS underwent stepping verticalization sessions after more than 30 days from brain injury and, unlike what can be seen with conventional tilt table sessions, they did not show syncope episodes. This improvement in terms of vagal side effects was probably linked to the leg stepping movement, which, by activating the muscle pump system, reduces blood pooling in the lower limbs, resulting in a subsequent increase in cardiac input and a reduction of orthostatic distress [12].

Instead, Krewer et al. compared the effects, on Coma Recovery Scale—revised (CRSr) scores, of 10 sessions of verticalization over 3 weeks with a standard tilt table

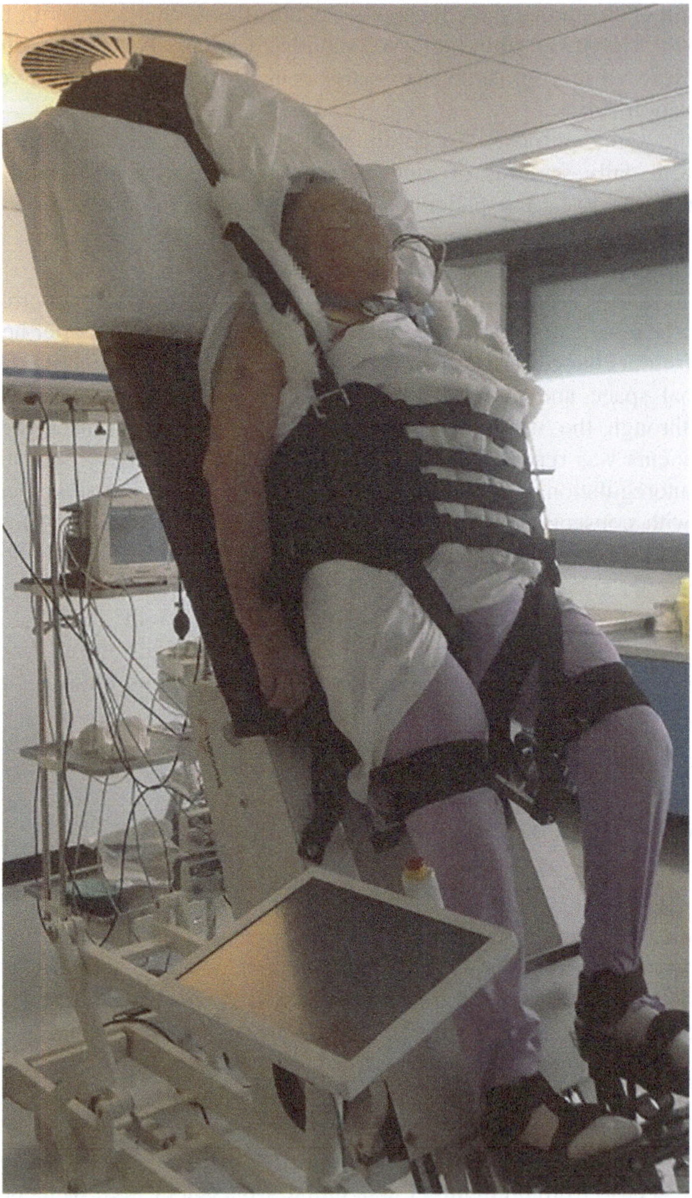

Fig. 1 "Stepping verticalization" using Erigo®

or a tilt table with an integrated stepping device in patients with VS or MCS. They enrolled patients at intervals of between 1 and 6 months from injury and assessed the CRSr scores at baseline, after the 3 weeks of treatment, and after 3 weeks of follow-up. Recovery was found to be better with the standard tilt table [13].

5 Safety and Feasibility of Early Verticalization

On the basis of these considerations, our group hypothesized that a rehabilitation program including "stepping verticalization" sessions from the acute phase of injury might lead to faster and better neurological improvements in VS or MCS patients.

However, given the critical conditions of patients in the acute phase of a brain injury, during which they are hospitalized in ICUs, the safety and feasibility of an intensive rehabilitation with a voluminous machine first needed to be evaluated.

For this purpose, we screened consecutive patients affected by severe acquired brain injury and related DOC. The inclusion criteria were: a GCS score ≤ 8 for 24 h from the event; a VS or MCS diagnosis on the third day after the injury (based on CRSr score); and admission to our neurological ICU within 24 h of the event. Patients who met these criteria and did not show respiratory, hemodynamic or intracranial instability, sedation, fractures or deep vein thrombosis were enrolled in the study [14].

The patients (mean basal CRSr score 3.6) underwent fifteen 30-minute sessions (5/week) of "stepping verticalization", starting between the 3rd and the 30th day after the injury-causing event, using a tilt table with integrated stepping device set up in the ICU room (Fig. 2). In our protocol the slope of the tilt table was gradually increased from 0° to 60° in a time span of 9 min, while the stepping frequency was set at 20 steps/min [14].

As safety outcomes, cardiovascular and respiratory parameters—mean arterial pressure (MAP), heart rate (HR), cardiac output (CO), arterial oxygen saturation—were continuously monitored and recorded every 20 s. The criteria for session interruption were MAP ≤ 70 mmHg, HR ≤ 40 or ≥ 150 bpm, oxygen saturation $\leq 90\%$ and traumatic dislodgement of a device (tracheal cannula, venous or arterial catheter, bladder catheter, external fixator). More severe events, such as

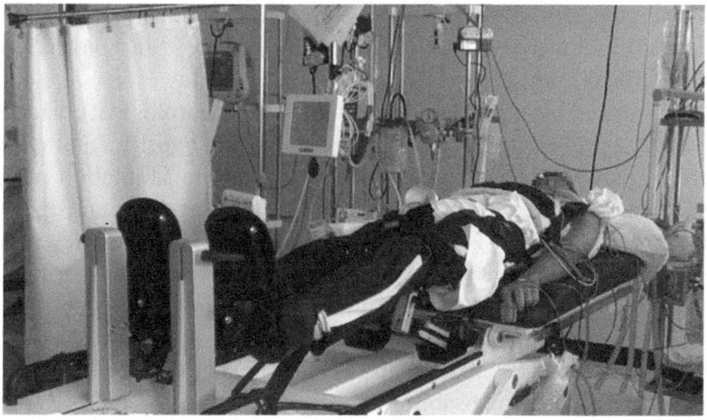

Fig. 2 Erigo® set up in the ICU room

neurological worsening or myocardial infarction, were conditions necessitating withdrawal of the patient from the study [14].

The patients showed various hemodynamic changes during the procedures (HR increase and MAP/CO decrease during the tilting phase, more pronounced at 60°), but all parameters stayed within the safety range (CO 3–12.3 l/min, HR 53–147 bpm, MAP 51–170 mmHg) and none of the patients experienced adverse reactions. Orthostatic hypotension and syncope were probably avoided thanks to the precocity of the intervention—the bed rest had not yet lasted long enough to alter autonomic and endocrine functions—and the rhythmic passive movement of the lower limbs, which helped to reduce fluctuation of cardiovascular parameters in the standing position.

As regards the feasibility of the intervention, the location of the tilt table in our ICU facilitated the organization of the sessions, and thus prevented time wasting. For each 30-minute treatment session, a further 15 min was needed for moving the patient (from the bed to the tilt table and back again) and for setting the cardiovascular monitoring apparatus, steps that were carried out by a nurse and a physiotherapist [14].

In conclusion, the study showed us that concerns over the safety of early verticalization of unconscious patients hospitalized in ICUs are exaggerated.

6 Efficacy of an Early "Stepping Verticalization" Program

Having verified the good tolerability of a very early "stepping verticalization" program, our group decided to investigate whether this same protocol might help to improve the functional and neurological outcomes of VS and MCS patients.

Consecutive patients were enrolled and randomized into two groups: the experimental group received fifteen 30-minute sessions of "stepping verticalization" as previously described, plus 30 min/day of conventional physiotherapy. Before the verticalization period only conventional in-bed physiotherapy was provided, for 60 min a day. Controls were treated only with conventional in-bed physiotherapy, for 60 min a day, throughout the ICU stay.

Once they showed clinical stability (general and neurological), and after completion of the "stepping verticalization" protocol in the experimental group, all the patients were moved from the ICU to our neurorehabilitation unit, where, throughout their stay, they received specialized nursing care and individualized rehabilitation treatment consisting of conventional physiotherapy, robotics (including "stepping verticalization" sessions), device weaning, speech/swallowing therapy, cognitive therapy and the best medical treatment [15].

We evaluated both short-term (end of ICU stay) and long-term (end of rehabilitation stay) outcome, calculating the improvement obtained from baseline on four outcome scales: GCS, Disability Rating Scale (DRS), CRSr and Levels of Cognitive Functioning (LCF). Each scale was assessed by a blinded investigator on the third day from the injury, at ICU discharge and at discharge from the rehabilitation unit [15].

A total of 40 patients were enrolled, but the final study population analyzed consisted of 31 patients. The two groups were comparable for sex, etiology, site of the main brain damage, comorbidities, LCF, DRS and CRSr scores at admission, and number of deaths during hospitalization. Patients in the early verticalization group started "stepping verticalization" 12.4 ± 7.3 days (between day 3 and day 30) after the brain injury [15].

As in the previous study, no adverse events during the "stepping verticalization" sessions were recorded. At the end of the ICU stay (short-term outcome) both groups showed significant improvements on all the tested scales ($p < 0.004$ all). However, when compared with standard physiotherapy care, early "stepping verticalization" was found to be associated with a greater improvement in the CRSr score ($p = 0.006$). The DRS improvement was also greater in the experimental group, but without reaching statistical significance. On the other hand, the GCS and LCF changes were not different, probably because of their lower range of scores that reduces their sensitivity in the context of neurological assessment [15].

The subsequent neurorehabilitation unit stay resulted in an additional improvement of all the parameters in both groups ($p < 0.004$ all), without any difference between them. The global improvement of the scores (between the first evaluation in the ICU and the evaluation at the end of the neurorehabilitation stay) was significant in both groups ($p < 0.001$ all). Nevertheless, we observed better long-term results in the experimental group, with significantly greater improvements on the CRSr ($p = 0.033$) and DRS ($p = 0.040$) and non-significant greater improvements on the GCS and LCF. Furthermore, at neurorehabilitation unit discharge we found that a greater number of patients in the experimental group recorded the CRS-r maximum score. On the basis of these findings, and in particular considering the absence of a between-groups difference in the improvement obtained in the neurorehabilitation phase, we assert that the initial gain obtained by the experimental group from the "stepping-verticalization" treatment in the ICU phase was retained until their discharge from the neurorehabilitation unit (on average 4 months later) [15].

In conclusion, our positive findings with regard to the long-term outcome of these patients support the use of a tilt table with robotic stepping device in the context of early rehabilitation of patients affected by disorders of consciousness.

References

1. The Multi-Society Task Force Report on PVS. Medical aspects of the persistent vegetative state. N Engl J Med. 1994;330:1499–508.
2. Laver K, Lannin NA, Bragge P, Hunter P, Holland AE, Tavender E, et al. Organising health care services for people with an acquired brain injury: an overview of systematic reviews and randomised controlled trials. BMC Health Serv Res. 2014;14(1):397.

3. Andelic N, Bautz-Holter E, Ronning P, Olafsen K, Sigurdardottir S, Schanke AK, et al. Does an early onset and continuous chain of rehabilitation improve the long-term functional outcome of patients with severe traumatic brain injury? J Neurotrauma. 2012;29:66–74.
4. Eifert B, Maurer-Karattup P, Schorl M. Integration of intensive care treatment and neurorehabilitation in patients with disorders of consciousness: a program description and case report. Arch Phys Med Rehabil. 2013;94(10):1924–33.
5. Elliott L, Walker L. Rehabilitation interventions for vegetative and minimally conscious patients. Neuropsychol Rehabil. 2005;15:480–93.
6. Castro–Avila AC, Serón P, Fan E, Gaete M, Mickan S. Effect of early rehabilitation during intensive care unit stay on functional status: systematic review and meta–analysis. PloS One. 2015;10(7):e0130722. Available at: www.journal.plos.org/plosone.
7. Elliot L, Coleman M, Shiel A, Wilson BA, Badwan D, Menon D, et al. Effect of posture on levels of arousal and awareness in vegetative and minimally conscious patients: a preliminary investigation. J Neurol Neurosurg Psychiatry. 2005;76(2):298–9.
8. Riberholt CG, Thorlund JB, Mehlsen J, Nordenbo AM. Patients with severe acquired brain injury show increased arousal in tilt–table training. Dan Med J. 2013;60(12):A4739. Available at: www.danmedj.dk.
9. Toccolini BF, Osaku EF, de Macedo Costa CR, Teixeira SN, Costa NL, Cândia MF, et al. Passive orthostatism (tilt table) in critical patients: clinicophysiologic evaluation. J Crit Care. 2015;30(3):655.e1–655.e6. Available at: www.jccjournal.org.
10. Schneider GH, von Helden GH, Franke R, Lanksch WR, Unterberg A. Influence of body position on jugular venous oxygen saturation, intracranial pressure and cerebral perfusion pressure. Acta Neurochir Suppl. 1993;59:107–12.
11. Blissitt PA, Mitchell PH, Newell DW, Woods SL, Belza B. Cerebrovascular dynamics with head–of–bed elevation in patients with mild or moderate vasospasm after aneurysmal subarachnoid hemorrhage. Am J Crit Care. 2006;15(2):206–16.
12. Luther MS, Krewer C, Muller F, Koenig E. Comparison of orthostatic reactions of patients still unconscious within the first three months of brain injury on a tilt table with and without integrated stepping. A prospective, randomized crossover pilot trial. Clin Rehabil. 2008;22 (12):1034–41.
13. Krewer C, Luther M, Koenig E, Muller F. Tilt table therapies for patients with severe disorders of consciousness: a randomized, controlled trial. PloS One. 2015;10(12):e0143180.
14. Frazzitta G, Valsecchi R, Zivi I, Sebastianelli L, Bonini S, Zarucchi A, et al. Safety and feasibility of a very early verticalization in patients with severe traumatic brain injury. J Head Trauma Rehabil. 2015;30(4):290–2.
15. Frazzitta G, Zivi I, Valsecchi R, Bonini S, Maffia S, Molatore K, et al. Effectiveness of a very early stepping verticalization protocol in severe acquired brain injured patients: a randomized pilot study in ICU. PloS One. 2016;11(7):e0158030. doi:https://doi.org/10.1371/journal.pone.0158030.

Functional Electrical Stimulation and Its Use During Cycling for the Rehabilitation of Individuals with Stroke

Elisabetta Peri, Eleonora Guanziroli, Simona Ferrante, Alessandra Pedrocchi and Franco Molteni

1 Introduction

Stroke is a neurological deficit due to an acute injury of the central nervous system with a vascular cause [1]. According to WHO data, it is one of the major causes of long-term disability, affecting 15 million people worldwide [2], of whom a third remains permanently disabled. Stroke therefore has a high social and economic impact on society [3]. Despite considerable efforts to reduce the most important risk factors (high blood pressure and smoking), the incidence of stroke is continuously increasing due to the aging of the population [2]. Most (77%) stroke survivors experience a reduction of motor function resulting in locomotion impairment and thus a reduced quality of life [4].

Some spontaneous recovery of motor activity occurs in the first weeks after stroke as adaptive mechanisms intervene to reinforce the existing pathways and bring about structural and functional changes [5]. In particular, a reorganization of the neural tissues (neuroplasticity) results in a new functional architecture that is different for each patient and crucial to the long-term success of any rehabilitation intervention [6]. Therefore, novel therapeutic strategies in stroke should be aimed primarily at interacting with the phenomenon of neuroplasticity to promote motor recovery.

E. Peri (✉) · S. Ferrante · A. Pedrocchi
NEARLab, Department of Electronic, Information and Bioengineering, Politecnico di Milano, Milan, Italy
e-mail: elisabetta.peri@polimi.it

E. Guanziroli · F. Molteni
Valduce Hospital, Villa Beretta Rehabilitation Center, Como, Italy

G. Sandrini et al. (eds.), *Advanced Technologies for the Rehabilitation of Gait and Balance Disorders*, Biosystems & Biorobotics 19,
https://doi.org/10.1007/978-3-319-72736-3_21

The use of technologically advanced tools to provide rehabilitation could be helpful to promote motor relearning and neuroplasticity. Functional electrical stimulation (FES), for example, is a technique that uses an electrical stimulus to induce a functional movement. The electrical pulse activates the axons of the intact lower motor neuron, producing an artificial muscular contraction. This system is used temporarily to facilitate recovery of muscle function and of voluntary control [7] in a large number of neurological diseases in which the lower motor neuron is intact, such as stroke [8–11], spinal cord injury (SCI) [12], multiple sclerosis [13] and cerebral palsy [14, 15]. Traditionally, it has been used to treat gait dysfunction in hemiplegic patients. This is because upper extremity FES systems have proven more difficult to employ than lower extremity systems designed to improve walking, which is a rhythmic activity with a standardized motor plan, largely controlled at spinal level [16]. Nevertheless, effective interventions on locomotion require extensive assistance during training because of the reduced balance, muscular strength and coordination of neurologically impaired patients.

A safe, inexpensive and easily controlled way to overcome these issues is to combine FES with the use of a cycle ergometer (FES-cycling). In this design, the stimulus is synchronized with the crank angle and the subject's residual voluntary effort can also be exploited.

FES-cycling is a means of obtaining intensive, goal-oriented, active and repetitive movement in the training of the paretic limb—all these features of the movement are recognized as key factors in facilitating motor relearning through neural reorganization and rewiring in the central nervous system [17].

Studies in post-stroke patients suggest that locomotion improvements can be achieved by means of cycling training [18, 19]. In fact, cycling and walking share certain peculiarities: both involve repetitive movements with coordinated activation of the lower limb muscles that alternate flexion and extension of the hip, knee and ankle in a predetermined way [20].

This chapter focuses on FES and FES-cycling systems used to promote motor recovery in post-stroke patients. It is divided into five sections: in the first, the neurophysiological principles of FES are described. The second focuses on the neuroplasticity changes occurring after a FES treatment; the third looks at cycling training as a means of regaining locomotion ability, and the fourth deals with the therapeutic effects that can be observed in the stroke population. The final section considers future directions in this field.

2 The Neurophysiological Basis of FES

FES is based on the delivery of an electrical volley to excitable tissue, which produces an artificial contraction of the corresponding motor unit [21]. The peculiarity of FES within the field of electrical stimulation techniques is the fact that the alternating sequences of artificial contractions serve to produce a functional movement [7].

Electrical stimulation is generally used to activate nerves rather than muscles, because the activation threshold of intact lower motor neuron axons is lower than that needed to directly activate muscle fibers [22]. Thus, FES can only be used to rehabilitate subjects whose lower motor neurons are intact from the anterior horns of the spinal cord to the neuromuscular junctions in the muscles that are to be activated. Thus, not all pathologies can be targeted with FES. Moreover, FES is effective when the lower motor neurons are excitable and the neuromuscular junction and muscle are healthy. Stroke, head injuries, SCI, cerebral palsy and multiple sclerosis usually meet these conditions [7].

When a current is delivered to a volume of tissue between two stimulation electrodes (an anode and a cathode), a localized electric field creates an ionic flux. In the vicinity of the cathode, a depolarization can be observed and, if its values are higher than a critical threshold, the migration of sodium ions from the extracellular space to the intracellular space generates an action potential that propagates in both directions from the stimulation site [7], as schematically shown in Fig. 1.

Since the majority of the axons are organized into sensory and motor fibers, the action potentials travel in both orthodromic and antidromic directions along the two types of fiber, as shown in Fig. 2. This means that there is an afferent volley that

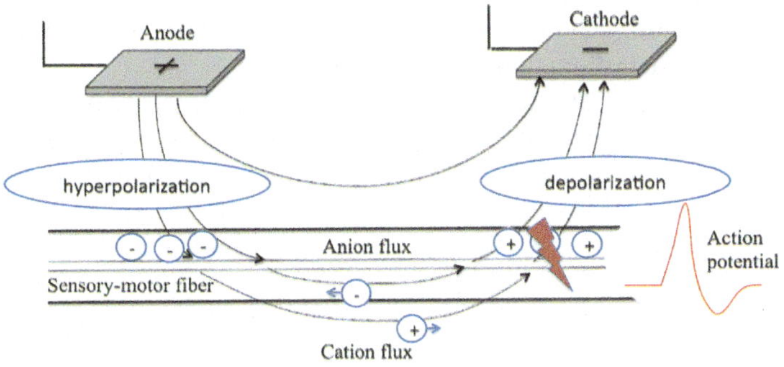

Fig. 1 Neurophysiological principles of FES

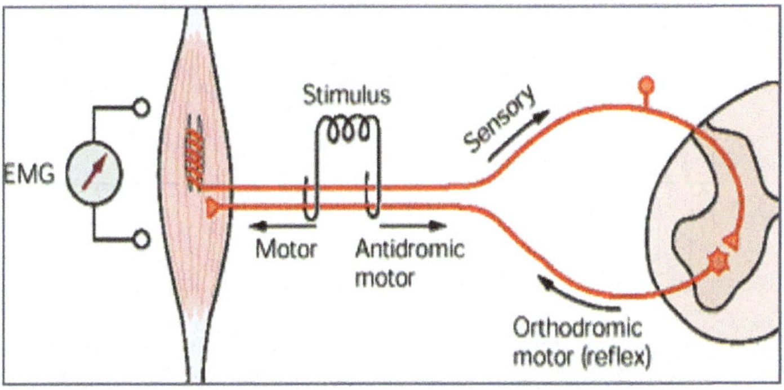

Fig. 2 Afferent and efferent stimuli induced by peripheral stimulation. Adapted from Kandel et al. [23]

reaches the spinal cord and the brain in parallel with an efferent volley that reaches the muscles. This effect is the basis of neuroplasticity facilitation, which is better described in the next paragraph.

When the current is delivered to the tissue, the order of recruitment of motor units is different from that occurring in physiological conditions. First of all, the orientation of the nerve fibers and their distance from the stimulation electrodes plays a major role: the sequence of activation seems to be from superficial to deep muscle layers, and this has the effect of reducing the physiological turnover of the motor units [24, 25]. This mechanism is called spatial summation. Second, the large-diameter axons (strong but not fatigue-resistant fibers), responsible for the larger motor units, are activated before the others at the same distance from the stimulation site, since they have a lower activation threshold than small axons (fine movement, fatigue-resistant fibers). This is due to the larger distance between nodes of Ranvier in large axons, which results in larger induced transmembrane voltage changes [7, 21]. This recruitment mechanism is the opposite of the physiological mechanism that, in accordance with the Henneman principle, ensures less muscle fatigue and a more accurate modulation of force [26]. Another difference compared with physiological contraction is due to the occurrence, at a certain stimulation frequency, of synchronous activation of the motor units which intervenes in the movement (temporal summation), limiting the natural turnover of the fibers. The results of these recruitment mechanisms is a the rapid onset of muscular fatigue, and this is one of the main limitations of FES [21, 27].

To reduce this effect, the waveform of the stimulus can play a role. In fact the FES is delivered with a train of pulses that can be defined through three parameters, as summarized in Fig. 3: the frequency (f), the amplitude (I), and the pulse width (PW). High stimulation frequency increases the rate of muscle fatigue because of the cumulative effect of the twitches occurring within a short period of time (temporal summation). This parameter should, in any case, be higher than the fusion frequency (typically 12.5 Hz) in order to obtain a smooth muscular contraction.

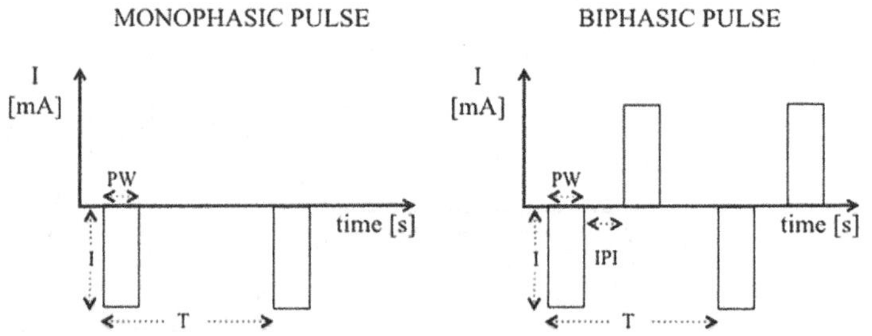

Fig. 3 Electrical stimulus waveform. Monophasic and biphasic pulses are reported in the left and right panel, respectively. The intensity (I), the inter-pulse interval (IPI), the pulse width and the period (T) (i.e. the inverse of the frequency f) are represented

Therefore, the strength of the muscular contraction is generally modulated via the PW and/or the I of the stimuli which act on the electric charge injected determining the spatial summation mechanism [7]. Typical working values are a frequency (f) of between 20 and 30 Hz, a current pulse width (PW) of between 100 and 500 μs, and an amplitude (I) of between 10 and 125 mA.

The pulses can be controlled in either voltage or current. The advantage of the voltage-controlled stimulator is that the current density is maintained below dangerous values in case of partial detachment of the electrodes. Instead, current-controlled stimulators are not affected by impedance variation due to the skin-electrode interface, thus they induce more reliable motor unit recruitment and are usually preferred in clinical applications [28].

Moreover, each waveform can have a biphasic or monophasic shape [7, 29], as shown in Fig. 3. Monophasic waveforms consist of repeated unidirectional pulses (usually cathodic), while biphasic waveforms comprise a cathodic pulse briefly followed by an anodic pulse. In this second configuration, the primary phase elicits axons located nearby, while the secondary positive pulse balances the charge injection of the primary pulse, preventing potential damage at the electrode-tissue interface. For this reason the biphasic configuration is usually preferred [7].

Surface, percutaneous and implanted electrodes can be used to deliver the electrical stimulus. Although surface electrodes have low selectivity for deep muscles [11], in rehabilitation applications they are commonly preferred thanks to their minimal invasiveness and the ease of donning and doffing [28]. For this reason, this chapter hereafter refers only to surface electrodes used for FES.

3 Neurological Changes Induced by FES for Rehabilitation Purposes

A core element of neurorehabilitation interventions is facilitation of cortical plasticity processes aimed at obtaining long-term potentiation of the motor cortex and motor recovery.

FES induces afferent and efferent pathway activation together with augmented proprioceptive and cutaneous inputs leading to augmented cortical and spinal activity. Combining these sensorimotor integration effects with goal-oriented, repetitive training could stimulate neural plasticity thus facilitating motor relearning [29].

Recent studies have looked at whether the motor recovery after FES-based rehabilitation could be, at least partially, ascribed to changes in cortical excitation and to brain reorganization mechanisms. A study in 10 healthy subjects showed a dose-response relationship between the stimulation intensity of FES delivered to the dominant quadriceps femoris muscle and the responses in sensorimotor brain regions contralateral to the stimulation [30]. Similar findings were obtained in a functional magnetic resonance imaging (fMRI)-based study in 12 healthy subjects in whom ankle dorsiflexion was induced by an active movement or by FES. During active dorsiflexion, greater activation in brain areas responsible for motor planning, execution and visual-motor coordination was shown, whereas the FES-induced movement produced greater activation in bilateral secondary somatosensory areas and in the insula. This finding is probably attributable both to increased sensory integration and to a nociceptive component due to the electrical stimulation [31].

The role, in motor relearning, of volitional effort concurrent with the movement induced by FES has also been widely investigated [29, 32]. These studies showed that volitional effort synchronized with an afferent volley produced by FES may produce some effects both at spinal [33] and cortical level [29, 32].

The spinal level was investigated by Rushton who hypothesized that the spinal cord anterior horn cells are Hebb-type cells, meaning that they are characterized by an increased firing rate if presynaptic and post-synaptic activities are coincident. Rushton suggested that the activity of Hebb-type synapses is significantly reduced after a brain injury because of the reduced descendent volley. Instead, when a neuromotor electrical stimulus is synchronized with the voluntary descendant volley, the antidromic pulses provide an artificial means of synchronizing presynaptic and post-synaptic activity, restoring the physiological synaptic condition [33] and providing a promising means of stimulating neuroplasticity.

At cortical level, Barsi and colleagues studied corticospinal excitability with transcranial magnetic stimulation (TMS) in a group of 25 healthy subjects who underwent three paradigms involving hand grasping: the first consisted of voluntary movement (VOL), the second exploited FES alone to accomplish the movement, while the third combined FES and voluntary movement (FES + VOL). Their findings showed that cortical excitability was increased by the FES + VOL paradigms much more than by FES or VOL alone, suggesting that the combination of voluntary effort and FES might have a greater potential to induce neuroplasticity [34]. Similarly, in a more recent study using fMRI during the same three paradigms in 17 healthy subjects, Iftime-Nielsen et al. showed that the cerebellum is better able to predict the sensory consequences of movement, reducing the subsequent activation in secondary somatosensory areas. This may reflect a better match between actual sensory feedback and an internal model [35]. With regard to the lower limb, ankle dorsiflexion was studied in four combinations: with and without volitional control and with or without FES. Both the primary motor cortex and primary somatosensory cortex showed a higher activation when the volitional control was combined with augmented proprioception due to FES, suggesting that this paradigm could promote the neuroplasticity changes at cortical level [36]. However, not all patients show carry-over effects. In a recent study on the neural correlates of FES, Gandolla et al. (2016) showed that only patients able to predict the movement and to perceive the stimulation as self-generated (sense of agency/body ownership) show carry-over effects, laying the basis for a prediction of carry-over effect in clinical settings [37].

4 Clinical Applications of FES and FES-Cycling

FES has consistently been shown to be beneficial for the rehabilitation of neuromotor-impaired subjects although no definite conclusions can be drawn concerning its superiority over other treatments [11, 38]. Patients seems to prefer it [11, 39].

A Cochrane review on the use of electrical stimulation for post-stroke rehabilitation which included 24 randomized controlled trials concluded that FES is an effective intervention to improve some aspects of functional motor ability and motor impairment and for promoting normality of movement. According to this review, FES was superior to conventional physical therapy only for the recovery of a few aspects of motor impairment. However, the authors underlined that no conclusion could be drawn due to the heterogeneity (in terms of type of electrical stimulation, dose of training and time since stroke) of the studies analyzed [38].

The main applications of FES for motor relearning in clinical practice can be divided into: FES during gait, electromyography-/biofeedback-mediated electrical stimulation and FES-cycling [29].

The very first use of FES for neuromotor impairment was in the form of a drop foot stimulator developed by Liberson and colleagues [40]. This application used single-channel stimulation of the peroneal nerve and a pressure sensor to detect the initial contact of the foot with the ground. In this context, repetitive movement training is carried out to accomplish a functional task that has a theoretical advantage with respect to conventional therapy. Nevertheless, it should be considered that in these applications the early onset of fatigue could dramatically reduce the dose of training and, consequently, the possibility of motor recovery. Bogataj and colleagues performed a 3-week controlled trial comparing the effects of a multichannel transcutaneous neuroprosthesis system (stimulation delivered to the soleus, hamstring, quadriceps femoris, gluteus maximus muscles) with respect to 3 weeks of conventional therapy. Significantly greater improvements in gait performance and motor functions were obtained by the FES group [41]. A more recent study (a multicenter, randomized, single-blinded trial) conducted in 197 post-stroke subjects compared the effect of 30 weeks' use of a foot drop stimulator or ankle-foot orthosis. The authors reported a significant improvement in gait speed in both groups, with no difference emerging from the between-group analysis [39].

Electromyography-/biofeedback-mediated electrical stimulation is based on the principle that combining afferent feedback with electrical stimulation-mediated repetitive training may stimulate corticospinal changes. EMG-triggered stimulation of the lower limb was delivered to 69 post-stroke patients who showed increases in voluntary EMG activity and mobility [42]. FES combined with biofeedback training was studied by Cozean and colleagues in 36 stroke patients who received 6 weeks of either control, FES, biofeedback or FES + biofeedback training. The authors reported that FES + biofeedback training was associated with improvements in knee and ankle joint angles during locomotion, velocity, and symmetry in stance [43]. It should be considered that these applications exploit patients' residual motor and cognitive ability. They may be not suitable for the most impaired subjects, especially during the post-acute phase of stroke when rehabilitation intervention is particularly important to trigger motor recovery.

FES-cycling is a safe, economical and widely accessible training method that combines a repetitive, goal-oriented task with sensorimotor information provided by FES, which thus facilitates neuroplasticity.

Motor impairments following a stroke often leave patients unable to walk. This is particularly true during the post-acute phase, when intensive intervention is recognized to be crucial to the subsequent motor outcomes. Functional training of patients with severe ambulatory limitations is often time consuming and costly, as extensive assistance is required during gait-related activities.

Studies suggest that pedaling could be a supplementary method for the recovery of walking. Indeed, it is safe, goal oriented and may avoid collateral risks due to the reduced motor activity (e.g. reduced cardiovascular performance and bone density). The pedaling motion in humans has been shown to activate some of the sensorimotor control mechanisms employed during locomotion [44] whose recovery is one of the main goals of post-stroke rehabilitation [8]. Moreover, as mentioned, cycling and walking share certain characteristics: both are rhythmic patterns that involve reciprocal flexion and extension of the hip, knee and ankles, with correct synchronization of agonist and antagonist muscles.

Studies in healthy subjects have shown that cycling training induces both short- and long-lasting changes in the spinal circuitry contributing to locomotion activity [44]. Similarly, it can be used to act on functional and motor abnormalities [44, 45], and to obtain improvements in aerobic fitness, balance and motor ability [46].

In this context, FES-cycling could be an effective intervention in post-stroke rehabilitation training. Severely impaired patients with no possibility of autonomous locomotion are eligible for a FES-cycling training, as it does not require residual motor activity and balance.

As described in Fig. 4, FES-cycling training can be delivered by means of a motorized cycle ergometer that imparts a smooth and safe pedaling motion to the patient' legs. The crank angle is used to deliver the stimulation synchronized with the pedaling phase in order to activate each muscle according to its physiological purpose (biomimetic stimulation strategy, Fig. 5), thereby promoting the motor relearning [9, 10]. Different stimulation paradigms can be used: FES during passive pedaling (during which the motorized cycle ergometer generates the movement) is widely used for the most impaired patients. FES-cycling can also be synchronized with a volitional effort that triggers the neuroplasticity facilitation mechanisms described above. Finally, patients can also be provided with visual biofeedback of the work produced by the two legs during volitional cycling augmented by FES. From a theoretical point of view, this should further enhance the neuroplasticity.

As can be seen in Fig. 4, the multichannel stimulation paradigms usually target different muscle groups that are massively involved both in walking and in cycling movements: the quadriceps femoris, the hamstrings, the gluteus maximus, the tibialis anterior and the gastrocnemius medialis or lateralis. The size of the stimulation electrodes placed over the muscle belly depends on the individual patient's

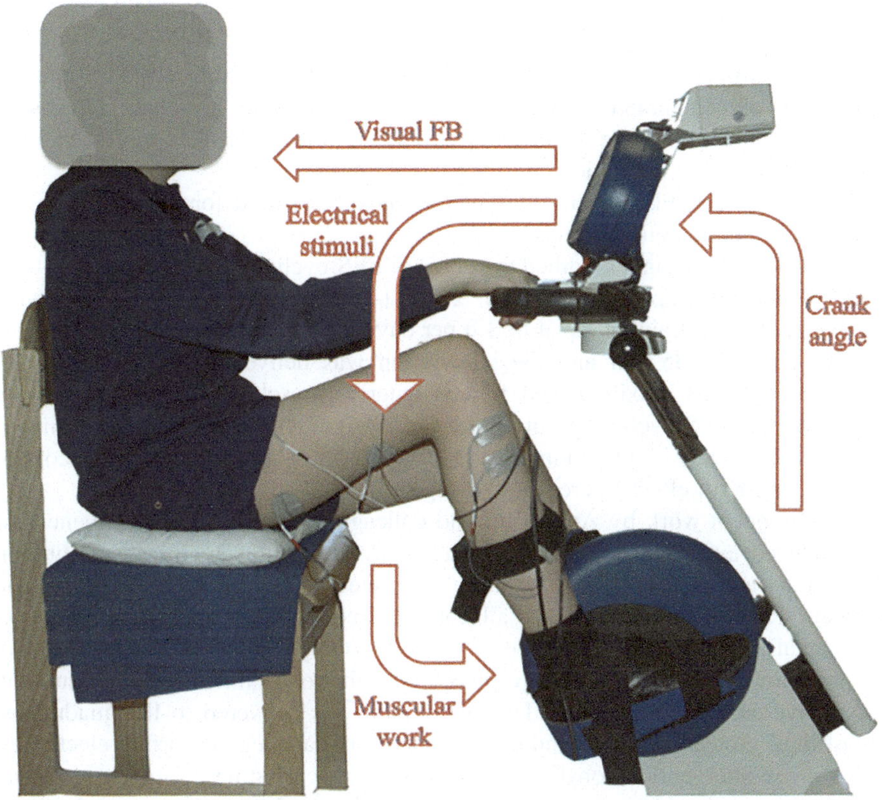

Fig. 4 A schematic representation of the FES-cycling, showing the cycle ergometer, the stimulator and the patient. The interactions between each block are also shown

Fig. 5 Stimulation ranges in a biomimetic strategy. 0: Corresponds to the maximal flexion of the hip. Q: Quadriceps. H: Hamstrings. T: Tibialis anterior. G: Gluteus maximus. Adapted from Ambrosini and colleagues [8]

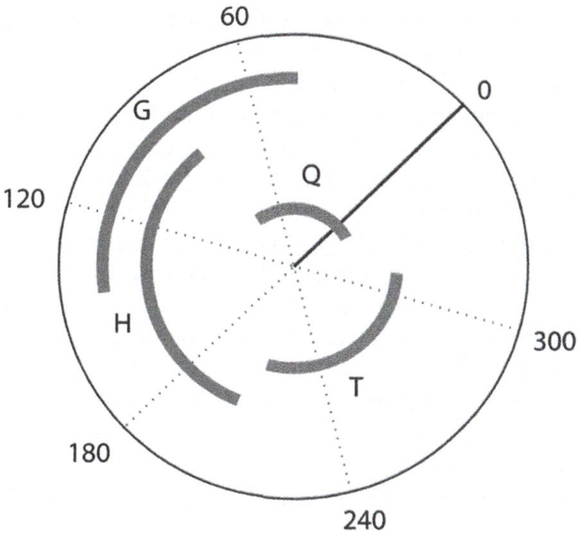

anthropological dimensions. They are typically between 2″ × 2″ and 2″ × 5″ for adult patients.

Some commercial devices are currently available to provide FES-cycling training in clinical practice. Among others, the RehaStim stimulator (Hasomed GmbH) together with the MOTOmed cycle ergometer (Reck GmbH) and the RT300 (Restorative Therapies, Inc.) are widely used.

In recent years, FES-cycling has increasingly been used for lower limb rehabilitation of hemiparetic subjects.

Ferrante and colleagues studied the effect of FES-cycling training compared with standard physiotherapy in a group of 20 post-acute stroke patients. Both groups received a dose of training equal to 3 h per day for 4 weeks. The FES-cycling was applied daily for 35 min and the stimulation was delivered to the quadriceps, hamstring, gluteus maximus and tibialis anterior muscles bilaterally. After the treatment the FES-cycling group produced a significantly increased maximum isometric voluntary contraction of the quadriceps, with respect to the control group. Long-term effects were not investigated [10].

A subsequent work by Ambrosini and colleagues assessed the effectiveness of FES-induced cycling with respect to passive cycling in lower limb rehabilitation through a randomized controlled trial conducted in 35 post-acute hemiparetic subjects. Patients were randomly allocated to receive FES-cycling training (experimental group) or an equal dose of passive cycling training with FES placebo, i.e. the stimulation electrodes were placed over the lower limb but no stimulation was delivered (placebo group). The stimulation was delivered to the quadriceps, hamstrings, gluteus maximus and tibialis anterior of each leg via surface electrodes. The 4-week intervention consisted of 20 sessions, each lasting 25 min, with 5 min of passing pedaling, 15 min of FES-cycling or placebo FES-cycling, and 5 min of passive pedaling.

The experimental group showed significant improvements in terms of the Motricity Index, Trunk Control Test, and the Upright Motor Control Test, as well as gait speed, mean work of the paretic leg and unbalance of mechanical work between healthy and paretic legs, both after training and at a 6-month follow-up assessment. Instead, none of the outcome measures demonstrated significant improvements after training in the placebo group, strongly suggesting that a four-week FES-cycling training intervention, more than cycling training alone, improves symmetry, mechanical work and motor coordination in post-acute hemiparetic patients [8, 9].

Although the volitional volley is recognized to play a role in enhancing neuroplasticity, producing long-term potentiation of the recovery, residual voluntary effort was not exploited in the two studies mentioned above. Differently, Alon and colleagues performed a study in 10 stroke subjects who were trained 3 times a week for 8 weeks with 30 min of FES-cycling training with voluntary effort. The quadriceps, hamstring and dorsal and plantar flexors were involved in the stimulation. The results showed an improved locomotor capability in terms of gait velocity and time to stand up, proceed to walk 3 m, turn around, walk back and sit down. Moreover the peak pedaling power increased during the intervention [47].

An attempt to exploit both biofeedback and cycling paradigms coupled with FES was made by Ferrante and colleagues. Patients were provided with information about their performance (i.e. the symmetry of work produced by the two legs during pedaling) in the form of online visual biofeedback. A case-series study in 3 post-stroke patients showed that this training paradigm could be promising, especially for patients with a strongly asymmetrical locomotion pattern and slow gait velocity. However, further studies should be performed to confirm these findings in a larger sample [19].

5 Conclusion and Future Perspectives

Evolving studies on central motor neuroplasticity support the role of goal-oriented, repetitive, voluntary training to obtain long-term potentiation in post-stroke rehabilitation.

Combining this kind of training with the augmented proprioceptive and cutaneous afferents mediated by FES, the motor relearning effect could be potentiated via both cortical and spinal mechanisms.

For the most impaired subjects, who are not able to walk autonomously, a safe and widely accessible means of providing FES training is to synchronize the stimulation with a cyclic movement imparted by a cycle ergometer.

Although some studies have already shown valuable short- and long-term results after exploiting FES in post-stroke patients, a definitive conclusion cannot yet be drawn. Furthermore, given the substantial lack of shared guidelines that might lead to the choice of intervention protocols customized to the single subject and/or pathology, the results of different studies are often not comparable. Establishing an evidence-based protocol could be a key factor in extending the use of FES in clinical practice.

Future investigations should take the form of large, multicenter, randomized clinical trials to evaluate long-term outcomes, maybe also including direct assessment of cortical changes (i.e. fMRI or TMS).

Furthermore, new technological advances should be sought in order to maximally exploit the benefits of FES. One of the most promising approaches is the use of the volitional residual muscle activation to trigger the FES-induced contraction (neuroprosthesis based on myocontrolled FES), for both rehabilitation and assistive purposes [28]. This paradigm ensures that the voluntary contribution is exploited, and it is thus particularly interesting from the perspective of long-term potentiation. However, its use is still limited because it is technologically challenging and also requires residual voluntary control, which makes it unsuitable for the most impaired patients. Another possible future research direction is the use of a robotic exoskeleton to assist and complete the movement where the patient is not able to achieve this. At present, however, this hybrid approach is still limited, partly because the technology is not yet sufficiently developed to guarantee optimal physical and cognitive interaction with patients, and partly because of portability and energy management issues [48].

References

1. Sacco RL, Kasner SE, Broderick JP, Caplan LR, Connors JJ, Culebras A, Elkind MSV, George MG, Hamdan AD, Higashida RT, Hoh BL, Janis LS, Kase CS, Kleindorfer DO, Lee JM, Moseley ME, Peterson ED, Turan TN, Valderrama AL, Vinters HV. An updated definition of stroke for the 21st century: a statement for healthcare professionals from the American heart association/American stroke association. Stroke. 2013;44(7):2064–89.
2. WHO. The atlas of heart disease and stroke. 2004.
3. Fattore G, Torbica A, Susi A, Giovanni A, Benelli G, Gozzo M, Toso V. The social and economic burden of stroke survivors in Italy: a prospective, incidence-based, multi-centre cost of illness study. BMC Neurol. 2012;12(1):137.
4. Bonita R, Beaglehole R, Bonita R, Beaglehole R. Recovery of motor function after stroke. Stroke. 1988;19:1497–500.
5. Brown JA. Recovery of motor function after stroke. Prog Brain Res. 2006;157:223–8.
6. Ward NS. Neural plasticity and recovery of function. Prog Brain Res. 2005;150:527–35.
7. Peckham PH, Knutson JS. Functional electrical stimulation for neuromuscular applications. Annu Rev Biomed Eng. 2005;7:327–60.
8. Ambrosini E, Ferrante S, Ferrigno G, Molteni F, Pedrocchi A. Cycling induced by electrical stimulation improves muscle activation and symmetry during pedaling in hemiparetic patients. IEEE Trans Neural Syst Rehabil Eng. 2012;20(3):320–30.
9. Ambrosini E, Ferrante S, Pedrocchi A, Ferrigno G, Molteni F. Cycling induced by electrical stimulation improves motor recovery in postacute hemiparetic patients: a randomized controlled trial. Stroke. 2011;42(4):1068–73.
10. Ferrante S, Pedrocchi A, Ferrigno G, Molteni F. Cycling induced by functional electrical stimulation improves the muscular strength and the motor control of individuals with post-acute stroke. Europa Medicophysica-SIMFER 2007 Award Winner. Eur J Phys Rehabil Med. 2008;44(2):159–67.
11. Kafri M, Laufer Y. Therapeutic effects of functional electrical stimulation on gait in individuals post-stroke. Ann Biomed Eng. 2015;43(2):451–66.
12. Gater DR, Dolbow D, Tsui B, Gorgey AS. Functional electrical stimulation therapies after spinal cord injury. NeuroRehabilitation. 2011;28(3):231–48.
13. Barrett CL, Mann GE, Taylor PN, Strike P. A randomized trial to investigate the effects of functional electrical stimulation and therapeutic exercise on walking performance for people with multiple sclerosis. Multiple Sclerosis J. 2009;15(4):493–504.
14. Peri E, Ambrosini E, Pedrocchi A, Pagliano E, Riva D, Baranello G, Arnoldi MT, Foscan M, Corlatti A, Marchi A, Ferrigno G, Ferrante S. Volitional cycling augmented by functional electrical stimulation in hemiparetic adolescents: a case series study. J Autom Control. 2013;21(1):37–42.
15. Trevisi E, Gualdi S, De Conti C, Salghetti A, Martinuzzi A, Pedrocchi A, Ferrante S. Cycling induced by functional electrical stimulation in children affected by cerebral palsy: case report. Eur J Phys Rehabil Med. 2012;48(1):135–45.
16. Singer B. Functional electrical stimulation of the extremities in the neurological patient: a review. Aust J Physiotherapy. 1987;33(1):33–42.
17. Harvey RL. Improving poststroke recovery: Neuroplasticity and task-oriented training. Curr Treat Options Cardiovasc Med. 2009;11(3):251–9.
18. Brown DA, Nagpal S, Chi S. Limb-loaded cycling program for locomotor intervention following stroke. Phys Ther. 2005;85(2):159–68.

19. Ferrante S, Ambrosini E, Ravelli P, Guanziroli E, Molteni F, Ferrigno G, Pedrocchi A. A biofeedback cycling training to improve locomotion: a case series study based on gait pattern classification of 153 chronic stroke patients. J Neuroeng Rehabil. 2011;8(1):47.
20. Burnfield JM, Shu Y, Buster T, Taylor A. Similarity of joint kinematics and muscle demands between elliptical training and walking: implications for practice. Phys Ther. 2010;90 (2):289–305.
21. Grill WM, Mortimer JT. Stimulus waveforms for selective neural stimulation. IEEE Eng Med Biol Mag. 1995;14(4):375–85.
22. McNeal DR. Analysis of a model for excitation of myelinated nerve. IEEE Trans Biomed Eng. 1976;BME-23(4):329–337.
23. Kandel ER, Schwartz JH, Jessell TM. Principles of neural science 4th ed. New York: McGraw-Hill, Health Professions Division. 2000.
24. Knaflitz M, Merletti R, De Luca CJ. Inference of motor unit recruitment order in voluntary and electrically elicited contractions. J Appl Physiol. 1990;68(4):1657–67.
25. Farina D, Blanchietti A, Pozzo M, Merletti R. M-wave properties during progressive motor unit activation by transcutaneous stimulation. J Appl Physiol. 2004;97(2):545–55.
26. Mortimer JT. Comprehensive physiology. Hoboken, NJ, USA: Wiley; 2011.
27. Bickel CS, Gregory CM, Dean JC. Motor unit recruitment during neuromuscular electrical stimulation: a critical appraisal. Eur J Appl Physiol. 2011;111(10):2399–407.
28. Ambrosini E, Ferrante S, Pedrocchi A. Design of myocontrolled neuroprosthesis: tricks and pitfalls. Appl Challenges Adv Electromyogr Signal Process. IGI Global, 2014;275–303.
29. Sheffler LR, Chae J. Neuromuscular electrical stimulation in neurorehabilitation. Muscle Nerve. 2007;35(5):562–90.
30. Smith GV, Alon G, Roys SR, Gullapalli RP. Functional MRI determination of a dose-response relationship to lower extremity neuromuscular electrical stimulation in healthy subjects. Exp Brain Res. 2003;150(1):33–9.
31. Francis S, Lin X, Aboushoushah S, White TP, Phillips M, Bowtell R, Constantinescu CS. fMRI analysis of active, passive and electrically stimulated ankle dorsiflexion. Neuroimage. 2009;44(2):469–79.
32. Krakauer JW. Motor learning: its relevance to stroke recovery and neurorehabilitation. Curr Opin Neurol. 2006;19(1):84–90.
33. Rushton DN. Functional electrical Stimulation and rehabilitation—an hypothesis. Med Eng Phys. 2003;25:75–8.
34. Barsi GI, Popovic DB, Tarkka IM, Sinkjær T, Grey MJ. Cortical excitability changes following grasping exercise augmented with electrical stimulation. Exp Brain Res. 2008;191 (1):57–66.
35. Iftime-Nielsen SD, Christensen MS, Vingborg RJ, Sinkjær T, Roepstorff A, Grey MJ. Interaction of electrical stimulation and voluntary hand movement in SII and the cerebellum during simulated therapeutic functional electrical stimulation in healthy adults. Hum Brain Mapp. 2012;33(1):40–9.
36. Gandolla M, Ferrante S, Molteni F, Guanziroli E, Frattini T, Martegani A, Ferrigno G, Friston K, Pedrocchi A, Ward NS. Re-thinking the role of motor cortex: context-sensitive motor outputs? Neuroimage. 2014;91:366–74.
37. Gandolla M, Ward NS, Molteni F, Guanziroli E, Ferrigno G, Pedrocchi A. The neural correlates of long-term carryover following functional electrical stimulation for stroke. 2016; (2016).
38. Pomeroy VM, King L, Pollock A, Baily-Hallam A, Langhorne P. Electrostimulation for promoting recovery of movement or functional ability after stroke. Cochrane Database Syst Rev. 2006; (2).
39. Kluding PM, Dunning K, O'Dell MW, Wu SS, Ginosian J, Feld J, McBride K. Foot drop stimulation versus ankle foot orthosis after stroke: 30-week outcomes. Stroke. 2013;44 (6):1660–9.

40. Liberson WT, Holmquest HJ, Scot D, Dow M. Functional electrotherapy: stimulation of the peroneal nerve synchronized with the swing phase of the gait of hemiplegic patients. Arch Phys Med Rehabil. 1961;42:101–5.
41. Bogataj U, Gros N, Kljajic M, Acimovic R, Malezic M. The rehabilitation of gait in patients with hemiplegia: a comparison between conventional therapy and multichannel functional electrical stimulation therapy. Phys Ther. 1995;75(6):490–502.
42. Fields RW. Electromyographically triggered electric muscle stimulation for chronic hemiplegia. Arch Phys Med Rehabil. 1987;68(7):407–14.
43. Cozean CD, Pease WS, Hubbell SL. Biofeedback and functional electric stimulation in stroke rehabilitation. Arch Phys Med Rehabil. 1988;69(6):401–5.
44. Mazzocchio R, Meunier S, Ferrante S, Molteni F, Cohen LG. Cycling, a tool for locomotor recovery after motor lesions? NeuroRehabilitation. 2008;23(1):67–80.
45. Meunier S, Kwon J, Russmann H, Ravindran S, Mazzocchio R, Cohen L. Spinal use-dependent plasticity of synaptic transmission in humans after a single cycling session. J Physiol. 2007;579(Pt 2):375–88.
46. Katz-Leurer M, Sender I, Keren O, Dvir Z. The influence of early cycling training on balance in stroke patients at the subacute stage. Results of a preliminary trial. Clin Rehabil. 2006;20(5):398–405.
47. Alon G, Conroy VM, Donner TW. Intensive training of subjects with chronic hemiparesis on a motorized cycle combined with functional electrical stimulation (FES): a feasibility and safety study. Physiother. Res. Int. 2011;16(2):81–91.
48. del-Ama AJ, Koutsou AD, Moreno JC, delos-Reyes A, Gil-Agudo N, Pons JL. Review of hybrid exoskeletons to restore gait following spinal cord injury. J Rehabil Res Dev. 2012;49(4):497.

Gait Training by FES

Thomas Schauer and Thomas Seel

1 Introduction

Stroke is among the leading causes of gait impairments. The prevalence of stroke events is expected to increase as the global population aged over 65 increases. In Europe, the number of stroke events per year is estimated to rise from 1.1 million in 2000 to 1.5 million by 2025 [1]. Worldwide, 15 million people experience a stroke each year; one third die and one third are left permanently disabled [2]. About 50–85% of stroke survivors are able to walk independently within six months after stroke [3, 4]. Although the majority of stroke patients achieve independent walking, chronic gait abnormalities persist, and many stroke survivors do not reach a walking level that enables them to perform all their daily activities. A walking speed of 0.8 m/s or less excludes most individuals from participating in walking-related activities in the community [5]. More than 50% of ambulatory stroke patients fall while walking or because of losing their balance due to muscle weakness or coordination problems [6].

Stroke patients experience a paresis of one side of the body (hemiparesis) and are not able to time and adjust muscle contractions appropriately. These impairments in conjunction with poor endurance and balance adversely affect walking. A few weeks after the stroke event, spasticity and changes in the mechanical properties of the muscles (e.g. stiffness in antagonistic muscles) often develop. Post-stroke hemiplegic gait is a mixture of deviations from normal joint kinematics and compensatory motion dictated by residual functions. This gait is often characterized by

T. Schauer (✉) · T. Seel
Control Systems Group, Technische Universität Berlin, Berlin, Germany
e-mail: schauer@control.tu-berlin.de

G. Sandrini et al. (eds.), *Advanced Technologies for the Rehabilitation of Gait and Balance Disorders*, Biosystems & Biorobotics 19,
https://doi.org/10.1007/978-3-319-72736-3_22

inability to flex the hip, knee and ankle joint of the paretic leg due to muscle weakness in the corresponding muscles and increased muscle activity in the antagonistic muscles. The resulting increased leg length causes toe dragging or circumduction of the leg (i.e. stiff-legged gait).

The limited ability to lift the inner (medial) or outer (lateral) edge of the foot, or both, by voluntary muscle activation is known as drop foot syndrome and it is present in about 20% of ambulatory chronic stroke patients [4]. In addition, there is often decreased hip and knee flexion at initial contact and mid-swing, while ankle plantar flexion is reduced at toe-off and increased at initial contact and during the swing phase. The pelvis of the hemiplegic side is mostly elevated (hip hike), and translation of the trunk occurs over the unaffected side to support foot clearance of the affected leg during the swing phase. Abnormal movement patterns can also be observed on the unaffected side, due to compensation movements in addition to muscle weakness.

Spinal cord injury (SCI) is another cause of gait impairment. The prevalence of traumatic SCI is highest in the United States of America (906 per million) [7]. The majority of studies reported by Singh et al. showed a high male-to-female ratio and an age at peak incidence younger than 30 years old. Traffic accidents were typically the most common cause of SCI, followed by falls in the elderly population. Depending on the completeness and level of the lesion, paresis and paralysis of the leg musculature will occur. A complete lesion above the thoracic level will cause a motor and sensory paralysis of both legs (paraplegia), resulting in immobilization of the patient and possible lifelong wheelchair dependence. A complete loss of bladder, bowel and sexual function is also common. These primary effects of SCI lead to a range of secondary medical complications, e.g. atrophy of the paralyzed muscles and decreased cardiovascular fitness.

In stroke patients or individuals with SCI, the signal pathway from the central nervous system (CNS) to the muscles is interrupted. However, the muscles themselves retain their ability to contract and produce force. Functional electrical stimulation (FES) applied to the still intact lower motor neurons can replace the missing signals from the CNS and can be used to generate muscle contractions. In combination with appropriate sensor technology and feedback control, this method can be exploited to elicit or support walking movements.

FES has a direct orthotic or prosthetic effect on walking and can also be used as an assistive technology in daily life. During rehabilitation in a clinical environment, FES is mostly applied to achieve a therapeutic (carry-over) effect. This includes an increase of muscle strength as well as improvements in endurance and cardiovascular fitness. The increased afferent feedback provided by FES is known to modulate motor cortex function and excitability. FES can also be used to give indications about the right timing of muscle activities to sensory-unimpaired patients during walking. Recent findings (Gandolla et al. [8], for example) advocate the use of FES co-incidentally with the voluntary drive to enhance the plasticity of the central nervous system, and thus further improve its therapeutic effects. A recent review of the therapeutic effects of FES on gait in stroke patients [9] provides a detailed discussion of FES-induced brain plasticity and motor learning.

This chapter is organized as follows. In Sect. 1.2, a general overview of technological aspects of FES-assisted gait training is given. Then, the state of the art in drop foot correction for chronic stroke patients is presented in Sect. 1.3. The use of multi-channel FES for gait therapy in clinical environments is investigated in Sect. 1.4. Finally, in Sect. 1.5 we describe the application of FES for the restoration of gait in SCI individuals.

2 Technological Aspects of FES-Assisted Gait

2.1 Real-Time Gait Phase Detection

The core element of any FES system for walking is a robust and reliable real-time gait phase detection (GPD). The early systems, which are still the most widely available on the market, use force-resistive switches below the heel to distinguish the stand and swing phases of gait. Recent work extended this approach by integrating knitted resistive strain sensors into socks to derive gait phases indirectly from the measured ankle joint angle [10]. Force/strain sensors generally require patient-specific calibration and have a limited lifespan due to the repeated loading. Therefore, many researchers investigated the use of accelerometers and gyroscopes for GPD (see, for example, Chia Bejarano et al. [11], Rueterbories et al. [12], Seel et al. [13, 14]). Such sensors can be attached to the shoe/foot and/or to the shank and facilitate more detailed GPD. Figure 1 shows a state automaton that describes the gait phases and gait events that can be detected by a full miniature inertial sensor (contains accelerometer and gyroscope, both 3D) placed on the instep of the foot [13, 14]. Current integration of electronics will soon yield wireless inertial sensors with the size of a coin, which can be placed inside the shoe or worn unnoticed under clothes. With implants, gait phases might also be derived from natural sources like nerve activity [15]. Taborri et al. provided a systematic overview of gait partitioning methods [16].

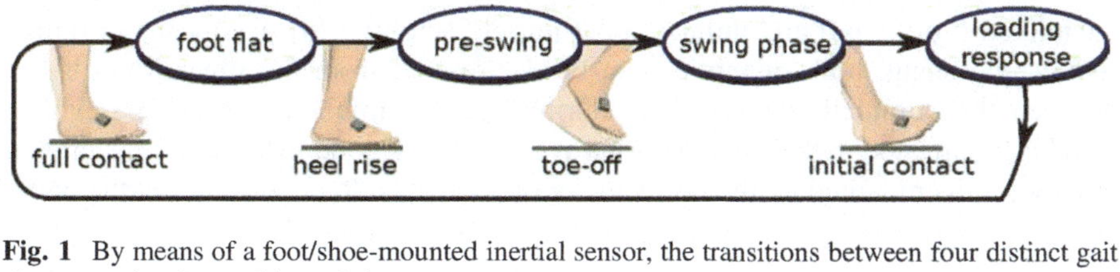

Fig. 1 By means of a foot/shoe-mounted inertial sensor, the transitions between four distinct gait phases can be detected in real time

2.2 Real-Time Assessment of Segment Orientations and Joint Angles

Wearable sensor technologies also enable real-time measurements of body segment orientation, e.g. the roll and pitch angle of the foot with respect to the ground, as well as walking velocity, stride lengths and joint angles. Such information can be used to adjust stimulation parameters during walking in order to improve the stimulation outcome, i.e. the motion of the patient. Knitted resistive strain sensors [10] and bio-impedance measurements [17] represent potential technologies for real-time assessment of joint angles. Both technologies can be integrated into textiles. Due to rapidly decreasing form factors, inertial sensors represent a particularly promising technology for ambulatory real-time motion analysis.

For example, by attaching an inertial sensor to each foot, shank and thigh, as well as an additional sensor to the hip, one can derive hip, knee and ankle joint angles with measurement accuracies that are comparable to those of optical motion capture systems. However, a few limitations remain. Precise placement of the inertial sensors or a sequence of predefined precise calibration movements is required, both of which can be challenging for motor-impaired patients. Another limiting factor is that many approaches require the use of magnetometers, which are known to be unreliable inside buildings and near ferromagnetic materials. Just recently, new methods have been proposed that overcome both of these limitations and enable automatic sensor-to-segment calibration of inertial sensor networks from arbitrary motions, including walking itself [18]. In view of these developments, future motion analysis systems are expected to be plug-and-play, in the sense that the sensors are attached in arbitrary orientation and calibrate automatically as the patient starts to walk [19].

2.3 Real-Time Assessment of Muscle Activity

Electromyography (EMG) can be used for multiple purposes in FES gait training. Figure 2 shows an example of a raw surface electromyography (sEMG) recording during active FES. When analyzing EMG signals, one has to distinguish between FES-evoked EMG and patient-induced EMG activity, where the latter includes both intentional (volitional) and unintentional muscle activity [20]. By means of online signal processing, both quantities can be determined from the raw EMG also in between the stimulation pulses, i.e. during active stimulation. The FES-evoked EMG is manifested in the so-called M-wave which is a good measure of the amount of motor units recruited by the last stimulation impulses. Recent studies in the upper

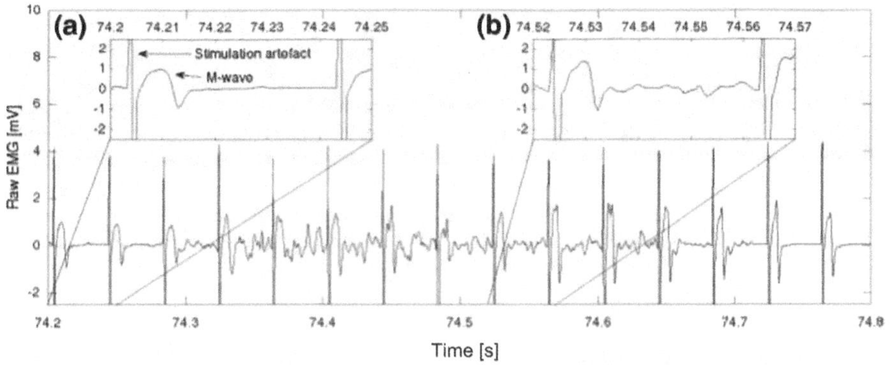

Fig. 2 EMG recording during active stimulation with a stimulation frequency of 25 Hz. **a** Stimulation period with almost no volitional muscle activity, **b** stimulation period with clearly visible volitional muscle activity

extremities show that feedback control of the M-wave magnitude compensates for the effects of muscular fatigue and maintains a desired stimulation effect (e.g. force production) [21, 22].

The EMG activity that is due to patient-induced muscle activity is much smaller than the M-wave. This rather noise-like signal with frequency components in the range of 30–300 Hz [23] can be separated from the M-wave about 20–30 ms after each stimulation pulse by high-pass filtering or by subtraction of an estimated/predicted M-wave (see, for example, Ambrosini et al. [24]). The patient's EMG can be used to trigger the stimulation onset, to modulate the intensity profile of stimulation or simply to monitor the effect of stimulation on the muscle activity and motor coordination of the patient. It has been demonstrated [25] that patient-induced muscle activity can be detected when using integrated stimulation and measurement electrodes. However, the simultaneous assessment of FES-induced and patient-induced muscle activity still requires the use of separate electrodes for stimulation and EMG monitoring.

2.4 Electrode and Stimulator Technology

Typically, charge-balanced bi-phasic stimulation impulses are delivered either via surface (skin) electrodes or via implanted electrodes to elicit action potentials in motor nerves of the target muscles. Surface electrodes are self-adhesive with a conductive hydro-gel and can be reused several times. Often, cuffs or body straps are used to improve the electrode-skin contact, whereas integration in trousers is less common. To overcome the poor selectivity of large surface electrodes and the

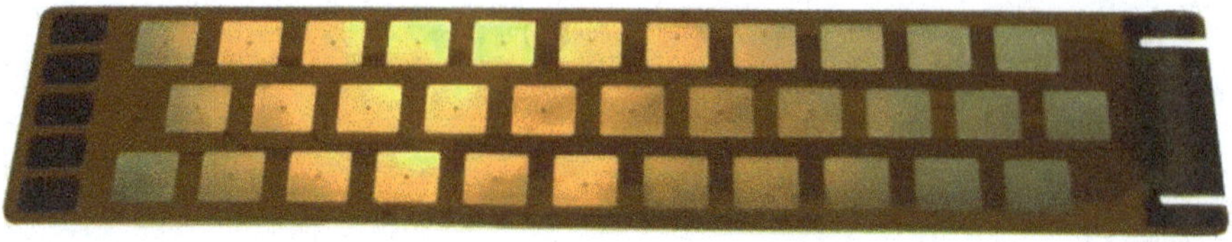

Fig. 3 Electrode arrays are used to overcome the requirement of precise placement and limited selectivity. Shown is a flexible electrode array for the stimulation of the peroneal nerve, as used e.g. in [29]. Each element of the array has a size of 8 mm $\times$ 8 mm

difficulties of electrode placement, the use of electrode arrays (multipad electrodes, see Fig. 3) has been proposed (see, for example, Heller et al. [26], Malesevic et al. [27, 28], Valtin et al. [29]). Such arrays contain many small electrodes and enable the formation of virtual electrodes consisting of a subset of these electrodes. Most arrays still use a common hydrogel layer below all electrodes [30]. This means that stimulation between two virtual electrodes inside one and the same array is not feasible. Instead, two arrays or one array and a conventional counter electrode are required to apply FES.

Stimulation with surface electrodes also excites pain receptors in the skin, which implies that stimulation intensities and producible forces are limited in patients with intact sensation. Percutaneous electrodes (inserted through the skin) or fully implanted electrodes cause less sensation and allow more selective muscle activation, also of more deeply located muscles. Implanted systems typically use nerve cuffs with a small array of multiple electrodes. To mitigate the problem of fast muscle fatigue in electrically stimulated muscles, alternating activation of these electrodes is performed to simulate the natural asynchronous muscle activation. The same effect is achieved with surface electrode arrays by alternating between virtual electrodes with similar stimulation outcome [31].

2.5 *Open-Loop and Closed-Loop Control*

Most FES systems control the timing of stimulation by detecting gait events, sensing volitional EMG activity or by hand-operated switches. Stimulation profiles are usually pre-programmed (feedforward control/open-loop control) and can only be changed manually. If the muscles fatigue or the muscle tone changes (spasticity), the FES parameters must be adjusted to obtain the same motion as before. Since repeated manual adjustments are undesirable, current research focuses on automatic adjustment of FES parameters to the current situation-dependent needs of the patient. Such closed-loop systems monitor the obtained motion and choose the stimulation intensities in such a way that the desired functional motion is obtained. At the same time, the onset of muscle fatigue can be delayed by avoiding over-stimulation.

Recently, wireless inertial sensors have increasingly been used to realize such closed-loop FES systems. The control algorithm that evaluates the measurements and decides how to adjust the FES parameters is typically implemented on a microcontroller. In conventional feedback control, the current stimulation intensity is adjusted on the basis of the current measurements. Since FES dynamics are slow and gait involves rather quick muscle contractions and motions, this conventional control approach was found to be of limited use. Learning control methods, like run-to-run control (see, for example, Veltink et al. [32]) or iterative learning control (see, for example, Seel et al. [14, 33]), are capable of exploiting the repetitive nature of gait by learning from the measurements obtained in previous strides. While run-to-run control typically aims at improving the amplitude of a stimulation window, iterative learning control can be used to optimize the entire time course of the FES intensities during each stride.

3 Drop Foot Stimulation

Liberson et al. [34] proposed the first clinical application of FES: stimulation of the peroneal nerve for correction of foot drop during the swing phase of gait. The peroneal nerve divides into a superficial and a deep branch, which innervate the m. fibularis longus and m. tibialis anterior, respectively. In a standard drop foot stimulator, both muscles are activated by positioning a pair of surface electrodes on the skin close to the head of fibula and on the insertion of the m. tibialis anterior. Both electrodes must be carefully placed to obtain a sufficient foot lift (dorsiflexion) without exaggerated eversion or inversion. The effect of stimulation is very sensitive to small ($\sim$1 cm) changes in the electrode positions and varies “from day to day due to a number of factors: changes in skin resistance due to sweating or dryness of the skin, condition of electrodes and fatigue and changes in resistance to dorsi-flexion caused by spasticity of the calf muscles” [35]. The review articles by Lyons et al. [36], Melo et al. [37] provide an excellent overview of drop foot stimulators in research and industry and classify them in several ways. Until now, all commercially available devices have been based solely on open-loop architectures, i.e. they only use sensors to time the stimulation [37]—typically a simple heel switch.

Several studies have shown the orthotic and therapeutic (carry-over) effects for both transcutaneous and implanted drop foot stimulation systems in terms of improved foot lift and walking speed, reduced Physiological Cost Index (PCI) and improved balance during walking (see, for example, Burridge et al. [35], Hausdorff and Ring [38], Kottink et al. [39, 40], Martin et al. [41], Ring et al. [42], Schiemanck et al. [43], Sheffler et al. [44]; Stein et al. [45], van Swigchem et al. [46], Taylor et al. [47, 48], Wilder et al. [49]). Many patients prefer drop foot stimulators to conventional ankle-foot orthoses [50, 51].

One of the best clinically evaluated systems is the Odstock dropped foot stimulator (ODFS) (Odstock Medical Ltd.). During the last two decades, several new systems have entered the marked, e.g. L300/L300plus/L300 Go (Bioness Inc.), WalkAide (Innovative Neurotronics Inc.), MyGait (Ottobock Healthcare GmbH) and ODFS Leg Cuff (Odstock Medical Ltd.). An important feature of these new systems is the integration of the stimulation device and electrodes in a leg cuff that is worn at the shank below the knee. Furthermore, the systems L300/L300plus, MyGait and ODFS Leg Cuff use a wireless heel switch. WalkAide does not rely on a heel switch at all—instead it uses an inclination sensor in the cuff to determine the gait phase [52]. An additional second stimulation channel for supporting plantar flexion, knee flexion, knee extension or hip extension is available in some of the systems.

In some patients, a desired foot motion cannot be achieved by transcutaneous stimulation, and some do not tolerate the stimulation intensities that are required for sufficient foot lift. Implantable dropped foot stimulators represent potential alternatives for these patients. Two systems have been developed: the two-channel implant Stimustep (Finetech Medical, UK) stimulates the n. peroneus profundus and the n. peroneus superficialis (both branches of the n. peroneus communis) to obtain better control over dorsiflexion and foot eversion/inversion [53]. The ActiGait system (Ottobock Healthcare GmbH) selectively activates the n. peroneus communis by means of a cuff electrode with four stimulation channels to achieve the same goal [54].

Besides these commercial systems, there are a number of promising novel systems being developed in research projects. Some recent contributions suggest the use of electrode arrays in combination with a search algorithm that finds the best position of a virtual electrode (see, for example, Heller et al. [26], Malesevic et al. [27], Prenton et al. [28], Valtin et al. [29]). At the current state of the art, however, this identification takes several minutes, and the virtual electrode is not adjusted when muscle tone or FES dynamics (and thus the induced foot motion) change during walking.

Also for transcutaneous stimulation, Seel et al. [33] proposed and investigated a three-electrode setup to manipulate the recruitment of the m. tibialis anterior and m. fibularis longus via two independent FES channels. Gait phase transitions as well as foot pitch and roll angles were assessed in real time by means of a shoe-mounted wireless inertial sensor. A decentralized iterative learning control scheme was used to adjust the stimulation intensity profiles to the current needs of the individual patient. Starting from conventional stimulation parameters, the controller automatically determined individual stimulation parameters and thereby achieved physiological foot pitch and roll angle trajectories within at most two strides in walking drop foot patients.

The application of EMG-derived stimulation intensity profiles has been investigated by Byrne et al. [55], Chen et al. [56], O'Keeffe and Lyons [57]. A stimulation proportional to the residual volitional activity of the m. tibialis anterior has been advocated by different authors [58–60]. Kesar et al. [61] suggested the use of variable-frequency pulse trains to enhance correction of foot drop compared with traditional FES systems that deliver constant-frequency pulse trains.

4 FES-Assisted Gait Therapy in Stroke Patients

Intensive FES training programs are often applied in clinics to restore and enhance gait patterns after stroke, both in sub-acute and chronic patients [9]. The meta-analysis by Teasell et al. [62] suggests FES as an adjunctive therapy in gait training. Another meta-analysis by Robbins et al. [63] showed a significant positive effect of FES on walking speed. A randomized controlled study even demonstrated recovery of coordinated gait in chronic stroke patients [64].

In clinical studies, the number of stimulation channels has been very diverse. In the study by Salisbury et al. [65], for example, a single-channel drop foot stimulator was employed for gait therapy of sub-acute stroke patients. By contrast, one of the first randomized studies with multi-channel FES considered heel-switch-triggered stimulation of the peroneal nerve as well as of the muscles triceps surae, hamstring, quadriceps femoris, gluteus maximus and triceps brachii [66]. Most clinical systems use transcutaneous stimulation, but the use of intramuscular (percutaneous) electrodes is also feasible, as demonstrated by Daly et al. [64].

The stimulation can be applied during level-ground walking, during treadmill walking (in possible combination with partial body weight support) (see, for example, Cho et al. [67], Daly et al. [64], Hesse et al. [68], Kesar et al. [69], Lindquist et al. [70], or in combination with a gravity-balanced orthosis [71], electromechanical gait trainers (e.g. [72]), or robotic locomotion devices (e.g. Dohring and Daly [73], McCabe et al. [74]). In the latter two cases, the timing of stimulation is usually derived from the mechanical support system and not by means of inertial sensors or heel switches. In order to better prepare non-ambulatory patients for gait training, FES cycling ergometers [75] or bed-side stimulation settings (for acute stroke patients) [76] can also be used.

Due to the necessary cabling effort, currently available clinical stimulation systems are cumbersome to apply—especially if many stimulation channels are used. In future, distributed wireless stimulation and sensor systems will enhance the usability of multichannel FES systems. The first prototypes have already been presented [77, 78].

5 FES-Assisted Ambulation After Spinal Cord Injury

The realization of standing and stepping in paraplegic individuals requires several stimulation channels. Bilateral stimulation of the m. quadriceps (for knee extension), peroneal nerve and, optionally, the m. gluteus maximus using surface electrodes represents a common approach [79]. To stand up and during standing, both quadriceps muscles are activated. To initiate a step, activation of the quadriceps stimulation is paused on one side, and the peroneal nerve is excited to elicit the withdrawal reflex (causing a flexion of the leg). The user will transfer his flexed leg forward by means of the upper body while holding on to a roller walker for balance. The initiation of steps is typically controlled by hand switches that are mounted on the handles of the walker. A commercially available system that uses this principle is the ParaStep system (Sigmedics, Inc.) [80, 81]. It is recommended for paraplegics with a lesion level between T4 and T12. The resulting stepping movement is not very physiological and not comparable to normal walking. Before using the system, a long-lasting and intensive program is required to build up fatigue-resistant muscles by electrical stimulation. A review of technical aspects of FES control of standing and stepping after SCI is provided by Braz et al. [82].

Implanted FES systems with up to 16 channels provide mobility in paraplegics [19, 83, 84, 85] and in individuals with incomplete spinal cord injury (iSCI) [86]. The use of implants reduces donning time and improves day-to-day repeatability compared to transcutaneous FES systems. Individuals with iSCI retain some control of the partially paralyzed muscles, which requires careful integration of FES. Dutta et al. [87] successfully exploited volitionally induced surface EMG activity to trigger stimulation via an implanted stimulation system in an iSCI individual.

The combination of FES with reciprocating gait orthoses (RGO) or powered exoskeletons offers hybrid solutions for the ambulation of SCI individuals. The mechanical structures stabilize the leg joints and trunk and provide good postural stability, while ambulation is supported by the artificially activated paralyzed muscles. Powered exoskeletons ensure precise movement execution by the motors even in the presence of time-varying muscle dynamics, providing consistent and repeatable gait. Hence, hybrid systems can combine the advantages of FES and orthoses/exoskeletons and thereby offer more advantages than the individual components alone. Examples of hybrid FES orthoses are described in papers by Durfee and Rivard [88], Kobetic et al. [89]. A good overview of hybrid FES-powered exoskeletons is given by del Ama et al. [90]. First results for the use of a hybrid FES-powered exoskeleton on three paraplegic subjects with motor-complete SCI are presented by Ha et al. [91]. For case studies with iSCI individuals using the hybrid Kinesis system (see Fig. 4) see del-Ama et al. [92], Del-Ama et al. [93].

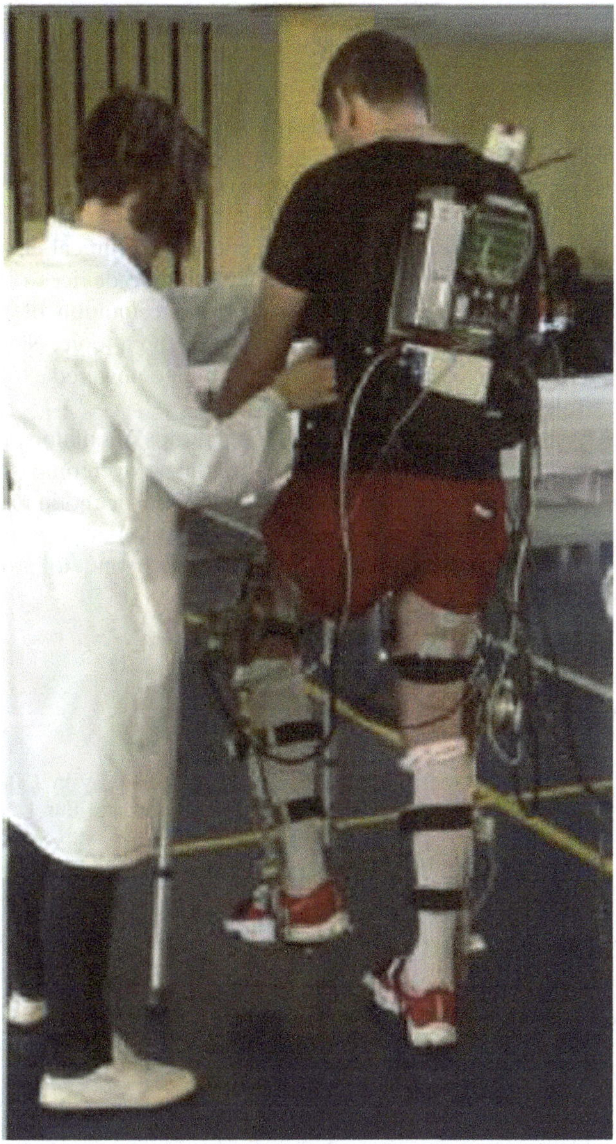

Fig. 4 Patient with incomplete spinal cord injury walking with the hybrid FES-powered exoskeleton Kinesis [92]

6 Conclusions

Functional electrical stimulation is a highly useful technology for the restoration and support of gait in stroke patients and spinal cord-injured individuals. Several studies have shown the orthotic and therapeutic (carry-over) effects for both transcutaneous and implanted drop foot stimulation systems.

Besides assistive systems for gait support of chronic drop foot patients, multi-channel FES systems are available for therapeutic use in clinical environments.

The latter might be used in combination with robotic devices or partial body weight support during walking on a treadmill. The restoration of gait in spinal cord-injured people, however, remains an ongoing research topic. New implantable stimulation systems and hybrid approaches that combine powered exoskeletons and FES are under investigation.

Remaining drawbacks and limitations of dropped foot stimulators, multi-channel FES systems and hybrid gait support systems might be overcome by present and future technological progress in the fields of inertial sensor motion analysis, electromyographic sensing and advanced feedback control. Future systems may be expected to adjust automatically to the individual user and to provide a more patient- and situation-specific gait support.

References

1. Truelsen T, Piechowski-Jozwiak B, Bonita R, Mathers C, Bogousslavsky J, Boysen G. Stroke incidence and prevalence in Europe: a review of available data. Eur J Neurol. 2006;13 (6):581–98.
2. Mackay J, Mensah GA, Mendis S, Greenlund K (2004) The atlas of heart disease and stroke. World Health Organization.
3. Jørgensen HS, Nakayama H, Raaschou HO, Olsen TS. Recovery of walking function in stroke patients: the Copenhagen Stroke study. Arch Phys Med Rehabil. 1995;76(1):27–32.
4. Wade DT, Wood VA, Heller A, Maggs J, Hewer RL. Walking after stroke. Measurement and recovery over the first 3 months. Scand J Rehabil Med. 1987;19(1):25–30.
5. Robinson CA, Shumway-Cook A, Matsuda PN, Ciol MA. Understanding physical factors associated with participation in community ambulation following stroke. Disabil Rehabil. 2011;33(12):1033–42.
6. Hyndman D, Ashburn A, Stack E. Fall events among people with stroke living in the community: circumstances of falls and characteristics of fallers. Arch Phys Med Rehabil. 2002;83(2):165–70.
7. Singh A, Tetreault L, Kalsi-Ryan S, Nouri A, Fehlings MG. Global prevalence and incidence of traumatic spinal cord injury. Clin Epidemiol. 2014;6:309–31.
8. Gandolla M, Ferrante S, Molteni F, Guanziroli E, Frattini T, Martegani A, Ferrigno G, Friston K, Pedrocchi A, Ward NS. Re-thinking the role of motor cortex: context-sensitive motor outputs? NeuroImage. 2014;91:366–74.
9. Kafri M, Laufer Y. Therapeutic effects of functional electrical stimulation on gait in individuals post-stroke. Ann Biomed Eng. 2015;43(2):451–66. https://doi.org/10.1007/s10439-014-1148-8.

10. Preece SJ, Kenney LP, Major MJ, Dias T, Lay E, Fernandes BT. Automatic identification of gait events using an instrumented sock. J Neuroengineering Rehabil. 2011;8(1):1.
11. Chia Bejarano N, Ambrosini E, Pedrocchi A, Ferrigno G, Monticone M, Ferrante S. A novel adaptive, real-time algorithm to detect gait events from wearable sensors. IEEE Trans Neural Syst Rehabil Eng. 2015;23(3):413–22. https://doi.org/10.1109/TNSRE.2014.2337914.
12. Rueterbories J, Spaich EG, Andersen OK. Gait event detection for use in FES rehabilitation by radial and tangential foot accelerations. Med Eng Phys. 2014;36(4):502–8.
13. Seel T, Escobar VC, Raisch J, Schauer T. Online gait phase detection with automatic adaption to gait velocity changes using accelerometers and gyroscopes. Biomed Eng/Biomed Techik. 2014;59(s1):S795–8. https://doi.org/10.1515/bmt-2014-5011.
14. Seel T, Werner C, Raisch J, Schauer T. Iterative learning control of a drop foot neuroprosthesis—generating physiological foot motion in paretic gait by automatic feedback control. Control Eng Pract. 2016;48:87–97.
15. Sinkjaer T, Haugland M, Inmann A, Hansen M, Nielsen KD. Biopotentials as command and feedback signals in functional electrical stimulation systems. Med Eng Phys. 2003;25 (1):29–40.
16. Taborri J, Palermo E, Rossi S, Cappa P. Gait partitioning methods: a systematic review. Sensors 16(1):66. http://doi.org/10.3390/s16010066.
17. Nahrstaedt H, Schauer T, Shalaby R, Hesse S, Raisch J. Automatic control of a drop foot stimulator based on angle measurement using bioimpedance. Artif Organs. 2008;32 (8):649–54.
18. Seel T, Raisch J, Schauer T. IMU-based joint angle measurement for gait analysis. Sensors. 2014;14(4):6891–909. https://doi.org/10.3390/s140406891.
19. Graurock D, Schauer T, Seel T. Automatic pairing of inertial sensors to lower limb segments – a plugand-play approach. Current Direct Biomed Eng. 2016;2:715–8. https://doi.org/10.1515/cdbme-2016-01552364-5504.
20. Merletti R, Knaflitz M, De Luca CJ. Electrically evoked myoelectric signals. Crit Rev Biomed Eng. 1992;19(4):293–340.
21. Klauer C, Raisch J, Schauer T. Linearisation of electrically stimulated muscles by feedback control of the muscular recruitment measured by evoked EMG. In: 2012 17th international conference on IEEE, Methods and Models in Automation and Robotics (MMAR); 2012. p. 108–13.
22. Klauer C, Ferrante S, Ambrosini E, Shiri U, Dahne F, Schmehl I, Pedrocchi A, Schauer T. A patient-controlled functional electrical stimulation system for arm weight relief. Med Eng Phys. 2016;38(11):1232–43.
23. De Luca CF, Knaflitz M. Surface electromyography, what's new?. Turin, Italy: CLUT Publishers; 1992.
24. Ambrosini E, Ferrante S, Schauer T, Klauer C, Gaffuri M, Ferrigno G, Pedrocchi A. A myocontrolled neuroprosthesis integrated with a passive exoskeleton to support upper limb activities. J Electromyogr Kinesiol. 2014;24(2):307–17. https://doi.org/10.1016/j.jelekin.2014.01.006.
25. Shalaby R, Schauer T, Liedecke W, Raisch J. Amplifier design for EMG recording from stimulation electrodes during functional electrical stimulation leg cycling ergometry. Biomed Technik Biomed Eng. 2011;56(1):23–33.
26. Heller BW, Clarke AJ, Good TR, Healey TJ, Nair S, Pratt EJ, Reeves ML, van der Meulen JM, Barker AT. Automated setup of functional electrical stimulation for drop foot using a novel 64 channel prototype stimulator and electrode array: results from a gait-lab based study. Med Eng Phys. 2013;35(1):74–81. https://doi.org/10.1016/j.medengphy.2012.03.012.
27. Malesevic J, Malesevic N, Bijelic G, Keller T, Konstantinovic L. Multi-pad stimulation device for treating foot drop: Case study. In: Annual conference of the Functional Electrical Stimulation Society (IFESS), IEEE, IEEE; 2014. p. 1–4.
28. Prenton S, Kenney LP, Stapleton C, Cooper G, Reeves ML, Heller BW, Sobuh M, Barker AT, Healey J, Good TR, et al. Feasibility study of a take-home array-based functional

electrical stimulation system with automated setup for current functional electrical stimulation users with foot-drop. Arch Phys Med Rehabil. 2014;95(10):1870–7.
29. Valtin M, Seel T, Raisch J, Schauer T. Iterative learning control of drop foot stimulation with array electrodes for selective muscle activation. In: Proceedings of the 19th IFAC World Congress; 2014. p. 6587–92.
30. Cooper G, Barker AT, Heller BW, Good T, Kenney LP, Howard D. The use of hydrogel as an electrode-skin interface for electrode array FES applications. Med Eng Phys. 2011;33 (8):967–72.
31. Sayenko DG, Nguyen R, Popovic MR, Masani K. Reducing muscle fatigue during transcutaneous neuromuscular electrical stimulation by spatially and sequentially distributing electrical stimulation sources. Eur J Appl Physiol. 2014;114(4):793–804.
32. Veltink PH, Slycke P, Hemssems J, Buschman R, Bultstra G, Hermens H. Three dimensional inertial sensing of foot movements for automatic tuning of a two-channel implantable drop-foot stimulator. Med Eng Phys. 2003;25(1):21–8.
33. Seel T, Werner C, Schauer T. The adaptive drop foot stimulator—multivariable learning control of foot pitch and roll motion in paretic gait. Med Eng Phys. 2016;38(11):1205–13.
34. Liberson W, Holmquest H, Scott M. Functional electrotherapy: stimulation of the common peroneal nerve synchronised with the swing phase of gait of hemiplegic subjects. Arch Phys Med Rehabil. 1961;42:202–5.
35. Burridge J, Taylor P, Hagan S, Wood DE, Swain ID. The effects of common peroneal stimulation on the effort and speed of walking: a randomized controlled trial with chronic hemiplegic patients. Clin Rehabil. 1997;11(3):201–10.
36. Lyons GM, Sinkjaer T, Burridge JH, Wilcox DJ. A review of portable FES-based neural orthoses for the correction of drop foot. IEEE Trans Neural Syst Rehabil Eng. 2002;10 (4):260–79.
37. Melo PL, Silva MT, Martins JM, Newman DJ. Technical developments of functional electrical stimulation to correct drop foot: sensing, actuation and control strategies. Clin Biomech. 2015;30(2):101–13. https://doi.org/10.1016/j.clinbiomech.2014.11.007.
38. Hausdorff JM, Ring H. Effects of a new radio frequency-controlled neuroprosthesis on gait symmetry and rhythmicity in patients with chronic hemiparesis. Am J Phys Med Rehabil. 2008;87(1):4–13. https://doi.org/10.1097/PHM.0b013e31815e6680.
39. Kottink AIR, Oostendorp LJM, Buurke JH, Nene AV, Hermens HJ. IJzerman MJ. The orthotic effect of functional electrical stimulation on the improvement of walking in stroke patients with a dropped foot: a systematic review. Artif Organs. 2004;28(6):577–86. https://doi.org/10.1111/j.1525-1594.2004.07310.x.
40. Kottink AIR, Hermens HJ, Nene AV, Tenniglo MJ, Groothuis-Oudshoorn CG. IJzerman MJ. Therapeutic effect of an implantable peroneal nerve stimulator in subjects with chronic stroke and footdrop: a randomized controlled trial. Phys Ther. 2008;88(4):437–48. https://doi.org/10.2522/ptj.20070035.
41. Martin KD, Polanski W, Schackert G, Sobottka SB. New therapeutic option for drop foot with the ActiGait peroneal nerve stimulator—a technical note. World Neurosurg. 2015;84 (6):2037–42. https://doi.org/10.1016/j.wneu.2015.06.074.
42. Ring H, Treger I, Gruendlinger L, Hausdorff JM. Neuroprosthesis for foot-drop compared with an ankle-foot orthosis: effects on postural control during walking. J Stroke Cerebrovasc Dis. 2009;18(1):41–7.
43. Schiemanck S, Berenpas F, van Swigchem R, van den Munckhof P, de Vries J, Beelen A, Nollet F, Geurts AC. Effects of implantable peroneal nerve stimulation on gait quality, energy expenditure, participation and user satisfaction in patients with post-stroke drop foot using an ankle-foot orthosis. Restorative Neurol Neurosci. 2015;33(6):795–807. https://doi.org/10.3233/rnn-150501.
44. Sheffler LR, Hennessey MT, Naples GG, Chae J. Peroneal nerve stimulation versus an ankle foot orthosis for correction of footdrop in stroke: impact on functional ambulation. Neurorehabilitation Neural Repair. 2006;20(3):355–60. https://doi.org/10.1177/1545968306287925.

45. Stein RB, Everaert DG, Thompson AK, Chong SL, Whittaker M, Robertson J, Kuether G. Long-term therapeutic and orthotic effects of a foot drop stimulator on walking performance in progressive and nonprogressive neurological disorders. Neurorehabil Neural Repair. 2010;24(2):152–67. https://doi.org/10.1177/1545968309347681.
46. van Swigchem R, Weerdesteyn V, van Duijnhoven HJ, den Boer J, Beems T, Geurts AC. Near-normal gait pattern with peroneal electrical stimulation as a neuroprosthesis in the chronic phase of stroke: a case report. Arch Phys Med Rehabil. 2011;92(2):320–4.
47. Taylor P, Humphreys L, Swain I. The long-term cost-effectiveness of the use of functional electrical stimulation for the correction of dropped foot due to upper motor neuron lesion. J Rehabil Med. 2013;45(2):154–60. https://doi.org/10.2340/16501977-1090.
48. Taylor PN, Burridge JH, Dunkerley AL, Wood DE, Norton JA, Singleton C, Swain ID. Clinical use of the odstock dropped foot stimulator: Its effect on the speed and effort of walking. Arch Phys Med Rehabil. 1999;80(12):1577–83. https://doi.org/10.1016/S0003-9993(99)90333-7.
49. Wilder RP, Wind TC, Jones EV, Crider BE, Edlich RF. Functional electrical stimulation for a dropped foot. J Long Term Eff Med Implants. 2002;12(3):149–59.
50. Bulley C, Shiels J, Wilkie K, Salisbury L. User experiences, preferences and choices relating to functional electrical stimulation and ankle foot orthoses for foot-drop after stroke. Physiotherapy. 2011;97(3):226–33. https://doi.org/10.1016/j.physio.2010.11.001.
51. van Swigchem R, Vloothuis J, den Boer J, Weerdesteyn V, Geurts AC. Is transcutaneous peroneal stimulation beneficial to patients with chronic stroke using an ankle-foot orthosis? A within-subjects study of patients' satisfaction, walking speed and physical activity level. J Rehabil Med. 2010;42(2):117–21.
52. Weber DJ, Stein RB, Chan KM, Loeb G, Richmond F, Rolf R, James K, Chong SL. BIONic WalkAide for correcting foot drop. IEEE Trans Neural Syst Rehabil Eng Publ IEEE Eng Med Biol Soc. 2005;13(2):242–6. https://doi.org/10.1109/TNSRE.2005.847385.
53. Kenney L, Bultstra G, Buschman R, Taylor P, Mann G, Hermens H, Holsheimer J, Nene A, Tenniglo M, van der Aa H, Hobby J. An implantable two channel drop foot stimulator: initial clinical results. Artif Organs. 2002;26(3):267–70.
54. Burridge JH, Haugland M, Larsen B, Svaneborg N, Iversen HK, Christensen PB, Pickering RM, Sinkjaer T. Patients' perceptions of the benefits and problems of using the ActiGait implanted drop-foot stimulator. J Rehabil Med. 2008;40(10):873–5. https://doi.org/10.2340/16501977-0268.
55. Byrne CA, O'Keeffe DT, Donnelly AE, Lyons GM. Effect of walking speed changes on tibialis anterior EMG during healthy gait for FES envelope design in drop foot correction. J Electromyogr Kinesiol. 2007;17(5):605–16. https://doi.org/10.1016/j.jelekin.2006.07.008.
56. Chen M, Wu B, Lou X, Zhao T, Li J, Xu Z, Hu X, Zheng X. A self- adaptive foot drop corrector using functional electrical stimulation (FES) modulated by tibialis anterior electromyography (EMG) dataset. Med Eng Phys. 2013;35(2):195–204. https://doi.org/10.1016/j.medengphy.2012.04.016.
57. O'Keeffe DT, Lyons GM. A versatile drop foot stimulator for research applications. Med Eng Phys. 2002;24(3):237–42.
58. Chen WL, Chen SC, Chen CC, Chou CH, Shih YY, Chen YL, Kuo TS. Patient-driven loop control for ambulation function restoration in a non-invasive functional electrical stimulation system. Dis Rehabil. 2010;32(1):65–71. https://doi.org/10.3109/09638280903026564.
59. Thorsen R, Ferrarin M, Veltink P. Enhancement of isometric ankle dorsiflex- ion by automyoelectrically controlled functional electrical stimulation on subjects with upper motor neuron lesions. Neuromodulation. 2002;5(4):256–63.
60. Yeom H, Chang YH. Autogenic EMG-controlled functional electrical stimulation for ankle dorsiflexion control. J Neurosci Methods. 2010;193(1):118–25. https://doi.org/10.1016/j.jneumeth.2010.08.011.
61. Kesar TM, Perumal R, Jancosko A, Reisman DS, Rudolph KS, Higginson JS, Binder-Macleod SA. Novel patterns of functional electrical stimulation have an immediate

effect on dorsiflexor muscle function during gait for people poststroke. Phys Ther. 2010;90 (1):55–66. https://doi.org/10.2522/ptj.20090140.
62. Teasell RW, Bhogal SK, Foley NC, Speechley MR. Gait retraining post stroke. Topics Stroke Rehabil. 2003;10(2):34–65. https://doi.org/10.1310/UDXE-MJFF-53V2-EAP0.
63. Robbins SM, Houghton PE, Woodbury MG, Brown JL. The therapeutic effect of functional and transcutaneous electric stimulation on improving gait speed in stroke patients: a meta-analysis. Arch Phys Med Rehabil. 2006;87(6):853–9.
64. Daly JJ, Zimbelman J, Roenigk KL, McCabe JP, Rogers JM, Butler K, Burdsall R, Holcomb JP, Marsolais EB, Ruff RL. Recovery of coordinated gait: randomized controlled stroke trial of functional electrical stimulation (FES) versus no FES, with weight-supported treadmill and over-ground training. Neurorehabilitation and Neural Repair. 2011;25(7):588–96. https://doi.org/10.1177/1545968311400092.
65. Salisbury L, Shiels J, Todd I, Dennis M. A feasibility study to investigate the clinical application of functional electrical stimulation (FES), for dropped foot, during the sub-acute phase of stroke—a randomized controlled trial. Physiotherapy Theor Pract. 2013;29(1):31–40. https://doi.org/10.3109/09593985.2012.674087.
66. Bogataj U, Gros N, Kljajic M, Acimovic R, Malezic M. The rehabilitation of gait in patients with hemiplegia: a comparison between conventional therapy and multichannel functional electrical stimulation therapy. Phys Ther. 1995;75(6):490–502.
67. Cho MK, Kim JH, Chung Y, Hwang S. Treadmill gait training combined with functional electrical stimulation on hip abductor and ankle dorsiflexor muscles for chronic hemiparesis. Gait Posture. 2015;42(1):73–8.
68. Hesse S, Malezic M, Schaffrin A, Mauritz K. Restoration of gait by combined treadmill training and multichannel electrical stimulation in non-ambulatory hemiparetic patients. Scand J Rehabil Med. 1995;27(4):199–204.
69. Kesar TM, Reisman DS, Perumal R, Jancosko AM, Higginson JS, Rudolph KS, Binder-Macleod SA. Combined effects of fast treadmill walking and functional electrical stimulation on post-stroke gait. Gait Posture. 2011;33(2):309–13. https://doi.org/10.1016/j.gaitpost.2010.11.019.
70. Lindquist AR, Prado CL, Barros RM, Mattioli R, Da Costa PHL, Salvini TF. Gait training combining partial body-weight support, a treadmill, and functional electrical stimulation: effects on poststroke gait. Phys Ther. 2007;87(9):1144–54.
71. Krishnamoorthy V, Hsu WL, Kesar TM, Benoit DL, Banala SK, Perumal R, Sangwan V, Binder-Macleod SA, Agrawal SK, Scholz JP. Gait training after stroke: a pilot study combining a gravity-balanced orthosis, functional electrical stimulation, and visual feedback. J Neurol Phys Ther JNPT. 2008;32(4):192–202. https://doi.org/10.1097/NPT.0b013e31818e8fc2.
72. Tong RK, Ng MF, Li LS. Effectiveness of gait training using an electromechanical gait trainer, with and without functional electric stimulation, in subacute stroke: a randomized controlled trial. Arch Phys Med Rehabil. 2006;87(10):1298–304. https://doi.org/10.1016/j.apmr.2006.06.016.
73. Dohring ME, Daly JJ. Automatic synchronization of functional electrical stimulation and robotic assisted treadmill training. IEEE Trans Neural Syst Rehabil Eng. 2008;16(3):310–3. https://doi.org/10.1109/TNSRE.2008.920081.
74. McCabe JP, Dohring ME, Marsolais EB, Rogers J, Burdsall R, Roenigk K, Pundik S, Daly JJ. Feasibility of combining gait robot and multichannel functional electrical stimulation with intramuscular electrodes. J Rehabil Res Dev. 2008;45(7):997–1006.
75. Ambrosini E, Ferrante S, Pedrocchi A, Ferrigno G, Molteni F. Cycling induced by electrical stimulation improves motor recovery in postacute hemiparetic patients a randomized controlled trial. Stroke. 2011;42(4):1068–73.
76. Yan T, Hui-Chan CW, Li LS. Functional electrical stimulation improves motor recovery of the lower extremity and walking ability of subjects with first acute stroke: A randomized placebo-controlled trial. Stroke. 2005;36(1):80–5.

77. Jovicic NS, Saranovac LV, Popovic DB. Wireless distributed functional electrical stimulation system. J Neuroengineering Rehabil. 2012;9:54.
78. Mecheraoui CA, Swain I, Cobb J. A distributed three-channel wireless Functional electrical stimulation system for automated triggering of stimulation to enable coordinated task execution by patients with neurological disease. Biomed Signal Proc Control. 2013;8(2):176–83. https://doi.org/10.1016/j.bspc.2012.08.006.
79. Kralj A, Bajd T, Turk R. Enhancement of gait restoration in spinal injured patients by functional electrical stimulation. Clin Orthop Relat Res. 1988;233:34–43.
80. Graupe D, Kohn KH. Functional neuromuscular stimulator for short-distance ambulation by certain thoracic-level spinal-cord-injured paraplegics. Surg Neurol. 1998;50(3):202–7.
81. Graupe D, Davis R, Kordylewski H, Kohn KH. Ambulation by traumatic t4–12 paraplegics using functional neuromuscular stimulation. Crit Rev Neurosurg. 1998;8(4):221–31.
82. Braz GP, Russold M, Davis GM. Functional electrical stimulation control of standing and stepping after spinal cord injury: a review of technical characteristics. Neuromodulation J Int Neuromodulation Soc. 2009;12(3):180–90. https://doi.org/10.1111/j.15251403.2009.00213.x.
83. Guiraud D, Stieglitz T, Koch KP, Divoux JL, Rabischong P. An implantable neuroprosthesis for standing and walking in paraplegia: 5-year patient follow-up. J Neural Eng. 2006;3 (4):268–75. https://doi.org/10.1088/1741-2560/3/4/003.
84. Guiraud D, Coste CA, Benoussaad M, Fattal C. Implanted functional electrical stimulation: case report of a paraplegic patient with complete sci after 9 years. J. Neuroengineering Rehabil. 2014;11:15.
85. Kobetic R, Triolo RJ, Uhlir JP, Bieri C, Wibowo M, Polando G, Marsolais EB, Davis JA Jr, Ferguson KA. Implanted functional electrical stimulation system for mobility in paraplegia: a follow-up case report. IEEE Trans Rehabil Eng. 1999;7(4):390–8.
86. von Wild K, Rabischong P, Brunelli G, Benichou M, Krishnan K. Computer added locomotion by implanted electrical stimulation in paraplegic patients (SUAW). Acta Neurochir Suppl. 2002;79:99–104.
87. Hardin E, Kobetic R, Murray L, Corado-Ahmed M, Pinault G, Sakai J, Bailey SN, Ho C, Triolo RJ. Walking after incomplete spinal cord injury using an implanted FES system: a case report. J Rehabil Res Dev. 2007;44(3):333–46.
88. Dutta A, Kobetic R, Triolo RJ. Ambulation after incomplete spinal cord injury with EMG-triggered functional electrical stimulation. IEEE Trans Bio-Med Eng. 2008;55(2 Pt 1):791–4. https://doi.org/10.1109/TBME.2007.902225.
89. Durfee WK, Rivard A. Design and simulation of a pneumatic, stored- energy, hybrid orthosis for gait restoration. J Biomech Eng. 2005;127(6):1014–9.
90. Kobetic R, To CS, Schnellenberger JR, Audu ML, Bulea TC, Gaudio R, Pinault G, Tashman S, Triolo RJ. Development of hybrid orthosis for standing, walking, and stair climbing after spinal cord injury. J Rehabil Res Dev. 2009;46(3):447–62.
91. del-Ama AJ, Koutsou AD, Moreno JC, de-los Reyes A, Gil-Agudo A, Pons JL. Review of hybrid exoskeletons to restore gait following spinal cord injury. J Rehabil Res Dev. 2012;49 (4):497–514.
92. Ha KH, Murray SA, Goldfarb M. An approach for the cooperative control of FES with a powered exoskeleton during level walking for persons with paraplegia. IEEE Trans Neural Syst Rehabil Eng. 2016;24(4):455–66. https://doi.org/10.1109/TNSRE.2015.2421052.
93. del-Ama AJ, Gil-Agudo A, Bravo-Esteban E, Perez-Nombela S, Pons JL, Moreno JC. Hybrid therapy of walking with kinesis overground robot for persons with incomplete spinal cord injury: a feasibility study. Robot Auton Syst. 2015;73:44–58.
94. Del-Ama AJ, Gil-Agudo A, Pons JL, Moreno JC. Hybrid gait training with an overground robot for people with incomplete spinal cord injury: a pilot study. Frontiers Hum Neurosci. 2014;8:298.

Gait Rehabilitation by Nociceptive Withdrawal Reflex-Based Functional Electrical Therapy

Ole Kæseler Andersen and Erika G. Spaich

1 Introduction

The nociceptive withdrawal reflex (NWR) can be used for supporting gait as the spinal stepping generator circuits can also be triggered by robust afferent input [36]. This has been utilised in many assistive functional electrical stimulation devices since the first reports by Liberson [32] who found a functional benefit when stimulating electrically the peroneal nerve during the swing phase. The NWR response is an integrated movement generated by a coordinated activation of several muscles in the limb when the body receives a potentially tissue damaging stimulus. The NWR is generated to ensure adequate and sufficient withdrawal while maintaining balance and ensuring continuation of the ongoing motor programs [4, 41, 49]. This obviously leads to involvement of the contralateral limb to ensure upright posture and balance control. During rhythmic movements like gait, the spinal pattern generators are involved in reflex modulation as the reflex responses are strongly modulated by the phases of the gait cycle [17, 56].

The NWR response depends also on the stimulation site in the sense that, for every muscle or group of synergistic muscles, a restricted skin area can be identified from which sufficiently strong input will lead to reflex activation in the muscle. This skin area has been termed the reflex receptive field (RRF) [2, 43]. Stimulation outside the RRF area may inhibit reflexes in the muscle [48]. The RRF is highly linked to the biomechanical function of the muscle so functionally, the muscle is activated when a contraction supports the effective withdrawal of the limb, e.g. dorsiflexion via activation of the tibialis anterior muscles when a stimulus is presented in the distal part of the sole of the foot [2, 25]. The stimulus site dependency is preserved during gait, however functionally modulated. Hence, the NWR

O. K. Andersen (✉) · E. G. Spaich
Integrative Neuroscience Group, SMI®, Department of Health Science and Technology, Aalborg University, Fredrik Bajersvej 7 D3, 9220 Aalborg, Denmark
e-mail: oka@hst.aau.dk

G. Sandrini et al. (eds.), *Advanced Technologies for the Rehabilitation of Gait and Balance Disorders*, Biosystems & Biorobotics 19,
https://doi.org/10.1007/978-3-319-72736-3_23

kinematic responses are stronger during the swing phase compared to the stance phase in healthy volunteers [49]. The stimulus site dependency and functional reflex modulation are also present during the relatively unstable gait initiation phase following stable symmetrical standing. Thus, the largest reflexes in the hip joint can be evoked at the initial heel off in the leading limb while at heel contact during the first step hip, reflexes are inhibited [39]. In general, larger reflex excitability is seen during gait initiation compared to static standing [45].

The spinal reflex pathways also include a gain mechanism via neuronal temporal summation. Hence, repetitive stimulation will lead to gradually larger NWR [5] most likely via enhanced firing of deep dorsal horn neurons [47]. Functionally, repetitive stimulation at frequencies up to 30 Hz leads to gradually increased reflex sizes for a short train duration (few seconds) [5, 50]. During gait, four stimulation pulses at a frequency of 15 Hz (total duration approximately 200 ms) at an intensity marginally above the pain threshold leads to strong muscle reflexes and hip joint reflexes exceeding 10° when delivered at heel off [50].

This chapter focuses on tailoring electrical stimulation of sensory afferents at the foot leading to gait support via spinal reflex pathways during post-stroke gait rehabilitation.

2 Nociceptive Withdrawal Reflex Modulation During the Hemiparetic Gait

After a brain injury, the supraspinal control of spinal reflexes is modified. Both the time course and the magnitude of the withdrawal reflex recorded in the most affected leg of stroke individuals shows changes compared to healthy individuals [14, 20, 22, 34, 35, 46]. Cyclic movements, and particularly gait, are known to modulate the reflex response [12, 18, 49], which is also modified in stroke individuals. The amplitude of the NWR in the ipsilateral tibialis anterior and soleus, and the contralateral vastus lateralis present a different phase modulation than in healthy individuals [51]. Hemiparetic individuals present for instance larger tibialis anterior responses at heel-off and during mid-swing than aged-matched healthy individuals (Fig. 1). Foot drop is characteristically present in the hemiparetic side after heel-off, it was suggested therefore, that the NWR response might have a functional meaning, i.e. to produce ankle dorsiflexion and consequently move the foot away from the noxious stimulus on the sole of the foot [51]. Ankle dorsiflexion, preceded by reduced plantarflexion, is indeed the primary kinematic reflex response at the ankle joint resulting in a swing phase more alike that of healthy individuals [51]. At the hip and knee joints, the withdrawal reflex response consisted of flexion resulting on unloading of the stimulated leg while maintaining balance and ensuring continuation of the ongoing motor program [51]. The typical site-modulation of the NWR is generally preserved after a stroke allowing for tailored NWR responses dependent on the stimulation site and the stimulation timing during the gait cycle.

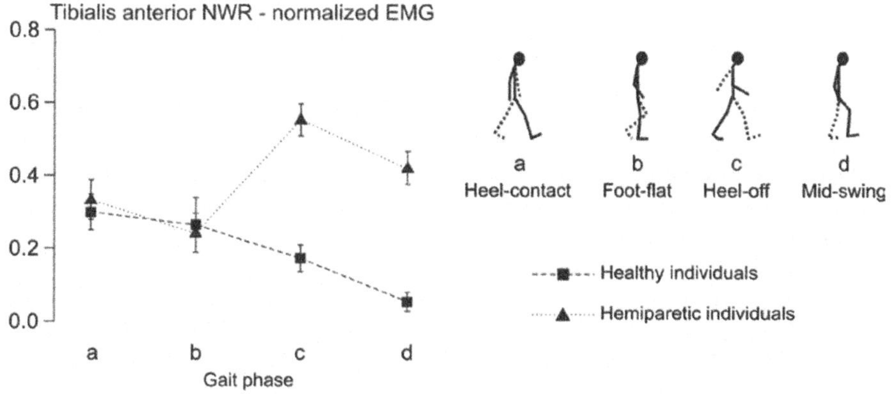

Fig. 1 Phase-modulation of Tibialis anterior NWR for hemiparetic and age-matched healthy individuals. The NWR is elicited by electrically stimulating the sole of the foot. The reflex responses are normalized to the peak activity recorded during control steps (hemiparetic individuals: 72 μV, healthy individuals: 136.5 μV)

3 Nociceptive Withdrawal Reflex-Based Gait Training

Some of the common gait deficiencies after stroke include reduced hip, knee, and ankle flexion during swing [37]. Facilitation of these movements follows the activation of the NWR [51], therefore, the NWR has been proposed as a therapeutic tool to facilitate gait training of hemiparetic individuals.

Gait training is an important aspect of rehabilitation programs as proper gait function is crucial for maintaining the quality of life after a stroke [9, 16]. This is a problem that affects a large part of the stroke population, since approximately 50% of the patients have initially no walking function and 12% need assistance to walk [28]. Training consists typically of a combination of different approaches including physiotherapy, lower extremity muscle strengthening, over ground walking combined with stepping and cycling, treadmill walking with and without weight support, and robot assisted walking [1, 30, 38, 42, 54]. Some of these techniques have been combined with functional electrical stimulation (FES) of selected leg muscles to facilitate the desired movements [8, 13]. In particular, FES applied during gait results on improvement of gait performance [8, 13, 53]. Inherent to this modality of stimulation is placing the stimulation electrodes on the motor points, adjusting the stimulation intensity, and synchronizing the stimulation onset and offset for each stimulation channel. This might result in a considerable donning time, especially for applications that require stimulating several muscle groups.

Alternatively, facilitation of gait related movements can be achieved by eliciting the NWR [51]. The NWR can thereby be used to initiate and facilitate the swing phase of the hemiparetic gait, by supporting the lift of the most affected leg and clearing the foot. The choice of stimulation site on the sole of the foot is not so sensitive to electrode location, since the NWR receptive field for different lower limb muscles spans to areas of several square centimeters [2]. This allows for some flexibility when placing the stimulation electrode (cathode). Additionally, the reflex receptive fields of several muscles overlap, which results on reflexes being elicited in different relevant muscles followed by complex, synergistic kinematic responses [2]. In the perspective of a gait training application, this means concretely that a multi-joint unloading response can be achieved by stimulating a single site on the sole of the foot. To elicit the NWR, stimulation intensities perceived as unpleasant or painful need to be used [3], which, in the context of a therapeutic approach, was not considered to be a problem by the patients [52].

Intensive physiotherapy-based gait training combined with activation of the NWR to initiate and support the swing phase is the basis of the NWR-based functional electrical therapy intervention [52]. The intervention is tailored individually by a physiotherapist and when administered in the sub-acute stroke phase, results in improved walking [52]. This is more evident for stroke subjects with severe walking impairment at inclusion time. The improvements include increased preferred and fast walking velocities, shortening of the gait cycle and lengthening of the stance phase on the affected side, and closer to normal stance time symmetry ratio (Fig. 2) [52]. The overall results suggest that the NWR-based therapy is useful to improve the outcomes of gait rehabilitation of subacute hemiparetic individuals.

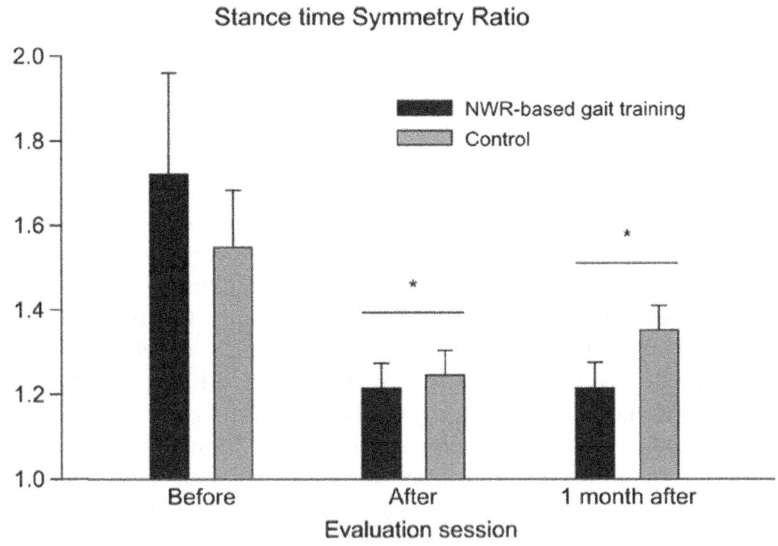

Fig. 2 Stance time Symmetry Ratio before training, immediately after completion of training, and 1 month after completion of training. The normative cut point for healthy individuals is 1.05. Asterisk indicates a statistically significant difference between groups after finishing treatment

One of the potential difficulties when using this technique is the habituation of the NWR, i.e. a gradual decay of the reflex responses following repetitive stimulation. This phenomenon can be minimized by changing the stimulus parameters [15, 31] and the inter-stimulus interval, which is naturally achieved when training with over ground walking.

4 Automatic Control of Reflex-Supported Systems for Gait Rehabilitation

Control strategies for automatic FES support of gait training have received most focus for training spinal cord injured subjects (SCI) [6, 24, 29, 33]. The common peroneal nerve has been the target for the production/support of the swing phase combined with activation of knee and ankle extensor muscles for the stance phase [7, 10]. Closed loop control of FES has been investigated with focus on knee extensor stimulation based on continuous measures of the knee joint angle and use of artificial neural networks (ANN) [21]. In another attempt, adaptive ANNs have been used for controlling electrical stimulation of the peroneal and femoral nerves to activate the swing phase in SCI combined with online learning of the ANN. This setup proved successful in a single patient with incomplete SCI [44]. ANNs have also been used in foot drop correction applications involving stimulation of the tibialis anterior muscle [26]. A closed loop FES system for SCI patients allowing both gait, stair climbing, and a program for sitting down was presented by Fuhr and colleagues [23]. This system also stimulated the peroneal nerve for producing the swing phase via reflex pathways.

Focusing on the swing phase, stimulation of the sole of the foot allows better control of the evoked reflex response by tailoring the stimulation site, timing and intensity according to the RRF concept and its modulation during the gait cycle. Such a neuromuscular system can be characterized as a Multiple Input Multiple Output (MIMO) system with coupled outputs since the joints are interconnected during all postures. This non-linear stochastic system is highly time variant because of the continuous neural integration of motor commands, central pattern generator activity, proprioceptive and sensory signals, fatigue, habituation, etc. To establish a deterministic model of such a plant is therefore not realistic and often the needed physiological knowledge is not even available. A model is needed to predict the state of the neuromuscular plant given a set of artificial sensor signals in order to create a closed loop system for automatic stimulation control [27, 40]. A numeric model of the NWR plant for the swing phase that is continuously updated has been suggested [19]. In this system, the NWR plant model describes the expected reflex based on stimulation site (four sites on the foot) and different stimulation onsets during the early swing phase of the gait cycle (three onsets). The model is continuously being updated from step cycle to step cycle during the training session. The model did not include variation in stimulus intensities.

Close loop control of the NWR within the gait cycle is difficult due to the long reflex latency compared to the duration of the gait cycle. Instead, control was designed to achieve a realistic joint angle target based on the present NWR model (in a sense a feed forward system within the individual gait cycle). This control scheme is called iterative learning control [55]. Adaptive closed loop control has been compared to a fixed control scheme in which the arch of the foot was stimulated in every step cycle during 10 min walking in chronic stroke patients [19]. This study clearly showed that automatic control of the swing phase support is possible in chronic stroke patients. For the short test period, the adaptive control system to a better degree reached the joint angle target and with a tendency for less habituation. The latter might reflect that variation in stimulus site by itself leads to less habituation [11].

5 Conclusion and Future Perspectives

The nociceptive withdrawal reflex is the net result of activity in a spinal reflex pathway. This pathway integrates afferent activity, descending control, and ongoing motor programs resulting in optimal withdrawal, balance control, and continuation of the movement. The reflex in a specific muscle has graded spatial sensitivity typically reflecting to effectiveness of the muscle to withdraw the stimulated skin area. Moreover, integration of afferent input over time (temporal summation) is pronounced and the reflex response is modulated during cyclic movements. For gait support after an injury, the spatial and temporal mechanisms can be exploited to tailor the desired functional movement. Following a cerebral stroke, the NWR is still present but with changes in the spatial and temporal characteristics during the gait cycle. Improved gait speed and better gait symmetry have been observed when gait training is supported by stimulation of the NWR at heel off in subacute stroke patients. Automatic control of functional electrical stimulation systems has been shown feasible. Specifically, for NWR-based gait therapy the closed-loop control must account for long delays in the reflex pathways compared to the gait cycle duration. Future perspectives could involve systematic studies of treatment duration, better control of stimulation parameters, and identification of patient types that benefit most from the NWR-based gait therapy.

References

1. Ada L, Dean CM, Hall JM, Bampton J, Crompton S. A treadmill and overground walking program improves walking in persons residing in the community after stroke: a placebo-controlled, randomized trial. Arch Phys Med Rehabil. 2003;84:1486–91.
2. Andersen OK, Sonnenborg FA, Arendt-Nielsen L. Modular organization of human leg withdrawal reflexes elicited by electrical stimulation of the foot sole. Muscle Nerve. 1999;22:1520–30.

3. Andersen OK, Sonnenborg FA, Arendt-Nielsen L. Reflex receptive fields for human withdrawal reflexes elicited by non-painful and painful electrical stimulation of the foot sole. Clin Neurophysiol. 2001;112(4):641–649.
4. Andersen OK. Studies of the organization of the human nociceptive withdrawal reflex. Focus on sensory convergence and stimulation site dependency. Acta Physiol 2007;189 Suppl;654: 1–35.
5. Arendt-Nielsen L, Sonnenborg FA, Andersen OK. Facilitation of the withdrawal reflex by repeated transcutaneous electrical stimulation: an experimental study on central integration in humans. Eur J Appl Physiol. 2000;81:165–73.
6. Bailey SN, Hardin EC, Kobetic R, Boggs LM, Pinault G, Triolo RJ. Neurotherapeutic and neuroprosthetic effects of implanted functional electrical stimulation for ambulation after incomplete spinal cord injury. J Rehabil Res Dev. 2010;47:7–16.
7. Bajd T, Kralj A, Karcnik T, Savrin R, Obreza P. Significance of FES-assisted plantarflexion during walking of incomplete SCI subjects. Gait Posture. 1994;2:5–10.
8. Bogataj U, Gros N, Kljajic M, Acimovic R, Malezic M. The rehabilitation of gait in patients with hemiplegia: a comparison between conventional therapy and multichannel functional electrical stimulation therapy. Phys Ther. 1995;75:490–502.
9. Bohannon RW, Horton MG, Wikholm JB. Importance of four variables of walking to patients with stroke. Int J Rehabil Res. 1991;14:246–50.
10. Braun Z, Mizrahi J, Najenson T, Graupe D. Activation of paraplegic patients by functional electrical stimulation: training and biomechanical evaluation. Scand J Rehabil Med Suppl. 1985;12(93–101):93–101.
11. Carstens E, Ansley D. Hindlimb flexion withdrawal evoked by noxious heat in conscious rats: magnitude measurement of stimulus-response function, suppression by morphine and habituation. J Neurophysiol. 1993;70:621–9.
12. Crenna P, Frigo C. Evidence of phase-dependent nociceptive reflexes during locomotion in man. Exp Neurol. 1984;85:336–45.
13. Daly JJ, Roenigk K, Holcomb J, Rogers JM, Butler K, Gansen J, McCabe J, Fredrickson E, Marsolais EB, Ruff RL. A randomized controlled trial of functional neuromuscular stimulation in chronic stroke subjects. Stroke. 2006;37:172–8.
14. Dimitrijevic MR. Withdrawal reflexes. In: Desmedt JE, editor. New developments in electromyography and clinical neurophysiology, vol. 3. Basel: Karger; 1973. p. 744–50.
15. Dimitrijevic MR, Faganel J, Gregoric M, Nathan PW, Trontelj JK. Habituation: effects of regular and stochastic stimulation. J Neurol Neurosurg Psychiat. 1972;35:234–42.
16. Dobkin BH. Clinical practice. Rehabilitation after stroke. N Engl J Med. 2005;352:1677–84.
17. Duysens J, De GF, Jonkers I. The flexion synergy, mother of all synergies and father of new models of gait. Front Comput Neurosci. 2013;7:14. https://doi.org/10.3389/fncom.2013.00014.eCollection;%2013.:14.
18. Duysens J, Tax AAM, Tripel M, Dietz V. Phase-dependent reversal of reflexly induced movements during human gait. Exp Brain Res. 1992;90:404–14.
19. Emborg J, Matjacic Z, Bendtsen JD, Spaich EG, Cikajlo I, Goljar N, Andersen OK. Design and test of a novel closed-loop system that exploits the nociceptive withdrawal reflex for swing-phase support of the hemiparetic gait. IEEE Trans Biomed Eng. 2011;58:960–70.
20. Faganel J. Electromyographic analysis of human flexion reflex components. In: Desmedt JE, editor. New developments in electromyography and clinical neurophysiology, vol. 3. Basel: Karger; 1973. p. 730–3.
21. Ferrante S, Pedrocchi A, Ianno M, De ME, Ferrarin M, Ferrigno G. Functional electrical stimulation controlled by artificial neural networks: pilot experiments with simple movements are promising for rehabilitation applications. Funct Neurol. 2004;19:243–52.
22. Fisher MA, Shahani BT, Young RR. Electrophysiologic analysis of the motor system after stroke: the "suppressive" effect of vibration. Arch Phys Med Rehabil. 1979;60:11–4.
23. Fuhr T, Quintern J, Riener R, Schmidt G. Walking with WALK! A cooperative, patient-driven neuroprosthetic system. IEEE Eng Med Biol Mag. 2008;27:38–48.

24. Granat MH, Ferguson AC, Andrews BJ, Delargy M. The role of functional electrical stimulation in the rehabilitation of patients with incomplete spinal cord injury—observed benefits during gait studies. Paraplegia. 1993;31:207–15.
25. Grimby L. Normal plantar response: Integration of flexor and extensor reflex components. J Neurol Neurosurg Psychiat. 1963;26:39–50.
26. Hansen M, Haugland MK. Adaptive fuzzy logic restriction rules for error correction and safe stimulation patterns during functional electrical stimulation. J Med Eng Technol. 2001;25:156–62.
27. Jonic S, Jankovic T, Gajic V, Popovic D. Three machine learning techniques for automatic determination of rules to control locomotion. IEEE Trans Biomed Eng. 1999;46:300–10.
28. Jorgensen HS, Nakayama H, Raaschou HO, Olsen TS. Recovery of walking function in stroke patients: the Copenhagen Stroke Study. Arch Phys Med Rehabil. 1995;76:27–32.
29. Kapadia N, Masani K, Catharine CB, Giangregorio LM, Hitzig SL, Richards K, Popovic MR. A randomized trial of functional electrical stimulation for walking in incomplete spinal cord injury: effects on walking competency. J Spinal Cord Med. 2014;37:511–24.
30. Laufer Y, Dickstein R, Chefez Y, Marcovitz E. The effect of treadmill training on the ambulation of stroke survivors in the early stages of rehabilitation: a randomized study. J Rehabil Res Dev. 2001;38:69–78.
31. Laursen CB, Gervasio S, Andersen OK, Hennings K, Spaich EG. Novel electrical stimulation paradigm to reduce habituation of the nociceptive withdrawal reflex: preliminary results. Soc Neurosci. 2015; 268.01/BB74 (Ref Type: Abstract).
32. Liberson WT, Holmquest HJ, Scot D, Dow M. Functional electrotherapy: stimulation of the peroneal nerve synchronized with the swing phase of the gait of hemiplegic patients. Arch Phys Med Rehabil. 1961;42:101–5.
33. Lynch CL, Popovic MR. A comparison of closed-loop control algorithms for regulating electrically stimulated knee movements in individuals with spinal cord injury. IEEE Trans Neural Syst Rehabil Eng. 2012;20:539–48.
34. Meinck H-M, Küster S, Benecke R, Conrad B. The flexor reflex—influence of stimulus parameters on the reflex response. Electroenceph clin Neurophysiol. 1985;61:287–98.
35. Milanov IG. Flexor reflex for assessment of common interneurone activity in spasticity. Electromyogr Clin Neurophysiol. 1992;32:621–9.
36. Nicol DJ, Granat MH, Baxendale RH, Tuson SJM. Evidence for a human spinal stepping generator. Brain Res. 1995;684:230–2.
37. Olney SJ, Richards C. Hemiparetic gait following stroke. Part I: Characteristics. Gait Posture. 1996;4:136–48.
38. Pohl M, Werner C, Holzgraefe M, Kroczek G, Mehrholz J, Wingendorf I, Hoolig G, Koch R, Hesse S. Repetitive locomotor training and physiotherapy improve walking and basic activities of daily living after stroke: a single-blind, randomized multicentre trial (DEutsche GAngtrainerStudie, DEGAS). Clin Rehabil. 2007;21:17–27.
39. Richard MA, Spaich EG, Serrao M, Andersen OK. Stimulation site and phase modulation of the withdrawal reflex during gait initiation. Clin Neurophysiol. 2015;126:2289.
40. Riener R, Fuhr T, Antico D, Quintern J. Modelling and control of the flexion withdrawal reflex for gait neuroprosthesis. In: Sinkjær T, Popovic D, Struijk JJ editors. Proceedings for the 5th annual conference of the international functional electrical stimulation society. Aalborg; 2000. p. 421–4.
41. Rietdyk S, Patla AE. Context-dependent reflex control: some insights into the role of balance. Exp Brain Res. 1998;119:251–9.
42. Salbach NM, Mayo NE, Wood-Dauphinee S, Hanley JA, Richards CL, Cote R. A task-orientated intervention enhances walking distance and speed in the first year post stroke: a randomized controlled trial. Clin Rehabil. 2004;18:509–19.
43. Schouenborg J, Kalliomäki J. Functional organization of the nociceptive withdrawal reflexes. I. Activation of hindlimb muscles in the rat. Exp Brain Res. 1990;83:67–78.

44. Sepulveda F, Granat MH, Cliquet AJ. Gait restoration in a spinal cord injured subject via neuromuscular electrical stimulation controlled by an artificial neural network. Int J Artif Organs. 1998;21:49–62.
45. Serrao M, Ranavolo A, Andersen OK, Conte C, Don R, Cortese F, Mari S, Draicchio F, Padua L, Sandrini G, Pierelli F. Adaptive behaviour of the spinal cord in the transition from quiet stance to walking. BMC Neurosci. 2012;13:80.
46. Shahani BT, Young RR. Human flexor reflexes. J Neurol Neurosurg Psychiat. 1971;34: 616–27.
47. Sivilotti LG, Thompson SWN, Woolf CJ. Rate of rise of the cumulative depolarization evoked by repetitive stimulation of small-caliber afferents is a predictor of action potential windup in rat spinal neurons in vitro. J Neurophysiol. 1993;69:1621–31.
48. Sonnenborg FA, Andersen OK, Arendt-Nielsen L. Modular organization of excitatory and inhibitory reflex receptive fields elicited by electrical stimulation of the foot sole in man. Clin Neurophysiol. 2000;111:2160–9.
49. Spaich EG, Arendt-Nielsen L, Andersen OK. Modulation of lower limb withdrawal reflexes during gait: a topographical study. J Neurophysiol. 2004;91:258–66.
50. Spaich EG, Emborg J, Collet T, Arendt-Nielsen L, Andersen OK. Withdrawal reflex responses evoked by repetitive painful stimulation delivered on the sole of the foot during late stance: site, phase, and frequency modulation. Exp Brain Res. 2009;194:359–68.
51. Spaich EG, Hinge HH, Arendt-Nielsen L, Andersen OK. Modulation of the withdrawal reflex during hemiplegic gait: effect of stimulation site and gait phase. Clin Neurophysiol. 2006;117:2482–95.
52. Spaich EG, Svaneborg N, Jorgensen HR, Andersen OK. Rehabilitation of the hemiparetic gait by nociceptive withdrawal reflex-based functional electrical therapy: a randomized, single-blinded study. J Neuroeng Rehabil. 2014;11:81.
53. Stanic U, Acimovic-Janezic R, Gros N, Trnkoczy A, Bajd T, Kljajic M. Multichannel electrical stimulation for correction of hemiplegic gait. methodology and preliminary results. Scand J Rehabil Med. 1978;10:75–92.
54. Teixeira-Salmela LF, Olney SJ, Nadeau S, Brouwer B. Muscle strengthening and physical conditioning to reduce impairment and disability in chronic stroke survivors. Arch Phys Med Rehabil. 1999;80:1211–8.
55. Xu J-X. The frontiers of iterative learning control —part II. Systems, control and information. 2002;46:233–43.
56. Zehr EP. Neural control of rhythmic human movement: the common core hypothesis. Exerc Sport Sci Rev. 2005;33:54–60.

Postural Rehabilitation Within the VRRS (Virtual Reality Rehabilitation System) Environment

Marco Pirini, Maria Cristina Bisi, Andrea Turolla, Michela Agostini, Denis Vidale, Alessio Fiorentin and Federico Piron

1 Introduction

Postural control has been defined as the ability to maintain, achieve or restore a state of balance during any posture or activity [1, 2]. Appropriate postural control is an absolute pre-requisite for activities of daily living and requires several different motor skills to be effective. To maintain a stable upright stance, with adaptive strategies for orientation and balance, information processed through the somatosensory (70%), visual (10%) and vestibular (20%) systems needs to be integrated [3, 4], and a complex interplay between sensory and motor systems [5] is required in order to control the multisegmental body system and interlimb coupling [6].

Thus, physiological conditions, including aging, that lead to disruption or alteration of proprioception, vision and/or vestibular transduction have a significant negative impact on postural control performance [7].

The most widely measured parameter to assess balance performance during quiet and/or perturbed standing is the center of pressure (CoP) [8]. As is well known, the CoP is the center of the distribution of the total force applied to the supporting surface; it is derived from force platform data and allows quantification of postural stability and evaluation of different postural strategies. The CoP is considered the neuromuscular response to imbalances in the body's center of gravity (CoG) [9]; it is an expression of movements on the floor generated by motor control dynamics for maintaining balance and/or for generating movement of the center of mass (CoM). The CoP reflects the

M. Pirini (✉) · D. Vidale · A. Fiorentin · F. Piron
Khymeia Group, Padua, Italy
e-mail: m.pirini@khymeia.com

M. C. Bisi
University of Bologna, Bologna, Italy

A. Turolla · M. Agostini
Kinematics and Robotics Laboratory, IRCCS Fondazione San Camillo, Venice, Italy

G. Sandrini et al. (eds.), *Advanced Technologies for the Rehabilitation of Gait and Balance Disorders*, Biosystems & Biorobotics 19,
https://doi.org/10.1007/978-3-319-72736-3_24

combined control of both left and right dorsiflexors/plantarflexors and invertors/evertors [10]. Through analysis of CoP excursion/trajectory together with the use of appropriate segmental models (from the simple inverted pendulum [10] to more complete multisegmental models [11–13]), it is possible to evaluate postural strategies used for the control of upright stance in the anteroposterior (AP) and mediolateral (ML) directions (i.e. ankle and hip strategies [14]).

Several different CoP variables can be extracted from raw CoP data to specifically analyze mechanisms involved in postural regulation [8]. In general, these variables have been found to be sensitive in comparing young with old individuals, and healthy subjects with neurologically impaired patients, allowing analysis and quantification of postural deficits (for a detailed description of these parameters see the review by Paillard and Noé [8]).

As with any motor skill, postural balance control can be usefully improved through training [7]. In this context, quantitative assessment of postural performance (e.g. through measurement of CoP during stance) can be a useful supportive tool both for assessing quantitatively the effects of interventions, and as a possible real-time biofeedback to be used in training with exergaming.

Exergaming (exercise + gaming) is a term used to describe computer applications that require players to physically move in response to game demands. The CoP has been used as input for controlling the game in different exercise applications, such as stepping on and off a board, or shifting weight [15, 16]. Exergaming has emerged as a promising means of facilitating balance improvements both in healthy and in clinical populations [16, 17], showing positive results in older adults [18], in patients with stroke [19, 20], cerebral palsy [21] and Parkinson's disease [22], and in people recovering from spinal cord injury or brain injury [23], allowing improvements in balance, gait and function.

Potential differences between the use of conventional balance training and exergaming have been evaluated in recent literature [16]. The two types of intervention were found to be comparable in terms of effects on balance and gait, but exergaming was found to be intrinsically more motivating than traditional balance training [16].

As an example, in the field of rehabilitation, conventional training with balance boards (or wobble boards) has been shown to be effective in many postural rehabilitation settings, such as the recovery of sport skills, the improvement of stability in the elderly, and the treatment of numerous postural dysfunctions [8, 24]. A multiaxial board challenges the postural control system and requires it to explore new schemas or to use different models developed and memorized during other experiences [24].

Even in this context, CoP measurement is useful for evaluating postural stability. For example, it allows quantitative analysis of oscillations along the AP and ML directions, and makes it possible to test whether the type of control observed during static upright stance is also used on the multiaxial board [24].

Exergaming offers great potential to further enhance this type of standard training through the use of an instrumented balance board, increasing the level of interest and enjoyment during the exercise [25]. Furthermore, given that proprioception is a fundamental component of quiet stance [5], the integration of proprioceptive input/feedback during training with a balance board can further enhance postural control rehabilitation.

Exergaming devices have shown several advantages over conventional exercises; in particular, in addition to their capacity to improve motivation to practice, they have been shown to reduce perception of effort [16]. Furthermore, the individual's attention is focused not on the actual production of movements, but rather on their outcome during performance of the game task [1, 25]; thus they produce a situation that is more similar to what happens in daily life, where attention is focused on the outcome of movements and not on the conscious control of balance [1].

2 VRRS Methodology. Description and Basic Principles

The VRRS (Virtual Reality Rehabilitation System) is a multi-domain and integrated ecosystem for rehabilitation. It is suitable for application in neurological, orthopedic, cognitive, speech, cardiorespiratory, and postural rehabilitation settings.

The VRRS methodology uses biofeedback and augmented feedback to promote functional recovery through cortical plasticity-based cortical reorganization, in the more general contexts of operant conditioning and reinforced learning.

Different VRRS devices are available, ranging in size and portability, and thus allowing both clinical and home-based implementations (see Fig. 1). Each VRRS is a class 1 medical device.

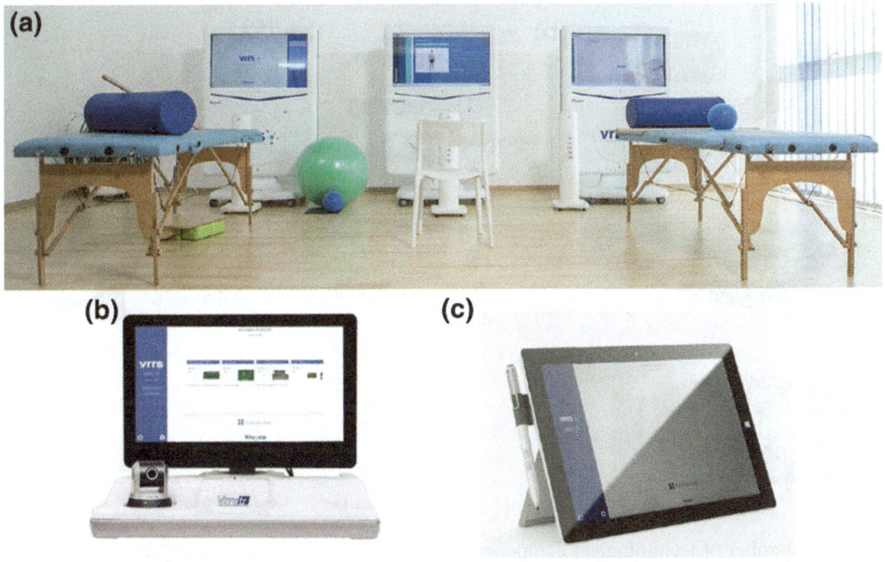

Fig. 1 Different VRRS devices are available for both clinical (**a**) and home-based (**b**, **c**) applications

2.1 VRRS Components

The typical VRRS includes:

- a computation unit, running the activities and generating feedback and indications for the patient;
- a means of measuring and capturing the postural behavior of the subject (see Fig. 2). Depending on the captured behavior, different rehabilitation applications can be proposed to the patient. The set of technologies that the system can currently integrate includes:
  - a kinematic tracking system based on magnetic technology which exploits wearable sensors for position and orientation tracking of hands, feet, upper arms, lower arms, trunk and head, and for kinematic tracking of joints (neurological, postural and orthopedic applications);
  - a kinematic tracking system based on IMUs (inertial motion units), allowing kinematic tracking of joints (neurological and orthopedic applications);
  - a 3D mouse emulator (cognitive and speech therapy applications);
  - posturographic and proprioceptive balance boards (neurological, postural and orthopedic applications);
  - a camera-based tracking device for fine hand and finger tracking (neurological and orthopedic applications focusing on the hand);
  - a spirometer to monitor and measure real-time inspiration and expiration flows (cardiorespiratory and speech therapy applications);

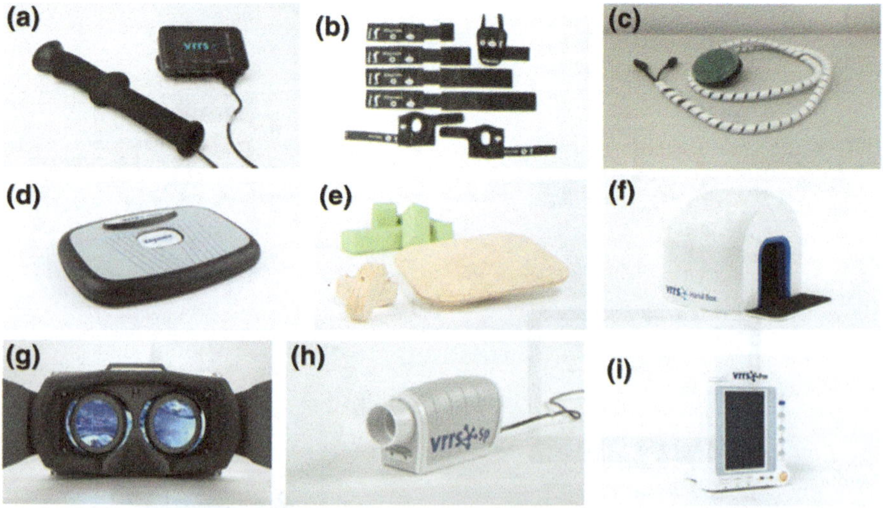

Fig. 2 A number of technological components and devices expand the capabilities of the VRRS, e.g. magnetic-based and IMU-based tracking systems, together with wearable bands and textiles to apply sensors to the patient's body (**a**, **b**, **c**); posturographic and proprioceptive boards (**d**, **e**); a camera-based tracking system for the hand (**f**); virtual reality headsets (**g**); and systems for tracking cardiorespiratory parameters and respiratory patterns (**h**, **i**)

In some activities, more than one device is needed to track the patient's behavior, while most activities require just one technological component. With the aim of expanding, as much as possible, the system's tracking capabilities, other devices will, in the future, be integrated and/or are currently under development.

- a feedback audio-visual device, by means of which the subject is immersed in non-immersive (screen; projector) or immersive (3D headset) and 2D or 3D scenarios, in which the task is proposed (see Fig. 3). Touch screen capabilities (for non-immersive applications) and hand and finger tracking (for the 3D immersive application) are available to the subject to allow multiple modes of interaction with the system.

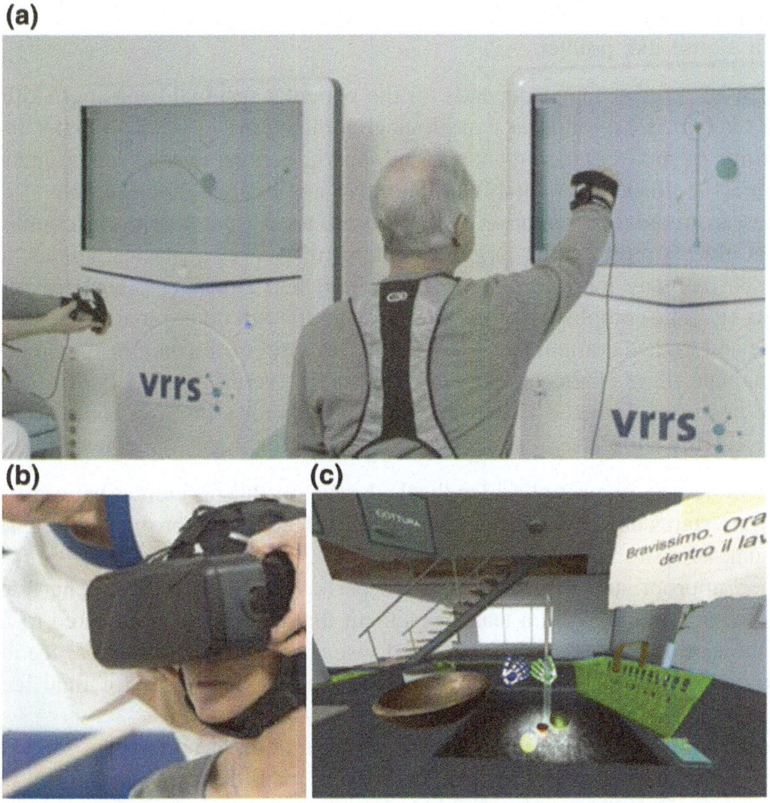

Fig. 3 The VRRS offers both non-immersive (**a**) and immersive (**b, c**) applications

2.2 VRRS Activities

Briefly, a VRRS activity is a task that the subject has to execute for a given number of repetitions and/or for a given amount of time. The inherent logic and complexity of the task depend on the application, and tasks thus range from very simple ones to more ecological tasks in rich environments. The key behavior of the patient, used to drive the task, is captured by a specific technological component, which depends on the exercise in question.

In general terms, the subject and his/her behavior can be represented in the virtual scenario in many different ways:

- as a realistic or abstract object;
- as a complete or partial avatar, which can be more or less realistic or game-like;
- as an abstract, game-like character;
- as a mouse-like pointer.

The type of representation depends on the patient's residual capacities/skills, thus higher realism is exploited in neurological applications in order to better promote re-learning of motor planning and execution, while more abstract representations of the subject's effector are suitable in cognitive applications, for example.

Apart from the representation of the subject, the virtual scenario is populated by abstract objects representing targets, points of reference, obstacles, guides, teacher elements, pathway indications and limits, start and stop areas, background components etc. The complexity of the exercise and the full determination of its various graphic and logical components are under the control of the therapist, who can alter and graduate these elements and even build new exercises using built-in editors.

The tasks are designed in order to promote learning through cortical reorganization. To this end, several strategies and key features are implemented:

- the subject is given online feedback, based on the difference between his/her current status and the desired behavior. This feedback is provided in the form of visual, acoustic and even verbal indications;
- when appropriate, the behavior to be performed in a 3D/2D scenario can be shown continuously by a teacher element that the patient is required to follow;
- at the end of the task, final vocal and visual (as percentage scores) feedback is provided; each exercise in each domain uses its own rules for final feedback computation and restitution;
- the difficulty of the task can be scaled, in order to tailor it to patient's capabilities at a given instant in time. Each exercise in each domain implements its own representation of complexity, and for the majority of exercises, automatic complexity adaptation algorithms can be activated;
- cognitive richness (i.e., the richness of the 3D/2D scenarios) varies enormously between exercises and tasks, thereby making it possible to tailor the cognitive workload to patient's possibilities in the course of his/her functional recovery;
- the subject's behavior relevant to the execution of the exercise can be scaled and magnified in the virtual environment. Such scaling represents another means of

providing the subject with augmented feedback; in addition, it represents an appropriate way to involve the subject in rehabilitation activities based on reinforcement learning; this applies even in cases where he/she is only able to execute small movements that, unless magnified, would not, per se, be capable of triggering significant feedback.

Together with the final global score and the single and repetition scores, each VRRS activity outputs specific parameters and metrics peculiar to its specific domain.

Nowadays, more than 300 activities have been implemented and integrated in the VRRS ecosystem. Each one has been co-developed and verified in clinical practice. Their representation of complexity, cognitive richness, rules for feedback restitution and score calculation, and difficulty and scaling are the result of combined research and development activities conducted, in conjunction, by clinical specialists, researchers and scientists.

2.3 *The VRRS Interface*

Each VRRS has a simplified user interface (see Fig. 4) that nevertheless allows a full set of capabilities. The VRRS interface:

- allows complete management of patient information;
- is a smart, single-screen interface, able to explore, select and launch activities;
- offers the possibility of modifying and creating new activities with built-in editors;
- offers the possibility of organizing activities in clinical protocols;
- incorporates an automated and integrated reporting system, able to produce both detailed and summary reports about the patient's activities and progress.

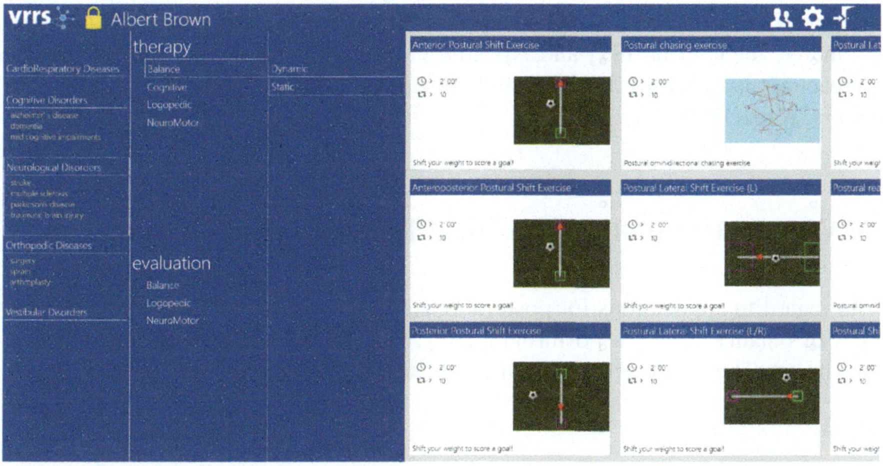

Fig. 4 The main VRRS interface

For home-based applications, the ICT-based VRRS technology has been integrated with audio-video teleconferencing and telecontrol capabilities. The VRRS user interface for home-based applications is obviously different from that implemented in clinical settings, being designed to have the patient as the primary user.

Thus, the VRRS ecosystem can be used to promote and implement home-based rehabilitation pathways without reducing or limiting proper therapeutic continuity with clinicians.

2.4 Clinical Validation

The VRRS methodology has been extensively validated and tested. The validity of the system and of its underlying methodology has been demonstrated in several publications.

Piron et al. [26] confirmed that therapy with VRRS improves upper limb motor performance after stroke more than conventional therapy does. Moreover, the kinematic results were coherent with the rationale based on the amplification of kinematic feedback to promote motor recovery; in fact, both motor function and kinematics of the upper limb improved concurrently. The same group [27] observed that the same results are achievable by remote control of the VRRS (i.e. telerehabilitation), thereby opening up, for the first time, the possibility of providing effective technology-based rehabilitation remotely.

Turolla et al. [28] and Kiper et al. [29] extended these findings to open populations of stroke inpatients, demonstrating that effectiveness is maintained, regardless of the etiology, across different baseline levels of motor impairment at admittance and different intervals from stroke onset. Thus, a diagnosis of stroke and the presence of residual voluntary motor activation of the upper limb are sufficient criteria to refer survivors for motor therapy with the VRRS. Luque-Moreno et al. [30] were the first to replicate results observed for the upper limb also in the lower limb.

Finally, Jelcic et al. [31] and Agostini et al. [32] demonstrated that the VRRS approach is also effective for the remote treatment of mild cognitive impairment and anomia, respectively.

3 VRRS Methodology. Postural Rehabilitation Devices

With regard to applications for postural rehabilitation, the VRRS uses two different types of balance board, a posturographic balance board and a proprioceptive balance board. These devices can be used for a wide range of activities.

3.1 Posturographic Balance Board

The posturographic balance board (POSTURO board) is a 80 cm × 55 cm planar device (see Fig. 5), connectable to the VRRS via USB, and able to detect:

- the total weight, Fz;
- the AP component of the CoP, Y_{COP};
- and the ML component of the CoP, X_{COP}

of a person standing on it.

3.1.1 Calibration and Output Measures

The key component of the POSTURO board is a set of 4 load cells. Signals from the load cells are acquired, amplified, and digitalized by a dedicated board, which acquires data at 120 fps and applies a 24-bit conversion. The calculation of Fz, Y_{COP}, and X_{COP} is performed though a dedicated software module.

The dedicated software module uses several calibration parameters obtained during a preliminary calibration procedure, performed on each board before its first use. Indeed, calibration is a critical step. The implementation of proper calibration procedures at the level of single load cells and at the level of the whole board has been described elsewhere [33].

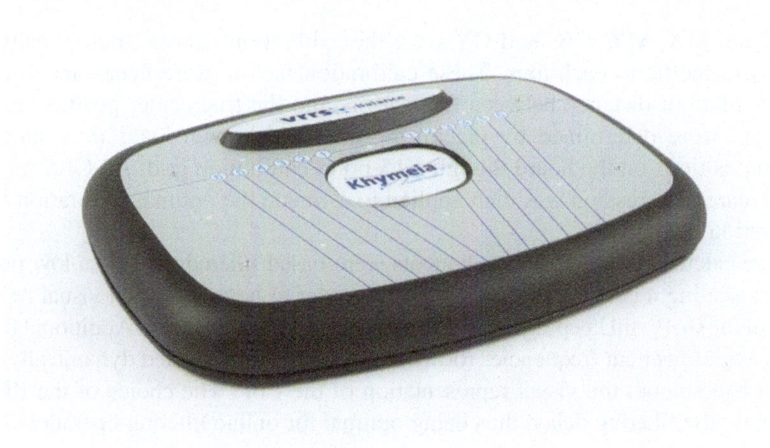

Fig. 5 The VRRS POSTURO board

The steps in the real-time calculation of Fz, Y_{COP}, and X_{COP} were, in the following order:

1. Calculation of the true force values (in N) for each load cell. Data from each of the four sensors were converted into true force values. To ensure the precision of these values a single cell calibration procedure was implemented (calibration step #1). This was performed by recording the raw data while applying different known loads to each of the sensors individually. The relationship between the increased load and the absolute value recorded for that sensor was linear (R2 > 0.999);
2. Offset of true force values for each load cell. The weight of the plate from the force value measured by the four sensors was subtracted from the true force values, such offsets being estimated during the calibration phase (calibration step #2); F_{BL}, F_{BR}, F_{TL} and F_{TR} were then calibrated;
3. Calculation of Fz (in N). Fz was determined by summing the calibrated values for each of the four sensors:
4. $FZ = F_{BL} + F_{BR} + F_{TL} + F_{TR}$;
5. Determination of the CoP coordinates (in mm). Y_{COP} and X_{COP} were determined using the equations:

$$X_{COP} = \frac{-F_{TL} - F_{BL} + F_{BR} + F_{TR}}{Fz} * MX + OX$$

$$Y_{COP} = \frac{-F_{BR} - F_{BL} + F_{TL} + F_{TR}}{FZ} * MY + OY$$

where and MX, MY, OX, and OY were the calibration factors (multiplicative and additive) specific to each axis. These calibration factors were necessary to correct for the different distance between the sensors and the true center position for each axis, and were determined by placing a variety of known loads at a number of known positions on the board though a 15-point calibration grid. An OLS (ordinary least squares) regression was then applied to estimate the optimal calibration factors (calibration step #3).

Once calculated, the COP components were based-filtered through a low pass IIR filter presenting a cut frequency at 20 Hz (in order to have a smooth visual representation of the CoP, still keeping the full bandwidth of the CoP signal). Additional filtering stages, with lower cut frequencies (down to 2 Hz) can be activated dynamically by the therapist to smooth the visual representation of the CoP. The choice of the IIR filter minimizes the filtering delay, thus being optimal for online filtering operations.

3.1.2 Limitations

The lack of detection of X and Y axes force values inherently removes a component of the true CoP equation [33], and, therefore, alters its correct estimation. Clark et al. [34] already addressed the issue of estimation of such errors. They compared the true CoP estimated through a force platform and the CoP estimated from data yielded by a commercial balance platform, in a number of standing posture activities (comparable to the VRRS postural activities performed using the balance platform). They found that the X and Y axis forces during such activities rarely exceeded 10 N. As expected, the magnitude of the X and Y axis forces during the standing balance tasks was much lower than the magnitude of the Z forces, and therefore this would have an only negligible influence (the correlation between the different CoP coordinate values exceeded R = 0.95). The authors concluded that the CoP calculated from the balance board is a reasonable representation of standing balance during tasks which do not have a large horizontal plane momentum component, while still concluding that due caution must be applied when comparing the absolute results of balance board CoP data with those obtained from a force platform.

3.1.3 Intended Modes of Usage

The balance board is designed to be used by a standing patient. However, supports like tripods or crutches can be used by the patient, and the caregiver can even support the patient if he/she presents postural standing issues. Obviously, CoP measurements, intended as the vertical projection of the CoM of a standing, unsupported, patient on the ground, become heavily modified in such cases; the tool can still be of use, however, for most of the exercise activities and also to augment the patient's confidence in his/her own CoP dynamics.

3.2 *Proprioceptive Balance Board*

The proprioceptive (PROPRIO) balance board is a 50 cm × 40 cm planar device (see Fig. 6), which has a semi-spherical element on the bottom. Thus, the PROPRIO board is an inherently unstable device.

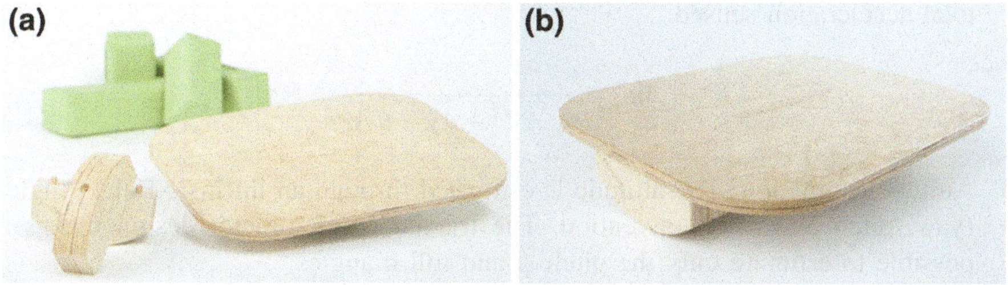

Fig. 6 The VRRS PROPRIO board. The board presents different components **a** that can be mounted in different ways—**b** shows a non-attenuated titling board in the anteroposterior direction

The PROPRIO board presents different removable inserts, allowing it to be used in multiple scenarios:

- two lateral semicircular inserts, with magnetic plugs, able to limit the instability to just the AP direction;
- four removable foam inserts, able to smooth the instability in all directions. Several sets of such foam inserts are available, each with a different grade of density. By varying the density of the foam, it is possible to grade the level of instability and the level of difficulty of the exercises.

Without inserts, the design of the board limits the AP tilt to ±30° and the ML tilt to ±25°.

3.2.1 Output Measures

The PROPRIO board integrates a triaxial accelerometer board whose center of coordinates is located precisely in the tilting center of the board. Therefore, the accelerations measured by the sensors are only minimally dependent on the cinematic accelerations and are dominated by the gravity-related component. The board outputs 3 digitized values (16-bit conversion) representing the accelerations sensed by the 3 sensors, Ax, Ay, and Az, in g units, at 120 samples/s.

Axis orientations of the accelerometers follow a right-hand convention, with:

- the Z axis being perpendicular to the plane of the platform and pointing upwards;
- and the X and Y axes being parallel to the plane of the platform and pointing towards the right (X) and towards the anterior direction (Y).

Estimation of the orientation of the platform is performed through a dedicated software module, which implements the following operations:

1. Filtering. Each sensor data stream An (n = x, y, z) is filtered with a low pass IIR filter at 10 Hz, which smooths the noisy signals from the accelerometers and increases the signal-to-noise ratio; the choice of the IIR filter minimizes the filtering delay, and is thus optimal for online filtering operations.
2. Normalization. Each filtered data stream An′ is normalized with respect to the total acceleration sensed:

$$An'' = \frac{An'}{\sqrt{Ax'^2 + Ay'^2 + Az'^2}}.$$

3. Attitude estimation. The attitude is estimated through an intrinsic Euler Angles (yaw, pitch and roll) convention. The triaxial accelerometer design makes it possible to estimate only the pitch φ and roll θ angles:

$$\varphi = atan2\left(Ay'', \sqrt{Ax''^2 + Az''^2}\right)$$

$$\theta = atan2(Ax'', Az'').$$

Attitude estimation of the board, as described above, allows a consistent and complete representation of a virtual board.

3.2.2 Intended Modes of Usage

The PROPRIO board is designed to be used by a standing patient, keeping one or both feet on it, or by a sitting patient, keeping one or both feet on it. However, supports like tripods or crutches can be used by the patient, and the therapist supports the patient if he/she presents postural standing issues. Due to the inherent instability of the PROPRIO board, the therapist helps and guides the patient during the initial phases of usage. This is usually crucial in order to guide the patient and help him/her become confident and familiar with the board, with his/her level of proprioceptive feedback, and with his/her own coping strategies in response to instability.

4 VRRS Methodology. Applications for Postural Rehabilitations

4.1 CoP Evalutation

CoP trace acquisition and parametric assessment during standing posture can be performed with the POSTURO board.

The application allows the tracking of several behavioral states of the subject—states relating to the eyes (open or closed), the arms (crossed, lying against the hips), and the feet (wide or narrow stance). Other aspects, like the presence of a foam layer to alter the proprioceptive channel, can also be recorded. Different pre-set durations of the acquisition can be chosen by the clinician. The CoP trajectory is hidden during the acquisition, so as not to alter the postural behavior of the subject.

The application (see Fig. 7) allows the calculation of the most common CoP parameters. In particular, the following parameters are automatically calculated, in accordance with Prieto et al. [35].

- The Distance measures: parameters associated with either the displacement of the CoP from the central point of the stabilogram, or the velocity of the CoP: mean CoP distance, AP and ML mean distances, rms (root mean square) CoP distance, AP and ML rms distances, total CoP excursion, total AP and ML excursions, mean CoP velocity, mean AP and ML velocities;

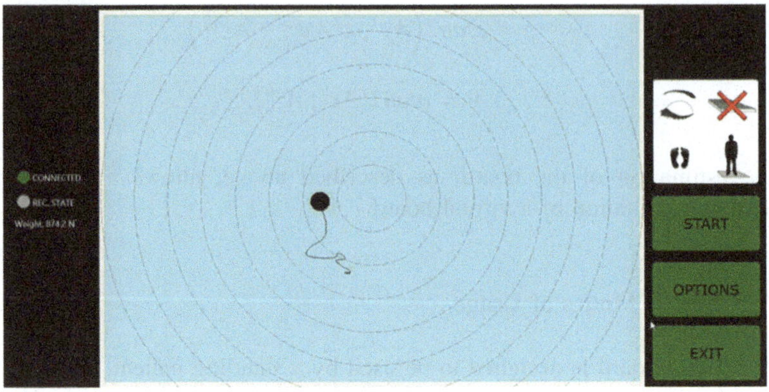

Fig. 7 The interface for CoP evaluation activity

- The Area measures: 95% confidence circle area, 95% confidence ellipse area (together with ellipse axes and orientation);
- The Hybrid measures: sway area, mean CoP frequency, mean ML and AP frequencies;
- The Frequency measures: total power, 50% power frequency, 95% power frequency, centroidal frequency, frequency dispersion.

4.2 *Load Asymmetry Evaluation*

The POSTURO board can be usefully used to evaluate the postural load asymmetry of the subject during standing posture. Load symmetry is affected in a number of situations, such as in cases of neurological insults or lower limb orthopedic surgery. Both hemiparetic stroke patients and orthopedic patients after a hip, knee or ankle surgery tend to distribute their weight asymmetrically, by loading more on the unaffected limb. Restoring proper weight load symmetry during standing posture is a key aim in neurological and orthopedic rehabilitation programs. Initial and ongoing evaluations of balance load asymmetry are, therefore, of primary importance.

In order to perform a load asymmetry evaluation, the key parameter to measure is the mean value of the ML component of the CoP, over a period of standing posture. As demonstrated by Genthon et al. [36], it is possible to estimate, with acceptable confidence, a 5% additional load asymmetry for each 10 mm lateral shift of the mean ML component of the CoP.

The POSTURO board, per se, does not allow such an evaluation. Indeed, while a two platform device could easily be used to perform the asymmetry evaluation, by having one platform placed under each foot, a single platform per se cannot

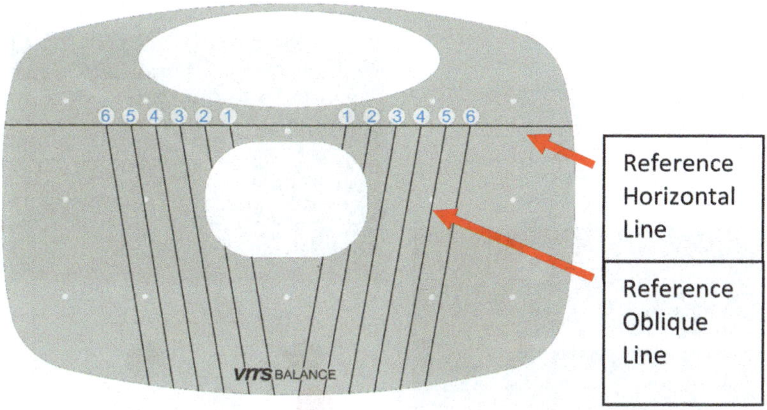

Fig. 8 The set of indications on the VRRS POSTURO board

distinguish between the ML shift component of the CoP due to load imbalance, and the one due merely to asymmetric positioning of the subject on the board. In order to address this issue, the POSTURO board has been equipped with a full set of indications on its surface (see Fig. 8), allowing the subject to place him/herself on it symmetrically with respect to the board's median line. As shown in the figure, to facilitate the positioning of the feet, several numbered lines, showing an opening angle of 18° (the typical feet opening angle during standing posture, as verified in [35]), are present on the POSTURO board.

After a standing posture acquisition (of settable duration, and tracking the behavioral states of the subject), the application outputs the percentage load asymmetry.

4.3 Exercises with the POSTURO Board

Several exercises use the POSTURO board as the primary tracking device and the CoP as the primary input signal (Fig. 9).

In all the exercises listed below, the CoP coordinates directly govern the position of an end-effector in 2D or 2.5D scenarios.

- Omni directional reaching exercise: the subject is required to shift his CoP from a central position to reach random targets placed around the central position, and then to return to the central position itself. The number of correct and erroneous hits, task durations, and path-to-target lengths are recorded and calculated. Vocal and visual feedback is provided, both during the execution of the task and at the end of each repetition. Complexity can be adjusted by setting the number of targets surrounding the central point (the higher the number of targets, the smaller their size and the higher the degree of precision required).

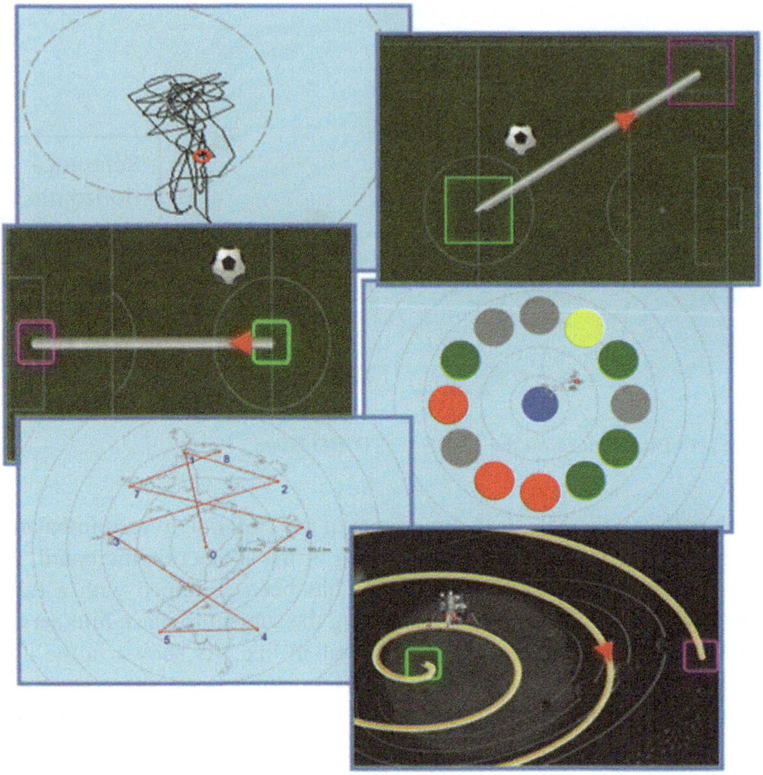

Fig. 9 Ensemble of some application interfaces for POSTURO board exercises

- Following exercise: the subject is required to shift his CoP in order to follow a movable circular target, randomly moving in a sequence of straight paths. Visual, acoustic and vocal feedback is provided, both during the execution of the task and at the end of each repetition. Complexity can be adjusted by setting the size and speed of the moving target. Parameters quantifying the distance between the target and the CoP paths are calculated.
- Path-following exercises; the subject is required to shift his CoP by moving it from a given position in order to reach a number of targets placed along a visible path. Visual, acoustic and vocal feedback is provided, both during the execution of the task and at the end of each repetition. Complexity can be adjusted by setting the number of targets along the path. Parameters quantifying the distance between the target and the CoP paths are calculated. Moreover, it is possible to place targets asymmetrically, in order to promote CoP control over, for example, the affected side.
- Left-right reaching exercise: this is a subfamily of the path-following exercise type. The subject is required to move his CoP to the right or to the left as indicated by randomly presented targets. Again, these exercises serve to promote CoP control relearning in patients presenting load imbalance.

Apart from the complexity which is specific for each exercise, there is, in each case, also the further possibility of grading the level of difficulty of the exercise by altering a gain parameter, representing the ratio between represented shift of the end-effector and the actual shift of the CoP. The higher the gain parameter, the faster and more sensitive the patient's perception of the end-effector dynamics will be; the lower the gain parameter, the smoother and slower this perception will be. Altering (increasing) the gain parameter is useful to promote gradual relearning of precise and accurate CoP control dynamics during the rehabilitation pathway.

4.4 Exercises with the PROPRIO Board

Several exercises use the PROPRIO board as the primary tracking device and its tilt measures as the primary input signals. In particular:

- Exercises are very similar to those available for the POSTURO board: the difference is related to the fact the end-effector position in the 2D or 2.5D scenario is determined by the pitch and roll tilting angles of the table, with the former governing the vertical coordinate of the end-effector and the latter governing its horizontal coordinate. Here, the gain parameter represents the ratio between represented shift of the end-effector and the actual tilting angles. The higher the gain parameter, the faster and more sensitive the patient's perception of the end-effector dynamics will be; the lower the gain parameter, the smoother and slower this perception will be. Altering (increasing) the gain parameter is useful to promote gradual relearning of precise and accurate control dynamics during the rehabilitation pathway.
- Exercises where the subject is required to keep the PROPRIO board as stable as possible. Such activities involve the use of a virtual end-effector that must be kept within a given area (typically circular), with visual, acoustic and vocal feedback provided to the patient both during and after completion of the task.

4.5 Governing Virtual Tables

Several exercises are available where the CoP and the tilt angles measured by the PROPRIO board are used to govern the tilt of a virtual board, rather than directly piloting a virtual end-effector. Such exercises typically involve the use of what we call an "indirect" end-effector, which is typically a spherical object having its own mass and inertia (see Fig. 10). By tilting the virtual board, the indirect end-effector moves according to the laws of dynamics. Exercises with virtual tables include exercises of the same main typologies listed above, and exercises where the virtual table presents a labyrinth that the patient has to solve by moving the end-effector from the initial position to the exit door.

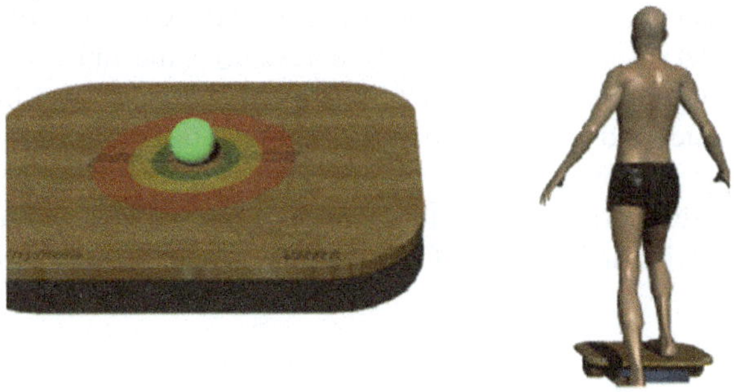

Fig. 10 Virtual table application with the PROPRIO board

4.6 Integration of the Boards as Secondary Input Devices

POSTURO and PROPRIO tables can be used as secondary input devices as well. They are used, in several activities in neurological and orthopedic rehabilitation settings, as devices measuring postural behavior, while magnetic sensors or IMUs measure the primary behavior. Examples include orthopedic and neurological exercises conducted with upper or lower limbs (e.g., reaching exercises with the upper limb, squat exercises), where it is important to have the subject recognize his postural behavior and balance shifts while performing the primary task. Such exercises usually present the CoP or the tilt angles in a portion of the screen (secondary end-effector), and the subject is instructed to perform the primary exercise while keeping the secondary end-effector within a given range. The ways in which the secondary end-effector influences the main task include the following:

- the primary task is blocked when the secondary end-effector exceeds set limits;
- the primary task is never blocked, but failure to perform the postural behavior influences (lowers) the final score;
- postural behavior and its dynamics alter the feedback profile given to the patient, which consists of dedicated feedback that may be visual (the aforementioned representation of CoP/tilt angles), acoustic (generally provided as positive punishments, e.g., unpleasant tones when limits are exceeded) or vocal (the subject is provided with context-dependent hints).

4.7 Further Developments

Research and development activities are currently being conducted to integrate magnetic sensors or IMUs into activities where the boards serve as the primary devices. Such integration would make it possible to measure, quantify, differentiate and condition the postural control strategies (i.e., ankle, knee, and hip strategies) employed by the patient during postural standing and during gait initiation. Such developments would greatly expand the array of rehabilitation strategies and opportunities available to therapists in the context of VRRS postural rehabilitation activities.

References

1. van Diest M, Lamoth CJC, Stegenga J, Verkerke GJ, Postema K. Exergaming for balance training of elderly: state of the art and future developments. J Neuroeng Rehabil. 2013;10:101. https://doi.org/10.1186/1743-0003-10-101.
2. Pollock AS, Durward BR, Rowe PJ, Paul JP. What is balance? Clin Rehabil. 2000;14:402–6.
3. Horak FB. Postural orientation and equilibrium: what do we need to know about neural control of balance to prevent falls? Age Ageing. 2006;35(Suppl 2):ii7–11. https://doi.org/10.1093/ageing/afl077.
4. Laughton CA, Slavin M, Katdare K, Nolan L, Bean JF, Kerrigan DC, Phillips E, Lipsitz LA, Collins JJ. Aging, muscle activity, and balance control: physiologic changes associated with balance impairment. Gait Posture. 2003;18:101–8.
5. Bekkers EMJ, Dockx K, Heremans E, Vercruysse S, Verschueren SMP, Mirelman A, Nieuwboer A. The contribution of proprioceptive information to postural control in elderly and patients with Parkinson's disease with a history of falls. Front Hum Neurosci. 2014;8:939. https://doi.org/10.3389/fnhum.2014.00939.
6. Jancová J. Measuring the balance control system—review. Acta Med Hradec Král Univ Carol Fac Med Hradec Král. 2008;51:129–37.
7. Li Y, Levine WS, Loeb GE. A two-joint human posture control model with realistic neural delays. IEEE Trans Neural Syst Rehabil Eng Publ IEEE Eng Med Biol Soc. 2012;20:738–48. https://doi.org/10.1109/TNSRE.2012.2199333.
8. Paillard T, Noé F. Techniques and methods for testing the postural function in healthy and pathological subjects. Biomed Res Int. 2015;2015:891390. https://doi.org/10.1155/2015/891390.
9. Winter DA. Biomechanics and motor control of human movement. Wiley; 2009.
10. Winter D. Human balance and posture control during standing and walking. Gait Posture. 1995;3:193–214. https://doi.org/10.1016/0966-6362(96)82849-9.
11. Horlings CGC, Küng UM, Honegger F, Van Engelen BGM, Van Alfen N, Bloem BR, Allum JHJ. Vestibular and proprioceptive influences on trunk movements during quiet standing. Neuroscience. 2009;161:904–14. https://doi.org/10.1016/j.neuroscience.2009.04.005.
12. Creath R, Kiemel T, Horak F, Peterka R, Jeka J. A unified view of quiet and perturbed stance: simultaneous co-existing excitable modes. Neurosci Lett. 2005;377:75–80. https://doi.org/10.1016/j.neulet.2004.11.071.
13. Pinter IJ, van Swigchem R, van Soest AJK, Rozendaal LA. The dynamics of postural sway cannot be captured using a one-segment inverted pendulum model: a PCA on segment rotations during unperturbed stance. J Neurophysiol. 2008;100:3197–208. https://doi.org/10.1152/jn.01312.2007.
14. Boonstra TA, Schouten AC, van der Kooij H. Identification of the contribution of the ankle and hip joints to multi-segmental balance control. J Neuroeng Rehabil. 2013;10:23. https://doi.org/10.1186/1743-0003-10-23.
15. Williams MA, Soiza RL, Jenkinson AM, Stewart A. EXercising with Computers in Later Life (EXCELL)—pilot and feasibility study of the acceptability of the Nintendo® WiiFit in

community-dwelling fallers. BMC Res Notes. 2010;3:238. https://doi.org/10.1186/1756-0500-3-238.
16. Robinson J, Dixon J, Macsween A, van Schaik P, Martin D. The effects of exergaming on balance, gait, technology acceptance and flow experience in people with multiple sclerosis: a randomized controlled trial. BMC Sports Sci Med Rehabil. 2015;7:8. https://doi.org/10.1186/s13102-015-0001-1.
17. Harris DM, Rantalainen T, Muthalib M, Johnson L, Teo W-P. Exergaming as a viable therapeutic tool to improve static and dynamic balance among older adults and people with iIdiopathic Parkinson's disease: a systematic review and meta-analysis. Front Aging Neurosci. 2015;7. https://doi.org/10.3389/fnagi.2015.00167.
18. Miller KJ, Adair BS, Pearce AJ, Said CM, Ozanne E, Morris MM. Effectiveness and feasibility of virtual reality and gaming system use at home by older adults for enabling physical activity to improve health-related domains: a systematic review. Age Ageing. 2014;43:188–95. https://doi.org/10.1093/ageing/aft194.
19. Kim JH, Jang SH, Kim CS, Jung JH, You JH. Use of virtual reality to enhance balance and ambulation in chronic stroke: a double-blind, randomized controlled study. Am J Phys Med Rehabil Assoc Acad Physiatr. 2009;88:693–701. https://doi.org/10.1097/PHM.0b013e3181b33350.
20. Hung J-W, Chou C-X, Hsieh Y-W, Wu W-C, Yu M-Y, Chen P-C, Chang H-F, Ding S-E. Randomized comparison trial of balance training by using exergaming and conventional weight-shift therapy in patients with chronic stroke. Arch Phys Med Rehabil. 2014;95:1629–37. https://doi.org/10.1016/j.apmr.2014.04.029.
21. Deutsch JE, Borbely M, Filler J, Huhn K, Guarrera-Bowlby P. Use of a low-cost, commercially available gaming console (Wii) for rehabilitation of an adolescent with cerebral palsy. Phys Ther. 2008;88:1196–207. https://doi.org/10.2522/ptj.20080062.
22. Esculier J-F, Vaudrin J, Bériault P, Gagnon K, Tremblay LE. Home-based balance training programme using Wii Fit with balance board for Parkinsons's disease: a pilot study. J Rehabil Med. 2012;44:144–50. https://doi.org/10.2340/16501977-0922.
23. Betker AL, Desai A, Nett C, Kapadia N, Szturm T. Game-based exercises for dynamic short-sitting balance rehabilitation of people with chronic spinal cord and traumatic brain injuries. Phys Ther. 2007;87:1389–98. https://doi.org/10.2522/ptj.20060229.
24. Valle MS, Casabona A, Cavallaro C, Castorina G, Cioni M. Learning upright standing on a multiaxial balance board. PLoS ONE. 2015;10:e0142423. https://doi.org/10.1371/journal.pone.0142423.
25. Fitzgerald D, Trakarnratanakul N, Smyth B, Caulfield B. Effects of a wobble board-based therapeutic exergaming system for balance training on dynamic postural stability and intrinsic motivation levels. J Orthop Sports Phys Ther. 2010;40:11–9. https://doi.org/10.2519/jospt.2010.3121.
26. Piron L, Turolla A, Agostini M, Zucconi CS, Ventura L, Tonin P, Dam M. Motor learning principles for rehabilitation: a pilot randomized controlled study in poststroke patients. Neurorehabil Neural Repair. 2010;24(6):501–8.
27. Piron L, Turolla A, Agostini M, Zucconi C, Cortese F, Zampolini M, Tonin P. Exercises for paretic upper limb after stroke: a combined virtual-reality and telemedicine approach. J Rehab Med. 2009;41(12):1016–20.
28. Turolla A, Dam M, Ventura L, Tonin P, Agostini M, Zucconi C, Kiper P, Cagnin A, Piron L. Virtual reality for the rehabilitation of the upper limb motor function after stroke: a prospective controlled trial. J Neuroeng Rehabil. 2013;1(10):85.
29. Kiper P, Agostini M, Luque-Moreno C, Tonin P, Turolla A. Reinforced feedback in virtual environment for rehabilitation of upper extremity dysfunction after stroke: preliminary data from a randomized controlled trial. Biomed Res Int. 2014;2014:752128.
30. Luque-Moreno C, Oliva-Pascual-Vaca A, Kiper P, Rodríguez-Blanco C, Agostini M, Turolla A. Virtual reality to assess and treat lower extremity disorders in post-stroke patients. Methods Inf Med. 2016;55(1):89–92.

31. Jelcic N, Cagnin A, Meneghello F, Turolla A, Ermani M, Dam M. Effects of lexical-semantic treatment on memory in early Alzheimer disease: an observer-blinded randomized controlled trial. Neurorehabil Neural Repair. 2012;26(8):949–56.
32. Agostini M, Garzon M, Benavides-Varela S, De Pellegrin S, Bencini G, Rossi G, Rosadoni S, Mancuso M, Turolla A, Meneghello F, Tonin P. Telerehabilitation in poststroke anomia. Biomed Res Int. 2014;2014:706909.
33. Bobbert MF, Schamhardt HC. Accuracy of determining the point of force application with piezoelectric force plates. J Biomech. 1990;23(7):705–10.
34. Clark RA, Bryant AL, Pua Y, McCrory P, Bennell K, Hunt M. Validity and reliability of the Nintendo Wii Balance Board for assessment of standing balance. Gait Posture. 2010;31 (3):307–10.
35. Prieto TE, Myklebust JB, Hoffmann RG, Lovett EG, Myklebust BM. Measures of postural steadiness: differences between healthy young and elderly adults. IEEE Trans Biomed Eng. 1996;43(9):956–66.
36. Genthon N, Gissot AS, Froger J, Rougier P, Pérennou D. Posturography in patients with stroke estimating the percentage of body weight on each foot from a single force platform. Stroke. 2008;39(2):489.

Cues and Body-Weight-Supported (BWS) Gait Training in Parkinson's Disease

Giorgio Sandrini, Cristina Tassorelli, Eliana Berra and Roberto De Icco

1 Cues in Gait Rehabilitation

Gait is one of the motor tasks most affected in Parkinson's disease (PD), due to a deficit of internal rhythmic signals that interferes with motor pathways [1].

Data from the literature show that external stimuli (acoustic, visual, somatosensory) can modulate motor patterns in PD, helping patients to start and maintain a rhythmic motor task [2]. Moreover each type of cue activates a different motor control strategy: auditory cues bypass the internal rhythm deficit [3], providing this rhythm on a voluntary basis; visual cues help the visual-cerebellar motor pathway to facilitate the generation of a better gait pattern [4]; sensory cues activate the dorsolateral pre-motor control system (voluntary), which bypasses the deficit of the supplementary motor area (involved in automatic movement) [5].

On the basis of these assertions, there has emerged a growing body of data and literature on the different aspects of rehabilitation involving cueing strategies.

In 1996, Thaut et al. tested the effects of rhythmic auditory stimulation (RAS) during a 3-week home-based gait training program for PD patients, comparing them with two control groups of PD subjects who either did not participate in any gait training, or underwent internally self-paced training. Patients trained with RAS showed significant changes in several gait parameters, their gait velocity improving by 25%, stride length by 12%, and step cadence by 10%; these improvements were more marked than those recorded in self-paced subjects [6].

McIntosh et al. (1997) studied the effect of RAS in 31 patients with idiopathic PD (21 in ON and 10 in OFF medication state) compared with 10 healthy elderly subjects: gait velocity, cadence, and stride length improved in 19 of the 21 ON patients. The same variables improved in all the OFF patients with the exception of stride

G. Sandrini · C. Tassorelli · E. Berra (✉) · R. De Icco
Neurological Rehabilitation Unit, Department of Brain and Behavioral Sciences, C. Mondino National Neurological Institute, University of Pavia, 27100 Pavia, Italy
e-mail: eliana_berra@yahoo.it

G. Sandrini et al. (eds.), *Advanced Technologies for the Rehabilitation of Gait and Balance Disorders*, Biosystems & Biorobotics 19,
https://doi.org/10.1007/978-3-319-72736-3_25

length in two of them, showing that patients with PD are still able to access rhythmic entrainment mechanisms, even in the absence of dopaminergic medication [7].

Marchese et al. (2000) devised a study to assess whether cues (visual, auditory or tactile stimulation) could potentiate a 6-week rehabilitation program. They compared two groups of patients with idiopathic PD differentiated by the use of external cues ("non-cued" vs. "cued"). A significant reduction in UPDRS scores (activities of daily living and motor sections) was present after the rehabilitation phase in both groups. However, while the mean UPDRS scores had returned to baseline 6 weeks after the rehabilitation in the non-cued group, these scores remained significantly reduced with respect to baseline in the cued group [8].

Lehman et al. (2005) set out to assess immediate and near-term (1 week and 4 weeks after training) effects of verbal instructional cues on gait parameters in patients with PD. They found that the instructional set was effective in improving parameters (significant increases in step length and gait velocity and a significant decrease in cadence) for at least 4 weeks. Moreover step length was significantly increased at all post-training time points, also in comparison with a control group that was not entrained with verbal instructions [9].

Lim et al., in 2005, provided the first systematic review of the literature. They stressed the efficacy of auditory cues in improving walking speed in patients with PD, while limited evidence precluded conclusions from being drawn with regard to their efficacy on stride length, cadence and the double support phase. Fewer data were available on visual and somatosensory cues, so the authors were not able to state a relationship between these and gait outcome measures [10].

In 2009, Arias et al. investigated the effect of rhythmic auditory stimulation on the gait of PD patients with freezing of gait during their end-of-dose periods. The number and duration of freezing episodes were measured by analysis of video footage; moreover freezing was also characterized by duration (less than 3 s; 3–10 s; more than 10 s). Furthermore, the authors compared gait velocity, cadence and step length with the same variables recorded in a second group of PD patients without freezing and in a third group of healthy controls. They reported significant reductions in the number and duration of freezing episodes in the presence of auditory stimulation. With regard to gait pattern, auditory cues reduced the time to turn, and improved cadence and increased velocity in all the three groups, without significant differences emerging between them [11].

Frazzitta et al. (2009) investigated the effectiveness of a 4-week rehabilitation program based on auditory and visual cues associated, or not associated, with treadmill training in patients affected by PD with freezing of gait. At the end of the rehabilitation the authors found improvements in clinical scale scores—UPDRS, Freezing of Gait Questionnaire (FoG), 6-minute walking test—speed of gait and stride cycle in both groups, with significantly more marked improvements in all outcomes being found in the group treated with both cues and treadmill training [12].

Rochester et al., in 2010, studied 153 subjects with PD who received 3 weeks of cued (auditory, visual and somatosensory) gait training as part of a randomized trial (the RESCUE trial). Gait performance was recorded with accelerometers after training and at 6 weeks of follow-up. The authors reported that cued gait training increased walking speed and step length, and that these effects were retained at follow-up. Given that these improvements were found to be retained by patients after training, transferred to non-cued gait and generalized across cue types, the authors speculated that cued training might enhance motor learning in PD [13].

In a questionnaire-based study conducted by Kadivar et al. in 2011, the authors enrolled 16 patients with PD and divided them into two groups: the first underwent 6 weeks of step training with external auditory pacing, while the second received step training without cueing. The patients were tested with the Dynamic Gait Index, UPDRS, Tinetti gait and balance test, Timed Up and Go test (TUG) and FoG at the end of training and at 1, 4 and 8 weeks thereafter. All the scale scores improved in both groups after rehabilitation, but the improvements were more marked in in the group entrained with cues. Moreover, these results were maintained until the 8-week follow-up only in patients treated with auditory pacing [14].

Mirelman et al., in 2011, published a pilot study conducted in 7 parkinsonian patients to describe the effects, on posture, sit-to-stand abilities and dynamic balance, of 6 weeks of training involving the use of an audio-biofeedback system (with feedback delivered through headphones). A significantly positive trend was observed in all measures of balance control after the end of the 6-week program. In particular, TUG scores improved by 11%; the time to perform sit-to-stand improved by 7.3%, while the Berg Balance Scale (BBS) and UPDRS significantly improved by 3 and 3.3% respectively. Moreover, TUG, BBS and UPDRS score changes were maintained at a 4-week follow-up [15].

Almeida et al., in 2012, compared two different methods of visual cueing (consisting of colored stripes on the ground perpendicular to gait direction) during traditional overground gait training or treadmill training in PD patients. Both groups were tested against a control group of matched PD patients, rehabilitated without cues. The two intervention groups showed improved step length and gait velocity and these improvements were maintained over the 6-week training, whereas the control group showed no changes over time. Only with the overground training was the TUG score found to decrease after the six-week intervention, while UPDRS scores improved only in patients rehabilitated with a treadmill [16].

El-Tamawy et al. (2012) investigated the influence of proprioceptive cues on gait parameters in PD. The authors divided a sample of PD patients with mild to moderate impairment into two groups in order to compare traditional physical therapy with treadmill training supplemented with vibratory stimuli applied to the feet plantar surfaces and proprioceptive neuromuscular facilitation. Cadence, stride length, speed and distance walked significantly improved in both groups, more markedly in patients who underwent proprioceptive cueing and treadmill training. It is important to note that hip and knee flexion increased at the end of rehabilitation only in patients who received physical therapy [17].

Spaulding et al., in 2012, published a meta-analysis conducted to compare the efficacy of visual versus acoustic cues on gait parameters in PD. Auditory cues were found to be efficient in improving cadence, stride length and gait velocity, while visual cues only improved stride length. Few studies investigated visual and acoustic cues used in combination, but those that did showed a positive effect on cadence. The authors therefore concluded that auditory cues, compared with visual ones, provide more consistent and positive effects on gait parameters in PD [18].

Lopez et al. (2014) provided evidence on how acoustic cues, used at home on a daily basis, can have a persistent effect on gait parameters in PD patients. They supplied patients with a portable pair of glasses able to produce 100 different sounds controlled by smartphone. All patients demonstrated a significant improvement in gait with the device turned on. In particular they showed improvements of 40.6% in walking speed, 30.2% in cadence, and 50.3% in stride length [19].

Rocha et al., in 2014, published a new systematic review of the literature on the effects of external cues on gait in PD. Overall, the use of cueing strategies results in improved gait speed, cadence and stride length. Visual cues seemed to be able to modulate speed, cadence and step length, while auditory cues influenced speed and step length. Sensory cues showed significant benefits on gait speed, cadence and stride length. Surprisingly none of the studies included in this review analyzed quality of life [20].

Vitòrio et al. (2014) studied the effects of visual cueing and exproprioception on gait in PD. The participants were required to walk over a carpet with horizontal lines while wearing or not wearing a blindfold, which served to remove exproprioceptive information from the environment. In both visual cueing conditions, patients with PD increased their step length and step time with respect to baseline. In addition when exproprioception was removed, all participants showed increased step length variability and decreased stride velocity [21].

As the previous paragraphs show, the medium-term effect of cueing on gait in PD has been extensively studied; conversely, strong data on the acute and long-term (over 8 weeks) effects of cues are lacking.

A study conducted in our institute investigated both the acute and direct effects of cues on gait parameters and their efficacy in the medium term (after four weeks of rehabilitation) and in the long term (at 3 months from hospital discharge). Sixty-eight PD patients were included in a randomized, controlled, parallel-groups study. They were divided randomly into three groups: the first group underwent intensive gait training with auditory stimulation (daily sessions), the second underwent intensive gait training centered on the use of visual stimulation (daily sessions), while the third group did overground gait training according to the traditional physiotherapy approach, without the use of cues (control group). Neurological evaluation and kinematic analysis of gait were performed at the beginning of the hospitalization (T0), after four weeks of neurorehabilitation (T1) and 3 months later (T2).

With regard to the acute effect of these treatments, we found significant increases in stride duration and stride length in the patients using acoustic cues, while the number of strides and the speed of gait were found to be reduced in patients trained with visual cues.

At the end of the rehabilitation program (T1), acoustic cues were associated with a decrease in the number of strides, and increases in stride length and gait speed, whereas visual cues were found to improve the number of strides, and the speed and pattern of gait. In patients undergoing traditional rehabilitation we saw improvements only in stride length and gait velocity. In accordance with other data from the literature, the gait parameter improvements achieved in all three groups were lost at three months. This finding could be explained by the progression of neurodegeneration typically seen in PD and by the well-known impairment of implicit learning in PD [22].

In conclusion, our study also supports the usefulness of cues in the rehabilitation of gait disorders in PD; the selective impact of different kinds of cues on gait parameters suggests that it would be useful to perform a gait analysis before starting a patient on a rehabilitation program, in order to optimize the choice of treatment.

2 Body-Weight-Supported Gait Training

Locomotor training on a treadmill with partial body-weight support (BWS), involving the use of an overhead harness, a pelvic belt and thigh straps (body-weight-supported treadmill training, BWSTT) is a promising therapeutic approach to help retrain neurological patients with motor impairments, and it is easy to replicate in any rehabilitation facility.

Several studies have shown that BWSTT is effective in improving the mobility outcome of patients with stroke [23], PD [24] and spinal cord injury (SCI) [25]. The association of a treadmill with BWS, originally adopted inpatients unable to walk independently, has the great advantages of keeping them in an upright posture with a redistribution of forces at the level of the trunk, and allowing the rehabilitation physiotherapist to concentrate on the quality of movement [26–28].

BWSTT is considered to be a safe method of training that helps patients to feel secure (with regard to falls), facilitates free leg movements compared with conventional treadmill training, and provides useful feedback from every step, which encourages self-correction of step length and enhances motor learning [29]. In addition, the provision of partial BWS has been shown to enable people with neurological conditions to walk for longer and with only minimally increased heart rates [30].

Other authors have already studied the use of treadmill training and BWS in gait rehabilitation in PD [24]. The added advantage of BWSTT in PD may result from the symmetrical continuous sensory stimuli coming from the moving treadmill, which could enhance locomotor pattern generators. An enhancement of the central pattern generator has been postulated as a mechanism underlying the efficacy of BWSTT also in the treatment of SCI [25] and stroke [23]. It has been supposed that these cueing strategies, by promoting the use of alternative pathways unaffected by PD, help to bypass the defective basal ganglia. Attention strategies, on the other hand, rely more on cognitive mechanisms of motor control and are therefore internally generated; they are therefore an alternative to external cues for helping to improve motor performance [31]. Other possible explanations for the efficacy of BWSTT include task-specific motor learning or improvements in postural reflexes

[32], exercise-induced and activity-dependent neural plasticity (i.e., neurogenesis, synaptogenesis and molecular adaptation) [33, 34], and normalization of cortico-motor excitability/cortical reorganization, especially in the supplementary motor area in persons with PD [35].

In a prospective crossover trial, Miyai et al. [24] studied ten patients randomized to receive either a 4-week program of BWSTT with up to 20% of their body weight supported, followed by 4 weeks of conventional physical therapy, or the same treatments in the opposite order. This study showed that BWSTT was superior to conventional physical therapy in improving short-term mobility, especially in patients with moderate gait difficulty whose gait speed was more than 8 s per 10 meters and whose number of steps was more than 15 per 10-meter walk [24].

Miyai et al. [26] also investigated the long-term effects of BWSTT, comparing functional outcomes of BWSTT and conventional physical therapy in a randomized controlled trial. Twenty-four PD patients were randomized to receive either a 45-minute session of BWSTT (up to 20% of their body weight supported) or conventional physical therapy 3 days a week for 1 month. In this study, BWSTT proved superior to conventional physical therapy in improving the short-step gait that characterizes PD. The improvements in clinical scale scores and gait parameters (speed and number of steps) lasted for 4 months. The authors underlined that all the patients initially tolerated a higher treadmill speed when walking with BWS rather than without, and they suggested that improvements in walking performance after BWSTT rehabilitation in patients with PD could be attributed to changes in gait control related to the activation of “internal cues” [26].

Ganesan et al. [36] investigated the role of BWSTT in improving balance in PD. Sixty patients were randomly assigned to three equally sized groups: a control group that only received a stable dosage of dopaminomimetic drugs, a conventional gait training (CGT) group that received dopaminomimetic drugs and conventional gait training, and a BWSTT group that received dopaminomimetic drugs plus BWSTT with unloading of 20% of body weight. The CGT and BWSTT groups underwent 30-minute sessions 4 days per week for 4 weeks (16 sessions). The UPDRS motor score and clinical scales investigating gait were all significantly better in the BWSTT group than in the control and CGT groups after the rehabilitation program, suggesting that BWSTT may be a better interventional choice than CGT for gait and balance rehabilitation in patients with PD.

The exact pathogenesis of postural instability in PD is still unknown, but it seems to be related to a combination of both dopaminergic and non-dopaminergic lesions. The influence of BWSTT on improvement of both L-DOPA-sensitive and L-DOPA-resistant components of balance has been speculated to play a role in improved balance [36].

The effect of BWSTT on balance may also be explained by the influence of this treatment on baroreflex sensitivity (BRS), as demonstrated by Ganesan et al. [37]. BRS is defined as a measure of sensitivity of the cardiac limb of the baroreflex and it is measured by the change in inter-beat interval per unit change in systolic pressure occurring either spontaneously or after a maneuver. Low blood pressure variability and a decrease in BRS significantly contribute to orthostatic hypotension in PD, leading to an increased risk of falling. In this study, four weeks of BWSTT significantly improved BRS in patients with PD. The authors concluded that BWSTT can be considered a non-invasive method of influencing BRS for the prevention of orthostatic hypotension in patients with PD [37].

A recent systematic Cochrane review [38] assessed the effectiveness and acceptability of treadmill training with and without BWS to enhance conventional gait rehabilitation for patients with PD. It included 18 trials involving a total of 623 participants. This systematic review provided evidence that treadmill training may improve clinically relevant gait parameters, such as gait speed and stride length, in patients with PD at Hoehn & Yahr stages one to three. However, walking distance and cadence were not found to improve significantly. Additionally, it is not known how long gait improvements after treadmill training may last. Adverse events and drop-outs did not occur more frequently in people receiving treadmill training versus control interventions and were not judged to be clinically serious adverse events. The authors concluded that, when treadmill training is available, this technology might be used in relatively young and fit people with PD to improve gait speed as one specific parameter of gait hypokinesia. However, a limit of this review is that the authors' conclusions are not specific for treadmill training with BWS [38].

Preliminary data about PD patients treated with BWSTT in our institute confirmed an improvement in motor functions, reflected both in clinical scale scores and in gait parameters recorded using an optokinetic gait analysis system. Thirty-six patients affected by PD, hospitalized in the Neurorehabilitation Unit of the C. Mondino National Neurological Institute in Pavia, Italy, were included in a randomized, controlled, parallel-group study. The subjects were randomly assigned to two groups: 14 patients to the BWSTT group and 22 to the control group. The patients underwent 5 daily rehabilitation sessions per week for 4 consecutive weeks. Each session lasted 60 min; the control group underwent 60 min of traditional rehabilitation treatment (physiokinesitherapy) while the BWSTT group performed 40 min of traditional treatment plus 20 min of BWSTT.

All patients were evaluated at the beginning of hospitalization (T0) and at the end of the 4-week neurorehabilitation period (T1). The clinical assessment consisted of administration of clinical scales, validated for the assessment of functional disability and clinical impairment, such as UPDRS-III and the Functional Independence Measure; instrumental assessment of gait was conducted with an optokinetic gait analysis system. At the end of treatment, both groups showed improvements on the clinical scales. From T0 to T1, the BWSTT group showed improved gait parameters: significant improvements in cadence and stride length, and reductions in stride duration, number of strides and double stance duration. However, the intergroup analysis between the BWSTT group and the control group revealed that double stance duration was significantly reduced only in the BWSTT group. In conclusion, our study showed that both BWSTT and traditional rehabilitation treatment with physiokinesitherapy improve motor function and gait parameters in PD patients.

Also on the basis of previous studies, BWSTT might be recommended, in particular, in the gait rehabilitation of PD patients with a significant risk of falling due to severe postural instability, freezing of gait and orthostatic hypotension.

References

1. Currà A, Berardelli A, Agostino R, et al. Performance of sequential arm movements with and without advance knowledge of motor pathways in Parkinson's disease. Mov Disord. 1997;12:646–54.
2. Majsak MJ, Kaminski T, Gentile AM, Glanagan JR. The reaching movements of patients with Parkinson's disease under self-determined maximal speed and visually cued conditions. Brain. 1998;121:755–66.
3. McIntosh GC, Brown SH, Rice RR, et al. Rhythmic auditory-motor facilitation of gait patterns in patients with Parkinson's disease. J Neurol Neurosurg Psychiatry. 1997;62:22–6.
4. Azulay JP, Mesure S, Amblard B, et al. Visual control of locomotion in Parkinson's disease. Brain. 1999;122:111–20.
5. Morris ME, Iansek R, Matyas TA, et al. Stride length regulation in Parkinson's disease. Normalization strategies and underlying mechanisms. Brain. 1996;119:551–68.
6. Thaut MH, McIntosh GC, Rice RR, Miller RA, Rathbun J, Brault JM. Rhythmic auditory stimulation in gait training for Parkinson's disease patients. Mov Disord. 1996;11(2): 193–200.
7. McIntosh GC, Brown SH, Rice RR, Thaut MH. Rhythmic auditory-motor facilitation of gait patterns in patients with Parkinson's disease. J Neurol Neurosurg Psychiatry. 1997;62(1): 22–6.
8. Marchese R, Diverio M, Zucchi F, Lentino C, Abbruzzese G. The role of sensory cues in the rehabilitation of parkinsonian patients: a comparison of two physical therapy protocols. Mov Disord. 2000;15(5):879–83.
9. Lehman DA, Toole T, Lofald D, Hirsch MA. Training with verbal instructional cues results in near-term improvement of gait in people with Parkinson disease. J Neurol Phys Ther. 2005;29 (1):2–8.
10. Lim I, van Wegen E, de Goede C, Deutekom M, Nieuwboer A, Willems A, Jones D, Rochester L, Kwakkel G. Effects of external rhythmical cueing on gait in patients with Parkinson's disease: a systematic review. Clin Rehabil. 2005;19(7):695–713.
11. Arias P, Cudeiro J. Effect of rhythmic auditory stimulation on gait in Parkinsonian patients with and without freezing of gait. PLoS ONE. 2010;5(3):e9675. https://doi.org/10.1371/journal.pone.0009675.
12. Frazzitta G, Maestri R, Uccellini D, Bertotti G, Abelli P. Rehabilitation treatment of gait in patients with Parkinson's disease with freezing: a comparison between two physical therapy protocols using visual and auditory cues with or without treadmill training. Mov Disord. 2009;24(8):1139–43.
13. Rochester L, Baker K, Hetherington V, Jones D, Willems AM, Kwakkel G, Van Wegen E, Lim I, Nieuwboer A. Evidence for motor learning in Parkinson's disease: acquisition, automaticity and retention of cued gait performance after training with external rhythmical cues. Brain Res. 2010;10(1319):103–11.
14. Kadivar Z, Corcos DM, Foto J, et al. Effect of step training and rhythmic auditory stimulation on functional performance in Parkinson patients. Neurorehabilitation Neural Repair. 2011;25:626–35.
15. Mirelman A, Herman T, Nicolai S, Zijlstra A, Zijlstra W, Becker C, Chiari L, Hausdorff JM. Audio-biofeedback training for posture and balance in patients with Parkinson's disease. J Neuroeng Rehabil. 2011;8:35.

16. Almeida QJ, Bhatt H. A manipulation of visual feedback during gait training in Parkinson's disease. Parkinsons Dis. 2012;2012:508720.
17. El-Tamawy MS, Darwish MH, Khallaf ME. Effects of augmented proprioceptive cues on the parameters of gait of individuals with Parkinson's disease. Ann Indian Acad Neurol. 2012;15 (4):267–72.
18. Spaulding SJ, Barber B, Colby M, Cormack B, Mick T, Jenkins ME. Cueing and gait improvement among people with Parkinson's disease: a meta-analysis. Arch Phys Med Rehabil. 2013;94(3):562–70.
19. Lopez WO, Higuera CA, Fonoff ET, SouzaCde O, Albicker U, Martinez JA. Listenmee and Listenmee smartphone application: synchronizing walking to rhythmic auditory cues to improve gait in Parkinson's disease. Hum Mov Sci. 2014;37:147–56.
20. Rocha PA, Porfírio GM, Ferraz HB, Trevisani VF. Effects of external cues on gait parameters of Parkinson's disease patients: a systematic review. Clin Neurol Neurosurg. 2014;124: 127–34.
21. Vitório R, Lirani-Silva E, Pieruccini-Faria F, Moraes R, Gobbi LT, Almeida QJ. Visual cues and gait improvement in Parkinson's disease: which piece of information is really important? Neuroscience. 2014;26(277):273–80.
22. De Icco R, Tassorelli C, Berra E, Bolla M, Pacchetti C, Sandrini G. Acute and chronic effect of acoustic and visual cues on gait training in Parkinson's disease: a randomized, controlled study. Parkinsons Dis. 2015;2015:978590.
23. Mehrholz J, Pohl M, Elsner B. Treadmill training and body weight support for walking after stroke. Cochrane Database Syst Rev. 2014;1.
24. Miyai I, Fujimoto Y, Ueda Y, Yamamoto H, Nozaki S, Saito T, Kang J. Treadmill training with body weight support: its effect on Parkinson's disease. Arch Phys Med Rehabil. 2000;81:849–52.
25. Morawietz C, Moffat F. Effects of locomotor training after incomplete spinal cord injury: a systematic review. Arch Phys Med Rehabil. 2013;94(11):2297–308.
26. Miyai I, Fujimoto Y, Yamamoto H, et al. Long-term effect of body weight-supported treadmill training in Parkinson's disease: a randomized controlled trial. Arch Phys Med Rehabil. 2002;83:1370–3.
27. Fisher BE, Wu AD, Salem GJ, et al. The effect of exercise training in improving motor performance and corticomotor excitability in persons with early Parkinson's disease. Arch Phys Med Rehabil. 2010; November: 22.
28. Rose MH, Løkkegaard A, Sonne-Holm S, et al. Improved clinical status, quality of life, and walking capacity in Parkinson's disease after body weight-supported high-intensity locomotor training. Arch Phys Med Rehabil. 2013;94:687–92.
29. Fernando CK, Basmajian JV. Biofeedback in physical medicine and rehabilitation. Biofeedback Self Regul. 1978;3:435–55.
30. Visintin M, Barbeau H. The effects of body weight support on the locomotor pattern of spastic paretic patients. Can J Neurol Sci. 1989;16:315–25.
31. Rubinstein TC, Giladi N, Hausdorff JM. The power of cueing to circumvent dopamine deficits: a review of physical therapy treatment of gait disturbances in Parkinson's disease. Mov Disord. 2002;17(6):1148–60.
32. Platz T, Brown RG, Marsden CD. Training improves the speed of aimed movements in Parkinson's disease. Brain. 1998;121:505–14.
33. Fisher BE, Petzinger GM, Nixon K, et al. Exercise-induced behavioral recovery and neuroplasticity in the 1-methyl-4-phenyl-1,2,3,6-tetrahydropyridine-lesioned mouse basal ganglia. J Neurosci Res. 2004;77:378–90.
34. Fox CM, Ramig LO, Ciucci MR, Sapir S, McFarland DH, Farley BG. The science and practice of LSVT/LOUD: neural plasticity-principled approach to treating individuals with Parkinson disease and otherneurological disorders. Semin Speech Lang. 2006;27:283–99.
35. Fisher B, Wu A, Salem G, et al. The effect of exercise training in improving motor performance and corticomotor excitability in people with early Parkinson's disease. Arch Phys Med Rehabil. 2008;89:1221–9.

36. Ganesan M, Sathyaprabha TN, Gupta A, Pal PK. Effect of partial weight-supported treadmill gait training on balance in patients with Parkinson disease. PM R. 2014;6(1):22–33.
37. Ganesan M, Pal PK, Gupta A, Sathyaprabha TN. Treadmill gait training improves baroreflex sensitivity in Parkinson's disease. Clin Auton Res. 2014; 24:111–118.
38. Mehrholz J, Kugler J, Storch A, Pohl M, Hirsch K, Elsner B. Treadmill training for patients with Parkinson's disease. Cochrane Database Syst Rev. 2015;9:CD007830.

Effects of Neuromodulation on Gait

Giuseppe Cosentino, Filippo Brighina, Enrico Alfonsi and Giorgio Sandrini

1 Non-invasive Modulation of Brain Activity: Transcranial Magnetic and Electrical Stimulation

Information processing in the brain is based on the generation and transmission of transient electrical pulses that travel along neurons and through synapses at high speeds [145]. The activity of neural networks can be modified through the use of transcranial brain stimulation. To date, transcranial magnetic stimulation (TMS) and transcranial electrical stimulation (TES) remain the two main techniques available for brain stimulation in humans. Collectively, they are referred to as "non-invasive brain stimulation" (NIBS), although this term has been recently been called into question [41].

Both TMS and TES involve the application of electric fields capable of modulating the dynamics of cortical networks. However, they differ in many important aspects. TMS consists of the application of brief magnetic pulses that easily cross the skull and induce electrical potentials in the brain. Even a single TMS pulse can induce massive depolarization of a neuron population and trigger action potentials [44]. TES, on the other hand, is a term that refers to different techniques based on the application of weak currents by means of a pair of electrodes placed on the

G. Cosentino (✉) · F. Brighina
Department of Experimental Biomedicine and Clinical Neurosciences (BioNeC), University of Palermo, Palermo, Italy
e-mail: gcosentino80@gmail.com

E. Alfonsi · G. Sandrini
C. Mondino National Neurological Institute, Pavia, Italy

G. Sandrini
Department of Brain and Behavioural Sciences, University of Pavia, Pavia, Italy

G. Sandrini et al. (eds.), *Advanced Technologies for the Rehabilitation of Gait and Balance Disorders*, Biosystems & Biorobotics 19,
https://doi.org/10.1007/978-3-319-72736-3_26

head, one (or both) of which over a target cortical area. In contrast to TMS, commonly used TES paradigms induce small subthreshold current flows unable to elicit neuron action potentials. Indeed, their effects on brain function are mainly based on a polarizing effect on the resting membrane potential and modification of spontaneous neuronal firing rates [121].

As illustrated below, the electrophysiological and behavioral effects of TMS and TES may vary greatly depending on various stimulation parameters (e.g., frequency, intensity and duration of stimulation). This explains why a number of different stimulation paradigms have been developed. Because of the complex interactions occurring between the electric currents induced in the brain and the cortical neuronal networks, composed of multiple layers of excitatory and inhibitory neurons that differ in function, size, localization and orientation, the exact physiological mechanisms by which NIBS techniques exert their action are still largely unclear [45].

In the last few decades, several NIBS techniques have been used to treat several neurological and psychiatric illnesses, giving encouraging preliminary results. The use of these techniques in the clinical setting is increasing, partly thanks to their excellent safety profile and, especially in the case of TES, the availability of relatively inexpensive stimulation devices.

In spite of these encouraging premises, some important considerations should be kept in mind when using NIBS for therapeutic purposes. The response to many NIBS paradigms may be small and relatively short-lasting, especially when stimulation is applied in single sessions. Moreover, there can be a marked intrasubject and intersubject variability of response linked to numerous factors, such as the synaptic activity history of the targeted region, and the genetic profile and age of the individual [144, 148]. It is also to be noted that, to date, the choice of stimulation parameters has tended to be based on clinical intuition and historical practices. In the future, NIBS is destined to become increasingly personalized and based, more and more, on new understanding of how brain networks generate activity patterns and how they interact with externally-induced perturbations.

1.1 Transcranial Magnetic Stimulation Paradigms

The effects of single magnetic pulses applied to the brain quickly disappear. Nevertheless, when TMS is delivered in trains of stimuli (repetitive TMS, rTMS), the modulatory effects on brain function outlast the stimulation period for a time ranging from several seconds to 30 min or more, depending on the frequency and intensity of the stimulation and the pattern of TMS delivery. Moreover, as with other NIBS techniques, including TES, cumulative effects may be induced by repeated sessions of rTMS, carried out on consecutive days (generally 5–10 days), which have been proven capable of inducing effects lasting more than one month.

Conventional rTMS protocols consist of trains of stimuli applied at either low (0.3–1 Hz) or high (5–30 Hz) frequency. A large number of studies supports the notion that low-frequency stimulation may induce a local decrease in cortical excitability, whereas high-frequency stimulation generally produces the opposite effect [32]. Direct evidence able to shed light on the mechanisms involved in the aftereffects of rTMS in humans is lacking. Several lines of evidence, however, suggest that these effects depend on modifications of synaptic efficacy similar to those characterizing the long-term depression (LTD) and long-term potentiation (LTP) of glutamatergic synapses observed in animals [33].

Recent studies have shown that the effects of low- and high-frequency rTMS may be different from, and even opposite to, those mentioned above, and that this depends mainly on stimulus parameters other than frequency (e.g., intensity and duration of stimulation) and also on the synaptic history. It is indeed well known that the tendency of a synapse to undergo depression or potentiation is strictly linked to its history of use [11, 17]. According to the Bienenstock-Cooper-Munro model, the threshold for induction of LTD and LTP is not fixed but continuously adjusted to the level of postsynaptic activity by homeostatic mechanisms collectively referred to as 'metaplasticity' [1]. That said, when the level of postsynaptic activity is high, oncoming stimuli will more readily promote LTD, rather than further potentiation. Conversely, LTP instead of LTD will be more easily induced when the background activity is low. Importantly, these concepts should be kept in mind when designing studies employing rTMS or other NIBS techniques for therapeutic purposes. Indeed, there is emerging evidence that homeostatic plasticity may be dysfunctioning or operate with different modalities in several pathological conditions, e.g. dystonia, migraine, Parkinson's disease, and different psychiatric disorders [37, 85, 94]. It is therefore crucial, when designing therapeutic protocols using NIBS in different pathological conditions, to know beforehand what the background cortical excitability state is, how homeostatic plasticity acts in that condition, and also whether concomitant treatment could influence these aspects [57, 131]. At the same time, it is also necessary to understand the possible pathophysiological implications (i.e., adaptive vs maladaptive) of an altered state of cortical excitability and/or homeostatic plasticity. All this information will be fundamental in order to choose the most appropriate stimulation parameters.

The disadvantages of traditional rTMS protocols include their length and also the need to use a relatively strong and unpleasant stimulus intensity. In the light of these problems, a new rTMS technique called theta burst stimulation (TBS) has been developed. TBS is based on a firing pattern recorded from the hippocampus of animals exploring a new environment [75, 76]. Unlike conventional rTMS, which uses regular stimulation frequencies, TBS paradigms consist of repeated high-frequency (50 Hz) bursts of stimuli delivered at theta (5 Hz) frequency and at lower stimulation intensities. Depending on the stimulus parameter settings (i.e., train duration and temporal spacing of the bursts), it is possible to either decrease (with continuous TBS) or increase (with intermittent TBS) cortical excitability for up to an hour after only seconds of stimulation. As with rTMS there is good evidence that changes in cortical excitability induced by TBS are mediated by LTD/

LTP-like mechanisms [76]. Considering the effective and powerful nature of this stimulation technique, TBS protocols are a more practical option than traditional rTMS for treating neuropsychiatric disorders.

Another TMS protocol able to produce LTD-/LTP-like phenomena in humans consists of repetitive electrical stimulation of the median nerve followed by TMS over the contralateral primary motor cortex. This technique is called "paired associative stimulation" (PAS) [155]. Its effects on motor cortical excitability depend strictly on the interval between the afferent and the magnetic stimulus during the intervention. Suppression is induced if the sensory stimulus is applied 10 ms before the magnetic pulse (PAS10); conversely, excitation is produced if a 25-ms interval (PAS25) is used.

It is important to note that PAS-induced aftereffects are to be considered synapse-specific, in contrast to synapse non-specific plasticity induced by other NIBS techniques. This because PAS depends on the cortico-cortical interactions that develop between the sensory afferents and the motor output of the homologous muscle.

1.2 Transcranial Electrical Stimulation Paradigms

TES is a term that covers various techniques, principally transcranial direct or alternating current stimulation (tDCS or tACS) and random noise stimulation (tRNS). To date, tDCS remains the most widely used technique both for evaluation of cortical function in healthy subjects and for therapeutic application in several neuropsychiatric disorders. Nitsche and Paulus [120] were the first to describe the efficacy of weak direct currents in modulating spontaneous cortical activity and inducing transient functional changes in the human brain. tDCS is delivered by a battery-driven constant current stimulator using a pair of rubber electrodes (usually 7 cm × 5 cm) housed in small synthetic sponges dampened with salt water to increase the electrode conductivity. The effects of tDCS on brain activity depend on a combination of different parameters, including the stimulation strength and duration, the size of the stimulated area, and the direction of the current flow. The latter is defined by the electrode positions and polarity, with anodal current enhancing cortical excitability and activity, and cathodal current having the reverse effect. The effects of tDCS on brain function are not restricted to the stimulation period but outlast it by minutes to hours depending on the intensity and duration of the stimulation itself [123]. Several studies conducted mainly on the motor and visual cortices, first in animals and subsequently in humans, have attempted to clarify the mechanisms of action of tDCS [18, 123, 142]. Anodal tDCS has been shown to enhance neuronal spontaneous firing rate by depolarizing neuronal membranes at a subthreshold level, whilst cathodal current produced the reverse effect, by hyperpolarizing neurons [121, 124]. The tDCS-induced shifts in membrane polarization depend on modulation of the conductance of sodium and calcium channels. The aftereffects have indeed been attributed mainly to changes in synaptic efficacy due to modulation of NMDA receptor activity [102, 122, 126, 127]. As we have seen, both rTMS and tDCS can produce bidirectional NMDA-mediated aftereffects on cortical excitability, depending on the stimulation parameters used. However, along with their different modes of action, the two methods differ in many other respects, too, including their spatial and temporal resolution. The spatial resolution of tDCS, which is usually applied through relatively wide rubber electrodes covering an equally wide cortical surface, is somewhat poorer than that of rTMS, whose hot-spot has a diameter of about 2 cm when a focal coil is employed. This can be either an advantage or a disadvantage, depending on whether it is necessary to modulate the activity of larger cortical areas or induce focally restricted changes. tDCS also has a lower temporal resolution with respect to single-pulse TMS, which is why TMS is more useful than tDCS for obtaining information about the involvement of a precise cortical area in the performance of a given task.

Transcranial alternating current stimulation (tACS) is less well studied, however an interesting aspect of this technique is the possibility of interaction with the intrinsic oscillatory activity of the brain [7]. tACS involves application of a constant low-intensity sinusoidal current via electrodes placed over the head, as for tDCS. The intuitive choice of a rhythmic brain stimulation is based on the growing evidence that changes in the rhythmic activity of cortical networks are essential for perceptual and behavioral functions. It has become clear that tACS-induced effects on cortical function crucially depend on the stimulation frequency: tACS applied at a 10 Hz frequency has been shown to facilitate motor learning [7], whilst at 20 Hz a slowing of movements has been observed [138]. Furthermore, tACS applied at a higher frequency, from 140 to 5 kHz, has been shown to be capable of increasing the motor cortical output as assessed by TMS [29, 112]. The possibility of using periodic stimulation patterns that can match and mismatch the endogenous cortical activity, to obtain, respectively, enhancement of physiological functioning and suppression of pathological activity, opens up interesting therapeutic perspectives, and some preliminary results seem to encourage this line of research [22, 110].

Transcranial random noise stimulation (tRNS) is one of the newest methods of electrical stimulation [163]. In the "noise" stimulation mode, the DC stimulator generates a normally distributed random level of current with a frequency spectrum generally ranging from 0.1 to 640 Hz. tRNS at a stimulation intensity of 1 mA induces a consistent increase in motor cortical excitability with aftereffects that may outlast those observed after tDCS stimulation. Instead, at a lower stimulation intensity of 0.4 mA, inhibitory aftereffects may be observed [113]. The mechanisms of action of tRNS differ from those of tDCS as they do not seem to be NMDA-dependent. The repeated opening of Na+ channels has been suggested to be a putative mechanism [30]. Another important aspect to consider is that tRNS, as well as tACS, has the advantage over tDCS of avoiding directional sensitivity, thus making it possible to modulate activity of the cortical areas covered by the two electrodes in the same way.

2 Neural Control of Gait: Potential Targets of NIBS in Gait Rehabilitation

Human bipedal locomotion depends on a complex dialogue between spinal networks and supraspinal locomotor centers including several cortical and subcortical regions (Fig. 1). Locomotion, understood as rhythmic movements of the legs, is based on automated spinal motor programs generated by networks of neurons spread over several spinal segments (Armstrong et al. 1988; [68]). Descending projections from supraspinal structures are fundamental in modifying the stereotyped locomotor movements generated by the spinal central pattern generators, and adapting them to specific task demands and environmental changes. The most important supraspinal regions involved in locomotion are the mesencephalic locomotor region (MLR), the pontomedullary reticular formation (PMRF), the basal ganglia, the cerebellar locomotor region (CLR), and the frontal cortical regions. It should be noted, too, that gait control also involves regulation of balance, i.e. of the postural axial tone that is fundamental in maintaining upright posture during

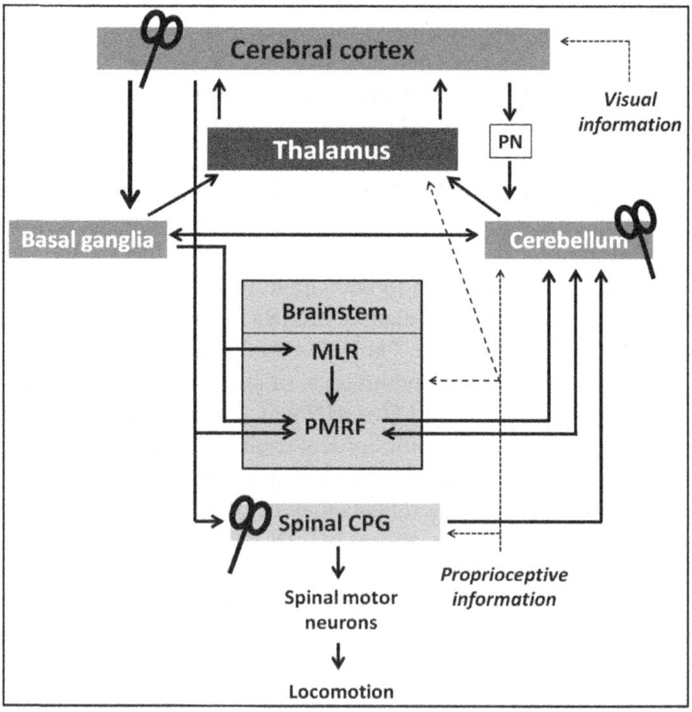

Fig. 1 Schematic representation of the circuitry involved in human locomotor activity. The TMS coil symbols indicate areas of the brain that could be possible targets of non-invasive brain stimulation. CPG: central pattern generator; MLR: mesencephalic locomotor region; PMRF: pontomedullary reticular formation; PN: pontine nuclei

walking. Balance and locomotion should not be considered purely motor phenomena, given that the afferent systems also play a crucial role by providing sensory feedback to the balance and gait generators. The whole complex picture of balance and locomotion regulation explains why dysfunctions in many different areas of the central nervous system can potentially be responsible for gait disturbances. It is extremely important to understand the pathophysiological processes underlying specific gait abnormalities in different pathological conditions, so as to be able to choose the best treatment strategy. In this regard, the use of new innovative treatment options based on NIBS techniques seems to be particularly attractive, for at least two different reasons: (1) different NIBS techniques may be applied, either to directly modulate the activity of cortical and/or cerebellar areas involved in gait control, or to induce functional changes in subcortical regions by means of cortical-subcortical projections, and (2) NIBS methods could be useful adjuvant strategies in neurorehabilitation of gait in a variety of clinical conditions, thanks to their ability to modulate brain plasticity in a controlled and specific manner.

2.1 Cortical Areas as a Target of Neuromodulation

Walking draws on different cognitive resources, including motivation, executive and attentional functions, visuospatial abilities and sensorimotor coordination, and should therefore be regarded as the result of global brain activity. Accordingly, several cortical areas are involved in the control of human gait. Among these, the supplementary motor area (SMA) plays a role in the initiation and termination of locomotion [39], while the premotor (PM) cortex may allow navigation of narrow spaces [129]. Both of these areas are part of a complex network that includes the primary motor and somatosensory cortices, the parahippocampal and fusiform gyri [79], and numerous subcortical regions [60, 69, 111]. Proprioceptive feedback processed within the somatosensory cortex is fundamental for motor programming and balance [10]. Visual information conveyed to the posterior parietal cortex also guides motor planning [97, 98], and is particularly critical when walking over and around obstacles, as this requires precise foot placement.

The frontal cortical areas appear to be the most promising target areas for neuromodulation therapies in patients with gait disturbances. The primary motor cortex, the PM cortex, and the SMA are all involved in stepping and postural adjustments [47, 86]. Furthermore, all of these areas directly influence the activity of the PMRF, the MLR and the spinal cord [47] by means of glutamatergic excitatory projections that counterbalance the inhibitory effect of the basal ganglia on the same brainstem and spinal networks. On the basis of these considerations, NIBS methods could be used to interfere with the balance between net excitation from the cerebral cortex and net inhibition from the basal ganglia, by modulating cortical activity. Depending on the stimulus parameters used, the activity of frontal areas could be either reduced or increased by different NIBS techniques in a hemispheric-specific fashion. However, to avoid painting an overly simplistic picture, it is also necessary to consider the mutual influences existing between the frontal cerebral cortex and basal ganglia that can be also influenced by cortical stimulation (see below).

Recent electrophysiological studies have raised awareness that distinct patterns of oscillatory activity involving several cortical areas underlie different aspects of gait control in humans [28, 171]. It has been shown that efficient motor activities are accompanied by suppression of μ (8–13 Hz) and β (13–35 Hz) oscillations in the sensorimotor and parietal cortex [134, 150]. Conversely, a β rhythm increase in the frontal-basal ganglia circuitry has been related to cognitive top-down gait control [25, 159]. The role played by altered brain oscillatory activity in different pathological conditions characterized by gait impairment deserves to be investigated in future studies as this knowledge could prove fundamental for the development of new treatment strategies, possibly based on the use of NIBS techniques, such as tACS, capable of modulating neuronal oscillations.

In addition to the frontal cerebral cortex, various sensory cortical areas could also be potential targets for neuromodulation. It is indeed well known that human gait can be heavily influenced by sensory signals of several kinds. Rhythmic auditory and visual cues have been shown to be capable of affecting the temporal dynamics of human walking, and this phenomenon has been considered of particular interest in neurorehabilitation [51]. In this regard, several studies have shown that different sensory cues, delivered in the form of continuous rhythmic patterns, may be useful in the rehabilitation of parkinsonian patients with freezing of gait [109]. Visual and proprioceptive feedback have also been used to improve gait in chronic stroke patients [100]. From this perspective, it is conceivable that NIBS methods, when applied to different sensory cortical areas, could potentially be used as an adjuvant to rehabilitation treatment of gait disorders.

2.2 The Cerebellum as a Target of Neuromodulation

The cerebellum is part of an integrated system, also including the cerebral cortex and the basal ganglia, that serves a wide range of motor and cognitive functions. In recent years, the classical view of the cerebellum as a nervous structure receiving inputs from multiple cortical regions and funneling these back almost exclusively to the primary motor cortex [5] has undergone considerable revision. It is now clear that the cerebellar efferents, via the thalamus, target widespread cortical areas that include, along with the primary motor cortex, also premotor, prefrontal and parietal cortical regions [26, 49]. Recent studies have also radically changed the idea that any interactions between cortico-cerebellar and cortico-basal ganglia loops occur primarily at the cortical level [72, 133]. Indeed, there is now experimental evidence that the cerebellum and the basal ganglia reciprocally interact by means of direct interconnections, thus providing the neural bases for the cerebellar involvement in pathological conditions typically associated with the basal ganglia, such as Parkinson's disease and dystonia [34, 72, 176].

All of the above explains why cerebellar neuromodulation has recently become a very appealing option in the fields of neuroscience and neurorehabilitation. Both TES and TMS have been used successfully for non-invasive transcranial cerebellar stimulation. In the earlier experiments TES was preferred over TMS, since both the round and the figure-of-eight magnetic coils normally used for motor cortical stimulation could be insufficient to activate deeper nervous structures such as the cerebellum. This problem was later solved by the use of the double-cone coil that proved to be more effective and reliable in stimulation both of the cerebellar hemispheres and of the deeper midline structures such as the vermis [67, 78, 168]. Ugawa et al. [167], using a paired-pulse TMS paradigm, were the first to show that the amplitude of a motor evoked potential elicited from the primary motor cortex (M1) is reduced by a conditioning stimulus applied over the contralateral cerebellar hemisphere 5–8 ms before cortical stimulation. This phenomenon, also referred to as cerebellar brain inhibition (CBI), has been attributed to activation of the Purkinje cells in the cerebellar cortex, which in turn can inhibit the dentate nucleus and its facilitatory output to the cerebral cortex. Different methods of NIBS have been proven capable of modulating CBI and/or inducing changes in motor cortical excitability, with effects outlasting the end of the stimulation itself due to induction of plastic changes. However, the effects of NIBS on cerebellar neurons remain poorly defined, and they are likely different from those involved in neuromodulation of the cerebral cortex, due to differences in functional organization and cytoarchitecture between the cerebellum and the neocortex. This also explains why mixed and contradictory results have been obtained in NIBS experiments targeting the cerebellum. A first study showed an increase in motor cortical excitability, as assessed by single-pulse TMS, after low-frequency (1–Hz) rTMS of the cerebellum [130]. This effect, not confirmed by a second rTMS study by Fierro et al. [56], was attributed to suppression of the Purkinje cells resulting in disinhibition of the facilitatory dentatothalamocortical pathway. In accordance with this interpretation, it was observed that "inhibitory" cathodal tDCS leads to a lasting inhibition of CBI, although, contrary to the findings of Oliveri et al., no changes in MEP amplitude were observed [61]. Conflicting results have also been given by TBS studies: "facilitatory" intermittent TBS applied to the cerebellum was, surprisingly, shown to induce motor cortical facilitation instead of inhibition, while conversely, "inhibitory" continuous TBS proved able to induce MEP suppression [93]. It has been hypothesized that these unexpected results could be a consequence of the opposite effects induced by intermittent TBS and continuous TBS on different populations of inhibitory GABAergic interneurons [93]. Very recently, tACS, too, was shown to induce cerebellar plasticity with weakening or strengthening effects on CBI depending on stimulation frequency, i.e. 50 and 300 Hz respectively [118].

It is well known that the cerebellum is involved at multiple levels in balance and gait control. Integrity of the cerebellum and its afferent and efferent connections with the cerebral cortex and the brainstem is critical for posture and motor coordination of locomotion [52, 104]. Accordingly, cerebellar impairment in humans results in instability of posture and gait (truncal and gait ataxia) [9]. The vermis and the paravermal cerebellar cortex are particularly important for balance and gait control in animals and humans thanks to their projections to the MLR via the fastigial nuclei and the CLR [8, 80]. This latter area, first described by Mori et al. [114] in a decerebrate cat, corresponds to a small area in the midline cerebellar white matter whose stimulation evokes well-coordinated locomotor patterns as the animal's feet come into contact with the moving surface of a treadmill. The MLR is connected to the PMRF, which in turn projects to the spinal cord. If the widespread connectivity of this network is interrupted at any level both the initiation and the maintenance of posture and walking are seriously impaired.

Many recent studies have investigated the involvement of the cerebellum in regulating synaptic plasticity in premotor and motor cortical networks [74, 132, 149], also providing evidence that the cerebellum contributes to the learning processes underlying motor adaptation [27, 62, 164]. The adaptation of locomotor patterns under certain contingent environmental conditions is extremely important in normal gait. Although the precise mechanisms underlying locomotor adaptation in humans are not fully understood, there is growing evidence that the cerebellum plays a pivotal role [82, 83]. Accordingly, altered adaptation of walking has been shown in ataxic patients with degenerative cerebellar diseases [116]. Further support for the potential therapeutic efficacy of cerebellar NIBS strategies in the neurorehabilitation of gait disorders has recently been provided by evidence that anodal tDCS applied over the cerebellum facilitated the acquisition of a new walking pattern, whilst cathodal tDCS resulted in the reverse effect [83]. These findings, however, seem to conflict with the concept that adaptive learning is promoted by LTD in Purkinje cells, which corresponds to a reduction of cerebellar inhibition [82]. Although several hypotheses have been proposed to explain these unexpected effects of anodal and cathodal cerebellar tDCS on motor learning, the question remains open and targeted studies will be required in order to clarify it.

3 Non-invasive Neuromodulation in Neurological Disorders with Gait Impairment: The State of the Art

In the following paragraphs, we provide a summary of the main findings from research pursuing new, non-invasive neuromodulation-based treatment strategies in gait disorders associated with neurological diseases.

3.1 Non-invasive Neuromodulation to Improve Gait and Balance in Parkinson's Disease

Gait impairment is a major impediment for patients with Parkinson's disease (PD), becoming, especially in the advanced phases of the disease, a major cause of disability [115, 117]. The current understanding is that locomotor abnormalities in PD are attributable, mainly, to a dysfunction in the cortico-basal ganglia pathway, in line with the concept that the basal ganglia contribute to the planning and execution of voluntary movements by means of bidirectional connections with the frontal cortex [4, 43, 166]. More recent findings, however, have challenged the exclusivity of this assumption. Specifically, it is now clear that the basal ganglia outflow is also directed at the brainstem motor networks involved in the regulation of postural muscle tone [71, 77, 161]. This basal ganglia-brainstem system is thought to play a pivotal role in integrating automatic and voluntary aspects of locomotor movements [162].

Deep brain stimulation (DBS) and lesional interventions targeting the basal ganglia have been shown to improve PD motor symptoms, including motor fluctuations, dyskinesia and refractory tremor. However, these interventions, in addition to carrying a risk of serious complications, have been shown to be largely ineffective in ameliorating postural instability and gait difficulties [15]. That is why there has been a growing interest in the use of NIBS as an alternative therapeutic tool.

Although the basal ganglia are not directly accessible to non-invasive stimulation methods, as they are located in the deeper parts of the brain, there is mounting evidence that the effects of cortical stimulation may spread widely across the cortico-basal ganglia-thalamocortical circuit. First, experimental studies in animals have shown that dopamine can be released under direct control of glutamatergic corticostriatal projections [119, 174]. Second, it has been shown that high-frequency rTMS of the frontal cortex may induce ipsilateral endogenous dopamine release in the striatum, both in healthy humans [156, 157] and in PD patients [158]. Furthermore, trans-synaptic effects of NIBS involving the basal ganglia have also been observed after cortical intermittent TBS in hemiparkinsonian rats [64] and after cortical tDCS in humans in vivo [139].

In the last decade or so, several sham-controlled studies have provided stimulating data regarding beneficial effects of NIBS on motor symptoms in Parkinson's disease (see Table 1). However, only a few studies have included assessment of gait as an outcome measure. As regards rTMS, Khedr et al. [89] recorded a long-lasting increase in the UPDRS motor scores and walking speed after 5 Hz rTMS applied bilaterally to the hand and leg motor cortex for 10 consecutive days. Subsequently, a study by Lomarev et al. [105] increased support for the therapeutic potential of high-frequency rTMS for gait impairment in PD; these authors showed that 25 Hz rTMS applied bilaterally to the motor and dorsolateral prefrontal cortex (DLPFC) over a 4-week period improved upper limb bradykinesia and reduced walking time, with effects lasting for at least 1 month after the treatment ended. Other authors [42] showed that high-frequency (10 Hz) rTMS applied over the DLPFC failed to improve hand movements and gait in PD, a finding which seems to suggest that the primary motor cortex is a more appropriate target for high-frequency rTMS than the DLPFC. This concept is also supported by a recent meta-analysis [35] showing that a motor improvement in PD may be observed both when high-frequency (≥ 5 Hz) rTMS is targeted at M1, and when low-frequency (≤ 1 Hz) rTMS is applied over other frontal regions.

Table 1 Sham-controlled studies evaluating the therapeutic potential of non-invasive brain stimulation in parkinsonian patients with gait impairment

	Neurostimulation paradigm	Patients	Targeted cortical area	Beneficial effects on gait and/or balance
Khedr et al. [89]	5 Hz rTMS at 120% of the RMT (2000 pulses) for 10 consecutive days	PD patients Off therapy	Primary motor cortex hot spot for lower limbs (first 1000 pulses) and for the hand, 500 pulses for each area of the two hemispheres (right then left hemisphere)	Increase in walking speed of about 15% after the end of the 10th session with beneficial effects still evident at 1-month follow-up
Lomarev et al. [105]	25 Hz rTMS at 100% of the RMT (1200 pulses); 8 stimulation sessions over a 4-week period	PD patients On therapy	Four cortical targets stimulated in each session: left and right hand motor cortex and DLPFC (300 pulses each)	Reduction in walking time of about 18% after the end of the 8th session with beneficial effects still evident at 1-month follow-up
del Olmo et al. [42]	10 Hz rTMS at 90% of the RMT, 450 pulses-day for 10 consecutive days	PD patients On therapy	DLPFC contralateral to the more affected side	No effects of rTMS on walking time either at preferred or at maximum speed (slight improvement due only to practice, as also observed after sham rTMS)
Benninger et al. [13]	Anodal tDCS at 2 mA for 20 min in 8 sessions within 2.5 weeks	PD patients On and off therapy	Anodes over the pre- and motor cortex or prefrontal cortex of both hemispheres in separate sessions (4 times each). Cathodes over the mastoids	Slight decrease in walking time one day after the end of the last tDCS intervention in patients in the off-state. No beneficial effects in patients stimulated in the on-medication state
Benninger et al. [14]	Intermittent TBS at stimulation intensity of 80% of the RMT; 8 sessions over 2 weeks	PD patients On and off therapy	Primary motor cortex and DLPFC of both hemispheres	No effects of intermittent TBS on gait in either the on- or off-medication state

(continued)

Table 1 (continued)

	Neurostimulation paradigm	Patients	Targeted cortical area	Beneficial effects on gait and/or balance
Verheyden et al. [170]	Cathodal tDCS at 1 mA for 15 min (single session)	PD patients On therapy	Primary motor cortex of the dominant hemisphere	Significant decrease in gait speed from the 10-m walk test
Yang et al. [177]	5 Hz rTMS (1200 pulses) at 100% of the RMT followed by treadmill training for 12 sessions over 4 weeks	PD patients On therapy	Leg area of the motor cortex contralaterally to the more affected side	Walking speed increased by 0.12 m/s after treadmill training only, and by 0.22 m/s after combined rTMS and treadmill training
Kaski et al. [88]	Anodal tDCS at 2 mA applied for 15 min during physical training in a single session	PD patients On therapy	Anode electrode (10 × 4 cm) positioned centrally across the scalp anterior to Cz. Cathode (4 × 4 cm) placed at the inion	tDCS enhanced the beneficial effects of physical training with mean increase in gait velocity of about 29.5% (vs 15.5% for physical training alone), and also improved balance by about 50.9% (vs. non-significant 1.5% for physical training alone) as assessed by the pull test (time of stability following the retropulsion stimulus)
Lee et al. [99]	10 Hz rTMS (20 trains of 5-sec) at 90% of the RMT in a single session. Double-cone coil used for stimulation of the primary motor cortex of the lower leg (dominant hemisphere)	Patients with PD, PPS, and vascular parkinsonism presenting FOG	Primary motor cortex of the lower leg, SMA, and DLPFC of the dominant hemisphere (in separate sessions)	Significant improvement in TUG test times, number of turn steps and turn time after stimulation of both the primary motor cortex and DLPFC, but not after stimulation of the SMA

(continued)

Table 1 (continued)

	Neurostimulation paradigm	Patients	Targeted cortical area	Beneficial effects on gait and/or balance
Valentino et al. [169]	Anodal tDCS at 2 mA applied for 20 min for 5 consecutive days	On-therapy PD patients with FOG persisting in the on-state	Primary motor cortex corresponding to the leg with which the patient usually started walking after a FOG episode	Reduction in number and duration of FOG episodes (by over 60% compared to baseline at 2 days after the end of the last intervention) and in number of steps and walking time as assessed by the SWS test. Beneficial effects still evident at 1-month follow-up
von Papen et al. (2014)	1 Hz rTMS (900 stimuli at 80% of the RMT) preconditioned by tDCS (10 min at 1 mA) in single sessions	PD patients On therapy	Reference electrode positioned over the primary motor cortex contralateral to the more affected body side	Improvement in gait kinematics after 1 Hz rTMS preconditioned by anodal but not cathodal and sham tDCS. Beneficial effects persisting for at least 30 min after the end of the stimulation
Costa-Ribeiro et al. (2015)	Anodal tDCS at 2 mA for 13 min followed by cueing gait training	PD patients On therapy	Anode positioned 2 cm anterior to Cz and cathode placed above the supraorbital area of the contralateral hemisphere of the more affected side	No additional beneficial effects of tDCS over cueing gait training alone, although improvement in gait velocity and TUG test was still evident at 1-month follow-up only when gait training was associated with tDCS

(continued)

Table 1 (continued)

	Neurostimulation paradigm	Patients	Targeted cortical area	Beneficial effects on gait and/or balance
Kim et al. [91]	10 Hz rTMS (1000 pulses) at 90% of the RMT for five sessions in a week	PD patients on therapy with FOG	Lower leg primary motor cortex of the dominant hemisphere	Significant improvements in the step required to complete the SS-180 test, FOG-Q, and TUG test with beneficial effects still evident at a 1-week follow-up

Abbreviations DLPFC: dorsolateral prefrontal cortex; dTMS: deep transcranial magnetic stimulation; FOG: freezing of gait; FOG-Q: freezing of gait questionnaire; NIBS: non-invasive brain stimulation; PD: Parkinson's disease; PPS: Parkinson-plus syndrome; RMT: resting motor threshold; rTMS: repetitive transcranial magnetic stimulation; SMA: supplementary motor area; tDCS: transcranial direct current stimulation; SS-180 test: Standing Start 180 test; SWS test: Stand Walk Sit test. TBS: theta burst stimulation; TUG test: Timed Up and Go test

The studies conducted to date are still too few to allow us to assert that tDCS has a significant therapeutic effect on gait disturbances in PD. Targeted studies are needed to clarify various issues concerning the application of tDCS for therapeutic purposes in PD, e.g. which cortical areas are the best targets, whether patients should be treated in the on- or the off-state, and even which clinical features should be considered, in individual patients, to guide the choice of the best stimulation parameters. Benninger et al. [13] showed that anodal tDCS applied to the motor and prefrontal cortex of both hemispheres in 8 sessions over a 2.5-week period only slightly improved, for a short time, some pathological aspects of gait in PD, whilst more evident and prolonged beneficial effects were observed on upper limb bradykinesia. Other authors [38, 88] have shown that anodal tDCS may improve gait and balance only when combined with physical therapy and not when applied alone, likely by virtue of the ability of anodal tDCS to enhance implicit motor learning [125] and thus the effects of the rehabilitation training.

One still poorly investigated pathophysiological aspect of PD is the asymmetry both in primary motor cortex excitability [95, 175] and in transcallosal interhemispheric inhibition, with reduced transcallosal inhibition of the less affected hemisphere, i.e. that contralateral to the less affected body side [101, 154]. Both of these features, which may reflect asymmetric impairment of the striato-frontal motor circuit, have been supposed to be involved in the asymmetric motor impairment that characterizes the disease. Notwithstanding this, to date, no targeted studies have been conducted to evaluate the therapeutic efficacy of different NIBS techniques when applied to one or the other hemisphere in PD patients with asymmetric motor symptoms. In this regard, interesting clues come from studies evaluating the therapeutic potential of tDCS in parkinsonian patients with freezing of gait (FOG), a disabling clinical phenomenon characterized by brief episodes of inability to generate effective stepping. FOG is associated with marked gait asymmetry [136], and a functional imbalance between homologous motor cortical areas has been suggested to play a pivotal role in the pathogenesis of this phenomenon [54, 84, 153, 169] showed a marked reduction in the number and duration of FOG episodes in PD when anodal tDCS was applied over the primary motor cortex corresponding to the leg with which the patient usually started walking after a FOG episode (i.e. the more affected leg). This result was interpreted as a possible expression of a rebalancing effect of tDCS on the activity of homologous motor cortical areas responsible for gait coordination. Lee et al. [99] and Kim et al. [91] have also shown gait improvement in parkinsonian patients with FOG by applying, respectively, anodal tDCS and 10 Hz rTMS to the frontal cortex. Even though these authors targeted the dominant hemisphere in all patients, regardless of which was the most affected leg, it should be noted that a prevalent involvement of the dominant hemisphere has been shown in PD patients with FOG, in line with clinical evidence that the right leg is usually the most affected one [58, 137, 169]. A study by Verheyden et al. [170] adds further support to the need to carefully choose the hemisphere to stimulate in NIBS experiments involving PD patients. These authors showed that cathodal tDCS applied to the M1 of the dominant hemisphere induced a worsening in walking speed. This was attributed to a possible imbalance between the two hemispheres induced or, if already present, worsened by tDCS. In particular, considering that the motor symptoms are more often predominant on the dominant hand side [151], "inhibitory" cathodal tDCS could have further destabilized an interhemispheric imbalance, unfavoring the dominant hemisphere [101, 154].

To our knowledge, only one TBS study, showing no significant improvement of walking, has been conducted in PD [14], while no studies involving the newest NIBS methods such as tACS and tRNS have yet been conducted. There is therefore a need for future research. Also, in the light of the evidence that homeostatic mechanisms regulating cortical activity can be exploited with therapeutic intent (von Papen et al. 2014), future studies should focus on evaluating the effect of different NIBS methods in combination.

3.2 *Non-invasive Neuromodulation to Improve Post-stroke Gait and Balance Impairment*

Gait and balance difficulties after stroke are a major impediment, making it difficult for patients to regain independence in daily living and quality of life. About 80% of stroke survivors have walking problems 3 months after onset [3] and, especially in the first year, there is a high risk of falls in post-stroke patients who are independently walking [173]. This explains why one of the main goals of post-stroke rehabilitation is to improve balance and restore/improve walking ability. Current rehabilitation protocols generally achieve only limited recovery of motor impairment after stroke. Thus, there is an obvious need to develop new methods capable of improving the effects of rehabilitation therapies. In this regard, NIBS methods are an attractive tool thanks to their ability to interfere with the neuroplastic changes underlying motor recovery and, potentially, to maximize the effects of physical rehabilitation.

It is well known that after an acute stroke several neuroplastic processes occur involving both the affected and the unaffected hemisphere. However, the extent to which these changes might be beneficial and promote motor recovery, or be maladaptive and prevent it, is still debated [107]. The large majority of studies conducted to test the potential therapeutic efficacy of NIBS in stroke patients were based on the concept of interhemispheric competition. It has been shown that a unilateral stroke alters the normal symmetry of interhemispheric corticomotor excitability [147]. In particular, increased excitability of the M1 of the undamaged hemisphere and enhanced interhemispheric inhibition of the M1 of the affected hemisphere have been shown [21, 92]. Such changes have been supposed to be maladaptive and unfavorable to recovery of the ipsilesional motor cortex [59, 165]. The evidence in this regard is stronger for the upper limbs [50, 70, 128], which have a more direct and unilateral cortico-motoneuronal representation [46]. There is growing evidence, however, that a functional balance between the two hemispheres is also critical in lower limb motor function [146]. In this regard it has been shown, in chronic stroke patients, that anodal tDCS is effective in increasing the activity of the leg corticospinal tract and decreasing contralesional motor cortical activity by enhancing transcallosal inhibition of the contralesional hemisphere [81]. On these bases, functional interhemispheric imbalance can be assumed to play a role in the pathophysiology of gait impairment in stroke patients.

A few studies have shown that NIBS may induce gait improvement in patients with unilateral stroke when applied with the aim of restoring more physiological symmetry of interhemispheric motor cortical excitability (see Table 2). Madhavan et al. [108] showed that anodal tDCS, when applied over the lower limb primary motor cortex of the affected hemisphere during tracking trials, enhanced tracking accuracy in chronic stroke patients. Conversely, application of anodal tDCS over the undamaged M1 had the opposite effect, i.e. it reduced tracking accuracy. In a study by Wang et al. [172], 1 Hz rTMS was applied over the lower limb motor cortex of the unaffected hemisphere with the aim of down-regulating activity in the contralesional hemisphere. The authors observed that low-frequency rTMS applied prior to task-oriented training increased symmetry in interhemispheric excitability as assessed by single-pulse TMS and, at the same time, improved walking ability and gait spatial symmetry.

In the majority of studies, neuromodulatory protocols have been used as potential adjuvants of gait rehabilitation. In a first study combining robot-assisted gait training with tDCS [63], there were no additional beneficial effects of tDCS when it was applied over the leg area of the lesioned hemisphere. Robot-assisted gait training may be more effective than traditional gait rehabilitation, and thus a ceiling effect may have been achieved following the rehabilitation treatment, thus precluding the possibility of further improvement. However, as the authors applied tDCS at 1.5 mA for only 7 min, it can also be hypothesized that more intensive transcranial stimulation currents might have been needed to produce additional

Table 2 Sham-controlled studies evaluating the therapeutic potential of non-invasive brain stimulation in stroke patients with gait impairment

	Neurostimulation paradigm	Patients	Targeted cortical area	Beneficial effects on gait and/or balance
Geroin et al. [63]	Anodal tDCS at 1.5 mA for 7 min combined with robot-assisted gait training or overground walking exercises (5 days a week for 2 consecutive weeks)	Chronic stroke patients	Leg area of the lesioned hemisphere	Robot-assisted training is more effective than conventional training in enhancing gait ability; anodal tDCS has no additional effects on robot-assisted training
Madhavan et al. [108]	Anodal tDCS for 15 min at 2 mA in combination with tracking trials (single session)	Chronic stroke patients	Lower limb primary motor cortex of the lesioned or the non-lesioned hemisphere	The practice effect observed after sham stimulation was enhanced by tDCS applied over the lesioned hemisphere and eliminated by tDCS applied over the non-lesioned hemisphere
Wang et al. [172]	1 Hz rTMS for 10 min followed by task-oriented training (30 min) for 10 sessions over 2 weeks	Chronic stroke patients	Leg area of the motor cortex of the unaffected hemisphere	Enhancement of the beneficial effect of training mainly due to improvement in spatial symmetry of gait
Danzl et al. [40]	Anodal tDCS for 20 min at 2 mA followed by training with a robot gait orthosis, 3 times per week for 4 weeks	Chronic stroke patients	Midline cortical motor areas	Although both the sham and active tDCS groups improved, a significantly greater improvement was observed for anodal tDCS as assessed by the FAC. The TUG, SIS-16 and 10 MWT also favored the active tDCS group but were non-significant

(continued)

Table 2 (continued)

	Neurostimulation paradigm	Patients	Targeted cortical area	Beneficial effects on gait and/or balance
Kaski et al. [87]	Anodal tDCS at 2 mA for 15 min applied during physical training (single session)	Patients with ischemic white matter lesions (leukoaraiosis)	Midline motor and premotor areas	Combining tDCS and training improves gait velocity (40% mean improvement), stride length, stride length variability and balance (58% mean reduction in the time to recovery on the retropulsion test); training without tDCS has no beneficial effects
Kim et al. [90]	1 Hz rTMS for 15 min for 5 consecutive days	Ataxic patients with posterior circulation stroke	Cerebellum	Significant improvement in the 10 MWT and BBS in the rTMS group. Percentage changes immediately after the last rTMS session for time in the 10 MWT, steps in the 10 MWT and BBS in the real vs sham group were: −16.7 versus 72.5%, −8.5 versus −0.3% and 46.4 versus 36.6%, respectively
Saeys et al. (2014)	tDCS for 20 min at 1.5 mA, 4 times a week for 4 week (16 sessions)	Stroke patients less than 4 months post-onset	Anode over the ipsilesional motor cortex and cathode on the contralesional side	Slight beneficial effect on balance and gait as assessed by the Tinetti test (significant effect only for the total score)

(continued)

Table 2 (continued)

	Neurostimulation paradigm	Patients	Targeted cortical area	Beneficial effects on gait and/or balance
Tahtis et al. [160]	Bi-cephalic tDCS at 2 mA for 15 min (single session)	Sub-acute stroke patients	Anode over the ipsilesional lower limb primary motor cortex and cathode over the contralesional leg motor cortex	Improvement in TUG test (mean reduction of about 4.6 s in the time to perform the test); no changes in POMA score
Chang et al. [31]	Anodal tDCS for 10 min at 2 mA (ten sessions over 2 weeks) in association with conventional physical therapy	Sub-acute stroke patients	Tibialis anterior area of the precentral gyrus in the affected hemisphere	Enhancement in cortical excitability and improvement in lower limb motor weakness were observed in the tDCS group in comparison with the sham group. However no significant changes were observed as regards standing and gait function
Picelli et al. [135]	Anodal tDCS (2 mA for 20 min) and cathodal tsDCS (2.5 mA for 20 min) during robot-assisted gait training (5 days a week for 2 consecutive weeks)	Chronic stroke patients	For tDCS: anode applied over the M1 of the affected hemisphere; for tsDCS: cathode placed over the spinous process of the tenth thoracic vertebra	Patients treated with anodal tDCS + cathodal tsDCS showed a significantly greater improvement in walking capacity and gait cadence than both the patients treated only with tDCS and those treated only with tsDCS

Abbreviations 10 MWT: 10 Meter Walk Test; BBS: Berg Balance Scale; FAC: Functional Ambulation Categories; iTBS: intermittent theta burst stimulation; POMA: Performance Oriented Mobility Assessment; rTMS: repetitive transcranial magnetic stimulation; tDCS: transcranial direct current stimulation; SIS-16: Stroke Impact Scale 16; tsDCS: transcutaneous spinal direct current stimulation; TUG test: Timed Up and Go test

effects on locomotion rehabilitation. This agrees with more recent findings by Picelli et al. [135], who showed that anodal tDCS, when applied over the M1 of the affected hemisphere at 2 mA intensity for 20 min, can enhance the improvement in walking capacity and gait cadence induced by robotic gait training. These authors, however, combined tDCS with cathodal transcutaneous spinal DCS (tsDCS), meaning that the improvement could also be attributable, at least partly, to an effect on the spinal cells. In particular, thoracic cathodal tsDCS is thought to make motoneurons more responsive to synaptic activation and, accordingly, there is evidence that it can improve motor unit recruitment in healthy people [19].

Two studies (Saeys et al. 2014; [160]) tested the therapeutic potential of bi-cephalic tDCS applied with the aim of restoring the interhemispheric balance that is disrupted after a unilateral stroke. Bi-cephalic tDCS is a useful paradigm for increasing activity in one cerebral hemisphere, while simultaneously decreasing activity in the other [23, 103]. The authors of both studies observed that tDCS improved walking, even though no significant improvements in gait and balance subscale scores were shown either on a performance-oriented mobility assessment [160] or on the Tinetti test (Saeys et al. 2014). Interestingly, Tahtis et al. [160] observed that of four subjects showing a greater than 20% improvement on the Timed Up and Go (TUG) test, three were patients with subcortical strokes without motor cortical involvement. This finding is consistent with the suggestion that patients with subcortical stroke may derive a greater beneficial effect from cortical stimulation than patients with cortical stroke [6]. Evidence further supporting this concept is that anodal tDCS over the motor and premotor cortices of both hemispheres may induce, even when applied in single sessions, a remarkable improvement in gait ability and balance in patients with leukoaraiosis, i.e. subcortical white matter lesions or small vessel disease [87].

Further studies are needed to evaluate the therapeutic potential of NIBS when targeting cerebral regions other than motor cortical areas in post-stroke patients. The brainstem, the cerebellar structures and the spinal networks involved in the automatic process of gait control are intact in more than 90% of total cerebral stroke cases. In subjects with chronic hemiparetic stroke, these structures are particularly active while walking [106, 178] and, thanks to their activity, gait can be still observed in some subjects even after complete lateral corticospinal tract injury [2]. On these bases, the hypothesis has been advanced that NIBS targeting the cerebellum or the spinal cord could improve gait in patients with hemispheric brain lesions and/or could potentiate the beneficial effects on walking observed with rehabilitation treatments activating subcortical neural networks [106].

Finally, and this brings us to a significant gap in the existing data, almost all previous studies evaluated patients with mono-hemispheric stroke. The therapeutic potential of NIBS in cerebellar stroke patients has been tested, giving encouraging preliminary results, only in a sham-controlled pilot study using 1 Hz rTMS [90] and in an open-label study using intermittent TBS over the injured cerebellar hemisphere [20].

Finally, in a single study using tACS, albeit not specifically targeted at improving gait disturbances, a beneficial effect on recovery of motor, sensory and speech functions in chronic stroke patients was observed [55].

3.3 Conclusions and Future Perspectives

In recent decades, the development of NIBS technologies has opened up the prospect of a broader therapeutic armamentarium for various psychiatric and neurological disorders. In this chapter we have provided an overview of some emerging concepts related to the use of NIBS in patients with balance and gait difficulties. The results of the studies presented, in addition to supporting the therapeutic potential of NIBS, provide important clues about the pathophysiological mechanisms underlying balance and gait impairment in different pathological conditions. Even though we have here focused on Parkinson's disease and stroke, which have been the most investigated diseases, it should be noted that encouraging preliminary results have also been reported in other pathological conditions characterized by body posture and gait impairment, such as cerebellar ataxia [16, 53, 140, 152], cerebral palsy in children [36, 48, 65, 66], multiple sclerosis [24], spinal cord injury [12, 73, 96, 141], and mitochondrial myopathy [143].

To conclude, it is important to underline a crucial point: given the different methodological approaches used and the considerable heterogeneity of the stimulation parameters employed (including stimulation sites, number of pulses and stimulation patterns for TMS, duration and intensity of stimulation for TES) and the number of sessions performed, it is very difficult to make comparisons between different studies. Therefore, further research efforts are needed in order to confirm current findings in larger patients groups, elucidate the mechanisms of action of the different NIBS methods, and identify which patients may benefit from NIBS in a meaningful manner and by what methodological approach.

References

1. Abraham WC, Bear MF. Metaplasticity: the plasticity of synaptic plasticity. Trends Neurosci. 1996;19(4):126–30.
2. Ahn YH, Ahn SH, Kim H, Hong JH, Jang SH. Can stroke patients walk after complete lateral corticospinal tract injury of the affected hemisphere? NeuroReport. 2006;17(10): 987–90.
3. Algurén B, Lundgren-Nilsson A, Sunnerhagen KS. Facilitators and barriers of stroke survivors in the early post-stroke phase. Disabil Rehabil. 2009;31(19):1584–91.
4. Alexander GE, Crutcher MD. Functional architecture of basal ganglia circuits: neural substrates of parallel processing. Trends Neurosci. 1990;13(7):266–71.
5. Allen GI, Tsukahara N. Cerebrocerebellar communication systems. Physiol Rev. 1974;54 (4):957–1006.
6. Ameli M, Grefkes C, Kemper F, Riegg FP, Rehme AK, Karbe H, Fink GR, Nowak DA. Differential effects of high-frequency repetitive transcranial magnetic stimulation over ipsilesional primary motor cortex in cortical and subcortical middle cerebral artery stroke. Ann Neurol. 2009;66(3):298–309.
7. Antal A, Boros K, Poreisz C, Chaieb L, Terney D, Paulus W. Comparatively weak after-effects of transcranial alternating current stimulation (tACS) on cortical excitability in humans. Brain Stimul. 2008;1(2):97–105.

8. Armstrong DM. The supraspinal control of mammalian locomotion. J Physiol. 1988; 405:1–37.
9. Bastian AJ, Martin TA, Keating JG, Thach WT. Cerebellar ataxia: abnormal control of interaction torques across multiple joints. J Neurophysiol. 1996;76(1):492–509.
10. Bastian AJ. Learning to predict the future: the cerebellum adapts feedforward movement control. Curr Opin Neurobiol. 2006;16(6):645–9.
11. Bear MF. Bidirectional synaptic plasticity: from theory to reality. Philos Trans R Soc Lond B Biol Sci. 2003;358(1432):649–55.
12. Benito J, Kumru H, Murillo N, Costa U, Medina J, Tormos JM, Pascual-Leone A, Vidal J. Motor and gait improvement in patients with incomplete spinal cord injury induced by high-frequency repetitive transcranial magnetic stimulation. Top Spinal Cord Inj Rehabil. 2012;18(2):106–12.
13. Benninger DH, Lomarev M, Lopez G, Wassermann EM, Li X, Considine E, Hallett M. Transcranial direct current stimulation for the treatment of Parkinson's disease. J Neurol Neurosurg Psychiatry. 2010;81(10):1105–11.
14. Benninger DH, Berman BD, Houdayer E, Pal N, Luckenbaugh DA, Schneider L, Miranda S, Hallett M. Intermittent theta-burst transcranial magnetic stimulation for treatment of Parkinson disease. Neurology. 2011;76(7):601–9.
15. Benninger DH. Parkinson's disease. Handb Clin Neurol. 2013;116:469–83.
16. Benussi A, Koch G, Cotelli M, Padovani A, Borroni B. Cerebellar transcranial direct current stimulation in patients with ataxia: a double-blind, randomized, sham-controlled study. Mov Disord. 2015;30(12):1701–5.
17. Bienenstock EL, Cooper LN, Munro PW. Theory for the development of neuron selectivity: orientation specificity and binocular interaction in visual cortex. J Neurosci. 1982;2(1): 32–48.
18. Bindman LJ, Lippold OC, Redfearn JW. The action of brief polarizing currents on the cerebral cortex of the rat (1) during current flow and (2) in the production of long-lasting after-effects. J Physiol. 1964;172:369–82.
19. Bocci T, Vannini B, Torzini A, Mazzatenta A, Vergari M, Cogiamanian F, Priori A, Sartucci F. Cathodal transcutaneous spinal direct current stimulation (tsDCS) improves motor unit recruitment in healthy subjects. Neurosci Lett. 2014;578:75–9.
20. Bonnì S, Ponzo V, Caltagirone C, Koch G. Cerebellar theta burst stimulation in stroke patients with ataxia. Funct Neurol. 2014;29(1):41–5.
21. Boylan LS, Sackeim HA. Magnetoelectric brain stimulation in the assessment of brain physiology and pathophysiology. Clin Neurophysiol. 2000;111(3):504–12.
22. Brittain JS, Probert-Smith P, Aziz TZ, Brown P. Tremor suppression by rhythmic transcranial current stimulation. Curr Biol. 2013;23(5):436–40.
23. Brunoni AR, Nitsche MA, Bolognini N, Bikson M, Wagner T, Merabet L, Edwards DJ, Valero-Cabre A, Rotenberg A, Pascual-Leone A, Ferrucci R, Priori A, Boggio PS, Fregni F. Clinical research with transcranial direct current stimulation (tDCS): challenges and future directions. Brain Stimul. 2012;5(3):175–95.
24. Burhan AM, Subramanian P, Pallaveshi L, Barnes B, Montero-Odasso M. Modulation of the left prefrontal cortex with high frequency repetitive transcranial magnetic stimulation facilitates gait in multiple sclerosis. Case Rep Neurol Med. 2015;2015:251829.
25. Buschman TJ, Denovellis EL, Diogo C, Bullock D, Miller EK. Synchronous oscillatory neural ensembles for rules in the prefrontal cortex. Neuron. 2012;76(4):838–46.
26. Caligiore D, Pezzulo G, Baldassarre G, Bostan AC, Strick PL, Doya K, Helmich RC, Dirkx M, Houk J, Jörntell H, Lago-Rodriguez A, Galea JM, Miall RC, Popa T, Kishore A, Verschure PF, Zucca R, Herreros I. Consensus paper: Towards a systems-level view of cerebellar function: the interplay between cerebellum, basal ganglia, and cortex. Cerebellum. 2016(Feb 13).
27. Cantarero G, Spampinato D, Reis J, Ajagbe L, Thompson T, Kulkarni K, Celnik P. Cerebellar direct current stimulation enhances on-line motor skill acquisition through an effect on accuracy. J Neurosci. 2015;35(7):3285–90.

28. Cevallos C, Zarka D, Hoellinger T, Leroy A, Dan B, Cheron G. Oscillations in the human brain during walking execution, imagination and observation. Neuropsychologia. 2015;79 (Pt B):223–32.
29. Chaieb L, Antal A, Paulus W. Transcranial alternating current stimulation in the low kHz range increases motor cortex excitability. Restor Neurol Neurosci. 2011;29(3):167–75.
30. Chaieb L, Antal A, Paulus W. Transcranial random noise stimulation-induced plasticity is NMDA-receptor independent but sodium-channel blocker and benzodiazepines sensitive. Front Neurosci. 2015;9:125.
31. Chang MC, Kim DY, Park DH. Enhancement of cortical excitability and lower limb motor function in patients with stroke by transcranial direct current stimulation. Brain Stimul. 2015;8(3):561–6.
32. Chen R. Studies of human motor physiology with transcranial magnetic stimulation. Muscle Nerve Suppl. 2000;9:S26–32.
33. Chen R, Udupa K. Measurement and modulation of plasticity of the motor system in humans using transcranial magnetic stimulation. Mot Control. 2009;13(4):442–53.
34. Chen CH, Fremont R, Arteaga-Bracho EE, Khodakhah K. Short latency cerebellar modulation of the basal ganglia. Nat Neurosci. 2014;17(12):1767–75.
35. Chou YH, Hickey PT, Sundman M, Song AW, Chen NK. Effects of repetitive transcranial magnetic stimulation on motor symptoms in Parkinson disease: a systematic review and meta-analysis. JAMA Neurol. 2015;72(4):432–40.
36. Collange Grecco LA, de Almeida Carvalho Duarte N, Mendonça ME, Galli M, Fregni F, Oliveira CS. Effects of anodal transcranial direct current stimulation combined with virtual reality for improving gait in children with spastic diparetic cerebral palsy: a pilot, randomized, controlled, double-blind, clinical trial. Clin Rehabil. 2015;29(12):1212–23.
37. Cosentino G, Fierro B, Vigneri S, Talamanca S, Paladino P, Baschi R, Indovino S, Maccora S, Valentino F, Fileccia E, Giglia G, Brighina F. Cyclical changes of cortical excitability and metaplasticity in migraine: evidence from a repetitive transcranial magnetic stimulation study. Pain. 2014;155(6):1070–8.
38. Costa-Ribeiro A, Maux A, Bosford T, Aoki Y, Castro R, Baltar A, Shirahige L, Filho AM, Nitsche MA, Monte-Silva K. Transcranial direct current stimulation associated with gait training in Parkinson's disease: a pilot randomized clinical trial. Dev Neurorehabil. 2016;10:1–8.
39. Crenna P, Frigo C. A motor programme for the initiation of forward-oriented movements in humans. J Physiol. 1991;437:635–53.
40. Danzl MM, Chelette KC, Lee K, Lykins D, Sawaki L. Brain stimulation paired with novel locomotor training with robotic gait orthosis in chronic stroke: a feasibility study. NeuroRehabilitation. 2013;33(1):67–76.
41. Davis NJ, van Koningsbruggen MG. "Non-invasive" brain stimulation is not non-invasive. Front Syst Neurosci. 2013;23(7):76.
42. del Olmo MF, Bello O, Cudeiro J. Transcranial magnetic stimulation over dorsolateral prefrontal cortex in Parkinson's disease. Clin Neurophysiol. 2007;118(1):131–9.
43. DeLong MR. Primate models of movement disorders of basal ganglia origin. Trends Neurosci. 1990;13(7):281–5.
44. Di Lazzaro V, Oliviero A, Pilato F, Saturno E, Dileone M, Mazzone P, Insola A, Tonali PA, Rothwell JC. The physiological basis of transcranial motor cortex stimulation in conscious humans. Clin Neurophysiol. 2004;115(2):255–66.
45. Di Lazzaro V. Biological effects of non-invasive brain stimulation. Handb Clin Neurol. 2013;116:367–74.
46. Dietz V. Do human bipeds use quadrupedal coordination? Trends Neurosci. 2002;25 (9):462–7.
47. Drew T, Prentice S, Schepens B. Cortical and brainstem control of locomotion. Prog Brain Res. 2004;143:251–61.
48. Duarte Nde A, Grecco LA, Galli M, Fregni F, Oliveira CS. Effect of transcranial direct-current stimulation combined with treadmill training on balance and functional

performance in children with cerebral palsy: a double-blind randomized controlled trial. PLoS ONE. 2014;9(8):e105777.
49. Dum RP, Strick PL. An unfolded map of the cerebellar dentate nucleus and its projections to the cerebral cortex. J Neurophysiol. 2003;89(1):634–9.
50. Edwards DJ, Krebs HI, Rykman A, Zipse J, Thickbroom GW, Mastaglia FL, Pascual-Leone A, Volpe BT. Raised corticomotor excitability of M1 forearm area following anodal tDCS is sustained during robotic wrist therapy in chronic stroke. Restor Neurol Neurosci. 2009;27 (3):199–207.
51. Sejdić E, Fu Y, Pak A, Fairley JA, Chau T. The effects of rhythmic sensory cues on the temporal dynamics of human gait. PLoS One. 2012;7(8):e43104.
52. Esposito MS, Capelli P, Arber S. Brainstem nucleus MdV mediates skilled forelimb motor tasks. Nature. 2014;508(7496):351–6.
53. Farzan F, Wu Y, Manor B, Anastasio EM, Lough M, Novak V, Greenstein PE, Pascual-Leone A. Cerebellar TMS in treatment of a patient with cerebellar ataxia: evidence from clinical, biomechanics and neurophysiological assessments. Cerebellum. 2013;12 (5):707–12.
54. Fasano A, Herzog J, Seifert E, et al. Modulation of gait coordination by subthalamic stimulation improves freezing of gait. Mov Disord. 2011;26:844–51.
55. Fedorov A, Chibisova Y, Szymaszek A, Alexandrov M, Gall C, Sabel BA. Non-invasive alternating current stimulation induces recovery from stroke. Restor Neurol Neurosci. 2010;28(6):825–33.
56. Fierro B, Giglia G, Palermo A, Pecoraro C, Scalia S, Brighina F. Modulatory effects of 1 Hz rTMS over the cerebellum on motor cortex excitability. Exp Brain Res. 2007;176(3):440–7.
57. Fierro B, Brighina F, D'Amelio M, Daniele O, Lupo I, Ragonese P, Palermo A, Savettieri G. Motor intracortical inhibition in PD: L-DOPA modulation of high-frequency rTMS effects. Exp Brain Res. 2008;184(4):521–8.
58. Frazzitta G, Pezzoli G, Bertotti G, Maestri R. Asymmetry and freezing of gait in parkinsonian patients. J Neurol. 2013;260(1):71–6.
59. Fregni F, Boggio PS, Mansur CG, Wagner T, Ferreira MJ, Lima MC, Rigonatti SP, Marcolin MA, Freedman SD, Nitsche MA, Pascual-Leone A. Transcranial direct current stimulation of the unaffected hemisphere in stroke patients. NeuroReport. 2005;16(14): 1551–5.
60. Fukuyama H, Ouchi Y, Matsuzaki S, Nagahama Y, Yamauchi H, Ogawa M, Kimura J, Shibasaki H. Brain functional activity during gait in normal subjects: a SPECT study. Neurosci Lett. 1997;228(3):183–6.
61. Galea JM, Jayaram G, Ajagbe L, Celnik P. Modulation of cerebellar excitability by polarity-specific noninvasive direct current stimulation. J Neurosci. 2009;29(28):9115–22.
62. Galea JM, Vazquez A, Pasricha N, de Xivry JJ, Celnik P. Dissociating the roles of the cerebellum and motor cortex during adaptive learning: the motor cortex retains what the cerebellum learns. Cereb Cortex. 2011;21(8):1761–70.
63. Geroin C, Picelli A, Munari D, Waldner A, Tomelleri C, Smania N. Combined transcranial direct current stimulation and robot-assisted gait training in patients with chronic stroke: a preliminary comparison. Clin Rehabil. 2011;25(6):537–48.
64. Ghiglieri V, Pendolino V, Sgobio C, Bagetta V, Picconi B, Calabresi P. Θ-burst stimulation and striatal plasticity in experimental parkinsonism. Exp Neurol. 2012;236(2):395–8.
65. Grecco LA, de Almeida Carvalho Duarte N, Mendonça ME, Cimolin V, Galli M, Fregni F, Santos Oliveira C. Transcranial direct current stimulation during treadmill training in children with cerebral palsy: a randomized controlled double-blind clinical trial. Res Dev Disabil. 2014a;35(11):2840–8.
66. Grecco LA, Duarte NA, Zanon N, Galli M, Fregni F, Oliveira CS. Effect of a single session of transcranial direct-current stimulation on balance and spatiotemporal gait variables in children with cerebral palsy: a randomized sham-controlled study. Braz J Phys Ther. 2014;18(5):419–27.
67. Groiss SJ, Ugawa Y. Cerebellar stimulation in ataxia. Cerebellum. 2012;11(2):440–2.

68. Guertin PA. The mammalian central pattern generator for locomotion. Brain Res Rev. 2009;62(1):45–56.
69. Hanakawa T, Katsumi Y, Fukuyama H, Honda M, Hayashi T, Kimura J, Shibasaki H. Mechanisms underlying gait disturbance in Parkinson's disease: a single photon emission computed tomography study. Brain. 1999;122(Pt 7):1271–82.
70. Hesse S, Werner C, Schonhardt EM, Bardeleben A, Jenrich W, Kirker SG. Combined transcranial direct current stimulation and robot-assisted arm training in subacute stroke patients: a pilot study. Restor Neurol Neurosci. 2007;25(1):9–15.
71. Hikosaka O, Takikawa Y, Kawagoe R. Role of the basal ganglia in the control of purposive saccadic eye movements. Physiol Rev. 2000;80(3):953–78.
72. Hoshi E, Tremblay L, Féger J, Carras PL, Strick PL. The cerebellum communicates with the basal ganglia. Nat Neurosci. 2005;8(11):1491–3.
73. Hou J, Nelson R, Nissim N, Parmer R, Thompson FJ, Bose P. Effect of combined treadmill training and magnetic stimulation on spasticity and gait impairments after cervical spinal cord injury. J Neurotrauma. 2014;31(12):1088–106.
74. Hua SE, Houk JC. Cerebellar guidance of premotor network development and sensorimotor learning. Learn Mem. 1997;4(1):63–76.
75. Huang YZ, Edwards MJ, Rounis E, Bhatia KP, Rothwell JC. Theta burst stimulation of the human motor cortex. Neuron. 2005;45(2):201–6.
76. Huang YZ, Chen RS, Rothwell JC, Wen HY. The after-effect of human theta burst stimulation is NMDA receptor dependent. Clin Neurophysiol. 2007;118(5):1028–32.
77. Inglis WL, Winn P. The pedunculopontine tegmental nucleus: where the striatum meets the reticular formation. Prog Neurobiol. 1995;47(1):1–29.
78. Iwata NK, Ugawa Y. The effects of cerebellar stimulation on the motor cortical excitability in neurological disorders: a review. Cerebellum. 2005;4(4):218–23.
79. Jahn K, Deutschländer A, Stephan T, Strupp M, Wiesmann M, Brandt T. Brain activation patterns during imagined stance and locomotion in functional magnetic resonance imaging. Neuroimage. 2004;22(4):1722–31.
80. Jahn K, Deutschländer A, Stephan T, Kalla R, Wiesmann M, Strupp M, Brandt T. Imaging human supraspinal locomotor centers in brainstem and cerebellum. Neuroimage. 2008;39 (2):786–92.
81. Jayaram G, Stinear JW. The effects of transcranial stimulation on paretic lower limb motor excitability during walking. J Clin Neurophysiol. 2009;26(4):272–9.
82. Jayaram G, Galea JM, Bastian AJ, Celnik P. Human locomotor adaptive learning is proportional to depression of cerebellar excitability. Cereb Cortex. 2011;21(8):1901–9.
83. Jayaram G, Tang B, Pallegadda R, Vasudevan EV, Celnik P, Bastian A. Modulating locomotor adaptation with cerebellar stimulation. J Neurophysiol. 2012;107(11):2950–7.
84. Johnsen EL, Mogensen PH, Sunde NA, Østergaard K. Improved asymmetry of gait in Parkinson's disease with DBS: gait and postural instability in Parkinson's disease treated with bilateral deep brain stimulation in the subthalamic nucleus. Mov Disord. 2009;24: 590–7.
85. Karabanov A, Ziemann U, Hamada M, George MS, Quartarone A, Classen J, Massimini M, Rothwell J, Siebner HR. Consensus paper: probing homeostatic plasticity of human cortex with non-invasive transcranial brain stimulation. Brain Stimul. 2015;8(5):993–1006.
86. Karayannidou A, Beloozerova IN, Zelenin PV, Stout EE, Sirota MG, Orlovsky GN, Deliagina TG. Activity of pyramidal tract neurons in the cat during standing and walking on an inclined plane. J Physiol. 2009;587(Pt 15):3795–811.
87. Kaski D, Dominguez RO, Allum JH, Bronstein AM. Improving gait and balance in patients with leukoaraiosis using transcranial direct current stimulation and physical training: an exploratory study. Neurorehabil Neural Repair. 2013;27(9):864–71.
88. Kaski D, Dominguez RO, Allum JH, Islam AF, Bronstein AM. Combining physical training with transcranial direct current stimulation to improve gait in Parkinson's disease: a pilot randomized controlled study. Clin Rehabil. 2014;28(11):1115–24.

89. Khedr EM, Farweez HM, Islam H. Therapeutic effect of repetitive transcranial magnetic stimulation on motor function in Parkinson's disease patients. Eur J Neurol. 2003;10(5): 567–72.
90. Kim WS, Jung SH, Oh MK, Min YS, Lim JY, Paik NJ. Effect of repetitive transcranial magnetic stimulation over the cerebellum on patients with ataxia after posterior circulation stroke: a pilot study. J Rehabil Med. 2014;46(5):418–23.
91. Kim MS, Hyuk Chang W, Cho JW, Youn J, Kim YK, Woong Kim S, Kim YH. Efficacy of cumulative high-frequency rTMS on freezing of gait in Parkinson's disease. Restor Neurol Neurosci. 2015;33(4):521–30.
92. Kobayashi M, Pascual-Leone A. Transcranial magnetic stimulation in neurology. Lancet Neurol. 2003;2(3):145–56.
93. Koch G, Mori F, Marconi B, Codecà C, Pecchioli C, Salerno S, Torriero S, Lo Gerfo E, Mir P, Oliveri M, Caltagirone C. Changes in intracortical circuits of the human motor cortex following theta burst stimulation of the lateral cerebellum. Clin Neurophysiol. 2008;119 (11):2559–69.
94. Koch G. Do studies on cortical plasticity provide a rationale for using non-invasive brain stimulation as a treatment for Parkinson's disease patients? Front Neurol. 2013 Nov 6;4:180.
95. Kojovic M, Bologna M, Kassavetis P, Murase N, Palomar FJ, Berardelli A, et al. Functional reorganization of sensorimotor cortex in early Parkinson disease. Neurology. 2012;78 (18):1441–8.
96. Kumru H, Benito J, Murillo N, Valls-Sole J, Valles M, Lopez-Blazquez R, Costa U, Tormos JM, Pascual-Leone A, Vidal J. Effects of high-frequency repetitive transcranial magnetic stimulation on motor and gait improvement in incomplete spinal cord injury patients. Neurorehabil Neural Repair. 2013;27(5):421–9.
97. Lajoie K, Drew T. Lesions of area 5 of the posterior parietal cortex in the cat produce errors in the accuracy of paw placement during visually guided locomotion. J Neurophysiol. 2007;97(3):2339–54.
98. Lajoie K, Bloomfield LW, Nelson FJ, Suh JJ, Marigold DS. The contribution of vision, proprioception, and efference copy in storing a neural representation for guiding trail leg trajectory over an obstacle. J Neurophysiol. 2012;107(8):2283–93.
99. Lee SY, Kim MS, Chang WH, Cho JW, Youn JY, Kim YH. Effects of repetitive transcranial magnetic stimulation on freezing of gait in patients with Parkinsonism. Restor Neurol Neurosci. 2014;32(6):743–53.
100. Lewek MD, Feasel J, Wentz E, Brooks FP Jr, Whitton MC. Use of visual and proprioceptive feedback to improve gait speed and spatiotemporal symmetry following chronic stroke: a case series. Phys Ther. 2012;92(5):748–56.
101. Li JY, Espay AJ, Gunraj CA, Pal PK, Cunic DI, Lang AE, Chen R. Interhemispheric and ipsilateral connections in Parkinson's disease: relation to mirror movements. Mov Disord. 2007;22(6):813–21.
102. Liebetanz D, Nitsche MA, Tergau F, Paulus W. Pharmacological approach to the mechanisms of transcranial DC-stimulation-induced after-effects of human motor cortex excitability. Brain. 2002;125(Pt 10):2238–47.
103. Lindenberg R, Renga V, Zhu LL, Nair D, Schlaug G. Bihemispheric brain stimulation facilitates motor recovery in chronic stroke patients. Neurology. 2010;75(24):2176–84.
104. Llinas R. Mechanisms of supraspinal actions upon spinal cord activities. Differences between reticular and cerebellar inhibitory actions upon alpha extensor motoneurons. J Neurophysiol. 1964;27:1117–26.
105. Lomarev MP, Kanchana S, Bara-Jimenez W, Iyer M, Wassermann EM, Hallett M. Placebo-controlled study of rTMS for the treatment of Parkinson's disease. Mov Disord. 2006;21 (3):325–31.
106. Luft AR, Macko RF, Forrester LW, Villagra F, Ivey F, Sorkin JD, Whitall J, McCombe-Waller S, Katzel L, Goldberg AP, Hanley DF. Treadmill exercise activates subcortical neural networks and improves walking after stroke: a randomized controlled trial. Stroke. 2008;39(12):3341–50.

107. Lum PS, Mulroy S, Amdur RL, Requejo P, Prilutsky BI, Dromerick AW. Gains in upper extremity function after stroke via recovery or compensation: Potential differential effects on amount of real-world limb use. Top Stroke Rehabil. 2009;16(4):237–53.
108. Madhavan S, Weber KA, Stinear JW. Non-invasive brain stimulation enhances fine motor control of the hemiparetic ankle: implications for rehabilitation. Exp Brain Res. 2011;209 (1):9–17.
109. Marchese R, Diverio M, Zucchi F, Lentino C, Abbruzzese G. The role of sensory cues in the rehabilitation of parkinsonian patients: a comparison of two physical therapy protocols. Mov Disord. 2000;15(5):879–83.
110. Mehta AR, Brittain JS, Brown P. The selective influence of rhythmic cortical versus cerebellar transcranial stimulation on human physiological tremor. J Neurosci. 2014;34 (22):7501–8.
111. Miyai I, Tanabe HC, Sase I, Eda H, Oda I, Konishi I, Tsunazawa Y, Suzuki T, Yanagida T, Kubota K. Cortical mapping of gait in humans: a near-infrared spectroscopic topography study. Neuroimage. 2001;14(5):1186–92.
112. Moliadze V, Antal A, Paulus W. Boosting brain excitability by transcranial high frequency stimulation in the ripple range. J Physiol. 2010;588(Pt 24):4891–904.
113. Moliadze V, Atalay D, Antal A, Paulus W. Close to threshold transcranial electrical stimulation preferentially activates inhibitory networks before switching to excitation with higher intensities. Brain Stimul. 2012;5(4):505–11.
114. Mori S, Matsui T, Kuze B, Asanome M, Nakajima K, Matsuyama K. Stimulation of a restricted region in the midline cerebellar white matter evokes coordinated quadrupedal locomotion in the decerebrate cat. J Neurophysiol. 1999;82(1):290–300.
115. Morris ME, Iansek R, Matyas TA, Summers JJ. The pathogenesis of gait hypokinesia in Parkinson's disease. Brain. 1994;117(Pt 5):1169–81.
116. Morton SM, Bastian AJ. Cerebellar contributions to locomotor adaptations during splitbelt treadmill walking. J Neurosci. 2006;26(36):9107–16.
117. Murray MP, Sepic SB, Gardner GM, Downs WJ. Walking patterns of men with parkinsonism. Am J Phys Med. 1978;57(6):278–94.
118. Naro A, Leo A, Russo M, Cannavò A, Milardi D, Bramanti P, Calabrò RS. Does transcranial alternating current stimulation induce cerebellum plasticity? Feasibility, safety and efficacy of a novel electrophysiological approach. Brain Stimul. 2016(Feb 12) (pii: S1935-861X(16) 30019-5).
119. Nieoullon A, Cheramy A, Glowinski J. Release of dopamine evoked by electrical stimulation of the motor and visual areas of the cerebral cortex in both caudate nuclei and in the substantia nigra in the cat. Brain Res. 1978;145(1):69–83.
120. Nitsche MA, Paulus W. Excitability changes induced in the human motor cortex by weak transcranial direct current stimulation. J Physiol. 2000;527(Pt 3):633–9.
121. Nitsche MA, Paulus W. Sustained excitability elevations induced by transcranial DC motor cortex stimulation in humans. Neurology. 2001;57(10):1899–901.
122. Nitsche MA, Fricke K, Henschke U, Schlitterlau A, Liebetanz D, Lang N, Henning S, Tergau F, Paulus W. Pharmacological modulation of cortical excitability shifts induced by transcranial direct current stimulation in humans. J Physiol. 2003;553(Pt 1):293–301.
123. Nitsche MA, Liebetanz D, Antal A, Lang N, Tergau F, Paulus W. Modulation of cortical excitability by weak direct current stimulation—technical, safety and functional aspects. Suppl Clin Neurophysiol. 2003;56:255–76.
124. Nitsche MA, Nitsche MS, Klein CC, Tergau F, Rothwell JC, Paulus W. Level of action of cathodal DC polarisation induced inhibition of the human motor cortex. Clin Neurophysiol. 2003;114(4):600–4.
125. Nitsche MA, Schauenburg A, Lang N, Liebetanz D, Exner C, Paulus W, Tergau F. Facilitation of implicit motor learning by weak transcranial direct current stimulation of the primary motor cortex in the human. J Cogn Neurosci. 2003;15(4):619–26.

126. Nitsche MA, Grundey J, Liebetanz D, Lang N, Tergau F, Paulus W. Catecholaminergic consolidation of motor cortical neuroplasticity in humans. Cereb Cortex. 2004;14(11): 1240–5.
127. Nitsche MA, Jaussi W, Liebetanz D, Lang N, Tergau F, Paulus W. Consolidation of human motor cortical neuroplasticity by D-cycloserine. Neuropsychopharmacology. 2004;29 (8):1573–8.
128. Nowak DA, Grefkes C, Ameli M, Fink GR. Interhemispheric competition after stroke: brain stimulation to enhance recovery of function of the affected hand. Neurorehabil Neural Repair. 2009;23(7):641–56.
129. Nutt JG, Marsden CD, Thompson PD. Human walking and higher-level gait disorders, particularly in the elderly. Neurology. 1993;43(2):268–79.
130. Oliveri M, Koch G, Torriero S, Caltagirone C. Increased facilitation of the primary motor cortex following 1 Hz repetitive transcranial magnetic stimulation of the contralateral cerebellum in normal humans. Neurosci Lett. 2005;376(3):188–93.
131. Palermo A, Fierro B, Giglia G, Cosentino G, Puma AR, Brighina F. Modulation of visual cortex excitability in migraine with aura: effects of valproate therapy. Neurosci Lett. 2009;467(1):26–9.
132. Penhune VB, Doyon J. Cerebellum and M1 interaction during early learning of timed motor sequences. Neuroimage. 2005;26(3):801–12.
133. Percheron G, François C, Talbi B, Yelnik J, Fénelon G. The primate motor thalamus. Brain Res Brain Res Rev. 1996;22(2):93–181.
134. Pfurtscheller G, Lopes da Silva FH. Event-related EEG/MEG synchronization and desynchronization: basic principles. Clin Neurophysiol. 1999;110(11):1842–57.
135. Picelli A, Chemello E, Castellazzi P, Roncari L, Waldner A, Saltuari L, Smania N. Combined effects of transcranial direct current stimulation (tDCS) and transcutaneous spinal direct current stimulation (tsDCS) on robot-assisted gait training in patients with chronic stroke: A pilot, double blind, randomized controlled trial. Restor Neurol Neurosci. 2015;33 (3):357–68.
136. Plotnik M, Giladi N, Balash Y, Peretz C, Hausdorff JM. Is freezing of gait in Parkinson's disease related to asymmetric motor function? Ann Neurol. 2005;57(5):656–63.
137. Plotnik M, Giladi N, Hausdorff JM. Bilateral coordination of walking and freezing of gait in Parkinson's disease. Eur J Neurosci. 2008;27(8):1999–2006.
138. Pogosyan A, Gaynor LD, Eusebio A, Brown P. Boosting cortical activity at Beta-band frequencies slows movement in humans. Curr Biol. 2009;19(19):1637–41.
139. Polanía R, Paulus W, Nitsche MA. Modulating cortico-striatal and thalamo-cortical functional connectivity with transcranial direct current stimulation. Hum Brain Mapp. 2012;33:2499–508.
140. Pozzi NG, Minafra B, Zangaglia R, De Marzi R, Sandrini G, Priori A, Pacchetti C. Transcranial direct current stimulation (tDCS) of the cortical motor areas in three cases of cerebellar ataxia. Cerebellum. 2014;13(1):109–12.
141. Priori A, Ciocca M, Parazzini M, Vergari M, Ferrucci R. Transcranial cerebellar direct current stimulation and transcutaneous spinal cord direct current stimulation as innovative tools for neuroscientists. J Physiol. 2014;592(16):3345–69.
142. Purpura DP, McMurtry JG. Intracellular activities and evoked potential changes during polarization of motor cortex. J Neurophysiol. 1965;28:166–85.
143. Rapinesi C, Janiri D, Kotzalidis GD, Serata D, Del Casale A, Scatena P, Dacquino C, Gentile G, Manfredi G, Danese E, Raccah RN, Brugnoli R, Callovini G, Ferri VR, Ferracuti S, Zangen A, Simmaco M, Angeletti G, Girardi P. Mitochondrial myopathy and comorbid major depressive disorder: effectiveness of dTMS on gait and mood symptoms. Gen Hosp Psychiatry. 2015;37(3):274.e7–9.
144. Ridding MC, Ziemann U. Determinants of the induction of cortical plasticity by non-invasive brain stimulation in healthy subjects. J Physiol. 2010;588(Pt 13):2291–304.
145. Rieke F. Spikes: exploring the neural code. Cambridge, MA: MIT Press; 1997.

146. Roche N, Lackmy A, Achache V, Bussel B, Katz R. Effects of anodal transcranial direct current stimulation over the leg motor area on lumbar spinal network excitability in healthy subjects. J Physiol. 2011;589(Pt 11):2813–26.
147. Rossini PM, Calautti C, Pauri F, Baron JC. Post-stroke plastic reorganisation in the adult brain. Lancet Neurol. 2003;2(8):493–502.
148. Sale MV, Ridding MC, Nordstrom MA. Factors influencing the magnitude and reproducibility of corticomotor excitability changes induced by paired associative stimulation. Exp Brain Res. 2007;181(4):615–26.
149. Schweighofer N, Arbib MA, Dominey PF. A model of the cerebellum in adaptive control of saccadic gain. I. The model and its biological substrate. Biol Cybern. 1996;75(1):19–28.
150. Seeber M, Scherer R, Wagner J, Solis-Escalante T, Müller-Putz GR. EEG beta suppression and low gamma modulation are different elements of human upright walking. Front Hum Neurosci. 2014;8:485.
151. Shi J, Liu J, Qu Q. Handedness and dominant side of symptoms in Parkinson's disease. Med Clin (Barc). 2014;142(4):141–4.
152. Shimizu H, Tsuda T, Shiga Y, Miyazawa K, Onodera Y, Matsuzaki M, Nakashima I, Furukawa K, Aoki M, Kato H, Yamazaki T, Itoyama Y. Therapeutic efficacy of transcranial magnetic stimulation for hereditary spinocerebellar degeneration. Tohoku J Exp Med. 1999;189(3):203–11.
153. Snijders AH, Leunissen I, Bakker M, et al. Gait-related cerebral alterations in patients with Parkinson's disease with freezing of gait. Brain. 2011;134:59–72.
154. Spagnolo F, Coppi E, Chieffo R, Straffi L, Fichera M, Nuara A. Interhemispheric balance in Parkinson's disease: a transcranial magnetic stimulation study. Brain Stimul. 2013;6(6): 892–7.
155. Stefan K, Kunesch E, Cohen LG, Benecke R, Classen J. Induction of plasticity in the human motor cortex by paired associative stimulation. Brain. 2000;123(Pt 3):572–84.
156. Strafella AP, Paus T, Barrett J, Dagher A. Repetitive transcranial magnetic stimulation of the human prefrontal cortex induces dopamine release in the caudate nucleus. J Neurosci. 2001;21:RC157 (4 pages).
157. Strafella AP, Paus T, Fraraccio M, Dagher A. Striatal dopamine release induced by repetitive transcranial magnetic stimulation of the human motor cortex. Brain. 2003;126:2609–15.
158. Strafella AP, Ko JH, Grant J, Fraraccio M, Monchi O. Corticostriatal functional interactions in Parkinson's disease: a rTMS/[11C]raclopride PET study. Eur J Neurosci. 2005;22: 2946–52.
159. Swann N, Tandon N, Canolty R, Ellmore TM, McEvoy LK, Dreyer S, DiSano M, Aron AR. Intracranial EEG reveals a time- and frequency-specific role for the right inferior frontal gyrus and primary motor cortex in stopping initiated responses. J Neurosci. 2009;29 (40):12675–85.
160. Tahtis V, Kaski D, Seemungal BM. The effect of single session bi-cephalic transcranial direct current stimulation on gait performance in sub-acute stroke: a pilot study. Restor Neurol Neurosci. 2014;32(4):527–32.
161. Takakusaki K, Habaguchi T, Ohtinata-Sugimoto J, Saitoh K, Sakamoto T. Basal ganglia efferents to the brainstem centers controlling postural muscle tone and locomotion: a new concept for understanding motor disorders in basal ganglia dysfunction. Neuroscience. 2003;119(1):293–308.
162. Takakusaki K, Saitoh K, Harada H, Kashiwayanagi M. Role of basal ganglia-brainstem pathways in the control of motor behaviors. Neurosci Res. 2004;50(2):137–51.
163. Terney D, Chaieb L, Moliadze V, Antal A, Paulus W. Increasing human brain excitability by transcranial high-frequency random noise stimulation. J Neurosci. 2008;28(52):14147–55.
164. Thoma P, Bellebaum C, Koch B, Schwarz M, Daum I. The cerebellum is involved in reward-based reversal learning. Cerebellum. 2008;7(3):433–43.
165. Traversa R, Cicinelli P, Pasqualetti P, Filippi M, Rossini PM. Follow-up of interhemispheric differences of motor evoked potentials from the 'affected' and 'unaffected' hemispheres in human stroke. Brain Res. 1998;803(1–2):1–8.

166. Turner RS, Anderson ME. Pallidal discharge related to the kinematics of reaching movements in two dimensions. J Neurophysiol. 1997;77(3):1051–74.
167. Ugawa Y, Day BL, Rothwell JC, Thompson PD, Merton PA, Marsden CD. Modulation of motor cortical excitability by electrical stimulation over the cerebellum in man. J Physiol. 1991;441:57–72.
168. Ugawa Y, Uesaka Y, Terao Y, Hanajima R, Kanazawa I. Magnetic stimulation over the cerebellum in humans. Ann Neurol. 1995;37(6):703–13.
169. Valentino F, Cosentino G, Brighina F, Pozzi NG, Sandrini G, Fierro B, Savettieri G, D'Amelio M, Pacchetti C. Transcranial direct current stimulation for treatment of freezing of gait: a cross-over study. Mov Disord. 2014;29(8):1064–9.
170. Verheyden G, Purdey J, Burnett M, Cole J, Ashburn A. Immediate effect of transcranial direct current stimulation on postural stability and functional mobility in Parkinsons disease. Mov Disord. 2013;28(14):2040–1.
171. Wagner J, Makeig S, Gola M, Neuper C, Müller-Putz G. Distinct β band oscillatory networks subserving motor and cognitive control during gait adaptation. J Neurosci. 2016;36 (7):2212–26.
172. Wang RY, Tseng HY, Liao KK, Wang CJ, Lai KL, Yang YR. rTMS combined with task-oriented training to improve symmetry of interhemispheric corticomotor excitability and gait performance after stroke: a randomized trial. Neurorehabil Neural Repair. 2012; 26(3):222–30.
173. Weerdesteyn V, de Niet M, van Duijnhoven HJ, Geurts AC. Falls in individuals with stroke. J Rehabil Res Dev. 2008;45(8):1195–213.
174. Whitton PS. Glutamatergic control over brain dopamine release in vivo and in vitro. Neurosci Biobehav Rev. 1997;21(4):481–8.
175. Wu AD, Petzinger GM, Lin CH, Kung M, Fisher B. Asymmetric corticomotor excitability correlations in early Parkinson's disease. Mov Disord. 2007;15;22(11):1587–93.
176. Wu T, Hallett M. The cerebellum in Parkinson's disease. Brain. 2013;136(Pt 3):696–709.
177. Yang YR, Tseng CY, Chiou SY, Liao KK, Cheng SJ, Lai KL, Wang RY. Combination of rTMS and treadmill training modulates corticomotor inhibition and improves walking in Parkinson disease: a randomized trial. Neurorehabil Neural Repair. 2013;27(1):79–86.
178. Yeo SS, Ahn SH, Choi BY, Chang CH, Lee J, Jang SH. Contribution of the pedunculopontine nucleus on walking in stroke patients. Eur Neurol. 2011;65(6):332–7.

Introducing a Surgical Procedure for an Implantable FES Device and Its Outcome

Kiriakos Daniilidis, Eike Jakubowitz and Daiwei Yao

1 Introduction

1.1 Causes of Drop Foot and Clinical Symptoms

The adult paralytic foot or drop foot is a secondary related foot deformity, which usually arises due to neurogenic damage [13, 26]. The lack of neural innervation of the muscles, which play a major role in ankle dorsiflexion—M. tibialis anterior, Mm. peronei, M. extensor digitorum longus, and M. extensor halluces longus—can cause a secondary malposition of the foot. As a dorsiflexion of the ankle cannot be actively provoked, this leads to a domination of the flexors and as a secondary outcome to a shortening of these muscles and their tendons. Similarly, it may also lead to a malposition in supination [16]. In general, an imbalance of agonist and antagonist can be expected, which can cause contractures and also subluxation in the bony foot architecture [4, 7]. It is vital to differentiate between contracture and a flexible deformity in the clinical examination, since this determines the subsequent therapeutic regimen [16]. The source for the neurological impairment can be central

K. Daniilidis (✉)
OTC Regensburg—Foot and Ankle Division, Paracelsusstrasse 2,
93053 Regensburg, Germany
e-mail: fusspraxisbayern@gmail.com

E. Jakubowitz
Laboratory for Biomechanics and Biomaterials (LBB) of the Orthopaedic Clinic
of the Medical School of Hannover, Hannover, Germany

D. Yao
Department of Orthopedic Surgery Diakovere Annastift, Medical School Hannover,
Hannover, Germany

G. Sandrini et al. (eds.), *Advanced Technologies for the Rehabilitation of Gait and Balance Disorders*, Biosystems & Biorobotics 19,
https://doi.org/10.1007/978-3-319-72736-3_27

or peripheral. Central lesions include stroke, multiple sclerosis, craniocerebral trauma or brain metastases [14]. All central lesions cause a motor deficit in the periphery. Injury of the pyramidal tract of the first motor neuron therefore produces spasticity of the muscles [8, 13, 14, 19, 26]. In contrast, flaccid paralysis impresses in the peripheral lesions. This circumstance is based on the damage to the lower motor neuron, which involves a damage location between the anterior horn cell of the spinal cord and the neuromuscular junction. Reasons for peripheral lesions include iatrogenic after surgery, post-polio syndrome or compartment syndrome. It is important to know that the peroneal nerve is still "active" in central lesions, but cannot be activated by missing signal transmission as the damage is located between the motor cortex and the spinal cord. Steppage gait is characteristic for foot drop. It is caused by missing foot dorsiflexion and the affected lower limb is relatively lengthened. This effects dragging toes along the ground and forces patients to lift their lower limb higher than usual to avoid stumbling. As a result an accommodative increased knee flexion and a circumductive leg swing during swing phase can be observed in affected patients (Fig. 1). Also a tiptoe walk on the opposite leg to equate the leg length may be characteristic for foot drop. All these circumstances induce an instable gait pattern, so that patients have to concentrate on walking while they looking at their feet to control each step.

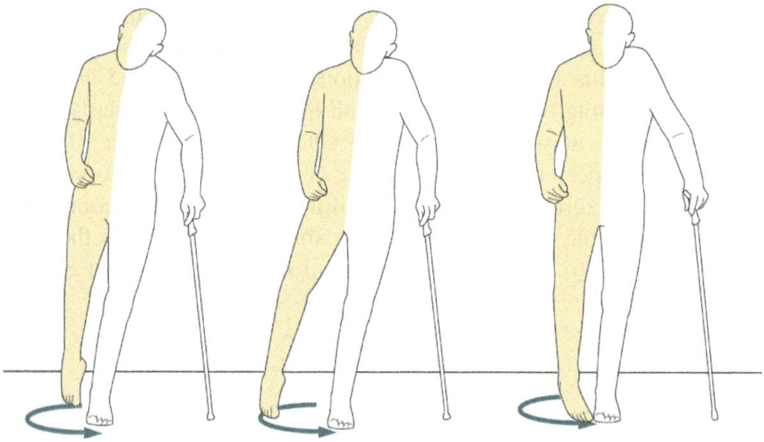

Fig. 1 In case of peroneal palsy a natural foot clearance and leg swing is not possible and the foot is remained in plantarflexion which increases the risk of stumbling or falling (left); During swing phase a higher knee flexion and/or an increased trunk deflection in order to raise the affected pelvis thus compensating the missing clearance can be observed. Likewise having the same purpose the leg is often just being moved forward with a circumductive compensating movement (middle). During stand phase ground contact usually can only be realized with either the forefoot or in plantigrade position at best (right)

1.2 Therapy Planning

The different therapeutic options must be decided individually for each patient according to existing spasticity, activity level, and patient's expectations. The factors mentioned here are essential for the entire postoperative outcome and also have a very strong influence on the patient's future life. In patients who are mobilized only in the domestic environment and spend the majority of time in a wheelchair or on crutches, conservative treatment should always the first choice. Surgical intervention can only make sense in these cases if, for example, the ability to stand is limited and the person concerned cannot execute transfer movements like from the wheelchair to the bed. Generally the aim of surgery is to produce an almost plantigrade position of the foot to the floor and restore walking ability. There are different surgical procedures ranging from the combination of soft tissue procedures and bony corrections through to implantation of neuroprostheses. It is vital substantial to make the correct indication in order to restore as much mobility as possible for the patients.

1.3 Former Therapy Concepts and Principle of FES

Treatment options for the reconstruction of dorsiflexion for drop foot are numerous. Earlier therapeutic concepts were based on the rigid resetting of the foot in the neutral position. The surgical treatment options include soft tissue procedures (e.g. tendon transfer), osteosynthetic intervention (e.g. arthrodesis) or combined methods. The classic conservative treatment of a drop foot is a treatment with an ankle-foot orthosis (AFO), which secures the foot in a plantigrade position. Most AFOs are made of a hard plastic brace. Incidentally, there are also orthoses with modifications, including those with a hinge joint in the ankle area. It could be shown that AFOs support dorsiflexion in the ankle during the swing phase and improve knee stability in early stance [9, 18]. However, AFOs cause essential disadvantages that include limited ankle mobility, favoring a contracture, and poor mobilization from sitting to standing [5, 10, 12]. Likewise aesthetic deficiencies, lack of comfort, and shoe conflict should not be ignored. Due to the rigid resetting of the foot in a plantigrade position no dynamic component adaptation of the foot to physiological motion sequences is possible with these therapeutic concepts. Functional electrical stimulation has been proven in the last 10 years as a new therapeutic approach [17, 22, 23, 25, 27]. The advantage of these systems is the dynamic treatment component by nerve stimulation, whereby the dorsiflexion can be trained intensely and constantly. Therefore the system can provide a positive feedback to the patients (biofeedback). Recent FES systems to treat drop foot consist of a heel switch and a cuff, which includes electrodes and stimulator. A cuff with surface electrodes is fitted to the lower leg, such that the electrodes are positioned over the nerve correctly. A wireless heel switch, worn in a special sock, is needed to differentiate between stance and swing phase during gait, and acts simply as an ON/OFF signal. It detects when the leg is lifted to take a step and correctly controls the timing of the stimulation. This signal is wirelessly transmitted to the battery-powered control unit and stimulator, held in the cuff. According to individually adjusted time parameters referenced to the switch signal, the stimulator emits the stimulation signal via the surface electrodes. In this way the muscles responsible for foot lift are activated and improve the walking pattern. Usually a wireless or other kind of remote control belongs to a recent FES system, which allows the user to adjust the settings to suit daily needs. Furthermore, current FES systems include a multi-channel electrode so that additional functional muscle groups can be stimulated (e.g. the knee or hip) to support a more natural gait.

1.4 Indication for FES and Implantable FES

An intact peroneal nerve in patients with a central lesion is extremely important to ensure a successful FES therapy. Therefore the nerve conduction and conduction velocity of the N. peroneus should be measured and assured in advance by a nerve conduction study. Furthermore, an increased tone or spasticity in the muscles opposite the anterior tibialis should be excluded or otherwise suitably treated with Achilles tendon lengthening or gastrocnemius release in order to obtain a good clinical outcome. The pulse for nerve stimulation is transmitted through the skin by electrodes, which are usually placed superficially in the in form of a sleeve. As a result external electrical stimulation may cause skin irritations. Another factor that should be considered is that patients with a central lesion often suffer from hemiplegia, whereby the independent use and handling of the device prove problematic in everyday life. One approach to this problem provides the surgical implantation of a neuroprosthesis. To the best of our knowledge only one recent device has been approved for clinical use, ActiGait® (Otto Bock, Duderstadt). The principle of this neuroprosthesis is related to the superficial functional electrical stimulation and is based on stimulation of the motor branch of the common peroneal nerve. It is a hybrid system consisting of internal and external components (Fig. 2). External components include a heel switch and a control unit. Implantable components of the ActiGait® system consist of a stimulator implanted in the lateral thigh subcutaneously and a cuff electrode placed around the peroneal nerve directly. Analogous to the surface FES the heel switch detects stance and swing phase during gait cycle by floor contact. This information is sent to the control unit. Unlike the surface FES, the control unit is usually worn on a waist belt. Based on this information the control unit sends a stimulation pulse according to individually adjusted time parameters to an induction coil fixated to the skin surface of the ipsilateral thigh. Due to the magnetic field this transmitter induces a pulse via antenna to the receiver of a subcutaneously implanted stimulation unit. This interface represents the connection between external and internal components. The stimulation unit with a multi-channel system consisting of twelve electrodes allows a direct and

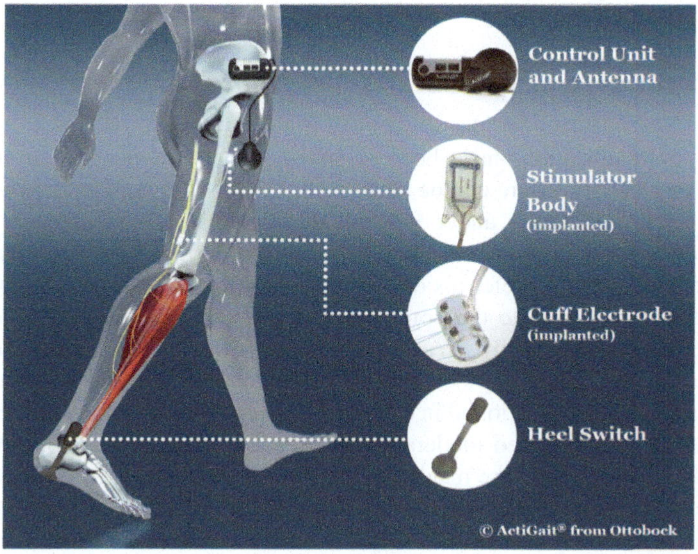

Fig. 2 Components of the drop foot stimulator: External components include the control unit with antenna and the heel switch. Internal components consist of the subcutaneously implanted stimulator and the stimulation cuff electrode (d) positioned directly to the peroneal nerve

differentiated stimulation of the motor branch of the peroneal nerve. In this way a balanced dorsiflexion with the correct amount of pronation and supination can be justified and lower amperage can be used in comparison to the surface FES. Besides preventing skin irritation, the implantation of the electrodes eliminates the difficult handling in daily life. As the principle of this neuroprosthesis is related to the superficial functional electrical stimulation, the following analogous indication criteria and contraindications exist for the use of an implantable neuroprosthesis (Table 1).

Table 1 Inclusion and exclusion criteria for an implantable FES

Inclusion criteria	Exclusion criteria
Drop foot by upper motor neuron disease	Peripheral nerve damage
Fully grown—older than 18	Pregnancy
Passive ROM of the affected ankle joint	Poorly controlled epilepsy
Ability to walk short distance without help of another person	Implanted defibrillators or pacemakers
Positive response to surface FES	Thickness of subcutaneous adipose layer in the thigh exceeding 40 mm

2 Surgical Procedure

2.1 Preparation of Patient and Landmarks

After all contraindications have been excluded and all preoperative arrangements done the surgical procedure can be performed. Usually the implantation of internal components is performed under general anesthesia. After the patient has been narcotized the lairing can be executed. An adequate lairing is essential for the later surgical procedure. We prefer a side lairing and softly padded operation table. For this the patient is turned to the non-surgical side so that the surgical side is positioned upwards and is easily accessible; especially the foot and ankle have to be laired in a way that guarantees enough space for motion. Hip and knee joint of the non-operated side are positioned in 0° till 10° flexion while hip and knee joint of the contralateral side are flexed moderately in circa 20°–30°. Furthermore, it must be ensured that critical spots are padded softly to prevent nerve or vessel damage due to incorrect lairing. Critical spots in our opinion are the lateral malleus and fibula head with N. peroneus of the non-surgical side, as well as the medial side of the surgical knee. To prevent lairing damage a gel pillow is put between both legs. Additionally a half soft roll is placed under the armpit of the non-surgical side to avoid plexus harm. To secure the side lairing, the back and the abdomen is fixed softly by padded kickstand. After a correct lairing has been confirmed and excess hair removed, the surgical leg including ankle and foot should be prepared sterilely with an approved disinfectant agent. Afterwards the non-surgical body parts are covered with sterile drapes, leaving the knee and lower thigh exposed and the surgical foot draped in transparent sterile foil.

Before making an incision it is essential to identify the landmarks needed for the surgery. First the fibula head should be found and indicated. Then the silhouette of the proximal edge of the tibia should be marked with a dotted line. Perpendicular to this line a second line with a length 8 cm has to be drafted parallel to the M. biceps femoris tendon in the proximal direction. The second line should be drafted with a gap of circa 1–2 cm medial to the M. biceps femoris tendon. It is absolutely crucial to identify the biceps femoris tendon correctly and not to mistake it for the tractus iliotibialis. This line marks the later skin incision. It is crucial that this skin incision should not be made too medial, as it will negatively affect the preparation and sight of the N. peroneus. In skinny patients the gap to the biceps tendon should be narrowed. If the incision line is extended by a further 4 cm proximally the landmark for the exit point of the tunneling will be obtained. The implantation position for the stimulator unit is 26 cm (if the stimulator is to be positioned upside down) or 28 cm away from the proximal tibia edge, at the middle third of the ventrolateral part of the thigh and should be marked.

2.2 Exposure of the Common Peroneal Nerve

After all marks are positioned correctly, the incision can be made along the incision line as mentioned above. It is important that the incision is made proximal to the knee fold and not through this fold. The skin edges are elevated with small hooks and the tissue is dissected along the biceps tendon. Next the thin subcutaneous fascia layer is opened and the peroneal nerve can be identified approximately 1–2 cm below the skin surface. A deep dissection is not recommended as the surgeon may reach the tibial nerve by mistake. If bleeding control is needed only bipolar coagulation should be used, as monopolar coagulation close to the nerve may induce permanent nerve lesions. Once the peroneal nerve has been identified distally in the operative field, a vessel loop should be placed around it. If magnification is used, the peroneal nerve can often be seen through the fascia layer of the biceps tendon, as this runs in a transverse fashion. Under slight retraction of the loop, the nerve can be followed and exposed with small scissors in a proximal direction, as the nerve runs along the biceps tendon. The nerve fuses into a larger trunk carrying motor fibers and one or two smaller sensory branches (N. cutaneus surae lateralis). If necessary, supplementary vessel loops can be placed on each branch to separate them. Now the common peroneal nerve can be cleaned from connective tissue flaps over a distance of 4–5 cm. The perineurium or epineurium should not be unnecessarily harmed during this step. If there are difficulties with identifying the peroneal nerve or distinguishing between sensory and motor fibers then it can be useful to apply electrical stimulation with an intraoperative nerve stimulator (GN 015; maximum 6 V, 10 mA, 2.5 Hz; Aesculap, Germany). Splitting the sensory branches of the common peroneal nerve is indicated, if it is not possible to exclude the sensory branches from the cuff, because including the sensory branch inside the cuff may lead to decreased stimulatory effectiveness or discomfort in the foot during stimulation. Microsurgical techniques should be applied in this part of the surgery. The reverse side of the nerve should certainly be checked as well. During preparation the nerve and operative field must be kept continuously moist with saline.

2.3 Selecting the Right Cuff Electrode Size

There are four cuff electrode sizes the with following diameters: 4.5, 5.4, 6.4 and 7.6 mm. A nerve measurement tool should be used to determine the right size. The tool is a plexiglass handle with a silicone tube attached perpendicularly at the tip. During measurement the nerve should be relaxed and not to be stretched. To determine the correct flap size, the measurement tool should be put underneath the common peroneal nerve and be wrapped around it. The flap edges should be closed gently. If the flap edges of the measurement tool close completely, the tool should be slid along the exposed part to ensure the correct size over the entire distance. The smallest nerve measurement tool that can close around the nerve determines the correct cuff size. Oversize in excess of 50% is only acceptable with the smallest cuff size. Choosing the right cuff is a crucial surgical step, as a too small cuff size can lead to nerve damage and an oversized cuff can lead to decreased stimulatory effectiveness.

2.4 Thigh Incision

The thigh incision should be marked correctly to ensure the cable is tension-free between the stimulator body and the cuff. Tractus iliotibialis is an important landmark in this surgical step. The thigh incision for the stimulator body should be made laterally on the thigh while being careful not to place the incision too anterior or too posterior to the tractus iliotibialis. A too anterior position may lead to excessive mechanical strain on the electrode cable. A too posterior position may lead to damage of the implant in sitting positions. As mentioned above, a maximum distance of 26 or 28 cm from the proximal tibia edge should be measured depending on the implanting position. Limiting the distance to 26 cm is recommended, if an upside- down implanting position is chosen. The final implant should be placed in a position that allows a slack, tension-free electrode cable path. Use of a demo implant is recommended to determine this position. The demo implant should therefore not exceed the marking in the proximal direction. Once the correct position has been determined, the incision should be marked. The incision length and location should allow the stimulator body to be fixed into place by stitching it to the fascia. After making the skin incision, a pocket for the stimulator body can be dissected with the index finger. For patients with a thicker layer of subcutaneous fat, the incision may be moved more distally or in a more anterior direction to get a position with subcutaneous fat layer no thicker than 4 cm, as the external transmitter antenna has a maximum operating range of 4 cm.

2.5 Tunneling

One of the key factors to a successful implantation is to ensure that the electrode cable follows a path parallel to the peroneus nerve in the cuff electrode vicinity. Due to anatomical constraints (biceps femoris muscle) this cannot be achieved with straight tunneling between the two incisions. The tunnel direction therefore needs to be controlled from both the distal and proximal incision and the tunneling path adapted accordingly. The distal end of the tunnel is about 4 cm proximal to the proximal end of the knee incision, which was used for preparing the common peroneal nerve. This point will guide the tunneling from the proximal direction. Next the boundary between the subcutaneous adipose tissue and the muscle fascia at the proximal end of the knee incision should be identified, and a distal tunnel between these layers should be prepared by inserting an index finger. The resulting tunnel should build a prolongation of the nerve path allowing a parallel routing of the electrode cable to the nerve within the knee incision. The final position of the fingertip may deviate from the mark set above. In this case aim for the fingertip. Now the insertion tool should be inserted into the thigh incision and led in between the muscle fascia and the subcutaneous adipose tissue oblique to the leg towards the tip of the finger in the distal tunnel end. Once the tip reaches the finger, the direction of the tunneling must be adapted so that the tunneling path becomes parallel to the nerve. Tunneling through the previously prepared distal tunnel should be continued towards the proximal end of the knee incision until few centimeters of the transparent tube is visible. After that the tip of the insertion tool should be eased and removed, leaving the insertion tube in the tunnel. In general, the outcome of tunneling should result in the tunnel exiting at the proximal end of the knee incision in order to allow the electrode cable to follow the peroneal nerve for about 10 cm proximally to the cuff and to cross the biceps femoris muscle following a smooth path.

2.6 Placing the Implant

The implant is passed through the tunnel by placing the electrode and electrode cable inside the wire guide with the sutures downwards at one end and the stimulator body on the other end. The cable must not be rotated at all during this step. Next the wire guide is led into the insertion tube beginning at the tight incision until the cuff electrode is visible at the knee incision. After that the wire guide should be removed distally, leaving the cuff and electrode cable in the insertion tube, visible at the knee incision. If the cuff and electrode cable are not visible then the entire implant should be removed from the insertion tube and the procedure repeated to ensure that no rotation or torsion of the cable has occurred. Finally, the insertion tube should be pulled out distally, leaving the electrode cable in the subcutaneous tunnel. Now the stimulator body should be inserted into the previously created subcutaneous pocket, with the curved side facing out towards the skin. The side showing the manufacturer and product name must face inwards. The cuff electrode on the peroneal nerve should be at least 10 mm from nerve branching and at least 25 mm from the tibial plateau. The cuff electrode is placed around the peroneal nerve by opening the cuff electrode and carefully pulling the sets of sutures on each side. Next the sutures of one side should be led under the nerve and the cuff should be placed around the nerve by carefully rotating it. Then the sutures should be closed by surgical knots. The two most distal sutures are therefore separated by cutting off the ends next to the knots. This set of sutures is tied with surgical double knot and the electrode edges are aligned and secured by three supplementary single knots. The suture ends are cut, leaving ca. 3 mm of free ends. This procedure is repeated until all sutures have been tied. During tying excessive force on the sutures should be avoided at all times as the sutures can be pulled out from the silicone. Once the sutures have been tied the knots of the electrode face outwards. Therefore the cuff should be turned around the nerve in such a way that the knots are buried deep under the nerve and the electrode cable exits on the side facing the skin, in a gentle curvature, following the path of the nerve as far as possible. As the leg is usually positioned in a bent position during surgery, a knee extension-flexion test must be performed to ensure a correctly positioned cuff electrode. During this procedure, the nerve is pulled through the cuff electrode by typically 5–10 mm. The knee should be slowly extended while the displacement of the cuff is observed. When extending the knee, the cuff electrode must not get trapped in a nerve bifurcation. If the initial positioning of the cuff is too close to the branching of the nerve, the electrode will end up hanging in it, which may lead to a nerve injury. It is important that no stress or tension is exerted on the nerve by the electrode cable once the device is in place. If necessary, cuff electrode and electrode cable should be repositioned. Once the correct position has been secured physiological saline should be injected into the cuff to ensure that no air or other tissue is trapped inside the cuff. This should preferably be done using a syringe.

2.7 Final Check and Closing the Incisions

The proper functioning of the implant should be tested before the implantation is completed and the skin closed. This is done by activating the stimulator with the control unit while the antenna is covered in sterile drape. During this step the control unit and antenna are held just above the stimulator body, inducing a cyclic training mode. This stimulation should provoke an ankle dorsiflexion and that demonstrates a perfect functioning. At this point how the foot moves is not relevant but a strong dorsiflexion should occur. If intraoperative testing is successful, the surgical procedure can be continued. However, if the testing is not successful, the cause of malfunction should be found and rectified. Possible reasons and proposed solutions are listed in Table 2.

After a perfect functioning is ensured the stimulator body can be fixed in the tight. Therefore not-resolvable 2-0 monofilament suture material should be used. The sutures should be placed through the suture holes and be stitched to the fascia. First, fix the stimulator body into place by suturing one single hole. Secondly, repeat the knee extension-flexion test. If the electrode cable still remains in a relaxed position during the knee extension-flexion test, the remaining holes can be secured by sutures. During fixation it is important to avoid damaging the silicone with the needle or very tight suturing. Depending on the particular operative situation and the patient's individual anatomy, it can be indicated to place sutures to create a small pocket of connective tissue. The stimulator body is thus sealed inside this pocket of connective tissue and is prevented from "floating" around. For closing the incisions a three-layer closure is recommended in the knee incision, as this decreases electrode cable kinking. Closing wound dead space by suture is

Table 2 Possible reasons for a malfunction and suggested solutions

Effect	Possible cause of malfunction	Suggested solution
No effect of stimulation	Transmitter antenna is too far away from implant	Antenna transmitting range must not exceed 4 cm. Probably implant is too deep under skin. Reduce the distance between stimulator and antenna and repeat testing again
No effect of stimulation	Implant malfunction	If the nerve can be stimulated by the intraoperative testing device and it is positively concluded that the control unit is active and the antenna transmitting range is correct, a malfunctioning implant is likely. In this case, remove implant and repeat surgical procedure
Poor effect of stimulation	Air or other tissue inside cuff and electrodes not isolated from the nerve	Flush the inside of the cuff with saline and repeat surgical step
No stimulation	Control unit does not transmit	Ensure correct control unit mode and correctly set stimulation parameters. All channels should preferably be set at maximum intensity
No dorsal flexion during stimulation	Cuff positioned on purely sensory nerve	Verify the nerve quality by using intraoperative nerve stimulator. If no foot movement is seen it is most likely a purely sensory nerve. Entire surgical procedure should be repeated and the motor nerve should be found
Plantar flexion	Cuff may have been placed on N. tibialis by mistake	Remove all of implant and repeat entire procedure of positioning cuff electrode around peroneal nerve

therefore endorsed. The subcutaneous layer should closed by using buried knots. Skin closure in knee and tight can be performed by intra-cutaneous closure or other comparable techniques. It is important to ensure that no cuff electrode or electrode cable are fixed with sutures.

2.8 Postoperative Care

In general, extreme knee flexion and excessive cable bending should be avoided until connective tissue ingrowth ensures cuff fixation. Repeated pull of the peroneal nerve in this period can result in nerve swelling and even compression neuropathy. In our department, patients are not allowed to bend the knee over 30° until the wounds are completely closed and sutures are removed, which equals a period of 12–14 days. Orthosis (0°) is therefore used during mobilization with a locked knee. Full weight bearing is allowed. Furthermore, knee flexion over 90° is not recommended for six weeks after surgery. Our patients have a mean clinical stay of about 5–6 days. During this period postoperative X-ray monitoring is performed. For this we usually use a radiograph of tight and knee in two planes. The proper positioning of the implant can be shown in a scaled X-ray image and is be 25–75 mm proximal to the tibial plateau. If a scaled radiograph is not possible, the cuff length can be taken as a reference. As a rule of thumb, the distal end of the cuff electrode should be placed between 1.5 and 3 cuff lengths proximal from the tibial plateau. Three weeks after surgery the implants are activated and adjustments are usually made with 1.1 mA, 20–30 Hz and an optimal impulse duration of 70 µs. Readjusting the impulse intensity with a patient programmer to produce a harmonious physiological gait pattern is performed over the course of time.

3 Outcome

3.1 *Own Findings*

As part of a retrospective study we investigated 21 patients (13 m/8 w) suffered from a chronic drop foot with at least six months duration who were treated with the implantable drop foot stimulator from June 2013 to August 2015. All patients showed a weak dorsiflexion due to a central lesion (stroke), a passive mobility of the ankle (at least ext./flex. 0°–5°–20°) and were able to walk a distance of at least 100 m with or without further walking aids. An external FES (Ness L300®, Bioness Inc. United States/MyGait®, OttoBock, Duderstadt, Germany) on the peroneal nerve was performed prior to surgery in order to ensure an unimpaired conductivity of the peroneal nerve and the indication of the implantable stimulator. Patient specific parameters at time of investigation can be taken from Table 3.

Table 3 Patient characteristics at screening

Characteristics				
	n	Mean	SD	Range
Age in years	21	52.8	9.3	33–73
Stroke onset in months	21	80.2	61.7	22–276
Follow up time in months	21	12.5	6.9	3–27
Gender				
Male	13			
Female	8			
Side of lesion				
Left	11			
Right	10			
Reason of lesion				
Ischemic	15			
Hemorrhagic	6			

All surgeries were done without any complications. A percutaneous Achilles tendon extension was necessary in four patients to ensure a sufficient dorsiflexion. To avoid stumbling two of them were additionally treated with an ipsilateral toe arthrodesis due to hallux malleus. None of the surgeries needed to be revised. We had no case of postoperative bleeding, although thrombosis prevention was performed in all patients with daily injections of Certoparin until full weight bearing was possible. Adjustments of the stimulator were performed without any complication 3 weeks after surgery. Usually, the channels 1 and/or 4 were used to stimulate motor fibers. Handling of the stimulator was always described as being uncomplicated during daily living. Up to date no technical failures of implanted components could be recognized within the cohort. In two cases the control units had to be replaced. One was lost and another one was destroyed during falling down by a closing car door. The external heel switch had to be replaced in 17 from 21 subjects due to broken protective rubber covers. Our patients reported a daily or at least every second day charging of the control unit.

After a mean follow up from 12.5 ± 6.9 months we measured walking speed, gait endurance and gait performance by the 10 m Walk Test (10 MWT), 6 min Walk Test (6 MWT) and the Emory Functional Ambulation Profile (EFAP), respectively. All tests were performed in turned-on and turned-off stimulation. In general, we could achieved significantly improvements in walking speed, gait endurance and gait performance by nearly 33, 45 and 40%, respectively. The results are listed in Table 4. Furthermore, we could note down a very high patient satisfaction. So 95% of the patient were satisfied or very satisfied with the postoperative situation, while 90% reported an improvement in quality of life.

Table 4 Test results with and without ActiGait® stimulation

Test results			
	Without ActiGait stimulation	With ActiGait stimulation	*P* Value
10 MWT (s)	11.8 ± 5.4 (5.4–19.9)	7.9 ± 3.4 (3.9–17.8)	0.007
6 MWT (m)	212.2 ± 75.5 (127.5–333)	306.4 ± 96.4 (174.5–487)	≤0.001
EFAP total (s)	105.9 ± 49.7 (49.4–194.7)	63.2 ± 31.3 (32.6–141.88)	≤0.001
EFAP floor time	11.5 ± 6.8 (5.3–26.9)	6.2 ± 2.3 (3.2–13.2)	≤0.001
EFAP carpet time	15.1 ± 9.1 (6.3–38.3)	8.2 ± 3.8 (4.2–15.9)	≤0.001
EFAP TUG	21.8 ± 10.2 (12.0–45.3)	14.3 ± 6.3 (7.8–32.4)	0.005
EFAP OC	36.6 ± 19.4 (15.5–73.4)	23.1 ± 10.1 (12.6–48.7)	0.011
EFAP stair time	20.7 ± 8.5 (10.2–40.9)	15.6 ± 6.9 (8.58–33.91)	0.038

Abbrevations 10 MWT: 10-meter Walk test; 6 MWT: 6-minute Walk test; EFAP: Emory Functional Ambulation Profile; TUG: Timed up and Go; OC: Obstacle Course

3.2 Comparison with Current Literature

Our findings confirmed the fact that the implantation of the neuroprosthesis is poor in intra- and postoperative complications as described in former studies [2, 3, 6, 15]. In our cohort only one postoperative hematoma was documented, unlike the studies from Burridge and Martin where also wound healing deficit and postoperative infection were described [2, 23]. Possible nerve injuries were not recorded fortunately.

With an increase of 49.4% the present study shows a significant improvement of the walking speed and therefore represents a comparable result with recent findings [1, 11, 24]. In their study with implantable stimulator Martin et al. described an improvement of walking speed by 47.2% [15]. In comparable studies regarding surface FES improvements of gait speed were described by Hausdorff and Ring with 34% after 8 weeks, by Bethoux et al. with 41.4% after 6 months and by Stein et al. with 37.8% after 11 months of use [1, 11, 24]. We achieved a mean walking speed with 1.27 m/s in activated stimulator which represented the highest walking speed in comparison to the above-mentioned studies and even surpassed the walking speed in the study from Martin by 0.23 m/s, while a walking speed over 0.9 m/s could not be assessed in the studies with surface FES [1, 15]. We explained this fact that a considerable orthotic effect with more physiological kinematics in the lower limb can better be achieved by an implantable stimulator due a direct positioned cuff electrode around the peroneal nerve which allows a more specific stimulation with more precise adjustability of the stimulation parameters compared with surface stimulation [15]. Furthermore we recorded the highest walking speed with 0.85 m/s in deactivated stimulation after a follow up time of 12.5 months. This circumstance can be interpreted that a persistent use of the stimulator may have a training impact of the gait pattern. As expected due better adaption to physiological gait pattern, gait endurance improved significantly by 44.4%, a comparable result to the findings from Martin et al. [15]. To the best of our knowledge, EFAP has not been performed for patients treated with implantable stimulator. Martin et al. assessed only the timed up-and-go test, which is a subtask in EFAP, in his study with a significant improvement by 48.2%. We assessed a 34.1% improvement which also meant significant enhancement. Related to the original study from Podsialo and Richardson our achieved time with an average of 14.34 s represented mild mobility impairment (11–19 s) [21]. Generally we documented a 40.3% improvement in EFAP total score, while only an improvement by 16.16% was described in the work from Bethoux et al. with surface FES after 6 months of use [1]. But it has to be mentioned that while Bethoux used multipliers in his work we measured without assistance factors [1]. Wolf et al. described a total time of 97.48 s without assistance factors although AFO and other assistive devices were allowed to use [28]. In comparison to this result we could achieve a 35.2% improvement with ActiGait® stimulation (63.17–97.48 s) and a marked convergence to the standard which was determined with 33.35 s in the control group [28].

The validity of our findings is limited due its retrospective study design. Because of the physical strain by exercising the clinical tests and the general limited fatigue of stroke patients it has to be considered that the presented results are depended to the daily physical activity at the time of examination. Furthermore it has to be noted that the examined patients had stroke related physical handicaps in different manifestation.

References

1. Bethoux F, Rogers HL, Nolan KJ, Abrams GM, Annaswamy TM, Brandstater M, et al. The effects of peroneal nerve functional electrical stimulation versus ankle-foot orthosis in patients with chronic stroke: a randomized controlled trial. Neurorehabil Neural Repair. 2014;28: 688–9.
2. Burridge JH, Haugland M, Larsen B, Svaneborg N, Iversen HK, Christensen PB, et al. Patients' perceptions of the benefits and problems of using the ActiGait implanted drop-foot stimulator. J Rehabil Med. 2008;40:873–5.
3. Burridge JH, Haugland M, Larsen B, Pickering RM, Svaneborg N, Iversen HK, et al. Phase II trial to evaluate the ActiGait implanted drop-foot stimulator in established hemiplegia. J Rehabil Med. 2007;39:212–8.
4. Cheng PT, Chen CL, Wang CM, Hong WH. Leg muscle activation patterns of sit-to-stand movement in stroke patients. Am J Phys Med Rehabil. 2004;83:10–6.
5. Doğan A, Mengüllüoğlu M, Özgirgin N. Evaluation of the effect of ankle-foot orthosis use on balance and mobility in hemiparetic stroke patients. Disabil Rehabil. 2011;33:1433–9.
6. Ernst J, Grundey J, Hewitt M, von Lewinski F, Kaus J, Schmalz T, et al. Towards physiological ankle movements with the ActiGait implantable drop foot stimulator in chronic stroke. Restor Neurol Neurosci. 2013;31:557–69.
7. Fatone S, Gard SA, Malas BS. Effect of ankle-foot orthosis alignment and foot-plate length on the gait of adults with poststroke hemiplegia. Arch Phys Med Rehabil. 2009;90:810–8.
8. Feigin VL, Lawes CM, Bennett DA, Barker-Collo SL, Paraq V. Worldwide stroke incidence and early case fatality reported in 56 population-based studies: a systematic review. Lancet Neurol. 2009;8:355–69.
9. Franceschini M, Massucci M, Ferrari L, Agosti M, Paroli C. Effects of an ankle-foot orthosis on spatiotemporal parameters and energy cost of hemiparetic gait. Clin Rehabil. 2003; 17:368–72.
10. Given JD, Dewald JP, Rymer WZ. Joint dependent passive stiffness in paretic and contralateral limbs of spastic patients with hemiparetic stroke. J Neurol Neurosurg Psychiatry. 1995;59:271–9.
11. Hausdorff JM, Ring H. Effects of a new radio frequency-controlled neuroprosthesis on gait symmetry and rhythmicity in patients with chronic hemiparesis. Am J Phys Med Rehabil. 2008;87:4–13.
12. Janssen WG, Bussmann HB, Stam HJ. Determinants of the sit-to-stand movement: a review. Phys Ther. 2002;82:866–79.
13. Kunst AE, Amiri M, Janssen F. The decline in stroke mortality. Exploration of future trends in 7 Western European countries. Stroke. 2011;42:2126–30.
14. Lozano R, Naghavi M, Foreman K, Lim S, Shibuya K, Aboyans V, et al. Global and regional mortality from 235 causes of death for 20 age groups in 1990 and 2010: a systematic analysis for the global burden of disease study. Lancet. 2010;380:2095–128.

15. Martin KD, Polanski WH, Schulz AK, Jöbges M, Hoff H, Schackert G, Pinzer T, Sobottka SB. Restoration of ankle movements with the ActiGait implantable drop foot stimulator: a safe and reliable treatment option for permanent central leg palsy. J Neurosurg. 2015;24:1–7.
16. Mayo Clinic. www.mayoclinic.org/diseases-conditions/foot-drop/basics/definition/con-20032918. Retrieved 14 Dec 2015.
17. Miller EL, Murray L, Richards L, Zorowitz RD, Bakas T, Clark P, et al. Comprehensive overview of nursing and interdisciplinary rehabilitation care of the stroke patient: a scientific statement from the American Heart Association. Stroke. 2010;41:2402–48.
18. Mulroy SJ, Eberly VJ, Gronely JK, Weiss W, Newsam CJ. Effect of AFO design on walking after stroke: impact of ankle plantar flexion ontracture. Prosthet Orthot Int. 2010;34:277–92.
19. Murray CJL, Vos T, Lozano R, Naghavi M, Flaxman AD, Michaud C, et al. Disability-adjusted life years (DALYs) for 291 diseases and injuries in 21 regions, 1990–2010: a systematic analysis for the Global Burden of Disease Study 2010. Lancet. 2012;380: 2197–223.
20. Neurodan A/S. Surgeon Manual—AcitGait Implantable Drop Foot Stimulator. Version 1.8/ 2015.
21. Podsiadlo D, Richardson S. The timed "Up & Go": a test of basic functional mobility for frail elderly persons. J Am Geriatr Soc. 1991;39:142–8.
22. Ring H, Treger I, Gruendlinger L, Hausdorff JM. Neuroprosthesis for footdrop compared with an ankle-foot orthosis: effects on postural control during walking. J Stroke Cerebrovasc Dis. 2009;18:41–7.
23. Sheffler LR, Hennessey MT, Naples GG, Chae J. Peroneal nerve stimulation versus an ankle foot orthosis for correction of footdrop in stroke: impact on functional ambulation. Neurorehabil Neural Repair. 2006;20:355–60.
24. Stein RB, Everaert DG, Thompson AK, et al. Long-term therapeutic and orthotic effects of a foot drop stimulator on walking performance in progressive and nonprogressive neurological disorders. Neurorehabil Neural Repair. 2010;24:152–67.
25. The Management of Stroke Rehabilitation Working Group. VA/DoD Clinical Practice Guideline for the Management of Stroke Rehabilitation. 2010;Version 2.0:150.4.
26. Truelsen T, Piechowski-Jozwiak B, Bonita R, Mathers C, Bogousslavsky J, Boysen G. Stroke incidence and revalence in Europe: a review of available data. Eur J Neurol. 2006;13:581–98.
27. van Swigchem R, Vloothuis J, den Boer J, Weerdesteyn V, Geurts AC. Is transcutaneous peroneal stimulation beneficial to patients with chronic stroke using an ankle-foot orthosis? A within-subjects study of patients' satisfaction, walking speed and physical activity level. J Rehabil Med. 2010;42:117–21.
28. Wolf SL, Catlin PA, Gage K, Gurucharri K, Robertson R, Stephen K. Establishing the reliability and validity of measurements of walking time using the Emory Functional Ambulation Profile. Phys Ther. 1999;79:1122–33.

Indications and Results of Implantable Functional Electrical Stimulation (FES) of the Peroneal Nerve

Michaela M. Pinter, Frank Berenpas and Alexander C. Geurts

1 Principles of FES

Drop foot is a common problem following neurological conditions such as stroke, multiple sclerosis (MS), traumatic brain injury (TBI), incomplete spinal cord injury (iSCI) and cerebral palsy (CP). Between 20 and 30% of patients entering neurological rehabilitation suffer from drop foot [1]. Typically, drop foot is caused by weakness of the ankle dorsiflexors leading to a lack of foot elevation during the swing phase of gait, which is often accompanied by a tendency towards varus deviation at the ankle due to muscular imbalance. In addition, spasticity of the ankle plantarflexors may worsen equinovarus deviation as a result of muscle stiffness, contracture and pathological co-contraction. Drop foot leads to an abnormal gait pattern, decreased walking speed, limited endurance walking and increased fall risk. All these factors can limit mobility, independence and social participation leading to reduced quality of life.

The principle of functional electrical stimulation (FES) applied to the common peroneal nerve during the swing phase of the gait cycle to treat drop foot was introduced in 1961 by Liberson et al. [2]. Peroneal nerve FES works by activating the ankle dorsiflexors and evertors to support foot elevation. Furthermore, peroneal nerve FES may reduce, through reciprocal inhibition, mild spasticity of the calf muscle, which facilitates dorsiflexion in the ankle joint [3].

In order to harmonize the gait pattern by FES, it is essential to adapt the stimulation parameters (rising ramp, plateau phase, extension time and falling ramp) to

M. M. Pinter (✉)
Department for Clinical Neurosciences and Preventive Medicine,
Center for Neurorehabilitation, Danube University Krems, Krems, Austria
e-mail: michaela.pinter@donau-uni.ac.at

F. Berenpas · A. C. Geurts
Department of Rehabilitation, Donders Centre for Neuroscience,
Radboud University Medical Centre, Nijmegen, The Netherlands

G. Sandrini et al. (eds.), *Advanced Technologies for the Rehabilitation of Gait and Balance Disorders*, Biosystems & Biorobotics 19,
https://doi.org/10.1007/978-3-319-72736-3_28

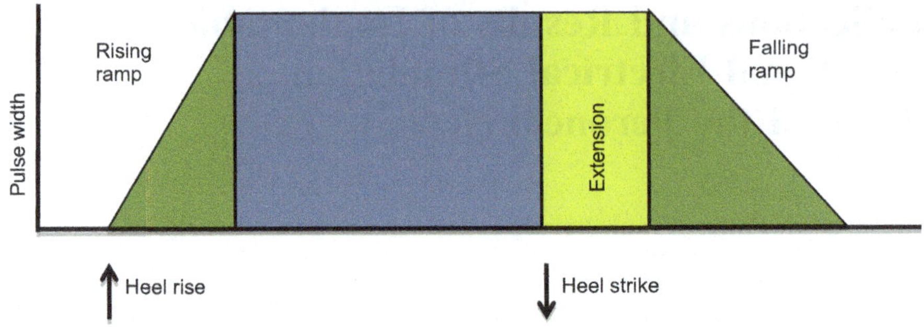

Fig. 1 This graph represents the general operation of FES devices. Along the bottom of the graph is time. Along the vertical axis is stimulation intensity (pulse width). Stimulation begins when the heel is lifted from the ground and continues until the heel strikes the ground. However, the stimulation is not stopped straight away, but continues for a short period called 'extension'. This helps to lower the foot to the ground and mimics the natural muscle activation pattern

the individual walking characteristics of the patient (Fig. 1). Rising ramp is the time taken for the pulse width to go from zero to the set pulse width after heel rise. A longer rising ramp means a slower ankle movement and slower stretch of the calf muscles, reducing the risk of evoking a stretch reflex or ankle clonus. The rising ramp typically coincides with the late stance phase of gait. After the swing phase (plateau phase), a period of extended stimulation can be added following heel strike (extension time), which provides an eccentric contraction of the tibialis anterior, lowering the foot to the ground and preventing foot slap. In this way, extension of the stimulation followed by the falling ramp (the time taken for the stimulation pulse width to reach zero) together stabilize the ankle during the loading phase of gait. The rising edge ramp and extension time are critical for adequate foot elevation, whereas the falling edge ramp is less critical. The faster the patient walks, the shorter the rising ramp and extension time must be.

2 FES with Surface Electrodes

Since Liberson et al. [2] first applied peroneal nerve FES, several studies have noted that subjects who used electrical stimulation improved their walking performance, even after the stimulation was turned off. This phenomenon received the name 'carryover effect', because it was initially reported as a short-lasting (minutes) effect of the electrical stimulation. Subsequent studies have shown that the so-called carryover effect may increase over time with long-term and repeated use [4–6] In more recent studies, the change in walking performance over time, measured while FES is *off*, has been referred to as a 'therapeutic' effect [7–9] a term that seems more appropriate for the changes associated with long-term FES use. The therapeutic effect of FES may occur independently of the 'orthotic' effect that occurs *during* the electrical stimulation.

The long-term orthotic and therapeutic effects of peroneal nerve FES on walking performance of subjects with progressive (e.g. MS) and non-progressive (e.g. stroke, TBI, iSCI) neurological disorders have been compared in the following study [10]. Forty-one subjects with non-progressive and thirty-two subjects with progressive conditions used a drop foot stimulator for 3–12 months while walking in the community. The primary outcome parameters were a 10 m walk test (walking speed), a 4-min figure-of-8 test (walking agility) and the physiological cost index (PCI), which is commonly used to measure walking effort. Subjects with progressive and non-progressive disorders had an orthotic benefit from FES up to 11 months. The therapeutic effect increased for 11 months in non-progressive disorders, but only for 3 months in progressive disorders. The combined effect remained significant and clinically relevant. Moreover, peroneal nerve FES has been shown to reduce fall incidence [11], to have a positive impact on activities of daily living [11–13] and on quality of life [13, 14], regardless of the underlying pathology.

The long-term effect of FES use on the correction of drop foot due to upper motor neuron syndrome of different etiology was shown in a recent study [15]. One hundred and twenty-six people with spastic drop foot (62 stroke, 39 MS, 7 iSCI, 3 CP, 15 others) were analyzed retrospectively. The median time of FES use was 3.6 years (mean 4.9, standard deviation (SD) 4.1, 95% CI 4.2–5.6). Thirty-three people still used FES after an average of 11.1 years. Since there was insufficient report of data for the other neurological conditions, only walking speed for 62 subjects with stroke and 39 subjects with MS was analyzed. People with stroke walked 0.08 m/s faster with FES ($p < 0.001$; 17% continuing orthotic effect) and also increased their walking speed without FES by 0.11 m/s ($p < 0.001$; 24% training effect), resulting in an overall increase in speed of 0.18 m/s ($p < 0.001$; 45% total effect), when compared to the start of treatment without FES. People with MS walked 0.09 m/s faster throughout a 100-day onwards period with FES ($p < 0.001$; 29% continuing orthotic effect), but did not show an overall training effect. Interestingly, approximately 10% of all patients—regardless of whether the condition was progressive or non-progressive—discontinued FES each year. Notably, stroke and MS patients showed similar patterns of drop out, but more people with MS dropped out because of deteriorating mobility, whereas people with stroke dropped out mainly because of co-morbidity or death [15].

The main drawbacks of a surface-based drop foot stimulator are the awkwardness in handling the external parts when putting it on, finding the right electrode position on the leg, and skin irritation due to stimulation [4]. In a study of 26 stroke patients, skin problems (n = 4), muscle soreness (n = 5) and discomfort below the knee (n = 7) were relatively common [16]. Nevertheless, participants were largely satisfied with the benefits of surface-based FES as compared to an ankle-foot orthosis (AFO) with regard to their gait quality, walking distance, and the stability and effort of walking. Because in this study the electrodes were embedded in an orthosis (Bioness L300®), ease of donning and doffing, ease of use and comfort to wear also scored better than AFO use.

3 Implantable 1-Channel and 2-Channel FES Systems

Already in the nineties implantable systems were tested to solve the above-mentioned problems. However, the first 1-channel systems were not suitable to provide a selective and balanced stimulation of the foot dorsiflexors and induced in some cases excessive inversion or eversion of the ankle joint [17]. Based on this experience, implantable 2-channel systems were developed to provide more selective stimulation of the peroneal nerve, resulting in a nearly normalized single stance and double support phase of the paretic limb [8].

In a randomized controlled trial, a 2-channel system (StimuStep®) was implanted in 29 patients with drop foot after stroke. The StimuStep® system was compared to a control group who continued using an AFO, orthopedic shoes or no device. FES resulted in a 23% improvement of walking speed measured with the 6-min Walk Test, whereas the improvement in the control group was only 3% ($p = 0.010$) [18]. In addition, FES was more effective to provide ankle dorsiflexion during the swing phase and normalized single stance and double support time of the paretic limb as well as single support time of the non-paretic limb in comparison to the control group [19]. A study evaluating the effects of StimuStep® in a group of 23 patients with MS also provided promising results. Improvement of gait performance was similar to using a surface-based stimulation system, while patients reported that they used the StimuStep® more days a week. The method of fixation, however, whereby the electrode was embedded within the epineurium, resulted in considerable adverse effects, with implant failure in four cases and pain in response to stimulation in two subjects. Pain was likely due to neuropraxia in one case and due to external pressure on the nerve from the external controller in another patient [20].

4 Indications for Implantable 4-Channel Drop Foot Stimulator

More recently, in 2007, an implantable 4-channel drop foot stimulator (ActiGait®, see Fig. 2), with the possibility of independent electrode adjustment resulting in more specific nerve stimulation, was officially approved for hemiplegia following stroke (see Table 1 for comparison with the approved indications for surface-based FES).

In recent studies on the clinical effects of ActiGait® all patients were over the age of 18 years and had a drop foot following a stroke at least 6 months prior to recruitment. All participants had at least 30° of passive ankle movement and were able to stand upright with their heels touching the floor when the hip and knee were in a neutral position. Walking capacity was defined either as the ability to walk 20 m in less than 2 min or the independent capacity to walk for 10 min without walking aids. Only patients with a positive response to surface-based electrical stimulation of the peroneal nerve resulting in muscle contraction leading to ankle dorsiflexion during the swing phase were eligible (see Table 2) [21–24].

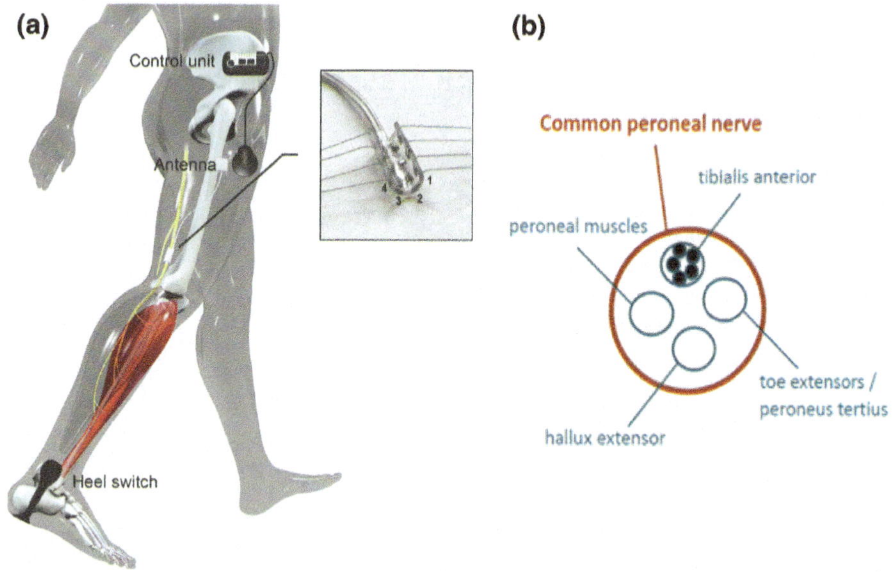

Fig. 2 **a** Illustration of the ActiGait® implantable 4-channel drop foot stimulator, copyright Otto Bock Group. The implanted part of the system consists of a stimulator body and an electrode cuff (4 channels) connected by a lead wire. The external parts consist of a heel switch (placed under the heel in a sock or shoe) and a control unit worn at the pelvis and connected to an antenna directly on the skin over the stimulator body, **b** schematic presentation of the common peroneal nerve. The electrode cuff, with 12 electrodes equally divided over 4 channels, is situated directly around the common peroneal nerve just above the knee joint allowing a selective, well balanced activation of the tibialis anterior muscle, toe extensors, and peroneal muscles

Table 1 Indications for functional electrical stimulation FES (Functional Electrical Stimulation); UMNS (Upper Motor Neuron Syndrome)

FES with surface electrodes	FES with ActiGait®
Stroke	Stroke
Multiple sclerosis	
Brain injury	
Spinal cord injury	
Infantile cerebral palsy	
Drop foot by other UMNS	

Interestingly, uncontrolled epilepsy, the presence of other implanted devices such as a cardiac pacemaker, unstable diagnosed psychological conditions, and pregnancy were reported as exclusion criteria in almost all studies. Only in the study by Burridge et al., were persons with limited walking capacity retained (see Table 3) [21]. Contraindications such as peripheral nerve damage, polyneuropathy, and a thickness of subcutaneous fat exceeding 3.5 cm in the region of the implant were only mentioned by Ernst et al. [22].

Table 2 Inclusion criteria for implantable electrical stimulation with ActiGait®

Inclusion criteria	Burridge et al. [21]	Ernst et al. [22]	Martin et al. [23]	Schiemanck et al. [24]
6 months post-stroke onset	x	x	x	x
Weakness of ankle dorsiflexors (MRC-Scale <5)	x	x	x	x
Passive range of ankle motion $\geq 30°$, with $\geq 0°$ ankle dorsiflexion while standing	x	x		x
Ability to stand upright, both heels touching the floor, hip and knee extended	x	x		
Muscle tone of ankle plantar flexors modified Ashworth scale ≤ 3				x
Independent walking capacity for 10 min without walking aids (except an AFO)		x	x	x
Ability to walk 20 m in less than 2 min	x			
Over the age of 18 years	x	x	x	
Age between 18 and 65 years				x
Positive response to surface-based peroneal nerve stimulation	x	x	x	x

MRC-Scale (Medical Research Council Scale); AFO (ankle-foot orthosis)

Table 3 Exclusion criteria for implantable electrical stimulation with ActiGait®

Exclusion criteria	Burridge et al. [21]	Ernst et al. [22]	Martin et al. [23]	Schiemanck et al. [24]
Uncontrolled epilepsy	x	x		
Presence of other implanted devices such as a cardiac pacemaker	x	x	x	
Peripheral nerve damage or polyneuropathy		x		
MRI to exclude any peripheral injury of the peroneal nerve			x	x
A thickness of subcutaneous fat exceeding 3.5 cm in the region of implant		x		
Unable to walk 100 m without stopping prior to their stroke	x		x	x
Walking faster than 1.2 m/s	x			
Severe cognitive deficits that might hamper informed consent	x			x
Psychiatric disorders that might hamper informed consent	x			x
Pregnancy	x	x		x

m/s (meters per second); cm (centimeter)

5 Clinical Results of FES with ActiGait®

Four studies reported clinical outcomes of ActiGait® use. All four studies presented gait speed and walking endurance (defined as the distance covered in a preset time) as outcomes. Compared to walking without stimulation, gait speed with ActiGait® was found to be increased by 19–47% [21–24] No differences in gait speed were found between ActiGait® and AFO in two studies [22, 24], but Martin et al. [23] did find a significant improvement of gait speed with ActiGait® compared to AFO as well as to surface-based FES. Walking endurance was tested either in a four-minute [21] or a six-minute [22–24] walking test. With stimulation, the distance covered was reported to be generally higher (8–105%) compared to walking without stimulation [21–23] However, compared to walking with an AFO, the covered distance with ActiGait® was not found to be improved nor was the energy expenditure as defined by oxygen consumption during the six-minute walking test [24]. Martin et al. [23] were the only group investigating the performance of additional functional gait tasks. They found a significant decrease in the timed-up-and-go test resulting in a transition of the impairment classification from 'functionally relevant mobility impairment' without stimulation to 'mild mobility impairment' with ActiGait® stimulation.

It has been suggested that the improvements in clinical outcomes with ActiGait® are due to restoration of ankle movements during gait. The groups of Ernst et al. [22] and Schiemanck et al. [24] performed a more thorough investigation of the effects of ActiGait® on the quality of walking. Using 3D-gait analysis, both groups presented improvements in paretic leg ankle kinematics with ActiGait®. Ernst et al. [22] reported a general normalization of the ankle angle with FES, with significantly improved initial dorsiflexion (9°) at heel strike and a significantly improved initial plantarflexion (7°) after heel strike compared to walking without stimulation. In contrast to Ernst et al. [22], who reported no statistical differences in ankle kinematics between ActiGait® and AFO, Schiemanck et al. [24] did find ActiGait® use to be statistically superior to AFO use. The latter study showed that during late stance, maximum plantarflexion was 5° larger with FES than with AFO. Importantly, this gain in late stance plantarflexion was believed to be utilized by residual calf muscle capacity as the peak plantarflexion power during late stance was also found to be improved (49%) with FES compared to AFO. This normalization of ankle kinematics and kinetics resulted in a reduction of step length asymmetry from 21% with AFO to 15% with ActiGait®.

Patient satisfaction with ActiGait® is generally good, favoring implanted FES over AFO and surface-based FES systems. Martin et al. [23] reported that after implantation a majority of patients reported a complete return to normal mobility (78%), normal social participation (67%) and normal quality of life (74%). Comparing ActiGait® with AFO, Schiemanck et al. [24] showed a significant benefit of ActiGait® in terms of 'comfort of wearing', 'appearance' and 'going up and down the stairs'. Finally, Burridge et al. [25] discussed an advantage of ActiGait® over surface-based FES, namely that the time needed for donning and doffing is less.

6 Extended Indications for ActiGait®

Since the ActiGait® system was officially approved in 2007 for hemiplegia following ischemic or hemorrhagic stroke, implantations for other conditions have been rare. The first report of successful implementation of FES applied directly to the peroneal nerve via an implanted 4-channel cuff electrode to aid dorsiflexion in two patients with MS was provided recently by Hausmann et al. [26]. Walking distance increased from 517 to 1884 m in one patient and from 52 to 506 m in another patient, while gait velocity changed significantly only in the latter patient from 0.6 to 0.8 m/s. Moreover, after 3 months of stimulation, maximum deviations of center of mass from the midline to each side while walking changed significantly compared to baseline, decreasing from 15 to 12 mm in the first patient and from 47 to 37 mm in the latter patient. Both patients experienced reduced pain and fatigue and benefits to quality of life. Adverse events did not occur during the observation period [26].

The long-term effect of the surface-based FES on the correction of drop foot due to upper motor neuron syndrome of different etiology was shown in a recent study [15]. Since no clinical differences were found between progressive and non-progressive neurological disorders, it is unlikely that the effects of implantable FES with the 4-channel drop foot stimulator will be different for conditions other than stroke. As for MS, only primary or secondary progressive MS patients with a maximum EDSS score [27] of 6 (EDSS 6 = ability to walk 100 m with intermittent or unilateral support) are indicated for treatment with ActiGait®.

7 Adverse Events Due to ActiGait® Stimulation

Surgical complications of ActiGait® implantation have only rarely been reported, such as hematomas at the side of the cuff placement, postoperative wound healing deficit (1 of 15 patients), and infections (2 of 15 patients) [21], but injury to the peroneal nerve may also occur [23, 24]. To avoid possible pitfalls of the surgical procedure and the perioperative care, a technical note was recently published [28].

8 Conclusion

Altogether, several (as yet uncontrolled) studies indicate that implantable FES with a 4-channel drop foot stimulator (ActiGait®) is most likely superior to surface-based FES in patients with drop foot after stroke, since a more precise and selective stimulation of the peroneal nerve can be achieved, leading to a well-balanced foot elevation [21]. Furthermore, with implantable FES, problems such as skin irritation and allergic skin reactions are avoided. In addition, it has been argued that implantable systems are technically more reliable than surface-based systems [23, 25]. Studies using implantable systems have shown evidence for improved gait quality, in particular more paretic ankle dorsiflexion during the swing phase and at initial contact [22], improved paretic ankle plantarflexion during the loading phase [22] and improved ankle power during the push-off phase [24]. Additionally, recent reports showed that the implantable device was easier to use than a surface stimulator [25]. Lastly, there are indications that long-term FES use may also lead to therapeutic effects in terms of improved motor output to the muscles of the lower leg [8].

Given these promising results, more studies are warranted to investigate the effects of implantable peroneal nerve FES after stroke, especially RCTs that make a direct comparison with surface-based FES and to AFO use. These studies should also be extended to other neurological conditions, including mild progressive diseases such as MS. Finally, we need more studies to identify the underlying mechanisms of any therapeutic (neuroplastic and neuromuscular) effects of long-term FES use, particularly in patients with stable neurological conditions such as stroke.

References

1. Karsinia A, Dillner S, Everfors I, Lundmark P. Why patients use or reject a peroneal muscle stimulator. Adv External Control Human Extremities 1990;251–60.
2. Liberson WT, Holmquest HJ, Scott D, Dow M. Functional electrotherapy, stimulation of the peroneal nerve synchronized with the swing phase of the gait of hemiplegic patients. Arch Phys Med Rehabil. 1961;42:101–5.
3. van Swigchem R, Weerdesteyn V, van Duijnhoven HJ, den Boer J, Beems T, Geurts AC. Near normal gait pattern with peroneal electrical stimulation as a neuroprosthesis in the chronic phase of stroke: a case report. Arch Phys Med Rehabil. 2011;92(2):320–4.
4. Taylor PN, Burridge JH, Dunkerley AL, Singleton C, Swain ID. Clinical use of the Odstock dropped foot stimulator: its effect on the speed and effort of walking. Arch Phys Med Rehabil. 1999;80:1577–83.
5. Ladouceur M, Barbeau H. Functional electrical stimulation-assisted walking for persons with incomplete spinal injuries: longitudinal changes in maximal overground walking speed. Scand J Rehabil Med. 2000;32:28–36.
6. Stein RB, Chong S, Everaert DG, Rolf R, Thompson AK, Whittaker M, Robertson J, Fung J, Preuss R, Momose K, Ihashi K. A multicenter trial of a footdrop stimulator controlled by a tilt sensor. Neurorehabil Neural Repair. 2006;20:371–9.
7. Burridge JH, Swain ID, Taylor PN. Functional electrical stimulation: a review of the literature published on common peroneal nerve stimulation for the correction of dropped foot. Rev Clin Gerontol. 1998;8:155–61.
8. Kottink AI, Hermens HJ, Nene AV, Tenniglo MJ, Groothuis-Oudshoorn CG, IJzerman MJ. Therapeutic effect of an implantable peroneal nerve stimulator in subjects with chronic stroke and footdrop: a randomized controlled trial. Phys Ther. 2008;88:437–48.
9. Stein RB, Everaert DG, Thompson AK, Chong SL, Whittaker M, Robertson J, Kuether G. Long-term therapeutic and orthotic effect of a foot drop stimulator on walking performance in progressive and nonprogressive neurological disorders. Neurorehabil Neural Repair. 2010;24 (2):152–67.

10. Taylor PN, Burridge JH, Wood DE, Norton J, Dunkerley A, Singleton C, Swain ID. Patient perceptions of the Odstock drop foot stimulator. Clin Rehabil. 1999;13:333–40.
11. Esnouf JE, Taylor PN, Mann GE, Barrett CL. Impact on falls and activities of daily living of use of a functional electrical stimulation (FES) device for correction of dropped foot in people with multiple sclerosis. Mult Scler. 2010;16:1141–7.
12. Bulley C, Shiels JE, Wilkie KM, Salisbury LG. User experiences, preferences and choices relating to functional electrical stimulation and ankle foot orthoses for foot-drop after stroke. Physiotherapy. 2011;97:226–33.
13. Barrett CL, Taylor PN. The effects of the Odstock drop foot stimulator on perceived quality of life for people with stroke and multiple sclerosis. Neuromodulation. 2010;13:58–64.
14. Wilkie KM, Shiels JE, Bulley C, Salisbury LG. "Functional electrical stimulation (FES) impacted on important aspects of my Life"—a qualitative exploration of chronic patients' and carers' perceptions of FES in the management of dropped foot. Physiother Theory Pract. 2011;28:1–9.
15. Taylor PN, Humphreys L, Swain I. The long-term cost-effectiveness of the use of functional electrical stimulation for the correction of dropped foot due to upper motor neuron lesion. J Rehabil Med. 2013;45:154–60.
16. Swigchem R, Vloothuis J, den Boer J, Weerdesteyn V, Geurts ACH. Is transcutaneous peroneal stimulation beneficial to patients with chronic stroke using an ankle-foot orthosis? A within-subjects study of patients' satisfaction, walking speed and physical activity level. J Rehabil Med. 2010;42:117–21.
17. Rozman J, Acimovic-Janiezic R, Tekavcic I, Kljajic M, Trelep M. Implantable stimulator for selective stimulation of the common peroneal nerve: a prelimary report. J Med Eng Tech. 1994;18:47–53.
18. Kottink AI, Hermens HJ, Nene AV, Tenniglo MJ, van der Aa HE, Buschman HP, IJzerman MJ. A randomized controlled trial of an implantable 2-channel peroneal nerve stimulator on walking speed and activity in poststroke hemiplegia. Arch Phys Med Rehabil. 2007;88(8):971–8.
19. Kottink AI, Tenniglo MJ, de Vries WH, Hermens HJ, van Buurke JH. Effects of an implantable two-channel peroneal nerve stimulator versus conventional walking device on spatiotemporal parameters and kinematics of hemiparetic gait. J Rehabil Med. 2012;44(1):51–7.
20. Taylor PN, Wilkinson IA, Khan MS, Slade-Sharman DEM. The correction of dropped foot due to multiple sclerosis using the STIMuSTEP implanted dropped foot stimulator. Int J MS Care. 2016, *preprint.* https://doi.org/10.7224/1537-2073.2015-038.
21. Burridge J, Haugland M, Larsen B, Pickering RM, Svaneborg N, Iversen HK, et al. Phase II trial to evaluate the ActiGait implanted drop-foot stimulator in established hemiplegia. J Rehabil Med. 2007;39:212–8.
22. Ernst J, Grundey J, Hewitt M, Von Lewinski F, Kaus J, Schmalz T, et al. Towards physiological ankle movements with the ActiGait implantable drop foot stimulator in chronic stroke. Restor Neurol Neurosci. 2013;31:557–69.
23. Martin KD, Polanski WH, Schulz AK, Joebges M, Hoff H, Schackert G, Pinzer T, Sobottka SB. Restoration of ankle movements with the ActiGait implantable drop foot stimulator is a safe and reliable treatment option for permanent central leg palsy. J Neurosurg. 2015. http://thejns.org/doi/abs/10.3171/2014.12.JNS142110.
24. Schiemanck S, Berenpas F, van Swigchem R, van den Munckhof P, de Vries J, Beelen A, Nollet F, Geurts AC. Effects of implantable peroneal nerve stimulation on gait quality, energy expenditure, participation and user satisfaction in patients with post-stroke drop foot using an ankle-foot orthosis. Restorative Neurol Neurosci. 2015;33:795–807.
25. Burridge JH, Haugland M, Larsen B, Svaneborg N, Iversen HK, Christensen PB, et al. Patients' perceptions of the benefits and problems of using the ActiGait implanted drop-foot stimulator. J Rehabil Med. 2008;40:873–5.
26. Hausmann J, Sweeney-Reed C, Sobieray U, Matzke M, Heinze HJ, Voges J, Buentjen L. Functional electrical stimulation through direct 4-channel nerve stimulation to improve gait in

multiple sclerosis: a feasibility study. J NeuroEngineering Rehabil. 2015;12:100. https://doi.org/10.1186/s12984-015-0096.
27. Kurtzke JF. Rating neurological impairment in MS: an expanded disability status scale (EDSS). Neurology. 1983;33:1444–52.
28. Martin KD, Polanski W, Schackert G, Sobottka SB. New therapeutic option for drop foot with the ActiGait peroneal nerve stimulator—a technical note. World Neurosurg. 2015;84 (6):2037–42. https://doi.org/10.1016/j.wneu.2015.06.074 Epub 2015 Jul 9.

Neuroprostheses: Significance in Gait Rehabilitation

Josefina Gutiérrez-Martínez

1 Introduction

1.1 The Nervous System

The nervous system is composed of billions of nerve cells arranged in patterns. It regulates and performs fundamental functions to control glands, organs, thought, emotion, behavior, movement and sensation. The central nervous system (CNS) and peripheral nervous system (PNS) form the entirety of the body's nervous system.

The CNS is the body's principal data control center, and it regulates everything from the functioning of organs to body movements. It engages in three main functions: gathering sensory information from external stimuli, organizing and synthesizing that information, and then providing instructions for motor output to the rest of the body. The main function of the PNS, on the other hand, is to connect the CNS to the limbs and organs, essentially serving as a communications relay, sending messages back and forth between the brain and spinal cord and the rest of the body [1, 2].

The CNS comprises the brain, brainstem and spinal cord. The brain, in turn, comprises the cerebrum and the cerebellum, which is located under the posterior side of the cerebrum. The main function of the cerebellum is to maintain coordination and govern balance and fine motor movements. The cerebrum has two hemispheres, each controlling the opposite side of the body; it regulates higher-level functions, such as motor functions and thought. Each hemisphere is divided into four separate lobes. In general, the frontal lobe controls motor functions, learning, planning and speech; the parietal lobe controls somatic or voluntary

J. Gutiérrez-Martínez (✉)
Division of Medical Engineering Research, Instituto Nacional de Rehabilitación LGII, Mexico City, Mexico
e-mail: josefina_gutierrez@hotmail.com

G. Sandrini et al. (eds.), *Advanced Technologies for the Rehabilitation of Gait and Balance Disorders*, Biosystems & Biorobotics 19,
https://doi.org/10.1007/978-3-319-72736-3_29

sensory functions; the occipital lobe controls vision, and the temporal lobe controls hearing and some other speech functions.

The brainstem includes the midbrain, pons and medulla oblongata, and continuing downward, it becomes the spinal cord. It controls many lower-level autonomic functions, such as respiration, heart rate, blood pressure and digestion. The spinal cord connects the brain and the body's main receptors, and not only serves as a conduit for sensory input and motor output, but also regulates all motor functions.

Sensory and motor neurons are highly specialized sensory receptors that travel through the brainstem. They connect the spinal cord and the cerebrum, allowing signals to be relayed between them.

Brain diseases, such as stroke, aneurysms, cancer, tumors, multiple sclerosis, spinal cord injury (SCI) and inflammation of the brain, as well as nerve impingement, can have a number of causes: changes in blood flow, lack of oxygen, blocked or broken blood vessels, or congenital disorders, but also automobile accidents, falls, acts of violence, and alcohol addiction. These lesions often result in permanent changes in strength, sensation and movement, and in other body functions such as speech, vision or hearing; they can also produce deficits in bowel, bladder and sexual function.

1.2 The Autonomic Nervous System

The functioning of many of our body's muscles, glands and organs, such as the heart, intestines and stomach, is regulated by a division of the PNS known as the autonomic nervous system (ANS). The ANS aids in maintaining homeostasis (internal stability and balance) through the coordination of various activities such as hormone secretion, circulation, respiration, digestion and excretion. The ANS is always "on" and functioning unconsciously; thus, we are unaware of the important tasks that it performs every waking (and sleeping) minute of every day [3].

Motor skills involve efferent systems (which carry information to the muscles) and afferent systems (which carry information to the nervous system) and they are the result of the integration of information at different hierarchical levels of the CNS and PNS. In persons with complete or incomplete SCI, interruption of or interference with these systems can result in paralysis of the upper and/or lower limbs. Consequently, impaired motor skills provoke secondary systemic problems, such as pressure ulcers or urinary incontinence [4]. Damage of the spinal cord and nerve roots occurring at the thoracic, lumbar and sacral levels results in paraplegia. It has been reported that some individuals with complete SCI actually retain some connectivity across the injury site; this could be represented by nonfunctioning myelin or denuded axons, which, in the presence of optimal activation, could potentially provide conductivity across the injury site [5].

1.3 Neuroplasticity

When a nervous system injury occurs, it triggers a cascade of rapid neurochemical/molecular changes at multiple subcortical as well as cortical locations. These may include functional alterations of normal excitation and inhibition, atrophy, and degeneration of normal structures, leading to the loss of relationships and connections between neighboring structures in central, peripheral, spinal and brainstem areas [6].

The fundamental properties [7] of the CNS include brain plasticity and excitability. Neural plasticity can be defined as the ability of the nervous system to modify (also through learning) its own structural and functional organization in response to endogenous and exogenous factors [8]. Remodeling is a dynamic process that leads to a new restructuring or reorganization of healthy structures [9].

Neural plasticity can be manifested at the macroscale level as changes in the spatiotemporal activation pattern of different brain regions, at the mesoscale level as alterations in long-range and local connections between distinct neuronal types, and at the microscale level as modifications of neurons and synapses at cellular and subcellular levels. Inappropriate or delayed neural plasticity may be due not only to numerous developmental, acquired and neurodegenerative brain disorders, but also to failure to implement a timely neurorehabilitation process.

The concept of neuroplasticity is not new. It first emerged in the 19th century with the studies of neurons conducted by brain researchers such as Ramón y Cajal in Spain [10], who highlighted the degenerative and regenerative capacities of brain tissue and the brain's malleability, i.e., its ability to gradually reorganize itself so as to take over some of the functions of destroyed cells. It is only in relatively recent times that it has become possible to measure and evaluate brain plasticity, a phenomenon whose effect is determined partially by the location and extension of the lesion.

Transcranial magnetic stimulation (TMS), quantitative electroencephalography (qEEG), magnetic resonance spectroscopy (MRS) and functional magnetic resonance imaging (fMRI) are techniques capable of disclosing the plastic ability of the brain [11]. TMS measures cortical excitability through a motor-evoked potential (MEP). The stimulation threshold and the type of electrical pulse applied to produce the MEP are parameters used to assess neuroplasticity [12]. qEEG provides objective measures (power spectra and coherence) of phase synchrony among EEG signals, reflecting functional interregional coupling and depending mainly on structural connections, such as interhemispheric and intrahemispheric coherence between the right and left hemisphere. EEG waves are linked with learning and plasticity processes both locally surrounding the lesion and within whole brain. Although EEG has good temporal resolution its spatial resolution is poor. MRS provides an index of metabolic changes of brain function [12]. fMRI images display brain reorganization following peripheral nerve injury, and allow brain activity to be measured by detecting associated changes in blood flow [13]. Within this same context, functional near-infrared spectroscopy (fNIRS) is emerging as an alternative method to fMRI for indirect and direct monitoring of brain activity [14].

1.4 Neurorehabilitation Goals

Recovering neural control of movement after a brain lesion does not mean replacing the destroyed brain tissue, since the brain has no way of creating new cells. However, there are now many novel technological alternatives for neurological rehabilitation that seek to promote reorganization of surviving brain tissue in order to create new neural pathways that will allow motor function to be regained. Neurorehabilitation can exploit the brain's ability to "relearn" the functions of paralyzed body segments [15].

Clinical application of neurorehabilitation with the aim of restoring or replacing lost functions of the nervous system demands in-depth knowledge of the structure and functioning of the nervous system, of the potential and limits of neuroplasticity, and of the changes that occur in response to a proposed stimulation strategy involving the use of devices. These changes can substitute for missing biological functions, i.e. take over motor, sensory or cognitive functions that have been impaired or lost as a result of injury or disease. The most important step for effective neurorehabilitation, able to reduce functional limitations, is to assess, in a timely manner, the size and extent of the lesion, the specificity of the loss of neural connections, and the degree of disability of the individual subject [16].

Physiotherapy is one of the most utilized methods for rehabilitation and it aims to improve motor function, stability of gait, balance, muscle weakness, depression, fatigue and walking capabilities. However, there is no convincing evidence that mechanical aids and physiotherapy treatments alone are able to produce effective, long-term recovery of lower limb functions in chronic patients after brain or spinal cord lesion.

Neurorehabilitation involves the use of various mechanical techniques to manipulate the CNS and PNS. These include equipment-supported training, treadmill exercises, robot-assisted gait training, constraint-induced movement therapy, proprioceptive neuromuscular facilitation, biofeedback, and mirror therapy. Studies, such as Szuhany's analysis, support the importance of exercise as a strategy for enhancing the brain-derived neurotrophic factor in human activity [17]. Van Praag et al., studying aged mice, found that spatial learning, neurogenesis and angiogenesis could be increased or even restored by exercise [18].

None of these techniques has demonstrated superiority over the others, which means that the appropriate method should be chosen on the basis of the capabilities and disabilities of the individual patient, but also the knowledge and resources of the rehabilitation team [19, 20].

Top-down strategies employing methodologies based on neurophysiological or metabolic brain feedback (i.e., the Bobath, Vojta and Brunkow therapies, proprioceptive neuromuscular stimulation, nerve stimulation with transcranial electric or magnetic stimulation, electromyogram-triggered neuromuscular stimulation, and robotic interactive therapies) may represent a promising approach to modulate brain reorganization and motor behavior by selectively enhancing preserved neural circuits or promoting the formation of new functional circuits in survivors of brain damage.

2 Neuroprostheses

A prosthesis is an artificial device that replaces a missing body part, which may have been lost due to injury, disease or congenital conditions. When the neural pathway is lost, or when there is neuromotor damage or sensory impairment of the nervous system, an artificial interface is required to substitute for the missing neural pathway. Such devices are named neuroprostheses (NPs) [21].

NPs are assistive devices based on functional electrostimulation at the neural level and controlled by biofeedback strategies. They play an important role in neurological rehabilitation because they may provide not only restoration of function in the short term, but also have the potential to increase the outcome of regeneration techniques [22].

NPs can assist in artificially replacing missing motor, sensory or cognitive functionality, or in controlling the activation of a function that is lost due to CNS disease or SCI. Their effect can be regulated, since the presence of denervation or neuropathic changes can be assessed, as can the conductivity of central and peripheral pathways, and the activity of reflexes can be localized [23]. Examples include devices to improve hearing, vision and motor and cognitive functions; this category also includes deep brain stimulators [24].

Neural mechanisms may be activated by electrical stimulation, which is directly applied to peripheral nerves or to the cerebral cortex, or even by inhibiting neural activity. Non-invasive cortical stimulation can consist of transcranial direct current stimulation (tDCS) or repetitive transcranial magnetic stimulation (rTMS). The latter is a painless method for modulating the functions of stimulated cortical regions or interconnected areas [21]; it has the effect of exciting the motor nerves to activate the muscles of the hand, leg and foot [25, 26]. tDCS and rTMS studies in healthy humans and in stroke survivors have demonstrated that different stimulation frequencies, pulse patterns and intensities will exert different effects on cortical and spinal cord excitability.

The success of NPs lies in three main factors: neuroplasticity, neural stimulation techniques and the neural substrate [21].

2.1 Functional Electrical Stimulation

Functional electrical stimulation (FES) is currently being investigated as a technique that may be used to elicit long-term neuroplasticity for motor cortical reorganization. FES refers to the use of electrical stimulation to activate a specific target muscle during a task, in order to train the affected muscles to mimic normal movements or functions, for example walking or grasping. FES is considered an ideal technique for use in combination with motor NPs.

FES can often produce useful clinical and functional outcomes, even though the basic physiological actions of NPs are often poorly understood", in the same way as many drug treatments, where the basic scientific understanding has often lagged far behind successful clinical application [22]. Emerging research indicates that systematic application of FES in patients with SCI provides a mechanism for optimizing the neural activity below the injury level, while reducing associated complications and improving overall health [5]. It is important to draw a clear distinction between paretic and paralyzed subjects: only paretic subjects have the potential in their neuromuscular system to be retrained using FES [15].

FES, which needs to be under the subject's control, should be available anytime and anywhere, rather than applied only at a specific time and place, such as a rehabilitation clinic. For these reasons, FES and NPs are very different from therapeutic electrical stimulation, whose main goal is to provide pain relief, improve muscle tone, bulk and strength, increase range of motion, reduce spasticity, and improve limb blood flow [27]. Functional electrical therapy is a combination of functional exercise and electrical therapy. The functional electrical therapy protocol comprises voluntary movement of the paretic limb in synchrony with the electrically assisted motor functions in order to perform typical daily activities [28, 15].

FES can be used with non-invasive or invasive NPs. Motor nerves may be stimulated using either surface (transcutaneous) or implanted (percutaneous) electrodes [29]. Surface FES systems (non-invasive) can be applied at a very early stage of the rehabilitation process, and can easily be removed if the patient is not comfortable with them. The transcutaneous stimulation is delivered via self-adhesive or non-adhesive electrodes that are placed on the subject's skin over nerve bundles.

These electrodes must have a sufficient surface area to guarantee electrical contact; they must be comfortable and must not irritate the skin (thanks to the use of hypoallergenic materials); they must also be easy to attach and should be able to stay in place for at least one active day. They should have a reliable means of connection to the stimulator. Finally, they should also be reusable, inexpensive, resistant to medical solvents and electrode gels, and offer low and stable electrical resistance [30]. The main disadvantages of the transcutaneous technique are the lack of stimulation selectivity, the impossibility of isolating deep muscles, and the poor reliability of muscle contraction due to the difficulty in localizing specific motor points; furthermore, the technique may be painful, and the electrodes have to be put on and taken off daily [31].

On the other hand, the percutaneous stimulation (invasive) system uses implanted electrodes that are attached to the nerves or to the muscles close to the nerves through surgical intervention. Implanted stimulation electrodes reliably and selectively activate deep muscles and avoid problems of cutaneous pain. In addition, once an implanted FES system is inserted, less time is required to put it on and to take it off compared with a surface stimulation system [29]. The use of implantable neuroprosthetic devices continues to be controversial because of a range of issues: medical complications, questions over the reliability and functional usefulness of the devices, the need for special care, as well as the fact that robust and fully implantable devices are limited [31].

Analysis of electrical behavior and thresholds has indicated that the surgical phase is crucial, due to the sensitivity of functional responses to electrode placement. Neural stimulation proved to be more efficient and more stable over time, compared with transcutaneous techniques. This mode requires less energy and provides more selective stimulation [32].

FES is a technique that employs bursts of short monophasic and biphasic current or voltage pulses applied to intact motor nerves to generate action potentials (APs), which are propagated along the axons towards the target muscle. When electrical pulses reach the muscle, they cause muscle contraction. To achieve a continuous muscle contraction, the FES system must induce at least 20 APs per second, otherwise, the muscle will not generate a steady output force, and instead will only twitch. Monophasic pulses can potentially cause skin burns and tissue damage due to the galvanic effect; therefore, the majority of FES systems use biphasic current pulses [29].

Intensity, pulse width and duty cycle, as well as output impedance of the current generator and impedance of the tissue-electrode interface, determine the electrical charge to be delivered to the stimulated neuromuscular structure. The electrical properties of the tissue, such as such impedance (ranging from 10 to 100 Ω), conductivity (0.04–0.14 S/m), and permittivity (1.5–40 M at 10 Hz), determine the pathways of current flow. Other important aspects to consider include the electrodes and the skin-electrode interface, whose resistive and capacitive properties can induce phase changes in the stimulation currents. In order to neglect the impedance changes, the current generator is selected as a constant or regulated voltage device with low-output impedance and precision control of the current supplied to the tissue; in these conditions, even if the voltage is high, it is not harmful [15].

Prior to beginning electrical stimulation treatment, it is important to evaluate the patient's medical history, and the potential risks and benefits in order to determine whether the patient is a suitable candidate for FES treatment. The following are critical issues and considerations:

- The desired peripheral nerve must be intact. The motor nerves of the targeted muscle must be intact for the APs to be propagated.
- The muscle and bone response to FES must be well studied for each patient.
- The success of surface stimulation can be limited; thus, alternative methods, such as the implantation of indwelling electrodes may need to be considered.
- The presence of active medical devices implanted in the subject, such as pacemakers, glucose monitors and infusion pumps, must be taken into account.
- The timing and strategy of the treatment must be carefully planned.

FES elicits contractions that lack a smooth, gradual onset, reflecting biased and asynchronous motor recruitment. Electrical stimulation recruits different motor units in comparison with a voluntary contraction. Contractions recruiting motor units depend on electrode size and proximity to the stimulation area. Fatigue occurs more rapidly in an electrically generated contraction because a greater portion of fatigable motor units are necessary for this type of contraction.

Combining voluntary contractions with FES produces the best and strongest contraction.

2.2 Control and Regulation Tasks

In addition to stimulating muscle, motor NPs must also fulfil other tasks normally performed by the nervous system in order to both control and regulate the artificial movements in the attempt to imitate natural gait [33].

The first control method used for this purpose was the feedforward (open-loop) method, in which the subject controlled the NP by pressing buttons and fixing the maximal level of electrical current that would be delivered to the muscles. The input of this system is entirely independent of its output, and final outcomes have no influence on input. Although many paraplegics can work with devices of this type, they require concentration; repeated button presses by thumbs can be uncomfortable and, in patients with complete SCI and reduced hand function, the use of manual switches may be precluded. Due to these limitations, the subject cannot manually perform a complete stimulation pattern in order to achieve the desired movement. The difference between actual movement and wanted movement is called an error signal of the system and it is very useful for correcting deviation in the NP output.

NPs that allow stimulation to be started and stopped voluntarily by the user (NP open-loop control systems) also must generate commands to create the basic pattern of motion. Adaptive feedforward control, as implemented in the cycle-to-cycle controller, has provided good compensation for the gradual decrease in performance observed with open-loop control [33].

Recently, automatic FES controllers have been developed. In these devices, the error signal comprises feedback to the input of the system in order to correct the tasks. As the input-to-output path and the error feedback path create a closed loop, this type of control system is referred to as a closed-loop control system. In current NP controllers (closed-loop control systems), movement is synthesized by iteratively modifying a basic time-varying stimulation pattern.

The control task has the function of driving the temporal patterns for muscle stimulation to produce the desired movements, and the regulation task is the modification of these patterns during use to correct for unanticipated changes (disturbances) in the stimulated muscles or in the environment. Figure 1 shows a general scheme of an NP control system, used to procure the temporal pattern of a particular desired movement.

An artificial neural network (ANN) has been used for adaptive control of gait swing generated by FES when stimulation was applied to the left femoral and peroneal nerves. The ANN inputs consisted of hip, knee and ankle angular data obtained utilizing a goniometer [34].

The temporal patterns of muscular activation (control), in addition to considering limb outcomes, must also take into account the nonlinear and dynamic relationships between stimulus parameters and muscle output. The most important dynamic properties include inertia of limb segments and the interval between stimulation of the muscle and generation of the force to accelerate or decelerate the limb [35].

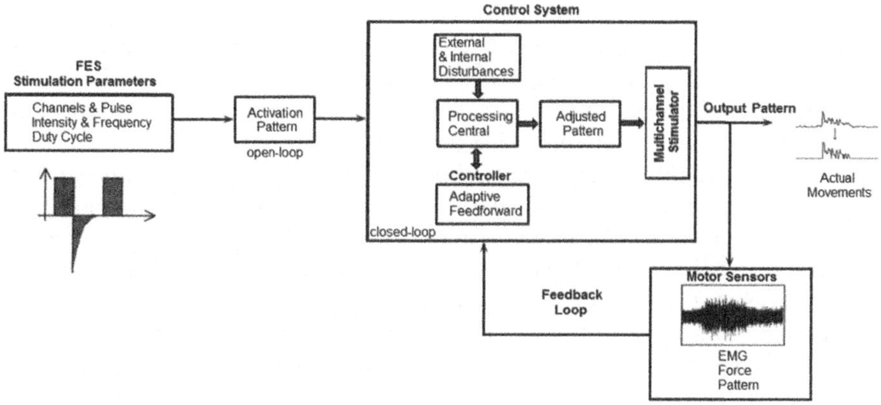

Fig. 1 Simplified blocks diagram of a control system for a neuroprosthesis. Open-loop and closed-loop view

2.3 *Motor Neuroprostheses*

Some patients with stroke, SCI, multiple sclerosis or traumatic brain injury can show lower-limb motor disabilities. Frequently, these patients can walk independently, but with gait abnormalities or impaired balance which limits their gait performance in daily activities and renders them more susceptible to injury [5].

NPs using FES to stimulate peripheral motor nerves (motor NPs), employing electrodes that may be implanted or placed on the surface of the skin, rely on activation of lower motor neurons. The main goal of these motor NPs is to restore an optimal degree of natural gait function to the damaged or paralyzed lower muscles by means of the application of extracellular electrical current patterns.

Brain injury survivors can derive significant benefit from short-term use of lower limb motor NPs, and their gait abilities, stability and balance can be improved to an even greater degree if they intensify their use of these devices.

2.3.1 Neuroprostheses for Gait

Several types of lower limb motor NP are available, for different purposes. The first and most popular is a stimulator that activates the fibular (usually called peroneal) nerve, sending low-level electrical impulses via surface electrodes to counteract foot drop. Foot drop is the inability to lift the foot and toes when walking. Liberson et al. [36], proposed that electrical stimulation of the peroneal nerve and the anterior tibial muscles may be coordinated with the gait cycle, thus improving gait quality in hemiplegic patients [36].

With conventional foot-drop NPs, surface electrodes are placed over the peroneal nerve (cathode) near the head of the fibula and above the tibialis anterior muscle (anode) [37]. Newer foot-drop NPs, such as the Walk Aide device, are controlled by a tilt sensor that is in radiofrequency communication with the stimulator. The tilt sensor is placed inside the shoe (or sole) so that it can detect and measure the pressure exerted by the heel on the ground, as well as the tilt of the leg, to allow tracking of the angle and speed of the leg. Essentially, when the lower leg is tilted back at the end of stance (between heel-off and toe-off), the tilt sensor triggers a train of stimuli. When the leg tilts forward immediately after the foot strikes the ground, the stimuli are interrupted [38].

Hausdorff et al. demonstrated that, even in the initial stages of applying the NESS L300 device, designed to relieve foot drop, patients showed improved stability and gait rhythmicity, and increased gait velocity [39]. The works of Hausdorff, as well as those of Weerdesteyn et al. [40], demonstrated that the number of falls was significantly reduced in hemiparetic patients who used FES to correct foot drop.

Since the 1990s, FES-assisted walking has been studied as a promising technology to correct spasticity and improve walking endurance, speed and lower-limb muscle strength [41].

Human walking motion involves stimulation of the lower-limb muscle groups, including the hip flexors and extensors, knee flexors and extensors, and ankle plantar flexors and dorsiflexors. The peroneal nerve is the main nerve stimulated. From a biomechanical point of view, FES of the ankle plantar flexors results in increased ground clearance of the lower limb. Additionally, FES-assisted lifting of the heel has been shown to result in elimination of extensor tone, thus shortening the swing time [42].

Walking performance evaluation and quantitative motion analysis are used as indicators to modify the intensity, frequency, duty cycle and timing of the stimulation, in order to customize the stimulation pattern to each subject. FES of the dorsiflexors is a well-accepted intervention that enables clinically meaningful changes in walking speed, leading to preserved or increased functional walking in persons with multiple sclerosis [43].

Open-loop NPs can cause excessive muscle fatigue. A gait closed-loop NP with a finite-state controller adapted to the individual knee was introduced to provide users with increased control over their desired movement; with this system, muscle activation of the knee extensors can be reduced by 50% compared with open-loop systems [35].

Some researchers found that single-channel FES is not sufficient to provide functional gait. Multi-channel NPs offer a strategy to assist gait therapy. The number of muscles to be targeted and the intensity, frequency and duty cycle of the FES-assisted gait training need to be determined, and these will depend on the single subject's residual functioning. An individual's suitability to undergo FES-assisted gait therapy also depends on his/her cardiovascular and neuromuscular capacity, in addition to psychological factors such as motivation [42].

2.3.2 Neuroprostheses for Vestibular Function

When vestibular function is lost, essential tasks such as postural control, gaze stabilization, and spatial orientation are limited; gait and balance are significantly affected. The peripheral vestibular system is composed of multi-dimensional motion sensors that provide information crucial to balance control. Despite intensive balance retraining, the majority of patients with bilateral vestibular function loss (BVL) do not show evidence of recovery of their long-term vestibular function.

The research consortium comprising the Service of Otorhinolaryngology and Head and Neck Surgery at Geneva University Hospitals, the Division of Balance Disorders of the Maastricht University Medical Center, and Translational Neural Engineering Laboratory of the École Polytechnique Fédérate de Lausanne, Switzerland, as well as the BioRobotics Institute of Pisa, Italy, investigated the potential of electrical stimulation of the ampullary branches of the vestibular nerve by means of a vestibular NP prototype consisting of a modified cochlear implant (MED-EL, Innsbruck, Austria) for the rehabilitation of patients with BVL [44].

These investigators reported that the vestibulo-ocular reflex (VOR) can be artificially restored in patients with BVL by means of a vestibular NP. VOR is a reflex eye movement that maintains the perception of a stable gaze. It is an important parameter in the assessment of vestibular function. These researchers conducted a study in three patients, and their results provide the first objective evidence that gaze stabilization mechanisms in patients with BVL can be restored using a vestibular NP, mimicking the stable gaze pattern, which is so important in daily locomotion [44].

2.3.3 Postural Neuroprostheses

Standing up, postural control (standing) and sitting down are highly complex motor activities. The stand-to-sit maneuver involves contraction of several muscles of the body [45]. Standing is a prerequisite for walking. Vertical posture is accomplished thanks to proprioceptive and cutaneous input deriving from the legs. Balance depends on bilaterally symmetrical responses to body perturbations [46]. For patients who cannot stand up by themselves, an external assistive system for the erect position is required. Some examples of external assistive systems are FES of joint extensors, knee-ankle-foot orthoses, and standing frames.

In lower-limb paralysis, vestibular function, anteroposterior stability, visual perception, and leg information are missing or modified. Muscles on the paretic and non-paretic side differ in strength, resulting in asymmetry. These asymmetrical weaknesses disrupt balance and make it difficult to manage postural disturbances [47]. Sixty percent of body weight is borne by the non-paretic limb [48], the paretic knee is slightly flexed, and the foot of the paretic limb is placed in front of the body's center of gravity (increasing the support base and moving the center of pressure to the forefoot zone of the non-paretic leg) [15].

Different closed-loop control strategies have been used for standing up and sitting down. The first devices comprised a proportional integral derivative controller (PID controller) for controlling FES in order to activate standing up and sitting down functions. Even though satisfactory control behavior was observed during standing up, paraplegic patients exhibited instability [49].

One implantable NP system providing support in standing and assisted walking consists of a multi-channel implanted receiver-stimulator, epimysial and surgically implanted intramuscular electrodes, and a programmable, wearable external controller; it is supported by associated software and clinical rehabilitation protocols [32].

Also, NP systems can improve balance, modulate spasticity, and reduce fatigue in standing and gait, but feedback on event detection is required to trigger transitions between stimulation sequences, as well as feedback to patients concerning the state of their lower limbs [50].

Current results indicate that NP stimulation strategy (patterns, sequences and control pulses) must be improved to achieve a more natural movement and to reduce the risk of injury during descent, minimizing impact and providing a gentle transition from standing to sitting [45].

3 Hybrid Neuroprosthesis Systems

A hybrid NP system is a neuroprosthesis coupled with another neurorehabilitation technology, such as a brain computer interface (BCI), based on an electroencephalography (EEG) signal or biofeedback by electromyography (EMG) signal, which has been developed as an NP control option. Similarly, orthotic, robotic or exoskeletal devices can be utilized to achieve normal motion patterns.

Chia et al. showed that gait training using an FES-based treadmill enhances walking abilities, increasing gait speed while lowering effort. This therapeutic intervention exhibited a significant additive effect on gait coordination when compared with that without FES [51].

A radiofrequency-controlled NP appears to enhance balance control during walking, thus more effectively managing foot drop in comparison with a standard ankle-foot orthosis without FES [52].

3.1 Electromyography Feedback

Movement achieved by specific patterns of stimulation is detected by placing EMG electrodes (surface or percutaneous) over target muscles. Processing of the EMG signal is carried out to determine the variance between the output EMG pattern and the physiological EMG pattern (desired movement). This difference serves as input for the NP controller, and allows adjustment of the FES stimulation pattern.

Patients normally use a switch to trigger each step manually and progress through the customized pattern of muscle activations required to achieve the walking function. Dutta et al. showed that using two-channel surface EMG signals to control an implantable FES device could produce cyclic movement of the lower limbs for ambulation. These authors demonstrated that myoelectric control commands can be selected accurately from surface EMG before a fully implantable EMG-triggered FES system for walking is implemented [53].

3.2 *Brain Computer Interface*

Current advances in NPs to restore walking focus on coupling these devices with BCIs, and on the use of motor cortical activity to control FES with the purpose of activating the paralyzed limb, bypassing the diseased neural pathway. Müller-Putz et al. [54], demonstrated that a patient was able to move a simple object from one place to another when an EEG-BCI was coupled with an implanted NP [54].

BCI systems aim to provide a non-muscular channel through which external devices are controlled by electrical activity of the brain. Ideally, a BCI accurately decodes the movement intention, i.e., imagined trajectories of body parts, in real time and transforms the information into a control signal to active an external device, e.g., a motor NP for restoring movement. This amounts to the establishment of a direct link between the intended movement and the stimulation pattern executed by the motor NP, facilitating natural and intuitive movement control.

There exist different strategies or paradigms in BCI technology. These paradigms determine the subject's intentions to move or communicate through the processing of electrical brain signals, typically, slow cortical potentials, visual evoked potentials, P300 potentials, or beta and mu rhythms, which are recorded on the scalp, or cortical neuronal activity recorded by electrodes implanted in the brain. BCI can be classified as dependent or independent according to whether or not physiological control is required.

A motor-imagery BCI comprises an independent promissory strategy that requires only decoding of the user's imagery of motor tasks, e.g., of right/left foot movement. The system is activated in response to visual cues or movement intention from the timeline, e.g. Graz paradigm [55]. Mu rhythms recorded in the sensorimotor cortex decrease their spectral power density when the user moves the limb. The same phenomenon occurs if the user imagines moving the paretic limb [56].

The subject performs actions (e.g., idling or foot dorsiflexion) to generate mu potentials in the sensorimotor cortex. Electrodes placed on the scalp pick up the underlying EEG, after which signal analysis is carried out by the BCI. During motor imagery tasks, multichannel EEG signals exhibit task-specific features in both spatial and temporal (or frequency) domains. Data processing consists of the extraction of discriminant spatio-spectral EEG features and classification of events. Finally, the classified signals are translated into meaningful commands that are sent to a microcontroller unit (MCU). The MCU controls the FES system, which sends the pattern of electrical stimulation to the subject's target muscles.

A BCI user needs to learn to generate motor imagery cortical patterns effectively in order to control the external device. This process is termed BCI learning, and it often requires significant effort and time. The fact that the BCI aims to elicit motor activity by providing afferent feedback to the sensorimotor cortex indicates that this method may also induce brain plasticity and sensory patterns [57].

Gender differences in EEG during motor tasks have been studied [58, 59]. In these papers, it was established that the calibration of a motor imagery BCI and of the subject's BCI learning can be improved if gender is taken into account. Carino et al. have shown that new algorithms for the classification of surface EEG signals, such as spiking neuron models (SNMs), with a time-varying encoding strategy, could increase the number of motor imagery BCI users. This is because the SNMs used the particle swarm optimization strategy, demonstrating high classification performance and low computational cost when the model was applied to identify the motor imagery time-frequency features of both stroke survivors and healthy subjects [60].

Figure 2 shows a typical BCI-controlled NP monitored with EMG. Sensors (which can be electrogoniometers, accelerometers, or electromyography electrodes)

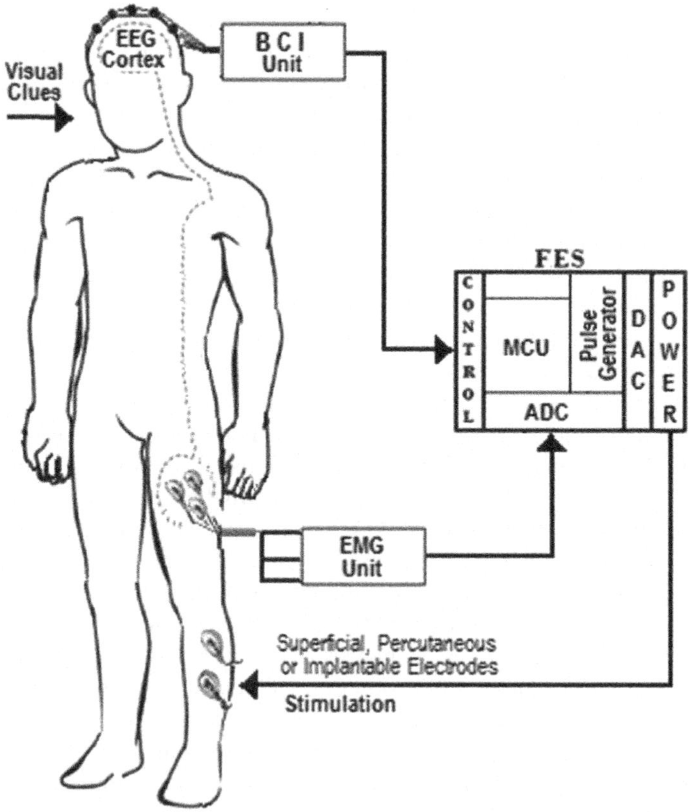

Fig. 2 Block diagram of a basic BCI-controlled neuroprosthesis with EMG muscle monitoring. When a deviation occurs, the FES pattern is adjusted or the stimulation electrodes are relocated

may be placed on the stimulated limb to verify the movement achieved. If a deviation occurs, the pattern is adjusted or the stimulation electrodes are relocated.

Invasive techniques to record the electrical signal within the brain (electrocorticography or deep recording) [61] have shown better success than non-invasive techniques based on surface EEG for decoding movement imagery to control devices. Nevertheless, the use of BCIs for non-invasive motor imagery has been growing, due to their low risk of complications (no surgical risk and minimal risk of infection), low cost, ease of use, and wide availability [62].

Only a few BCIs have used hemodynamic signals to control lower-limb prostheses. Frontal premotor and posterior parietal activations could be detected by fNIRS during preparation of hip movement, balance and posture retention during standing and walking. Recent developments in fNIRS-BCI suggest that these systems are more suitable for the rehabilitation of lower limb movement since the occurrence of head motion artifacts corrupting the fNIRS signal is not such an issue [63].

3.3 *Neuroprosthesis-Assisted Gait Training*

SCI and stroke survivors present gross muscular atrophy, altered muscle molecular phenotype, impaired cardiovascular endurance, increased intramuscular fat, elevated tissue inflammatory markers, bone loss, and diminished peripheral blood flow dynamics in the paretic leg. The incidence of hip fracture, which is the most frequent fracture following stroke, can be 2–4 times higher in stroke patients than in the reference population. Therefore, voluntary exercise combined with FES exercise has been shown not only to improve motor function, but also to increase cardiovascular fitness and reduce bone loss and fat.

NP-assisted gait training comprises muscle activation by FES, conventional physiotherapy, and equipment-supported training, using equipment such as treadmills, rowing devices and robot-assisted equipment. This rehabilitation methodology has shown the additive effects of FES in terms of reducing spasticity and improving dorsiflexor strength, walking ability and metabolic fitness. Davoodi and Andrews presented a rowing machine adapted for FES control. Rowing therapy is initiated by voluntary movement of the upper limbs and FES generates movement of the paralyzed legs. To achieve a smooth maneuver, coordinated rowing exercise, and less muscle energy expenditure, the authors proposed the use of a fuzzy logic control system [64].

The intensity and frequency of this rehabilitation program may aid in improving motor and cardiovascular functions. Also, NP-assisted gait training should be started as soon as the patient becomes clinically stable, since early intervention has been shown to give better functional outcomes and better survival rates, and to reduce the duration of therapy required.

4 Conclusion

Neuroprostheses implemented to restore or enhance motor functions are aimed at improving the health, independence and quality of life of persons living with the effects of brain injury, SCI, or neurodegenerative diseases. Neuroprosthetic technology employing FES offers great potential, not only because it is safe and efficacious, but also because it may help to enhance motor and cardiovascular functions by restoring and improving the ability to stand, transfer and exercise [32].

NP technology application depends on the development of hardware and novel signal processing algorithms, including implantable devices, electrode-tissue interfaces, advances in the understanding of physiological adaptations to closed-loop interactions with neural devices, and refinement of stimulation methods for precise activation of neural tissue [65].

Top-down strategies utilizing methodologies based on neurophysiological or metabolic brain feedback in conjunction with conventional physiotherapy and mechanical devices may represent a promising approach to modulate brain reorganization and motor behavior by selectively enhancing preserved neural circuits or promoting the formation of new functional circuits in individuals with brain damage. Limitations following brain lesions are varied, and include gait dysfunction, fall risk, limitations in activities of daily living, swallowing difficulties, reduced lower limb function, and impaired communication, among others.

FES-assisted leg training using devices such as ergometers, treadmills and rowing machines bring about improvements in muscle size, strength and composition. The increase in fiber area and in capillary number improves fatigue resistance and oxidative capacities, as does the conversion from type IIB to type IIA and type I muscle fibers.

Task-specific FES-assisted gait therapy may drive functionally relevant neuroplastic changes in the brain, exert an influence on cerebral reorganization, and consequently improve volitional gait in order to reach a plateau for therapeutic benefits without adverse effects.

Gait therapy needs to be tailored to each individual condition in accordance with the World Health Organization (WHO) International Classification of Functioning (ICF). The WHO-ICF model recommends intervention at multiple levels, for example, consideration of the individual's capacity for functional recovery, metabolic proficiency and cardiovascular fitness, as well as functional gait analysis to select the paretic muscles to be assisted with FES. The WHO-ICF model may help us to clarify the response to FES-assisted gait therapy at each level and also the relationships between different levels, for the benefit of future rehabilitation strategies.

NP-BCI training supported by EMG is expected to induce or enhance motor recovery, through improvement of brain plasticity at the sensorimotor cortical area near the lesion.

This potential benefit is often associated with afferent feedback.

Novel methods are emerging for optical and magnetic stimulation of the nervous system to supplement the electrical stimulation techniques currently used with NPs. Combining neural stimulation and recording technologies may result in intuitive closed-loop controlled assistive NPs that address the need to control and modify the stimulation pattern [64].

The clinical application of NPs demands close and long-term collaboration between scientists, engineers and clinicians. The lack of accessible, well-equipped rehabilitation facilities is due to their high costs; overcoming this deficiency is a current challenge. Full restoration of function with hybrid NP systems is unlikely in the near future, but constant research and development in this field will likely result in substantial improvements in the quality of life of disabled individuals.

References

1. Van Dijk J. On the interaction between the central nervous system and the peripheral motor system. Biol Cybern. 1978;30(4):195–208.
2. Jacobson M. Beginnings of the nervous system. In: Rao M, Jacobson M, editors. Developmental neurobiology. US: Springer; 2005. p. 365–413.
3. Janig W. Autonomic nervous system. In: Schmidt R, Thews G, editors. Human physiology. New York, NY: Springer; 1989. P. 333–70.
4. Rodriguez MR, Clemente FAR. Avaliação das disfunções do controle motor. Universitas Ciências da Saúde. 2008;2(2):259–67.
5. Martin R, Sadowsky C, Obst K, Meyer B, McDonald J. Functional electrical stimulation in spinal cord injury: from theory to practice. Top Spinal Cord Inj Rehabil. 2012;18(1):28–33.
6. Wall J, Xu J, Wang X. Human brain plasticity: an emerging view of the multiple substrates and X sensory inputs from the body. Brain Res Rev. 2002;39(2):181–215.
7. Portera-Sánchez A, Toffano G. Neuroplasticity: a new therapeutic tool in the CNS pathology. Berlin: Springer; 1987. p. 9–30.
8. Aguilar-Rebolledo F. Plasticidad cerebral: antecedentes cientificos y perspectivas de desarrollo. Bol Med Hosp Infant Mex. 1998;55(9):514–25.
9. Young J, Tolentino M. Neuroplasticity and its applications for rehabilitation. Am J Ther. 2011;18(1):70–80.
10. Stahnisch FW, Nitsch R. Santiago Ramón y Cajal's concept of neuronal plasticity: the ambiguity lives on. Trends Neurosci. 2002;25(11):589–91.
11. Massimini M, Tononi G, Huber R. Slow waves, synaptic plasticity and information processing: insights from transcranial magnetic stimulation and high-density EEG experiments. Eur J Neurosci. 2009;29(9):1761–70.
12. Auriat AM, Neva JL, Peters S, Ferris JK, Boyd LA. A review of transcranial magnetic stimulation and multimodal neuroimaging to characterize post-stroke neuroplasticity. Front Neurol. 2015;6:226.
13. Pawela Ch, Biswal B, Hudetz A, Li R, Jones S, Cho Y, Matloub H, Hyde J. Interhemispheric neuroplasticity following limb deafferentation detected by resting-state functional connectivity magnetic resonance imaging (fcMRI) and functional magnetic resonance imaging (fMRI). NeuroImage. 2010;49(3):2467–78.
14. Irani F, Platek SM, Bunce S, Ruocco AC, Chute D. Functional near infrared spectroscopy (fNIRS): an emerging neuroimaging technology with important applications for the study of brain disorders. Clin Neuropsychol. 2007;21(1):9–37.

15. Popovic D, Sinkjaer T. Restoring movement state of the art (Chapter 4). In: Control of movement for the physically disabled: control for rehabilitation technology. Berlin: Springer Science & Business Media; 2012. p. 171–313.
16. Popović DB. Principles of command and control for neuroprostheses. In: Kilgore K, editors. Implantable neuroprostheses for restoring function. Cambridge: Woodhead Publishing Elsevier; 2015. p. 45–55.
17. Szuhany K, Bugatti M, Otto M. A meta-analytic review of the effects of exercise on brain-derived neurotrophic factor. J Psychiatr Res. 2015;60:56–64.
18. Van Praag H, Shubert T, Zhao Ch, Gage F. Exercise enhances learning and hippocampal neurogenesis in aged mice. J Neurosci. 2005;25(38):8680–5.
19. Stephenson R. A review of neuroplasticity: some implications for physiotherapy in the treatment of lesions of the brain. Physiotherapy. 1993;79(10):699–704.
20. Flachenecker P. Clinical implications of neuroplasticity—the role of rehabilitation in multiple sclerosis. Front Neurol. 2015;6:36–40.
21. Wang W, Collinger J, Perez M, Tyler E, Cohen L, Birbaumer N, et al. Neural interface technology for rehabilitation: exploiting and promoting neuroplasticity. Phys Med Rehabil Clin N Am. 2010;21(1):157–78.
22. Prochazka A, Mushahwar V, McCreery D. Neural prostheses. J Physiol. 2001;533(Pt 1): 99–109.
23. Rushton D. Functional neurostimulation in rehabilitation. In: Greenwood R, Barnes M, McMillan T, Ward C, editors. Handbook of neurological rehabilitation, 2nd ed. Psychology Press Taylor & Francis Group; 2003. p. 245–60.
24. Kasten M, Ievins A, Moritz C. Neural prostheses. New York: Wiley; 2001. Published Online: 27 Jan 2015.
25. Perez MA, Lungholt BK, Nielsen JB. Short-term adaptations in spinal cord circuits evoked by repetitive transcranial magnetic stimulation: possible underlying mechanisms. Exp Brain Res. 2005;162:202.
26. Zuur AT, Cristensen MS, Sinkjaer T, et al. Tibials anterios stretch reflex in early stance is suppressed by repetitive transcranial magnetic stimulation. J Physiol. 2009;587:1669.
27. Sujit OK. Functional electrical stimulation in neurological disorders. Eur J Neurol. 2008;15:437–44.
28. Popovic MB, Popovic DB, Schwirtlich L, Sinkjaer T. Functional electrical therapy (FET): clinical trial in chronic hemiplegic subjects. Neuromodulation. 2004;7(2):133–40.
29. Popovic MR, Curt A, Keller T, Dietz V. Functional electrical stimulation for grasping and walking: indications and limitations. Spinal Cord. 2001;39:403–12.
30. Bajd T, Marinček Č, Munih M. Functional electrical stimulation with surface electrodes. J Autom Control. 2008;18(2):3–9.
31. Bhadra N, Chae J. Implantable neuroprosthetic technology. NeuroRehabilitation. 2009;25: 69–83.
32. Davis J, Triolo R, Uhlir J, Bieri C, Rohde L, Lissy D, Kukke S. Preliminary performance of a surgically implanted neuroprosthesis for standing and transfers—where do we stand? J Rehabil Res Dev. 2001;38(6):609–17.
33. Crago P, Lan N, Veltink P, Abbas J, Kantor C. New control strategies for neuroprosthetic systems. J Rehabil Res Dev. 1996;33(2):158–72.
34. Sepulveda F, Granat MH, Cliquet A. Two artificial neural systems for generation of gait swing by means of neuromuscular electrical stimulation. Med Eng Phys. 1997;19(1):21–8.
35. Fuhr T, Quintern J, Riener R, Schmidt G. Closed-loop control of a gait neuroprosthesis. European Control Conference. 2001;2001:3939–44.
36. Liberson WT, Holmquest HJ, Scot D, Dow M. Functional electrotherapy: stimulation of the peroneal nerve synchronized with the swing phase of the gait of hemiplegic patients. Arch Phys Med Rehabil. 1961;42:101–5.
37. Dai R, Stein RB, Andrews BJ, James KB, Wieler M. Application of tilt sensors in functional electrical stimulation. IEEE Trans Rehabil Eng. 1996;4:63–72.

38. Stein R, Chong S, Everaert D, Rolf R, Thompson A, Whittaker M, Robertson J, Fung J, Preuss R, Momose K, Ihashi K. A multicenter trial of a footdrop stimulator controlled by a tilt sensor. Neurorehabilitation Neural Repair. 2006;20(3):371–9.
39. Hausdorff J, Ring H. The effect on the NESS L300 neuroprosthesis on gait stability and symmetry. J Neurologic Physical Therapy. 2006;30(4):198.
40. Weerdesteyn V, De Niet M, Van Duijnhoven H, Geurts A. Falls in individuals with stroke. J Rehabil Res Dev. 2008;45(8):1195–213.
41. Granat M, Maxwell D, Ferguson A, Lees K, Barbenel J. Peroneal stimulator: evaluation for the correction of spastic drop foot in hemiplegia. Arch Phys Med Rehabil. 1996;77(1):19–24.
42. Khattar B, Banerjee A, Reddi R, Dutta A. Feasibility of functional electrical stimulation-assisted neurorehabilitation following stroke in India: a case series. Case reports in neurological medicine, vol. 2012. Article ID 830873, 7 p.
43. Street T, Taylor P, Swain I. Effectiveness of functional electrical stimulation on walking speed, functional walking category, and clinically meaningful changes for people with multiple sclerosis. Arch Phys Med Rehabil. 2015;96:667–72.
44. Perez A, Guinand N, van de Berg R, Stokroos R, Micera S, Kingma H, Pelizzone M, Guyot JP. Artificial balance: restoration of the vestíbulo-ocular reflex in human with a prototype vestibular neuroprosthesis. Front Neurol. 2014;5(66):1–11.
45. Chang S, Kobetic R, Triolo R. Understanding stand-to-sit maneuver: implications for motor system neuroprostheses after paralysis. J Rehabil Res Dev. 2014;51(9):1339–52.
46. Horak FB, Nashner LM, Diener HC. Postural strategies associated with somatosensory and vestibular loss. Exp Brain Res. 1990;82:167–77.
47. Hamrin E, Eklund G, Hillgren AK, Borges O, Hall J, Hellström O. Muscle strength and balance in post-stroke patients. Ups J Med Sci. 1982;87(1):11–26.
48. Bohannon RW, Larkin PA. Passive ankle dorsiflexion increases in patients after a regimen of tilt table-wedge board standing. A clinical report. Phys Ther. 1985;65(11):1676–8.
49. Riener R, Boll M, Pavan E, Ferrarin M, Frigo C. Neuroprosthesis for standing-up and sitting-down: experimental results. In: Proceedings of the first joint BMES/EMBS conference serving humanity, advancing technology 1999. p. 603.
50. Guiraud D, Stieglitz T, Koch KP, Divoux JL, Rabischong P. An implantable neuroprosthesis for standing and walking in paraplegia: 5-year patient follow-up. J Neural Eng. 2006;3 (4):268–75.
51. Chia N, Ambrosini E, Baccinelli W, Nardone A, Monticone M, Ferrigno G, Pedrocchi A, Ferrante S. A multi-channel biomimetic neuroprosthesis to support treadmill gait training in stroke patients. In: 37th annual international conference of the IEEE engineering in medicine and biology society 2015. p. 7159–62.
52. Ring H, Treger I, Gruendlinger L, Hausdorff J. Neuroprosthesis for footdrop compared with an ankle-foot orthosis: effects on postural control during walking. J Stroke Cerebrovasc Dis. 2009;18(1):41–7.
53. Dutta A, Kobetic R, Triolo R. An objective method for selecting command sources for myoelectrically triggered lower-limb neuroprostheses. J Rehabil Dev. 2011;48(8):935–48.
54. Müller-Putz GR, Scherer R, Pfurtscheller G, Rupp R. EEG-based neuroprosthesis control: a step towards clinical practice. Neurosci Lett. 2005;382(1–2):169–74.
55. Pfurtscheller G, Neuper C. Motor imagery and direct brain-computer communication. Proc IEEE. 2001;89(7):1123–34.
56. Gutiérrez J, Cantillo J, Cariño R, Elías D. Los sistemas de interfaz cerebro-computadora: una herramienta para apoyar la rehabilitación de pacientes con discapacidad motora. Investigación en Discapacidad. 2013;2(2):62–9.
57. Wander J, Blakely T, Miller K, Weaver K, Johnson L, et al. Distributed cortical adaptation during learning of a brain–computer interface task. Proc Nat Acad Sci USA. 2013;110 (26):10818–23.
58. Cantillo J, Gutiérrez J, Carino R, Carrillo P, Elías D. An approach to improve the performance of subject-independent BCIs-based on motor imagery allocating subjects by gender. Biomed Eng Online. 2014;13:158.

59. Cantillo J, Carino R, Carrillo P, Flores T, Elías D, Gutiérrez J. Gender differences in quantitative electroencephalogram during a simple hand movement task in young adults. Revista de Investigación Clinica. 2016;68:245–55.
60. Carino R, Cantillo J, Gutiérrez J, Vazquez R. Classification of motor imagery electroencephalography signals using spiking neurons with different input encoding strategies. In: Neural computing and applications 2016. Online ISSN: 0941–0643.
61. Hiremath S, Chen W, Wang W, Foldes S, Yang Y, Tyler-Kabar E, Collinger J, Boninger M. Brain computer interface learning for systems based on electrocorticography and intracortical microelectrode arrays. Front Integr Neurosci. 2015; 9(Article 40):1–10.
62. Cincotti F, Mattia D, Aloise F, Bufalari S, Schalmk G, Oriolo G, et al. Non-invasive brain-computer interface system: towards its application as assistive technology. Brain Res Bull. 2008;75(6):796–803.
63. Rea M, Rana M, Lugato N, Terekhin P, Gizzi L, Brötz D, Fallgatter A, Birbaumer N, Sitaram R, Caria A. Lower limb movement preparation in chronic stroke: a pilot study towards an fNIRS-BCI for gait rehabilitation. Neurorehabil Neural Repair. 2014;28(6): 564–75.
64. Davoodi R, Andrews B. Fussy logic control of FES rowing exercise in paraplegia. IEEE Trans Biomed Eng. 2004;51(3):541–3.
65. Moritz Ch, Ruther P, Goering S, Stett A, Ball T, Burgard W, Chudler E, RaoNew R. Perspectives on neuroengineering and neurotechnologies: NSF-DFG workshop report. IEEE Trans Biomed Eng. 2016;63(7):1354–67.

Part IV
Spasticity and Gait Rehabilitation

Pathophysiology of Spasticity and Therapeutic Approach

Jörg Wissel

1 Introduction

It is well known that with a delay a lesion of the central nervous system (CNS) involving senso-motor networks in the brain or cervical or thoracic spinal cord will lead to an Upper Motor Neuron Syndrome (UMNS) caudal of the lesion. Clinically UMNS could be detected by increased resistance against passive movement during rest position (defined by Lance [22]), enhanced tendon reflexes [12, 28, 38], pyramidal signs and flexor-reflexes [12, 28], Co-contraction [12, 38], spastic dystonia [12, 38], and result in disturbed posture, slowed motor performance with decreased dexterity and coordination difficulties named spastic movement disorder (SMD, [13]).

In every day communication clinicians use the term "spasticity" as a collective to describes a motor syndrome that include positive and negative symptoms reflecting the UMNS of which spasticity defined by Lance [23] is only one part. The Lance 1980 definition describes the phenomenon only with its reflex features during rest, and that is not enough to reflect the burden of SMD.

Therefore it is of major importance to include all positive features of UMNS that may be part of SMD during voluntary and involuntary movements in the definition to allow those as targets for future management or training programs to better reduce motor coordination difficulties and slowing of voluntary movement as main activity limitation features of SMD [14].

J. Wissel (✉)
Department of Neurology, Department Neurological Rehabilitation and Physical Therapy, Vivantes Hospital Spandau, Neue Bergstrasse 6, 13585 Berlin, Germany
e-mail: Joerg.Wissel@vivantes.de

G. Sandrini et al. (eds.), *Advanced Technologies for the Rehabilitation of Gait and Balance Disorders*, Biosystems & Biorobotics 19,
https://doi.org/10.1007/978-3-319-72736-3_30

It is estimated that at this time point more than 12 million people worldwide suffer from SMD of different severity [21, 55]. In those people UMNS can be caused by a variety of diseases such as ischemic stroke of the brain or spinal cord, brain or spine hematomas, traumatic brain (TBI) or spinal cord injury (SCI), brain or spinal cord tumors, multiple sclerosis (MS), inflammation or infection of the brain or spinal cord, spastic cerebral palsy (CP), neurodegenerative diseases like Amyotrophic Lateral Sklerosis (ALS) or hereditary disorders like Hereditary Spastic Paraplegia (HSP).

With respect to ongoing discussion on how we should handle spasticity in early stages of diseases common ground in clinical neurology is that acute causal treatment of underlying disease should be completed or finished (e.g. systematic thrombolysis in stroke or antibiotics or virostatic treatment in encephalitis), causal treatment should be on an established therapeutic level (e.g. immune modulation in MS) or not available (e.g. in HSP) to allow the team to focus with therapeutic intervention on the management of SMD only. Nowadays in most patients with lesions of the CNS (e.g. more than one week following stroke, TBI, SCI) there is no option of further causal treatment of the remaining symptoms, but it is of major importance to introduce preventive measures to avoid another stroke like secondary prevention following stroke (e.g. introducing anticoagulation in cardiogenic stroke) or treat risk factors for further insults (e.g. treat cardiac valve defects, metabolic disease or arterial hypertension) or avoid consequences of chronic sequelae (like contractures or skin damage from severe spasticity).

The exact prevalence of UMNS with clinically relevant positive features that can be classified as spasticity is not known. However, it is estimated that up to 40% of stroke [51] survivors and more than 50% of patients with MS and CP are affected by increased resistance against passive movement during rest position [23] throughout the cause of their disease. This implies that in industrialized countries—with increasing numbers of elderly inhabitants and increasing numbers of stroke and cancer survivors and countries with well organized intensive care units with higher numbers of survivors of severe CNS lesions (TBI and SCI)—the consequences of spasticity create an increasing social and economical burden and triggers increased efforts to better understand and manage SMD [55].

2 Clinical Signs and Definition of Spasticity

Unfortunately in the last 30 years the term spasticity has been inconsistently defined [27]. Nowadays consensus among specialists in basic science and clinical management in the field of spasticity research is that spastic muscle tone defined as increased resistance against passive movement during rest position is only one of several components of the UMNS that form the clinical syndrome spasticity [13, 32].

Spasticity definition by Lance [23] focuses on spinal reflexes during rest position and not on disturbed voluntary movement performance in UMNS and defines spasticity as a motor disorder, characterized by a velocity-dependent increase in tonic stretch reflexes with exaggerated tendon jerks, resulting from hyper-excitability of the stretch reflex as one component of the UMNS during rest position. Passive stretch of a spastic muscle during rest position, if monitored by surface electromyography (sEMG), produces increased sEMG activity while slow stretch velocities than in normal controls or compared to sEMG recordings in the same condition (angle velocity constant) from non affected muscles [43]. Therefore in case of spasticity defined by Lance [23] and the other positive symptoms/signs of the UMNS like clonus, co-contraction of antagonists or spastic dystonia higher amounts of sEMG activity can be registered from involved movement segments (antagonistic muscles) than in segments that are not affected from UMNS when passively stretched.

Other positive features of UMNS than velcocity-dependent increase in muscle tone are hyperreflexia (increased amplitude of tendon reflexes and increased area where the tendon reflexes can be elicit), muscle hypertonia (increased baseline muscle tone/activity), co-contraction of antagonistic muscles (disturbed antagonistic coordination, mainly inhibition of antagonist is diminished), associated reactions and disinhibited movement synergies [14].

The SPASM Consortium (European Thematic Network to Develop Standardized Measures of Spasticity [32]) put together 2005 a new definition: Spasticity is defined as a disordered sensorimotor control, resulting from an upper motor neuron (UMN) lesion, presenting as intermittent or sustained involuntary activation of muscle. That definition excluded all negative features from UMNS (see above) and secondary changes like soft tissue shortening, contracture and bony changes from definition of spasticity. Therefore as described above spasticity represents only involuntary muscle activation that could be induced by stretch, voluntary movement or other triggers. Those spastic activity could be spontaneous—intermittent (like spastic dystonia without trigger [12, 38], or e.g. sustained muscle activity following stretch (with trigger, e.g. pyramidal signs and flexor-reflexes [12, 28]) or Co-contraction [12, 38], that create spastic posture or movements in body segments affected from the UMNS.

Based on this definition it is possible to clinically classify the topical distribution of spasticity over the different body segments affected from UMNS [50]. With respect to the topical distribution of involuntary muscle activity that fulfill the SPASM definition a focal (one hand, one foot or elbow) or multi-focal (hand and foot) distribution can be differentiated from segmental spasticity (two or more focal areas beside to each other are affected e.g. segmental arm-spasticity: hand and forearm with elbow or segmental leg-spasticity: toes, ankle, knee and hip is involved) or multi-segmental (both legs: para- or leg and arm on one side: hemi-spastic), and generalized distribution of spasticity (e.g. all four limbs and body is affected) [50].

Using neurophysiological measures with poly-s-EMG (surface-Electromyography) to monitor muscle activity at standardized electrode position over multiple muscles (poly-s-EMG) at upper and lower limb and core muscles during different body positions and action it is possible to document SMD [54]. While recordings at rest, when eliciting mono- and polysynaptic reflexes, and during a protocol of standard passive and active motor tests/tasks e.g. alternating passive and active extension and flexion of joints, in the body segment affected from UMNS the negative and positive symptoms of the UMNS could be registered as increased and/or un-coordinated tonic or phasic EMG activity in antagonistic muscles (for method see Brain Motor Control Assessment = BMCA) [39]. This highly standardized evaluation procedure BMCA with poly-sEMG recordings allow to classify the different spastic motor patterns and positive clinical features of UMNS on the basis of poly-sEMG registration in cerebral and spinal lesions.

In case of instrumented gait analysis with poly-sEMG of leg muscles and additional registration of kinematic parameters of hip, knee and ankle and kinetic parameters (force platform) it allows to classify spastic gait pattern (e.g. co-contracting activation pattern of rectus femoris during swing phase in stiff knee gait pattern) [5].

Biomechanical changes of muscle properties in the region affected from UMNS are believed to begin with delay from the CNS lesion [13]. Over time body segments affected from spasticity show muscle atrophy and increased muscle stiffness (increased inertia of the muscle) as well as soft tissue (fascias and tendons) shortening that ends up in muscles and soft tissue contractures that are clinically named spastic contractures. Spastic contracture can begin few hours after the onset of immobilization following CNS lesion [14]. Progressive shrinking of muscles and soft tissue may result in restriction in passive and active Range of Motion (pROM and aROM) of joints and whole limbs involved which add to the spastic movement patterns and spastic postures and limbs disfigurements [50].

Muscle atrophy may be due to loss of voluntary activation [31] or by reduced stretching and loss of sarcomers that was found in muscle biopsy [25].

Negative features of the UMNS are muscle weakness or paresis (reduced ability to voluntarily develop adequate muscle force in intended—selected muscles), generalized fatique (loss of ability to produce adequate levels of motor activity), loss of dexterity (incoordination of fine motor tasks), loss of flexibility (inability to fast react with senso-motor system to external irritations) and disturbed fine motor tasks or falls coordination of movements [13, 14].

Features of these negative symptoms of the UMNS like e.g. paresis, fatique and disturbed coordination of fine motor tasks result in the opposite features in sEMG compared to those of the positive features of the UMNS. Usually in paretic muscles less amount of voluntary sEMG activity could be generated by the patient in movement segments involved in UMNS and less well coordinated sEMG activity can be registered in case of multi-sEMG recordings from antagonistic muscles affected from the UMNS compared to multi-sEMG recordings from movement segments non involved in an UMNS [5, 39].

In case of spastic paresis or SMD voluntary single joint movements are characterized by a combination of weak force generation (paresis, measured clinically with the Medical Research Council scale, MRC scale) and changes in movement coordination (disturbed reciprocal inhibition) which can be described in kinematics as disturbed (reduced velocity and coordination) intended trajectories compared with trajectories produced by normal controls [1].

Typical changes in kinematic parameter of ballistic single- or multi-joint movements in patients with SMD compared with normal controls are performed in a reduced movement velocity and disturbed velocity and acceleration profile representing and mirroring the clinical impression of uncoordinated and slowing of fine motor task performances in patients with spastic limbs and SMD.

In SMD movements directed against the direction of increased spastic muscle tone (spasticity defined by Lance [23]) are altered by a higher quantitative resistance around the joint that should be moved than usually generated in normal movement without spasticity. This increased resistance could result from joint stiffness from neural origin, e.g. from hyper-reflexia or increased muscle tone (Lance [23] definition) and/or non-neural origin, e.g. increased tissue visco-elastic resistance and contractures resulting from soft tissue or muscle shortening [7].

The primary neuronal network features of the UMNS as well as the secondary changes e.g. contractures are the driving factors that cause decreasing ability to manage daily activities and mobility, reduced comfort while sitting and promote spasticity-associated pain. Therefore beside paresis, which always is focused by patients, caregivers and sociaty (negative feature of the UMNS) spasticity defined by Pandyan et al. [32] and spastic contractures (shortening of muscles and soft tissue involved) has a substantial negative impact on patients' and caregivers' quality of life [50].

Coming from a patient centric approach in neurorehabilitation spasticity should be characterized as an individual combination or mixture of positive symptoms of the UMNS in certain topical distribution that causes a characteristic SMD. Nowadays it is consensus among physicians and therapists in the multiprofessional team that the way of staging the different symptoms and consequences of spasticity is to use reliable and valid clinical measures like scales or scores and if possible (patient or caregiver agreement) to videotape the individual SMD during standard motor tasks (e.g. sitting, standing, walking, reaching an object and drinking from a cup of water) [8, 50]. It is recommended to capture beside the personal goals for treatment [46] the level of impairment (e.g. p- and a-ROM, muscle tone with AS, REPAS or MAS, spasticity and co-contraction with Tardiue scale in every movement segment involved in spasticity), the level of activity limitations in the upper limbs (UL) and lower limbs (LL) and evaluate of quality of life (QoL) with established questionnaires as well as carer burden (if any) and participation to fulfill the standards of the International Classification of Functioning (ICF) [50].

The minimum standard of communication in between specialized centers should include upper limb (UL) and lower limb (LL) muscle tone (AS/MAS/REPAS), paresis (graded with BMC scale) and p-ROM (Neutral-0-Methode) as well as evaluation of voluntary movement capacity (a-ROM and defined motor tasks in standardized test manuals, e.g. nine-howl-peg-test or the box and block test) in limbs involved in UMNS, activities of daily living (ADL scales e.g. the Barthel or FIM) as well as quality of life information (QoL, e.g. EQ5D or SF36) and in a descriptive way social and professional participation.

3 Pathophysiology of Spastic Paresis

It is believed that reflex features of spasticity and disordered motor control in SMD result from altered balance of inputs from reticulo-spinal and sub-cortical descending pathways supplying the anterior horn cells pool (Sherrington path) and inter-neuronal circuits at spinal cord levels and not from isolated lesion located in the primary motor cortex that origin the cortico-spinal or pyramidal tract [37].

The absence or disturbance of cortico-spinal tract information that project directly to anterior horn cells (tractus corticospinalis anterior and lateralis) also seems to be of major importance in the concept of a dysbalance and loss of descending tonic or phasic excitatory and inhibitory inputs projecting to the spinal sensorimotor networks and therefore alter segmental spinal balance of excitatory and inhibitory control from supraspinal drive [4].

A CNS lesion involving sensorimotor cortical and subcortical motor areas and tracts of the brain or brainstem may disturb the balance of supra-spinal inhibitory and excitatory input to the segmental and multi-segmental spinal mono- and polysynaptic reflexes and anterior horn cells and may produce spontaneous muscle activation or co-contraction (spastic dystonia) of antagonistic muscles as well as disturbed reciprocal inhibition of antagonistic muscles and create with a certain delay from the start following the lesion a so called cerebral spasticity pattern [13, 14].

Altered abnormal efferent drive from residual motor areas or tracts often result in characteristic spastic co-contraction from disturbed reciprocal inhibition or dysbalance of efferent motor drive to antagonistic muscles. Therefore this spastic co-contraction is a phenomenon of supraspinal origin and is defined as an excessive degree of antagonistic activation in response to voluntary agonist command [47]. This pathological co-contraction originates from the lesion in the brain or is compensatory and produces misdirection of supraspinal descending pathways, particularly from the brainstem region, resulting in pathologically co-activation of antagonistic muscles [13, 14].

The dysbalance of supra-spinal input to segmental interneuron network supplying anterior motor horn cells is producing a state of disorganization of voluntary activation and disinhibition of the spinal reflexes. These include the stretch reflex, the nociceptive polysynaptic reflexes and the withdrawal reflexes and extensor reflexes. This disinhibition of mono- and polysynaptic reflexes create a disabling situation of hyperactive spinal reflexes (e.g. increased sensitivity of tendon-reflexes, decreased inhibition of nociceptive reflexes and increased reflex amplitudes of mono and polysynaptic reflexes), while other positive symptoms are related to disordered control of voluntary movement from abnormal efferent motor drive to the anterior motor horn cells. With respect to the performance of voluntary movements it seems that a major factor is the overall involvement of antagonist coordination, especially the aspect of disturbed reciprocal inhibition and the resulting resistance to voluntary movements [4].

Typical limb postures in chronic spasticity e.g. following stroke are coined as spastic patterns and in more than 90% of these patients with post stroke spasticity show spastic flexion pattern in the UL (spastic flexion of the elbow and wrist) [18] and spastic extension pattern in the LL (spastic stiff knee and pes equines). Spastic dystonia is of supra-spinal origin and the main driver of such spastic postures and contribute to contracture, pain and deformities [15].

Spastic dystonia is characterized by tonic muscle activation of antagonistic muscles around joints and the amount of muscle mass involved add to typical postures (muscle mass of flexors in UL and extensors in LL is bigger than antagonists). These spastic limb pattern has negative consequences on body image and self perception, and patients tend to desire a more natural and relaxed limb position in public and consider this as a relevant goal for focal spasticity treatment e.g. with Botulinum Neurotoxin [50].

In patients with spinal cord lesions e.g. in the cervical and upper thoracic levels these disturbance included dysbalance of supra-spinal inhibitory and excitatory inputs to the spinal reflexes and caudal from lesion a dis-inhibition of spinal automatisms e.g. so called stepping automatism from a spinal stepping generator in the disconnected lower thoraco-lumbal myelon. This may be an additional feature of spinal cord lesions compared to cerebral disconnecting features and justify naming this somewhat different clinical picture as spinal spasticity [7].

Disturbance of active movements in SMD (spastic movement disorder) result in major parts from disturbed antagonistic coordination and not from paresis. Active movements against spastic force (from an spastic antagonist) generated from an agonist directed against the spastic antagonist are disturbed by a lack of inhibitory command to the spastic antagonist muscle resulting from a falls coordination of motor commands on the spinal level that originate from falls supra-spinal commands that origin from the damage of cortical, subcortical or spinal sensorimotor areas or tracts. Other positive symptoms that result from this dysbalance on spinal level in the UMNS also include muscle tendon hyperreflexia and clonus, increased tonic stretch reflexes (muscle tone increase), the clasp-knife phenomenon, flexor and extensor spasms, and spastic co-contractions, associated reactions and spastic dystonia [15].

Negative symptoms result from lesion of the motor cortex, sub-cortical ganglia and descending motor tracts (pyramidal and para-pyramidal tracts) in the brain and spinal cord that result in lack of directed excitatory activity to targeted anterior horn cell cohorts for intended movements and create an unbalanced excitatory and inhibitory descending command to sensorimotor spinal networks and result in weakness (paresis), central fatique and lack of motor co-ordination.

Positive and negative symptoms of the UMNS are caused by a CNS lesion, whereas it is believed that biomechanical changes are secondary and occur with delay from the insult. It is well known that every individual with an UMNS show an individual combination of direct consequences from CNS lesion called positive and negative features and secondary changes as a result of spontaneous remission and management of the symptoms and complications that can occur during the chronic phase of spasticity.

4 Therapeutic Approach

The primary goal for management of spasticity is maximal independence in life for patients affected from SMD. Therefore especially in the acute and post-acute phase of the management of spasticity (during the neurorehabilitation phase) a combination of different symptomatic non-pharmacological and adequate pharmacological treatments with low risk of side effects and an individualized self-stretching and re-learning program of basic motor skills that allow improved mobility (such as standing, transfer, walking) and self care (such as washing themselves, eating and dressing) should be applied. The ultimate goal for managing the chronic phase of spasticity would be to gain the best improvements in activities of daily living as possible to reach maximal quality of life and best re-integration into prior professional and social life possible. As each patient has individual disease and specific combination of positive and negative symptoms of the UMNS and complications (muscle shortening, contractures) the management program should aim for SMART-goals (S = specific for the patient, M = measurable, A = attainable and action orientated, R = realistic and relevant, T = time sensitive, time bound) [50].

Adequate management of spasticity requires multi-professional team of specialized therapists (physio- and occupational, language and swallowing therapists, sports- and training therapists, rehabilitation nurses and social workers) in an adequate setting (in- or out-patient facilities) under supervision and lead of a specialized head-physician with education in neurorehabilitation, neurology or physical medicine and rehabilitation and long standing experience in the management of spasticity. An additional team of adjunctive specialized physicians (neurosurgeon, orthopedic or plastic surgeon, ENT-physician, ophthalmologist and so on) should also be available and if needed part of the specialized spasticity management team [8, 50].

In the beginning of the management process it is of major importance to include patient and if adequate caregivers in the process of appropriate goal setting for the treatment. Appropriate treatment goals should be SMART (see above) and should help to reinforce communication in between patient and the multi-professional team. Such SMART goals allow to bring patient and multiprofessional team activities to synergistic rehabilitation efforts and allows to adapt spasticity management strategies according to the patients abilities to overcome restrictions from SMD [45, 48].

4.1 Management Strategies

A variety of treatment options for spasticity are available. Selection and sequence of the specific treatment measures for individual patient suffering from UMNS should be based on thorough clinical evaluation and multiprofessional—and if adequate interdisciplinary—team decision. Clinical experience has shown that a so called parallel multi-modal approach to spasticity management using different measures/ tools in the same time frame for treatment of SMD has many benefits for the patients, e.g. combining physical therapy with pharmacological and/or surgical treatments [8, 26, 49, 50].

4.2 Assess Spasticity to Implement Individualized Management Strategy

To implement an optimal individualized management program first step is accurate assessment of muscle tone, range of motion, spasticity features and functional impairment. Nowadays it is consensus among physicians and multiprofessional team that the best way of staging the different symptoms and consequences of spasticity is to use reliable and valid scores and scales and to videotape the SMD if patient agrees and gives informed consent for it. It is recommended to document on the different levels of the ICF and gain information on the level of impairment (pROM, Modified Ashworth scale, Tardiue Scale), level of activity limitation and dexterity as well as quality of life (QoL) and participation levels. It is of major importance to cover all levels and domains of the International Classification of Functioning (ICF) [8, 50]. Several scales are introduced to assess SMD.

4.3 Muscle Tone

Ashworth Score (AS) [3], Modified Ashworth Sore (MAS) [2] and the Resistance to Passive Stretch scale (REPAS) [34] are well established to communicate the degree of muscle tone increase among clinicians. They are widely used in epi-demiological and interventional studies to clinically score this feature of SMD. In this scores (AS, MAS and REPAS) higher numbers of the score values represent more marked muscle tone increase when passively stretch muscles of a movement segment/joint during rest position. AS and MAS counts from 0 to 4, with additional +1 in between 1 and 2 in the MAS. 0 represents no, and 4 the maxim of muscle tone increase (severe increase in muscle tone). A highly standardized form of scoring muscle tone increase in all limbs at one time point is established with the Resistance to Passive Stretch scale (REPAS scale). This scale allows documentation of the distribution of muscle tone increase and therefore takes topical aspects of spasticity distribution over the different body segments (e.g. focal, segmental, hemi-, para-, generalized spasticity pattern) into account and allows to detect changes in muscle tone distribution following interventions in regions that was not focally treated [34]. However, AS, MAS and REPAS only measures muscle tone increase and not disturbance of active movement from spasticity and the impacts on loss of activity and function from spasticity, that affects patient's lives. To measure consequences on activity and participation from UMNS other instruments have to be used [33].

4.4 Range of Motion

In normal controls every single joint of the body could be moved in a passive and active manner to a certain degree. Every joint with normal anatomical conditions of bones, joint capsula, ligaments and muscles as well as soft tissue can be moved in a certain range of motion (ROM: normal values for every joint available in the literature). Therefore these ROM could be clinically evaluated with respect to its passive range of motion (p-ROM) or active range of motion (a-ROM).

An established form of documentation of the p-ROM and a-ROM (e.g. the elbow joint) is the Neutral-0-Methode. Intrapersonally the p- and a-ROM usually is the same as the muscles are physiologically strong enough to move the howl range of motion and therefore no contractures can be established (e.g. for the elbow a normal ROM would be described as 10° extension and 130° flexion of the elbow. Documentation of ROM with respect to rules of the Neutral-0-Methode: 10/0/130). In a patient with e.g. acute paresis of the elbow flexors due to stroke (minus symptom of the UMNS) a-ROM could be less for elbow flexion than p-ROM (e.g. p-ROM 10/0/130 and a-ROM 10/0/90: Paresis result in decrease of active elbow flexion from p-ROM 130° to a-ROM 90°). In a patient with chronic spastic paresis and established contractures (chronic spasticity) in extension and flexion movement of the elbow a- and p-ROM could be reduced compared to normal values (e.g. p-ROM 0/10/90: 10° extension movement is not possible/no 0° passively reached, maximum passive extension—stretching is 10° flexion/maximum flexion 90° flexion; a-ROM 0/40/60: active extension only to 40° of flexion position and active flexion to 60° flexion of the elbow, no 0° reached).

Unfortunately in chronic phase of spasticity many patients develop shortening of muscles and soft tissue in joints/movement segments involved in SMD. E.g. in post stroke spasticity (PSS) more than half of the patients affected from spasticity developed at least one restriction in passive range of motion (p-ROM) of joints involved. Restricted ROM from spasticity result in immobility and discomfort when sitting and sleeping, and create difficulties with skin care and hygiene that may lead to skin lesions and pressure source [8, 50]. Reduced ROM in combination with clinical features of the UMNS in the same joint should form the clinical diagnosis of spastic contracture. If contractures include multiple joints of spastic limbs this may result in typical spastic upper limb deformities [18] or spastic gait patterns [5].

4.5 *Spastic Paresis: Muscle Force Decrease and Disturbed Reciprocal Inhibition*

With respect to the performance of voluntary movements it seems that one major component of the SMD is the overall involvement of antagonist coordination, especially the aspect of disturbed reciprocal inhibition and the resulting resistance to voluntary movements against a spastic antagonist. The most adequate scale to cover this aspects of the positive features of the UMNS is the Tardieu Scale (TS). A systematic review of the value of the Tardieu Scale for the measurement of spasticity confirmed that statement [17].

To cover the aspect of paresis it is recommended to test muscle force of involved body segments and include the Medical Research Council scale (MRC scale) for scoring of paresis in all movement segments included in spastic paresis. In case of SMD voluntary single- or multi-joint movements are characterized by a combination of weak force generation (paresis from decreased ability to activate adequate number of anterior horn cells, measured clinically with the MRC scale) and disturbed coordination of muscles involved in terms of disturbed reciprocal inhibition and disturbed synergistic muscle activation (scored clinically with the Tardiue scale).

Movement performance in SMD can be captured and quantified by kinematic analysis of single- or multi-joint movements. Typical changes in kinematic parameter of ballistic single—or multi-joint movements in patients with SMD compared with normal controls show reduced movement velocity and disturbed velocity and acceleration profiles (increased numbers of velocity and acceleration changes per trajectory/stroke) representing and mirroring the clinical impression of slow un-coordinated (discontinuous) motor task performances [9]. As a consequence of UMNS voluntary movement of the agonist (e.g. extensors of the wrist) directed against the resistance of increased spastic muscle tone produced by the antagonist (e.g. flexors of the wrist and fingers) due to loss of antagonistic inhibition or due to resistance from other neuronal (e.g. clonus, disinhibition of tendon reflexes [13, 14]) or non-neuronal joint stiffness (e.g. increased visco-elastic resistance of muscles and soft tissue [25, 31]) the numbers of changes in velocity and acceleration in the profile for spastic movements against spastic antagonists increases and reflect the loss in dexterity and coordination of fine motor tasks.

Spastic paresis with all these neuronal network features of the UMNS (paresis and disturbed reciprocal inhibition) as well as secondary changes e.g. contractures are the most driving factors for reducing levels in activities of daily activities (ADL) and participation and create more need for caregiver assistance and decrease levels of mobility and promote spasticity-associated pain. Therefore beside paresis, which always is the focus of the patients and caregivers (negative feature of

UMNS) spasticity (all positive features of UMNS) and spastic contractures (consequence of spasticity with shortening of muscles and soft tissue combined with spastic features in the same movement segment) has a substantial negative impact on patients' and caregivers' quality of life [55].

4.6 Spastic Contracture

Using the terminology spastic contracture for restriction in p-ROM in the context of an UMNS does not allow to differentiate whether the spastic contracture is caused by increase in muscle tone, co-contraction, spastic dystonia or disinhibited movement synergists and associated reactions or whether the contracture result from paresis of agonist muscles or chronic false positioning of the limb [13, 14].

As a result from the individual CNS lesion that create an individual mixture of positive and negative features of the UMNS and spontaneous (as a result of the UMNS) or correlated with additional factors, like e.g. neuropathic pain or shoulder hand syndrome (complex regional pain syndrom) visco-elastic changes in spastic muscles and surrounding soft tissue arises and create a certain force of a spastic torque imbalance around the spastic joint involved and lead to spastic joint position. With time and without positioning in stretched position shrinking of soft tissue increases to spastic contractures (loss in normal stretched positions, normal pROM) and may result in spastic upper and lower limb deformities, e.g. called typical spastic upper limb pattern following stroke [18].

4.7 Prerequisite Before Starting Symptomatic Spasticity Treatment

Before specific treatment for spasticity should be initiated the absence of so called spasticity triggers or triggering factors that promote spasticity (e.g. local skin irritation, local pain or pressure ulcer, bladder infection, and so on) should be confirmed or excluded [49]. If no trigger factors can be identified start of the management should be made by an adequate nursing regime with positioning of the spastic limbs in mild stretch position [50].

4.8 Physical Treatment Modalities

The most important physical management strategy is lengthening of muscles involved in spasticity. Stretching activity for at least 30 min a day should be started as soon as possible following CNS lesion to avoid spastic contractures [44]. If spasticity and restriction in p-ROM is evident long lasting stretching is recommended (minimum 6 h a day [1]), therefore positioning techniques in bed or wheelchair, splinting, casting or bracing of spastic limbs are recommended to increase time in adequate stretching position. Beside passive, active stretching by activation of antagonist muscles and stretching from postures (standing in a tilt table or a frame) or positioning of limbs in standardized positions are also recommended as self training or training activities with relatives or care givers [15].

The role of physical treatment measures (physio-, sports- and occupational therapy, training therapy and robot based movement therapy) alone or in combination with Botulinum Neurotoxin injections (see below) in the management of post stroke spasticity (PSS) is established in national and international guidelines and form the basis for meaningful improvements in the management of patients suffering from spasticity features and their consequences in every day clinical practice [8, 50].

The combined treatment approach of physical treatment in physio- and occupational therapy or robot-based repetitive training of agonist muscles and Botulinum Neurotoxin injections of spastic antagonistic muscles with the option of re-training of reciprocal inhibition should include alternating movements of different velocities in maximal amplitude to reduce muscle co-contraction and therefore re-educate motor-coordination [50]. This repetitive performance may help to reduce spasticity, avoid contractures and re-establish reciprocal activation and inhibition on a spinal level. Intensity and repetition rate of exercises can be enhanced effectively by using robotic devices or support motivation with virtual reality. This may allow more active movements and increase therefore repetition rate per day [24].

With respect to gait training following e.g. incomplete spinal cord injury or brain lesions (e.g. stroke) it is evident from controlled studies (see Chapter) that increasing number of steps per day above a certain level (level that should be reached seems to be more than 500 steps per day) and introducing training in real context of walking (verticalisation together with coordinated leg movements) results in faster re-learning of walking capacity [19]. Current data on available technological approaches that use high-intensity and repetitive task-specific practice with high number of movement repetitions indicate that better results of re-learning of active movements are achieved in the lower leg and the arm than in the hand [24].

Virtual reality (VR) rehabilitation-based therapy has also shown to promote improvements in SMD by using simple computer games representative of daily activities of self-support. This new therapies applied in a multiprofessional team approach for spastic paresis has demonstrated clinical value, although the underlying changes in neuronal reorganisation supported by VR are still not clear.

Therefore if positive features of UMNS occur and alters physical therapy or robot-based training or VR rehabilitation injection of Botulinum Neurotoxin Type A (BoNT-A, see below) may help to decrease restrictions in training from increased muscle tone in certain antagonistic muscles and improve co-ordination of antagonists and will allow the patient to continue with high intensity repetition training using robotic or VR devices or a self rehabilitation training approach.

4.9 Botulinum Neurotoxin Treatment of Focal and Segmental Spasticity

BoNT-A is treatment of choice for focal, multifocal and segmental spasticity [40, 42]. BoNT-A has a grade A recommendation from the American Academy of Neurology for the treatment of focal spasticity in adults and children. There is ample evidence that BoNT-A significantly decreases muscle tone and improves passive function. The demonstration of functional gains in terms of active function has proved to be more difficult but reached statistical significant levels in a systematic review for the spastic upper limb [11] and could be nicely shown in a controlled randomized trial in chronic stroke patients published by Gracies [15, 16]. However, combining toxin injections with active physical therapy has shown functional improvements, lending support to the concept that the howl management of spastic paresis should be part of a comprehensive spasticity service and included in a multi-professional team approach [8, 50].

4.10 Mechanism of Action Botulinum Neurotoxin

The chlostridial toxin named Botulinum Neurotoxin Type A and B (BoNT-A and -B) acts in vertebrates at the level of the synapses (e.g. connecting point between the nerves and the muscles: motor endplate). Following intake into the body of a vertebrate (e.g. intramuscular injection) BoNT-A enters the cholinerge neuron in the region of the terminal axon membrane. By blocking the ability to fuse intracellular vesicals filled up with Acetylcholine with the synaptic membrane BoNT-A induces in intoxicated neurons a dose dependent blockade of cholinergic transmission and led to a clinically flaccid paresis by so called chemodenervation of cholinergic motor endplates to both extrafusal and intrafusal muscle fibers.

Nowadays the molecular mechanism is much better understood. Following entering the body e.g. BoNT-A is bound to specific receptors called SV-2 that are exposed at the outer surface of the nerve cell when vesicles are fused with the membrane. If BoNT-A is bound to the SV-2 receptor it enters the terminal axon by transportation into the cytoplasma and blocks specific proteins (SNAP-25) necessary for further vesicle fusion.

Accidental oral intake (eating of poisoned food) with clostridial BoNT usually led to generalized flaccid paresis of all voluntary muscles within hours and causes severe respiratory failure that usually led to respirator ventilation and intensive care unit therapy for 3 month (Botulism). On the opposite therapeutic intramuscular injection of defined amounts of BoNT-A or -B (products available, doses are calculated in so called Mouse Units = MU) led to a dose dependent paresis (blockade of muscle contraction) of the muscles injected. BoNT-A blocks Achetylcholin release at the motor endplates and therefore stops voluntary and involuntary muscle contraction follow intramuscular injection of the drugs available. Only the BoNT-A products are licensed to be used in focal spasticity treatment [42]. To be sure to inject BoNT A in the muscles intended, e.g. in small and deep seated muscles, injection guidance techniques (ultrasound-, electrical stimulation- or electromyographic-guidance methods) should be used to inject the toxin diluted in normal saline accurately [50].

A single spastic muscle is rarely treated solely and it is important that the individual spastic pattern of muscle under- and over-activity, at rest and while moving, is correctly understood by the evaluating therapists and injection physicians, so that all relevant muscles can be treated appropriately. To optimize the uptake rate of BoNT-A the injected muscles should be activated following injection e.g. by electrical stimulation or by inducing spasticity with e.g. stretching of the spastic muscles to enhance SV2-receptor exposure and therefore the binding and consecutive uptake of the BoNT injected [19].

Beside blocking voluntary and involuntary muscle activity BoNT injections also induces changes in afferent input to spinal sensomotor networks via denervation of the intra-fusal muscle fibres and therefore reduces changes in afferent IA input. In addition, BoNT-A injections into the shorter of the co-contracting antagonistic muscles in spastic dystonia around the joint will augment stretching activities and allow to actively train antagonistic coordination.

Following injection of an adequate dose of BoNT-A into a spastic muscle it requires 24–72 h to detect reduction in muscle force. The peak effect on force occurs within 10 days to 4 weeks. Clinical improvements in SMD can be expected from BoNT-A injections for up to 12–24 weeks [40].

Clinical experience and published studies with the different BoNT-A drugs has shown that all products licensed for spasticity treatment are well tolerated and associated with few adverse events across all regions injected for spasticity treatment [40]. Local adverse effects (AE) are caused by local diffusion of BoNT-A from the target muscle into adjacent muscles or tissues. Systemic AE occur in tissues distant from the injection site and based upon BoNT-A transport within the lymphatic or blood circulation. AE of the different drugs occur in a typical latency about one week after injection of the toxin. Severity and duration of local and systemic AE depend on the local or total dose of the different products applied. Therefore concerning latency of AE all BoNT-A drugs have similar AE profiles. Neutralising antibodies seems to be no longer a problem in spasticity treatment for incobotulinumtoxinA and onabotulinumtoxinA. With more than a million injections of incobotulinumtoxinA never ever secondary non-response due to neutralising antibodies was proofen and with the reformulation of onabotulinumtoxin A in 1997 the rate of antibodies in onabotulinumtoxinA treated patients was calculated below a rate of 1%. The incidence of neutralising antibodies following repetitive abobotulinumtoxin A injections is calculated from published studies with 3–5%.

It is evident from controlled studies that in order to induce an optimal uptake of the toxin following injection within muscles with diffuse endplate distribution injected volume per muscle should be distributed in more injection sites and this is particularly important in larger muscles, whereas in muscles with endplate bands the dose of toxin should be divided across this defined endplate region at one or two sites.

It must be recognised and included in the sequence of the management plan in spasticity that BoNT-A treatment effects are temporary. With respect to combination of different treatment approaches it could be used to opening a so called "window of opportunity" or "therapeutic window" with less spastic muscle tone and allow for a better combination of neurorehabilitative treatment approaches by reducing muscle tone increase with BoNT-A and allow to better re-establish antagonistic coordination. Reversibility of BoNT-A effects may lead to repeated treatment in post-acute and chronic spastic paresis with muscle tone increase, muscle overactivity, spastic dystonia and disturbed reciprocal inhibition, but may perhaps modify the course of muscle overactivity in early post-stroke intervention. Nowadays we know from controlled studies in the post-acute phase of stroke rehabilitation (less than 3 month following stroke) that BoNT-A injected before spasticity become chronic doses injected can be lower and improvements on impairment and passive function level tend to be more pronounced and longer lasting [36].

Several studies have investigated the effect of BoNT-A on post-stroke upper limb function and mobility, usually combined with an exercise programmes and adjunctive treatments. Treatment with BoNT-A gave a notable improvement in hand function, and hence improvements in self-care tasks and other activities of daily living, and alleviated pain [29]. Reaching and grasping functions were improved in individuals but not significantly in the verum groups in most controlled trials. The optimal time to administer BoNT-A may be when muscle overactivity becomes evident and bothersome to the rehabilitation program of the individual patient, resulting in impairment of active and passive functions, hinders active training programs or robot based training and therefore increased disability and associated reactions, or when it induces pain [35].

As mentioned above early single-dose BoNT-A treatments (<3 months after stroke) of spasticity has been investigated in three upper limb [6, 20, 35] and in one in the lower limb studies [10]. Main result of this studies was compared with placebo a significant and sustained reduction in muscle tone observed for 6 months following a single fixed dose of BoNT-A. Early use of BoNT-A therefore may extend the time window for motor re-learning with active motor traing by decreasing overactive of extrafusal muscle fibres (spasticity) and afferences from intrafusal muscle fibres to spinal sensomotor networks through chemodenervation of extra and intrafusal muscle fibres. With this the early BoNT-A intervention paradigm may potentially modify the natural progress of spasticity, may prevent spasticity and spastic dystonia-related complications in SMD.

BoNT-A drugs available are different and not interchangeable. The most important difference in BoNT drugs available refers to the serotype used. So far, only BoNT-A and BoNT-B are commercially available, whereas BoNT-C and BoNT-F have been tried in humans in studies in dystonia only.

The currently available BoNT-A drugs in Europe and North America are: Botox® (onabotulinumtoxin A; Allergan Inc, Irvine, CA, USA), Dysport® (abobotulinumtoxin A; Ipsen Ltd, Slough, Berks, UK), Xeomin® (incobotulinumtoxin A; Merz Pharmaceuticals, Frankfurt/M, Germany).

Neurobloc® (rimabotulinumtoxin B; Eisai Europe Limited, London, UK) is the only type B drug that is available in Europe. In the US and in some other countries

NeuroBloc® is distributed as Myobloc® (rimabotulinumtoxin B; Solstice Neurosciences Inc, Malvern, PA, USA).

Botox® was the first BoNT drug to be registered in 1989, whereas Dysport® was registered in 1991, Hengli® in 1993, NeuroBloc®/Myobloc® in 2000 and Xeomin® in 2005. For all BoNT-A drugs instead incobotulinumtoxinA special storage temperatures are required. Xeomin® is the only drug which can be stored at room temperature. Additional BoNT drugs are the Chinese Hengli® (Lanzhou Institute of Biological Products, Lanzhou, Gansu Province, China) which is based upon BoNT type A. It is distributed in some Asian and South American countries (e.g. Brazil) as Prosigne®. Neuronox® (Medy-Tox, Ochang, South Korea) is another BoNT-A drug available in South Korea and in some other Asian countries too.

Dosages of the BoNT-A drugs that are licensed in European countries and North America for the treatment of spasticity are given in the Summary of Product Characteristics (SPC) of each drug, however the doses and muscles licensed in the different countries of each drug vary in between different countries.

Apart from that it is important that dosing should be determined by the individual patient's condition (e.g. body weight, muscle mass, sever of spasticity) and the goals of treatment and can be reassessed according to the response to treatment. It is common clinical practice to initiate BoNT type A therapy at low, but effective, doses and titrate upwards as effects become evident. Therapeutic dosages of BoNT-A drugs in spasticity vary more widely than with almost any other drug. Whereas minimum therapeutic BoNT A doses used for intrinsic hand muscles as low as 10–15 MU inco-or onabotulinumtoxin A, maximum reported BoNT A doses used for severe spasticity with involvement of upper and lower limbs can reach 1500 MU abobotulinumtoxinA [16], 600 MU onabotulinumtoxinA [50] or 800 MU incobotulinumtoxin A [53]. When incobotulinumtoxinA are used in high doses per injection session (up to 800 MU) in a setting including adequate dosing per muscle (according the published we move recommendations) and injection site (not more than 50 MU onabotulinumtoxinA and incobotulinumtoxinA per site) and inclusion of injection guidance for deep seated or small muscles (muscle ultrasound or electrical stimulation injection guidance) local and systemic motor and autonomic adverse effects are reported very rarely [53]. Same is true when using abobotulinumtoxin A in doses of 1500 MU [16].

4.11 Management of Severe Multisegmental and Generalized Spasticity and Spastic Contractures

Oral antispastic drugs are licensed for systemic treatment of spasticity, most drugs available without any restriction on distribution of spasticity or etiology of spasticity (exclusion for Tolperison and Sativex: Tolperison is licensed for PSS only and Sativex for pain and spasticity in MS only) [26, 31]. Still these oral antispastic drugs are used widely. Specially baclofen (Gamma-Aminoacid-[GABA-] B-Agonist) and tizanidin (central Alpha2-Agonist) are well known by GPs and non-neurologists and are given widely without specific goals when clinical signs of spasticity appear. Other antispastic oral drugs are also in use like Benzodiazepines (GABA-A-Agonisten) and Dantrolen (pheripheral acting muscle relaxans that inhibit Ca-Ions at the level oft he muscle), tolperison (central acting inhibitor of Na-influx at neurons, licensed in Germany only in stroke spasticity) and gabapentine.

Sativex is the only oromucosal spray available to treat spasticity and painful spasms consisting of 2 Cannabis-components: tetrahydrocannabinol (THC) and cannabidiol (CBD, licenced for pain, spasms and spasticity management in MS) [26].

Central acting drugs directed against positive symptoms of UMNS (e.g. muscle tone increase, spastic dystonia, spasms, and spasticity) are introducing inhibition in cortical level or spinal interneuron pool and therefore not only inhibit the different features of the UMNS but also block voluntary muscle activity and core muscle tone, as well as cognitive activity and vigilance. Dantrole as well is not a selective inhibitor of spastic muscle tone and it acts directly in the muscle and is known to be hepatotoxic. Beside this negative impact of oral antispastics on voluntary muscle force (and core stability and breathing volume) all central acting oral agents are known to frequently cause side effects like sedation, vertigo, dry mouth and cognitive impairment and therefore are not recommended to be introduced as first line treatment in focal, segmental and multi-segmental cerebral spasticity [26, 49].

As well in a controlled "head to head" comparison Simpson et al. [41] where able to show that patients with post-stroke spasticity profit much more (antispastic effect much better in size and less side effects) from focal treatment with BoNT A with respect to their focal and segmental spasticity than from systemic oral treatment with Tizanidin [41]. On the contrary many specialists in spinal cord rehabilitation recommend to first line—start with orals in spinal spasticity before moving to other spasticity management regimes.

The first line recommendation of intrathecal baclofen (ITB) management in severe multisegmental and generalized forms of spasticity from SCI, TBI, MS and CP is based on well designed studies that showed significant improvement in positive signs of UMNS and no weakening on residual muscle force in non-affected body segments when dose of ITB is titrated upward and programming mode of the implanted pump is used in managing individual spasticity of the patients implanted with a pump. As the pump for ITB has to be implanted and many components of the implanted system has to function smooth side effect frequency compared to conventional treatment with oral drugs is higher in ITB spasticity management. Therefore following concent of patient and/or caregiver it is recommended to use this concept in severe segmental and generalized forms of UMNS and to combine treatment as recommended with physical measures and if necessary additional focal treatment with BoNT-A [26].

If spasticity is accompanied by neuropathic pain syndroms (e.g. as often the case in thalamic stroke, TBI or SCI) it is recommended to add to antispastic local management with BoNT-A in the beginning antineuropathic—analgesic drugs like GABA-analoga Gabapentin or Pregabalin (central Na-blocker, licensed as antiepileptic and anxiolytic drug) and pain modulators (antidepressive agents). If indicated also oromucosal spray of THC and CBD (Sativex) or other cannabis derivates (THC and THC/CBD oil) or canaboids (Nabilone) are effective symptomatic drugs in treating combinations of severe pain and severe spasticity [26, 52].

In case of no response to antispasticity management and major impairment and activity limitations from spastic contractures plastic-orthopedic surgical procedure like fasciotomia, tendon lengthening or complex tendon-muscle-bony-surgery should be discussed to gain improved activity and pain levels. As well reconstructive surgery with tendon or muscle transfers is an option to reach mobility and dexterity goals and overcome activity and participation limitations from severe spastic paresis [8, 50].

References

1. Ada L, Vattanasilp W, O'Dwyer NJ, et al. Does spasticity contribute to walking dysfunction after stroke? J Neurol Neurosurg Psychiatry. 1998;64(5):628–35.
2. Ansari NN, Naghdi S, Arab TK, Jalaie S. The interrater and intrarater reliability of the modified Ashworth scale in the assessment of muscle spasticity: limb and muscle group effect. NeuroRehabilitation. 2008;23(3):231–7.
3. Ashworth B. Preliminary trial of carisoprodol in multiple sclerosis. Practitioner. 1964;192:540–2.
4. Burke D, Wissel J, Donnan GA. Pathophysiology of spasticity in stroke, *Neurology*, 2013; 80(3)(suppl 2):S20–6.
5. Caty GD, Detrembleur C, Bleyenheuft C, et al. Effect of simultaneous botulinum toxin injections into several muscles on impairment, activity, participation, and quality of life among stroke patients presenting with a stiff knee gait. Stroke. 2008;39(10):2803–8.
6. Cousins E, Ward A, Roffe C, et al. Does low-dose botulinum toxin help the recovery of arm function when given early after stroke? A phase II randomized controlled pilot study to estimate effect size. Clin Rehabil. 2010;24:501–13.
7. Dietz V, Sinkjaer T. Spastic movement disorder: impaired reflex function and altered muscle mechanics. Lancet Neurol. 2007;6:725–33.
8. Esquenazi A, Novak I, Sheean G, et al. International consensus statement for the use of botulinum toxin treatment in adults and children with neurological impairments–introduction. Eur J Neurol. 2010;17(Suppl 2):1–8.
9. Flash T, Hogan N. The coordination of arm movements: an experimentally confirmed mathematical model. J Neurosci. 1985;5(7):1688–703.
10. Fietzek UM, Kossmehl P, Schelosky L, et al. Early botulinum toxin treatment for spastic pes equinovarus—a randomized double-blind placebo-controlled study. Eur J Neurol. 2014;21 (8):1089–95.
11. Foley N, Pereira S, Salter K, et al. Treatment with botulinum toxin improves upper-extremity function post stroke: a systematic review and meta-analysis. Arch Phys Med Rehabil. 2013;94:977–89.
12. Gracies JM. Pathophysiology of impairment in patients with spasticity and use of stretch as a treatment of spastic hypertonia. Physical Med Rehabil Clin N Am. 2001;12:747–68.
13. Gracies JM. Pathophysiology of spastic paresis. I: paresis and soft tissue changes. Muscle Nerve. 2005;31(5):535–51.
14. Gracies JM. Pathophysiology of spastic paresis. II: emergence of muscle overactivity. Muscle Nerve. 2005;31(5):552–71.

15. Gracies J-M. Coefficients of impairment in deforming spastic paresis. Ann Phys Rehabil Med. 2015;58(3):173–8.
16. Gracies JM, Brashear A, Jech R, et al. Safety and efficacy of abobotulinumtoxinA for hemiparesis in adults with upper limb spasticity after stroke or traumatic brain injury: a double-blind randomized controlled trail. Lancet Neurol. 2015;14:992–1001.
17. Haugh AB, Pandyan AD. Johnson GR A systematic review of the Tardieu Scale for the measurement of spasticity. Disabil Research. 2006;28(15):899–907.
18. Hefter H, Jost WH, Reißig A, et al. Classification of posture in poststroke upper limb spasticity: a potential decision tool for botulinum toxin A treatment. Int J Rehabil Res. 2012;35:227–33.
19. Hesse S. Recovery of gait and other motor functions after stroke. Restaurative Neurol Neurosci. 22(2004):359–69.
20. Hesse S, Mach H, Fröhlich S, et al. An early botulinum toxin A treatment in subacute stroke patients may prevent a disabling finger flexor stiffness six months later: a randomized controlled trial. Clin Rehabil. 2012;26:237–45.
21. Kwah LK, Harvey LA, Diong JH, et al. Half of the adults who present to hospital with stroke develop at least one contracture within six months: an observational study. J Physiother. 2012;58(1):41–7.
22. Lance JW. Pathophysiology of spasticity and clinical experience with baclofen. 185–220. In: Feldman R, Young R, Koella W, editors. Spasticity: disordered motor control. Chicago: Yearbook Medical Publishers; 1980. p. 185–220.
23. Lance JW. The control of muscle tone, reflexes, and movement: Robert Wartenberg lecture. Neurology. 1980;30(12):1303–13.
24. Lee KW, Kim SB, Lee JH, et al. Effect of upper extremity Robot-assisted exercise on spasticity in stroke patients. Ann Rehabil Med. 2016;40(6):961–71.
25. Lieber RL, Steinman S, Barash IA, et al. Structural and functional changes in spastic skeletal muscle. Muscle Nerve. 2004;29(5):615–27.
26. Liepert J. Therapie des spastischen Syndroms. Aus: Hans-Christoph Diener, Christian Weimar (Hrsg.) Leitlinien für Diagnostik und Therapie in der Neurologie. Herausgegeben von der Kommission "Leitlinien" der Deutschen Gesellschaft für Neurologie. Thieme Verlag, Stuttgart; 2012.
27. Malhotra S, Pandyan AD, Day CR, et al. Spasticity, an impairment that is poorly defined and poorly measured. Clin Rehabil. 2009;23(7):651–8.
28. Mayer NH. Clinicophysiologic concepts of spasticity and motor dysfunction in adults with upper motoneuron lesion. Muscle Nerv. 1997;20(suppl 6):S1–13.
29. Mills PB, Finlayson H, Sudol M, et al. Systematic review of adjunct therapies to improve outcomes following botulinum toxin injection for treatment of limb spasticity. Clinical Rehabil. 2016; 0269215515593783.
30. Olsson MC, Krüger M, Meyer L-H, et al. Fibre type-specific increase in passive muscle tension in spinal cord-injured subjects with spasticity. J Physiol. 2006;577(Pt 1):339–52.
31. Olvey EL, Armstrong EP, Grizzle AJ. Contemporary pharmacologic treatments for spasticity of the upper limb after stroke: a systematic review. Clin Ther. 2010;32:2282–303.
32. Pandyan AD, Gregoric M, Barnes MP, et al. Spasticity: clinical perceptions, neurological realities and meaningful measurement. Disabil Rehabil. 2005;27:2–6.
33. Platz T, Eickhof C, Nuyens G, Vuadens P. Clinical scales for the assessment of spasticity, associated phenomena, and function: a systematic review of the literature. Disabil Rehabil. 2005;27:7–18.
34. Platz T, Vuadeus P, Eickhof C, et al. REPAS, a summary rating scale for resistance to passive movement: item selection, reliability and validity. Disabil Rehabil. 2008;30(1):44–53.
35. Rosales R, Botulinum toxin therapy as an early intervention for post-stroke spasticity: beyond a functional viewpoint. J Neurol Sciences. 2017; 382:187–8.
36. Rosales RL, Kong KH, Goh KJ, et al. Botulinum toxin injection for hypertonicity of the upper extremity within 12 weeks after stroke: a randomized controlled trial. Neurorehabil Neural Repair. 2012;26:812–21.

37. Sheean G. The pathophysiology of spasticity, Eur J Neurol. 2002;9(s1)(suppl 1):3–9, 53–61.
38. Sheean G. Botulinum toxin treatment of adult spasticity. Expert Rev Neurotherapeutics. 2003;3, 773–85.
39. Sherwood AM, Mc Kay WB, Dimitrijevic MR. Motor control after spinal cord injury: assessment using surface EMG. Muscle Nerve. 1996;19(8):966–79.
40. Simpson DM, Gracies JM, Graham HK, et al. Assessment: Botulinum neurotoxin for the treatment of spasticity (an evidence-based review): report of the therapeutics and Technology Assessment Subcommittee of the American Academy of Neurology. Neurology. 2008;70:1691–8.
41. Simpson DM, Gracies JM, Yablon SA, et al. BoNT/TZD Study Team: Botulinum neurotoxin versus tizanidine in upper limb spasticity: a placebo-controlled study. J Neurol Neurosurg Psychiatry. 2009;80:380–5.
42. Simpson DM, Hallett M, Ashman EJ, et al. Practice guideline update summary: botulinum neurotoxin for the treatment of blepharospasm, cervical dystonia, adult spasticity, and headache: Report of the Guideline Development Subcommittee of the American Academy of Neurology. Neurology. 2016;86(19):1818–26.
43. Thilmann AF, Fellows SJ, Gams E. The mechanism of spastic muscle tone. Variation in reflex gain over the time course of spasticity. Brain. 1991;14:233–44.
44. Turner-Stokes L, Ward A. Botulinum toxin in the management of spasticity in adults. Clin Med. 2002;2:128–30.
45. Turner-Stokes L. Goal attainment scaling (GAS) in rehabilitation: a practical guide. Clin Rehabil. 2009;23:362–70.
46. Turner-Stokes L, Williams H, Johnson J. Goal attainment scaling: does it provide added value as a person-centred measure for evaluation of outcome in neurorehabilitation following acquired brain injury? J Rehabil Med. 2009;41:528–35.
47. Vinti M, Couillandre A, Hausselle J, et al. Influence of effort intensity and gastrocnemius stretch on co-contraction and torque production in the healthy and paretic ankle. Clin Neurophysiol. 2013;124(3):528–35.
48. Ward AB, Wissel J, Borg J, et al. Functional goal achievement in post-stroke spasticity patients: the BOTOX(R) Economic Spasticity Trial (BEST). J Rehabil Med. 2014;46:504–13.
49. Winter T, Wissel J. Behandlung der Spastizität nach Schlaganfall. Konsultationsfassung der DGNR-Leitlinie. Neurologie und Rehabilitation. 2013;19:285–309.
50. Wissel J, Ward AB, Erztgaard P, et al. European consensus table on the use of botulinum toxin type A in adult spasticity. J Rehabil Med. 2009;41:13–25.
51. Wissel J, Manack A, Brainin M. Toward an epidemiology of poststroke spasticity. Neurology. 2013;80(Suppl 2):S13–9.
52. Wissel J, Ganapathy V, Ward AB, et al. OnabotulinumtoxinA improves pain in patients with post-stroke spasticity: findings from a randomized, double-blind. Placebo-controlled Trial. J Pain Sympt Manag. 2016;52(1):17–26.
53. Wissel J, Djamel Bensmail D, Ferreira JJ et al. Safety and efficacy of IncobotulinumtoxinA doses up to 800 U in limb spasticity: the TOWER study. Neurology. 2017.
54. Yanagisawa N, Shindo M, Morita H. Spinal mechanisms of spasticity. Electroencephalogr Clin Neurophysiol Suppl. 1999;50:190–4.
55. Zorowitz RD, Gillard PJ, Brainin M. Poststroke spasticity: sequelae and burden on stroke survivors and caregivers, Neurology, 2013;80(3)(suppl 2):S45–52.

Gait Analysis in the Context of Spasticity Management

L. Jorge Jacinto and Miguel Reis Silva

1 Introduction

Spasticity is a motor disorder characterized by a velocity-dependent increase in tonic stretch reflexes with exaggerated tendon jerks, caused by hyperexcitability of the stretch reflex [1]. It is a common entity that is estimated to affect 35% of people post stroke [2], 40% of people post spinal cord injury [3], and 50% of people post traumatic brain injury [4]. It is also a condition associated with high morbidity that increases pain/discomfort levels, impairs daily living functioning, self-image and self-esteem, and, most of all, impairs mobility and gait.

This chapter presents a pragmatic, gait analysis-based approach to spasticity treatment that focuses on everyday clinical challenges and aims to answer precise questions relevant to patients' quality of life.

2 Brief Historical Perspective

Nowadays, gait analysis is associated with complex hardware, numbers, graphic illustrations and three-dimensional digital graphic reconstructions. However, simple visual analysis of the locomotion of a human body is an approach as ancient as Aristotle (384–322 BC), who first described the vertical oscillating movement of the head during walking.

L. J. Jacinto (✉)
Serviço de Reabilitação de Adultos 3, Centro de Medicina de Reabilitação de Alcoitão, Alcabideche, Portugal
e-mail: jor.jacinto@netcabo.pt

M. Reis Silva
Serviço de MFR, Centro Hospitalar de Lisboa Central, Lisboa, Portugal

G. Sandrini et al. (eds.), *Advanced Technologies for the Rehabilitation of Gait and Balance Disorders*, Biosystems & Biorobotics 19,
https://doi.org/10.1007/978-3-319-72736-3_31

However, it was only in the XVII and XVIII centuries that the contributions of Galileo Galilei to modern scientific methods and Isaac Newton to the principles of mechanics opened the way for the first descriptions of human locomotion, which were provided by a number of French physiologists.

The first objective descriptions of pathological gait, by Duchenne and Trendelenburg, date back to the XIX century, while the first description of a correct gait cycle, by Gaston Carlet, appeared at the end of that same century. It was also during this period that the first photographic and three-dimensional gait analyses were performed, by Georges Demeny and Willhelm Braune, respectively [5].

In the XX century, gait analysis essentially assumed its present form, thanks to the development of the first biomechanical laboratories with force plates, introduced by Jules Amar, and electromyography, introduced by Jacqueline Perry, and the addition of synchronized films, by David Sutherland [6].

3 The Spastic Muscle

Even though spasticity is commonly approached as a pure neurological entity, research shows that there are also profound alterations of the musculoskeletal system in the affected anatomical areas. Spastic muscle presents cell atrophy and fiber type transformation [7]. The sarcomeres are decreased in length and there are marked alterations of muscle and viscoelastic properties of the extracellular matrix [8]. Even gene expression of spastic muscle is different from what is observed on the non-affected side, with alterations in signal transduction pathways, cell cycle progression, muscle metabolism and contractile proteins [9].

It is important to note that soft tissue changes and shortening may contribute to increased muscle tone by up to 50%, and can therefore be significantly responsible for physical impairment and activity limitations, including reduced walking capacity. Soft tissue shortening is a phenomenon that also extends to joint capsules, ligaments and tendons, making it difficult to distinguish where the line lies between spasticity and rigidity in some spastic patients. In recent years, selective nerve blocks, which involve quickly and temporarily switching off muscle hyperactivity to allow evaluation of the degree of contracture, have been used as a useful procedure for differentiating spasticity from morphological changes of the spastic areas.

Spastic muscle may be evaluated in several ways. Clinical measurement tools such as the modified Ashworth Scale, the Penn Spasm Frequency Scale, Associated Reaction Rating Scale, clonus and spasm scores [10] or the Tardieu Scale are simple and efficient ways of measuring spasticity-related phenomena. Biomechanical methods, such as goniometry or resistance to passive movement, albeit more time consuming, are also commonly used. Neurophysiological measurements, such as EMG and H-reflex, only used for this purpose in research settings, are other possible ways of measuring spasticity.

It is important to note that the finding of spastic muscles, per se, does not necessarily demand therapeutic intervention. Patients with spasticity commonly complain of stiffness, pain, heaviness, tightness, spasms, clonus and difficulties in sitting, sleeping, performing activities of daily living and, frequently, walking. The way each patient experiences their symptoms is unique and dependent on a myriad of factors, such as genetic predisposition, cultural background, level of education, past functional level, or even expectations for the future. Consequently, the therapeutic intervention should address the specific needs and expectations of the single patient and/or his/her carers, rather than simply aiming to bring about changes in scores on universal clinical scales.

4 Approaches to Spasticity and Gait

From the specific cellular level to the broader environmental level, there are several steps through which we can evaluate any disease or condition, and spasticity is no exception.

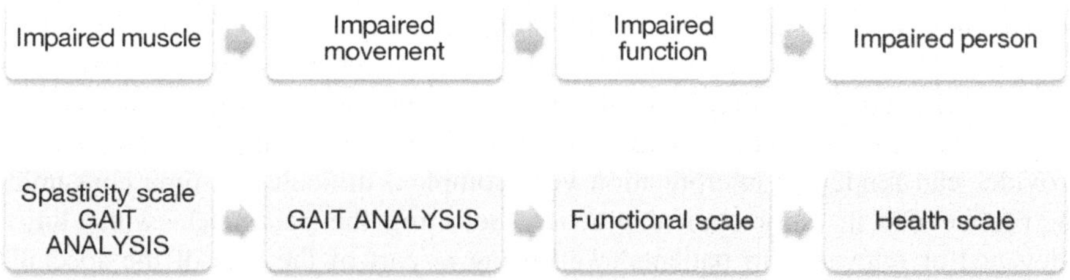

At the first, physiological, level, we may measure spasticity using the Modified Ashworth Scale, the Tardieu Scale and the Penn Spasm Frequency Scale. Additionally, any spasticity-derived symptom may be quantified by the widely used visual analog scales and Likert-like scales. This is an important premise, since these symptoms are frequently the main and most impairing factors, both for patients and carers. Consequently, when important to patients/carers and amenable to clinical interventions, they should become the "treatment goals". These goals should be individually tailored, meet the SMART criteria (i.e. be specific, measurable, attainable, realistic, timed), and each be measured using tools that reflect the magnitude of the change produced by the treatment interventions.

At the second level, there exist several clinical scales developed to evaluate the impact of the spasticity on gait, namely the Waterloo Gait Profile Form, the Rancho Los Amigos System, the Rivermead Visual Gait Assessment, the Rivermead Mobility Index, the Physician Rating Scale and the Salford Gait Tool.

If we adopt a Gestalt approach, we can choose functional scales for the upper limbs, such as the Nine-Hole Peg Test, the Frenchay Arm Test, the PRS (Physician Rating Scale), the Fugl-Meyer Assessment, the Action Research Arm Test and the

Leeds Adult Spasticity Impact Scale, or for the lower limbs, such as the Functional Ambulatory Categories, 10 m walking test, 6-min walking test, PRS, Paper Walkway, and Timed Up & Go Test. As global functional performance scales, we can use the Barthel Index and the Functional Independence Measure. To measure success in achieving treatment goals, there is the Goal Attainment Scaling (GAS) methodology [11]. Health-related quality of life scales can be used for broader evaluation of the impact of the condition, although to date there is no health-related quality of life scale that is specific for people with spasticity.

Instrumented gait analysis falls within the first two steps as it is a specific method for evaluating spasticity: it identifies the impaired muscles by electromyography (EMG) (in-phase or out-of-phase activation during the gait cycle) and the effect of the spasticity on movement by spatiotemporal parameters, kinematics and kinetics of gait.

5 Gait Analysis

Gait analysis is the systematic study of animal locomotion, more specifically of human motion, using the eye and the brain of observers, augmented by instrumentation for measuring body movements, body mechanics, and the activity of muscles [12]. From this definition alone, its usefulness in the clinical management of spasticity appears quite obvious. However, the wide range of parameters it provides can render its interpretation very complex, difficult and time consuming for routine use in daily clinical practice. Selecting the parameters with clinical relevance or relevance to patients' well-being is part of the role of the specialist clinician within the gait analysis laboratory team in a clinical setting.

Naked-eye gait analysis is the first and also the simplest and fastest way of analyzing gait. However, it has too many drawbacks, such as the limited capacity of the human eye to register images and the multitude of events occurring at the same time in three dimensions, the limitations of human memory, attention and concentration, which are not sufficient to register all the relevant features, the limited capacity of patients to repeat the task over and over again, and the inter-individual variability of any subjective measurement tool.

Instead, instrumented gait analysis is able to provide valuable information that cannot be obtained by any other means: slow-motion video analysis provides information that cannot be gathered in real time, the spatiotemporal parameters allow objective quantification of multiple function-related parameters, the EMG analysis identifies and quantifies muscle activity in the different phases of the gait cycle, and the kinematic/kinetic analysis shows multiple joint angles, forces, moments and powers that characterize the effects of spasticity on movement and the forms of compensation adopted, as well as their effectiveness and efficiency.

Gait analysis gains relevance as a measurement tool after an initial evaluation that will answer specific questions, on which depend the future therapeutic actions. It may also be a tool for objective measurement of the outcomes of therapeutic

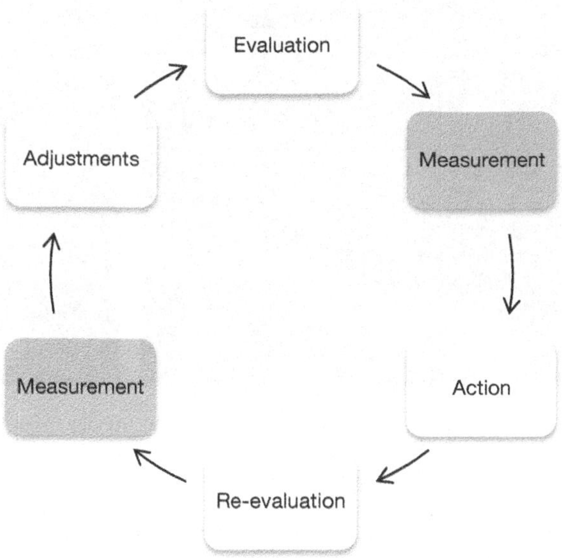

Fig. 1 The usefulness of gait analysis in clinical practice

actions taken, and thus prompt adjustments. These data have profound clinical implications, since gait analysis findings may change up to 81% of botulinum toxin injection plans, 37% of orthotic choices, and 32% of physiotherapy programs [13] (Fig. 1).

6 Hardware

The construction of a gait analysis laboratory is an expensive process, due to the amount of different technologies that need to be synchronized.

Video cameras, usually two, operating respectively in a lateral view and in a front/back view, are a basic requirement. In fact, even just simple interpretation of the slow-motion video can provide important information.

Infrared cameras are used to collect the live three-dimensional positions of reflective markers that are placed on the patient's body in standard anatomical reference positions (specific to each 3D motion analysis system). From this information, the processors can build three-dimensional reconstructions (Fig. 2).

Dynamic EMG processors collect the information from surface or fine wire EMG electrodes placed on the target muscles. The chosen muscles vary according to the clinical situation and purpose of the examination.

Force plates, placed on the ground, ideally in a seamless way, sense the forces (anteroposterior, medial-lateral and vertical) that are applied to the ground during the stance phase. The forces measured are of the same magnitude, but opposite in direction, to the ones coming from the ground (ground reaction forces), which

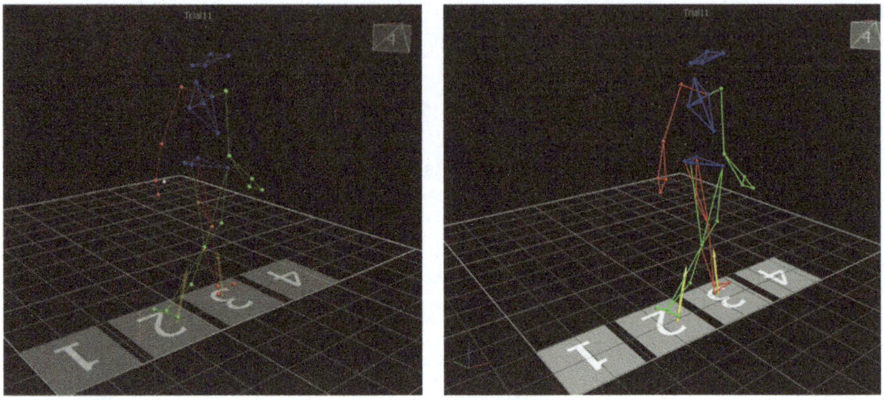

Fig. 2 Construction of a three-dimensional model from the reflective markers placed in anatomical reference positions

determine by inverse dynamics the moments and powers produced in each joint at any instant of the gait cycle.

Computers using specific software perform the synchronization and integration of all the input data. This is actually what allows the system to do the inverse dynamics calculations, as well as graphically represent which muscles are "on" and which ones are "off" in each phase of the gait cycle (Fig. 3).

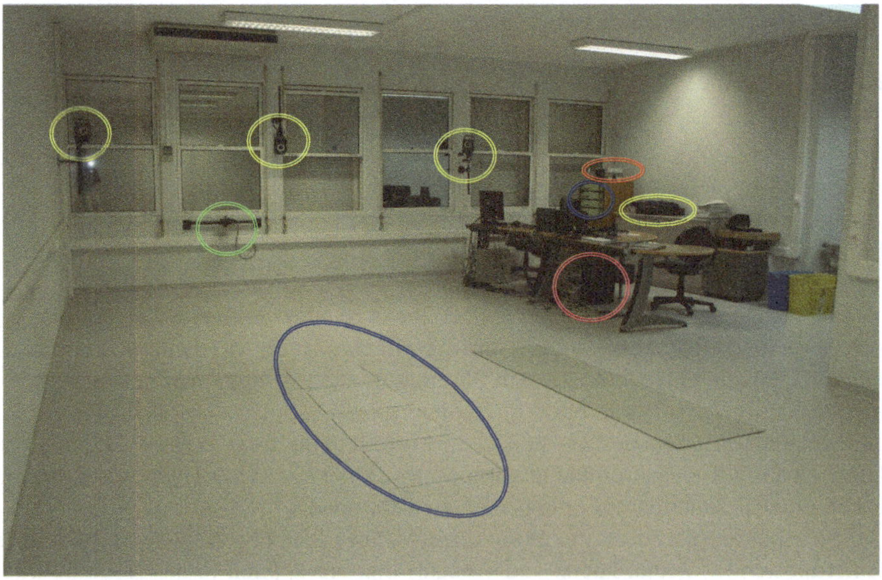

Fig. 3 Gait analysis laboratory at Centro de Medicina de Reabilitação de Alcoitão. (yellow—infrared cameras; green—video camera; orange—EMG processor; blue—force plates; pink—computer processors)

7 Gait Analysis Parameters

Data obtained from gait analysis are important in the management of spastic patients since they make it possible to perform, in an objective way, parameter quantification, characterization and quantification of deviations from normal, measurement of the results of therapeutic interventions, and comparisons with baseline situations and between different subjects. They can also shed light on the mechanisms underlying a certain type of movement, as well as distinguish primary deficits from compensatory phenomena, and establish whether or not the latter are effective.

By simply viewing the videos it is possible to subjectively identify the main deficits of the stance and swing phases.

The spatiotemporal parameters are usually the first parameters analyzed. Speed, measured in meters per second, is one of the most important parameters, with functional implications, influencing all other parameters and ultimately defining the efficacy of gait. Functional ambulatory gait for a community dweller has a minimum speed of approximately 0.7 m/s. Step/stride lengths and cadence are determinants of speed (step/stride length × cadence = velocity of gait). The percentage of the gait cycle corresponding to double support/single support/swing for each limb, the percentage of the gait cycle when foot-off occurs, the limp index (the contact time of the ipsilateral foot, divided by the contact time of the opposite foot), and the times when opposite foot contact and foot-off occur also provide important information about gait symmetry (Fig. 4).

	Left	Right
Average Cadence	121 steps/min	
Cadence	122 steps/min	121 steps/min
Double Support	0.20 s	0.20 s
Foot Off	59.8 %	60.0 %
Limp Index	0.99	1.00
Opposite Foot Contact	49.4 %	50.1 %
Opposite Foot Off	9.76 %	10.3 %
Single Support	0.39 s	0.40 s
Step Length	0.57 m	0.58 m
Step Time	0.50 s	0.50 s
Step Width	0.22 m	0.23 m
Stride Length	1.15 m	1.15 m
Stride Time	0.98 s	0.99 s
Walking Speed	1.17 m/s	1.16 m/s

Fig. 4 Spatiotemporal parameters that are usually automatically provided by the system with the biomechanics report after data processing (normal patient)

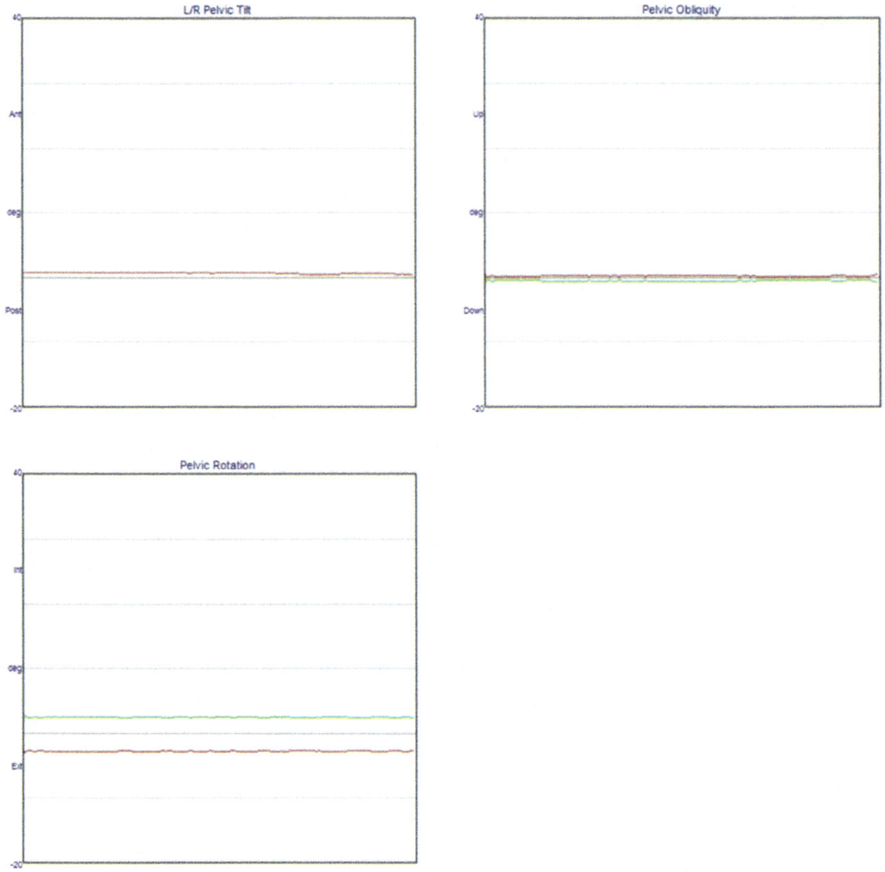

Fig. 5 Static examination of the pelvis of a normal patient. Note the symmetry in the three-dimensional axis that is not seen in a spastic patient (red line—left; green line—right)

The static position of the patient is always captured before the dynamic trials, as it provides relevant information and frequently has implications for both the biomechanical and the clinical analysis (Fig. 5).

The kinematic information collected should consist of 3D (frontal, sagittal and coronal) data regarding the pelvis, hip, knee and ankle. However, since the associated reactions of the upper body and upper limb usually have a significant impact on gait, including its velocity, in selected cases, these segments should also be analyzed. The information regarding kinematics is usually shown in a time/angle graphic illustration.

Force plates (evaluating kinetics), placed on the ground, provide information about anterior-posterior, medial-lateral and vertical forces (the ground reaction forces). Anterior-posterior forces (the minimum for the first trough and maximum of the last peak of stance) give information about the capacity to brake at initial contact, and to accelerate at foot-off. Vertical forces (maximum values for the first and second peak of stance phase) give information about the amount of weight bearing that the patient is applying on the limb as well as the capacity to push at foot-off. The percentage of the gait cycle in which the first peak of vertical forces occurs determines the time until the other foot can initiate swing, therefore it determines cadence and affects the efficacy of gait (velocity = cadence × step length). The possibility to record data regarding ground reaction forces and, simultaneously, kinematic data allows the system to determine joint moments (angular accelerations), which provide indirect information about the muscle groups that are predominant in each instant of the gait cycle for each joint and in three dimensions. It also allows the calculation of joint powers, i.e., whether a certain joint is producing or absorbing energy, and how much, in each instant of the gait cycle.

Dynamic EMG collects data on the electrical activity, at the skin (surface EMG) or within the muscle tissue (fine wire EMG), produced by muscle activation. The clinical interpretation of EMG findings can be simplified by visually classifying the activity of each muscle during each phase of the gait cycle as "on" or "off". Once again, patient characteristics, the clinical situation, and the question one is trying to answer determine which muscles are selected for study. According to whether they are located superficially (gluteus maximus, quadriceps, hamstrings, triceps surae, tibialis anterior, extensor halluces, etc.) or deeply (tibialis posterior, flexor digitorum longus, flexor hallucis longus, gluteus medius, etc.), surface or fine wire EMG electrodes are used respectively.

Taking into account the patient being studied and the clinical question that prompted the request for the examination, biomechanical findings are clinically interpreted and reported, to be correlated with other clinical findings, therapeutic goals and both the patient's and clinicians' expectations with regard to disease progression and/or predicted outcome of interventions (Fig. 6).

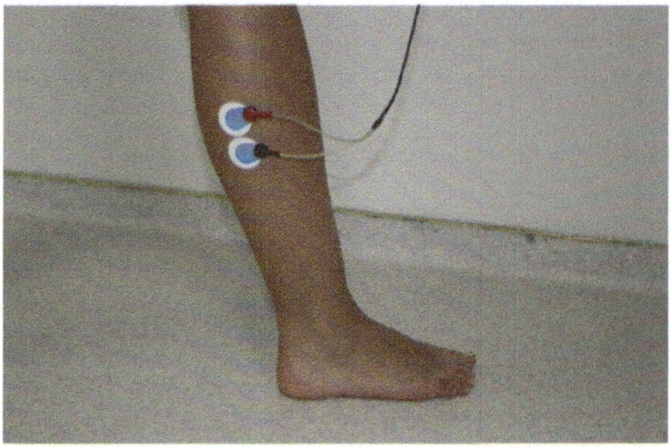

Fig. 6 Surface EMG electrodes

8 The Goal Attainment Scaling and Gait Parameters

One of the biggest challenges in rehabilitation is to define clear and specific patient-centered and real-life-based therapeutic goals for each individual. In fact, what is important to patient A may mean nothing to patient B, due to differences in their disease/disability type and severity, cultural backgrounds, lifestyles and aspirations. Consequently, a patient-centered approach has gained importance in recent years.

The GAS methodology involves negotiation and definition of goals and measurement of success in reaching them within the expected time frame, and offers the possibility of translating the degree of success into a numerical score that can be treated statistically for research purposes. Used in such way, GAS can be expected to be useful in determining the extent to which goals have been attained and thus allow more comprehensive evaluation of the effectiveness of the treatments used to attain them, and of the impact of the outcomes in everyday life for each subject [14].

Using GAS, the patient/carers are involved in goal setting: they let the clinician/rehabilitation team know about their problems and expectations regarding the treatment and, on the basis of the predicted outcomes (both their magnitude and the time frame envisioned for achieving them), can accept or refuse it.

After goal definition, the goals need to be prioritized and stated in clinical records according to the SMART rule, which requires that they be: specific, measurable, attainable, realistic and timed. The next step is the weighting of the goals. The weight of each goal is defined as the importance attached to it by the patient/carers × the difficulty, as rated by the clinician/rehabilitation team, as follows:

Importance	Difficulty
0: Not important at all	0: Not difficult at all
1: A little important	1: A little difficult
2: Moderately important	2: Moderately difficult
3: Very important	3: Very difficult

The GAS score for each goal is defined as follows:

Achievement scores
−2: Goal nowhere near achieved/much less than expected
−1: No change/goal not quite achieved/a little less than expected
0: Goal achieved as expected
1: Goal slightly exceeded/a little more than expected
2: Goal greatly exceeded/much more than expected

The last step of GAS is the calculation of baseline and outcome scores. This is done by entering the weight of each goal, the baseline score and the attainment score in a complex formula, widely available in the form of computerized spreadsheets. Changes in GAS scores provide an objective quantification of the success of any therapeutic intervention in terms of meeting the patient's/carers' expectations of it.

Gait analysis provides objective values that may be used as parameters to measure the outcomes of therapeutic goals, and thus feed the GAS assessment. The gait goals commonly measured through gait analysis are:

- to increase gait velocity by a certain percentage
- to increase right/left step length by a certain percentage
- to obtain right/left flat-foot or heel initial contact
- to improve left/right knee extension during stance by a certain percentage
- to increase left/right limb weight bearing during stance by a certain percentage
- to achieve walking, without aids, at a certain velocity measured in m/s.

9 Gait Analysis as a Tool for Measuring the Impact of Spasticity on Gait

9.1 Normal Gait

Gait is the means by which humans displace themselves between any two points in space, by changing in an alternate way the position of the feet, while always keeping at least one of the feet in contact with the ground. To describe the gait of an individual subject, whether normal or a pathological, we have to divide it into several events (phases and sub-phases), which are repeated in time as the subject walks (the gait cycle).

The main division of gait sees it split into the stance phase (foot in contact with the ground) and the swing phase (aerial phase), which normally account for 2/3 and 1/3 of the gait cycle, respectively. The stance phase consists of four sub-phases: Loading response—from the initial contact to opposite foot-off, Mid-stance—until heel rise, Terminal stance—until opposite initial contact, and Pre-swing—until toe-off. The swing phase is divided into three sub-phases: Initial swing—from toe-off to feet adjacent, Mid-swing—until tibia vertical, and Terminal swing—until initial contact [15] (Fig. 7).

In clinical or instrumental gait analysis, the phases and sub-phases are important for the interpretation of the findings according to the different parameters measured: spatiotemporal parameters, kinematics, kinetics and dynamic EMG.

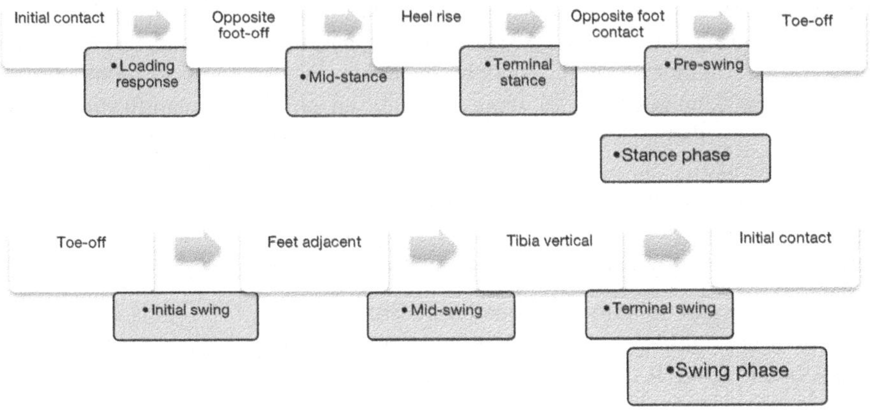

Fig. 7 Phases and sub-phases of the gait cycle

9.2 Spastic Gait

A muscle connects two bony surfaces which usually have at least one joint between them. In the presence of a spastic muscle, the voluntary and involuntary movements of the joint in question will be impaired. Consequently, the patient will develop forms of compensation in order to retain the capacity to perform gait.

Spastic gait is usually asymmetrical, slower than normal and laborious, characterized by uncoordinated limb movements, synergies of stereotypical movements and patterns of movements, and alternation deficits. Compensations adopted to mitigate the disability generally lead to one or more of the following: inadequate impact absorption at initial contact; lack of control of joint moments during the stance phase; lack of capacity to generate force for push-off; and inadequate limb excursion during the swing phase.

It is important to adopt a systematic and synthetic approach in order to get an initial overall idea of the problems and compensations presented. In a spastic patient, during the stance phase, it is important to assess support, stability and propulsion, whereas in the swing phase it is more important is to assess the aerial progression of the limb.

Simple slow-motion video analysis alone is sufficient to describe the type of foot contact (forefoot, flat-foot, heel, etc.) and evaluate the major kinematic asymmetries and compensations shown.

With regard to spatiotemporal parameters, spastic patients usually have slower gait, with a shorter paretic limb stance time.

With regard to kinematic aspects, the results depend on the patient's pattern of spasticity. It is necessary to focus on the three main joints of the lower limb, always comparing the affected and non-affected sides and measuring the deviation from the expected values for non-pathological gait. In a spastic patient, we should be concerned with the aspects listed below:

- Pelvis. In the static examination, anterior pelvic tilt and pelvic obliquity will commonly be found. The latter orientation depends on the patient's spastic pattern: a patient with a flexed hip, knee or ankle will have an obliquity in the direction of the paretic limb, whereas a patient with a hyperextended hip or ankle will have an obliquity in the direction of the normal limb. In the dynamic examination, a higher pelvic obliquity during the swing phase is a common form of compensation for a lack of lower-limb triple flexion during the swing phase, and serves to prevent tripping during this phase. A larger pelvic rotation is also common, serving to compensate for a shorter hip excursion.
- Hip. Sagittal excursion of the hip is highly correlated with gait speed, as is its maximum extension during the stance phase. A higher hip abduction during the swing phase is a common form of compensation for a stiff knee and/or equinus foot, allowing adequate clearance and aerial limb progression. External hip rotation during the swing phase is a common compensation for weaker hip flexors; this position produces anterior projection of the limb with activation of the hip adductor muscles, hence helping in the swing phase.
- Knee. Excursion of the knee is important mainly in two phases: during the swing phase, to allow aerial progression of the limb without foot contact with the ground, and during single support in the stance phase, to allow the anterior projection of the body. In the static examination, knee hyperextension may be an indirect sign of ankle plantarflexion. In the dynamic examination, during the stance phase, hyperextension of the knee, commonly referred to as "locking knee" or "recurvatum", can be due to spasticity of the quadriceps, triceps surae, or serve to compensate for weakness of the quadriceps muscle.
- Ankle. Excursion of the ankle is important during the swing phase (dorsiflexion), in order to prevent foot contact with the ground. It is also important during initial foot contact, in order to allow heel strike. On the other hand, plantarflexion is most important during the second half of the stance phase, serving to push from the ground ("push-off") and project the body upward and forward. In fact, the power of the ankle at terminal stance is positively correlated with gait velocity (efficacy). Some patients compensate for reduced hip and knee flexion during the swing phase through hyperextension of the contralateral ankle at the end of the stance phase; this compensatory phenomenon, named "vaulting", helps them to avoid tripping.
- Kinetics. The magnitude of the curves is usually reduced (especially at the second peaks due to the lack of ankle power at the end of stance); the reaching of the first peaks of the vertical and anteroposterior components is delayed (difficulty in load acceptance and weight bearing).

10 A Useful Tool for Spasticity Management with Botulinum Toxin

10.1 Effect of Botulinum Toxin on Spastic Muscle

Botulinum toxin is a potent presynaptic acetylcholine release blocker whose action can be divided into four steps: binding to the presynaptic membrane, internalization into the nerve ending, inhibition of acetylcholine release, and recovery by neural plasticity. The main effects produced by botulinum toxin on spastic muscle are: reduction of muscle tone, facilitation of active or passive mobilization and stretching, reduction of associated symptoms such as pain, spasms or clonus, and reduction of involuntary movements and associated reactions.

I. Identification of Target Muscles

Even though kinematic, kinetic and video analysis allow us to predict the affected muscles, dynamic EMG remains the gold standard for the precise identification of muscles that are activated out of phase (agonist-antagonist co-contaction). By knowing the normal activation pattern of the different muscles during the gait cycle, we can correlate the activation of spastic muscles with the kinematic and kinetic repercussions.

Commonly evaluated muscles are:

- the tibialis anterior, in order to assess its contribution to ankle dorsiflexion during the swing phase. This is one of the most commonly used muscles in neuro-orthopedic surgical treatment of spastic equinus foot;
- the extensor hallucis longus, mainly used in potential candidates for surgical treatment. When it is activated during the swing phase as an agonist of the tibialis anterior, its transposition to the mid-foot as an ankle dorsiflexor can be beneficial;
- the tibialis posterior, a difficult muscle to assess with surface EMG due to its deeper position, but easy to evaluate with fine wire EMG. If activated during the swing phase it should be treated with botulinum toxin. Another possibility is to use it as a dorsiflexor by transposing it to the dorsal aspect of the tarsum. When there is no out-of-phase activation and the varus deformity is due to its shortening, a tenotomy can be performed to release the ankle/foot, allowing for a plantigrade stance phase and adequate clearance during swing (by allowing either active dorsiflexion or the effective use of an ankle-foot orthosis);
- The soleus and gastrocnemius medialis and lateralis, which have major implications for gait functionality. Their differential assessment may help in the selection of the target muscle for botulinum toxin treatment in spastic equinus foot and/or hyperextended knee in stance;
- The hamstrings, which are usually assessed when out-of-phase activation (swing phase) and/or shortening are suspected on the basis of naked-eye observation. They may be responsible for reduced hip flexion in the swing phase, as well as hyperextension of the knee during the stance phase;

- The quadriceps, which can be a contributor to stiff-knee gait. EMG activity during the first half of the swing phase may identify this muscle as the source of knee flexion impairment during swing, hence making it a target for botulinum toxin treatment.

11 An Assessment Tool for Possible Candidates for Surgical Neuro-orthopedic Treatment

Other than for simpler therapeutic interventions, for which the use of laboratory gait analysis is perhaps debatable, the ambiguities and limitations of visual observation, especially prior to costly or invasive treatments, should certainly be recognized [16]. In fact, in equinovarus foot surgery, instrumental gait analysis data, as opposed to visual gait analysis findings, may change up to 2/3 of surgery protocols [17]. In post-stroke patients, laboratory gait analysis changes 73% of the surgical plans, making it an essential pre-surgery subsidiary diagnostic examination [13].

The surgeries most frequently based on the findings of an instrumented gait analysis, which should be analyzed by the clinician who interprets the data and draws up a clinical report, include:

- Achilles tendon lengthening, to correct equinus deformity, when there are fixed ankle contractures associated with functional deficits.
- Split anterior tibialis tendon transfer, to correct varus deformity, when there is tibialis anterior activation during the swing phase, with concomitant activation of the extensor hallucis longus and a weak extensor digitorium comunis. The lateral portion of the split tendon, inserted in the outer and dorsal aspect of the foot, helps to balance the supination of the forefoot during the swing phase.
- Extensor hallucis longus transfer to the neck of the first metatarsal (Jones suspension), when it is adequately activated during the swing phase, in the absence of tibialis anterior activation [18], or as described in the previous point. This transfer transforms a finger extensor into an ankle dorsiflexor during the swing phase.
- Tibialis posterior transfer to the dorsum of the foot in order to correct varus deformity and aid foot dorsiflexion during the swing phase.
- Peroneus longus splitting and transfer to the tibialis anterior tendon and peroneus tertius tendon, in order to aid ankle dorsiflexion during the swing phase [19].

12 What to Report

Any laboratory gait analysis report should cover the main spatiotemporal parameters that have functional implications, such as velocity, cadence and foot contact time. In the kinematic analysis, the main asymmetries should also be described, as well as the main findings from the analysis of ground reaction forces and joint moments and powers.

As with any complementary examination, the gait analysis report should end by answering the specific question that motivated it. The answers may be as diversified as the clinical questions, examples of which are given below:

- The examination was motivated by the need to detect specific spastic muscles e.g. soleus vs. gastrocnemius):
  - In this case, the muscle activity ("on" or "off") in the different phases of the gait cycle should be described together with remarks on the implications for the affected joint. The activity of other adjacent muscles, which could also impair the same joint, should also be described.
- The examination was performed to establish whether a patient is a suitable candidate for surgical treatment (tendon lengthening, transposition or tenotomy):
  - As previously mentioned, the pattern of muscle activation should be described, and suggestions should be given regarding the muscles that could be transposed. A final comment should summarize the potential benefit of the surgery for the single patient, in view of the other gait analysis parameters.
- The examination was performed to establish whether a patient walks more effectively with a specific walking aid:
  - A comparison of functionally relevant parameters, and a description of the main differences found between gait with and without the walking aid, should be given.
- The examination was performed to assess the effect of a lower limb orthosis on gait:
  - The comparison of functionally relevant parameters, and a description of the main differences found between the gait pattern with and without the use of the orthosis, should be given. The conclusion should end with a comment on the effect of the use of the orthosis on gait.
- The examination was performed to objectively measure the effect of a therapeutic intervention on gait performance:
  - Functionally relevant parameters that can be related to the specific intervention (e.g. a specific physiotherapy program, exoskeleton gait training, a pharmacological intervention) should be described and their impact measured.

References

1. Lance J. Spasticity: disordered motor control. In: Feldman RG, Young RP, Koella WP, editors. Symposium synopsis. Miami, FL: Year Book Medical Publishers; 1980.
2. Welmer AK, Von Arbin M, Holmqvist LW, Sommerfeld DK. Spasticity and its association with functioning and health-related quality of life 18 months after stroke. Cerebrovasc Dis. 2006;21(4):247–53.
3. Noreau L, Proulx P, Gagnon L, Drolet M, Laramee MT. Secondary impairments after spinal cord injury: a population-based study. Am J Phys Med Rehabil [Internet]. 2000;79(6):526–35. Available from: http://www.ncbi.nlm.nih.gov/entrez/query.fcgi?cmd=Retrieve&db=PubMed&dopt=Citation&list_uids=11083303.
4. Wedekind C, Lippert-Grüner M. Long-term outcome in severe traumatic brain injury is significantly influenced by brainstem involvement. Brain Inj [Internet]. 2005;19(9):681–4. Available from: http://www.ncbi.nlm.nih.gov/pubmed/16195181.
5. Al-Zahrani KS, Bakheit MO. A historical review of gait analysis. Neurosciences. 2008; 13:105–8.
6. Baker R. The history of gait analysis before the advent of modern computers. Gait Posture. 2007;26:331–42.
7. Fridén J, Lieber RL. Spastic muscle cells are shorter and stiffer than normal cells. Muscle Nerve. 2003;26(2):157–64.
8. Dietz V, Ketelsen UP, Berger W, Quintern J. Motor unit involvement in spastic paresis. Relationship between leg muscle activation and histochemistry. J Neurol Sci. 1986;75(1): 89–103.
9. McKenzie MJ, Yu S, Macko RF, McLenithan JC, Hafer-Macko CE. Human genome comparison of paretic and nonparetic vastus lateralis muscle in patients with hemiparetic stroke. J Rehabil Res Dev. 2008;45(2):273–81.
10. Smith C, Birnbaum G, Carlter JL, et al. Tizanidine treatment of spasticity caused by multiple sclerosis:results of a double-blind, placebo-controlled trial. US Tizanidine Study Group Neurol. 1994;44:S34–42.
11. Turner-Stokes L. Goal attainment scaling (GAS) in rehabilitation: a practical guide. Clin Rehabil [Internet]. 2009;23(4):362–70. Available from: http://journals.sagepub.com/doi/10.1177/0269215508101742.
12. Whittle M. Gait analysis: an introduction. Butterworth: Heinemann; 1991.
13. Ferrarin M, Rabuffetti M, Bacchini M, Casiraghi A, Castagna A, Pizzi A, et al. Does gait analysis change clinical decision-making in poststroke patients? Results from a pragmatic prospective observational study. Eur J Phys Rehabil Med. 2015;51(2):171–84.
14. Kiresuk T, Sherman R. Goal attainment scaling: a general method for evaluating comprehensive community mental health programs. Community Ment Health J. 1968;4(6):443–53.
15. Levine D, Richards J, Whittle M. Gait analysis. Churchill: Livingstone; 2012.
16. Gitter A, Mcanelly R. The value of information resulting from instrumented gait analysis: the physiatrist. Gait Anal Sci Rehabil. 1998;69:75.
17. Fuller DA, Keenan MAE, Esquenazi A, Whyte J, Mayer NH, Fidler-Sheppard R. The impact of instrumented gait analysis on surgical planning: treatment of spastic equinovarus deformity of the foot and ankle. Foot Ankle Int. 2002;23(8):738–43.
18. Carda S, Molteni F, Bertoni M, Zerbinati P, Invernizzi M, Cisari C. Extensor hallucis longus transfer as an alternative to split transfer of the tibialis anterior tendon to correct equinovarus foot in hemiplegic patients without overactivity of tibialis anterior. J Bone Jt Surg. 2010;1262–6.
19. Banks A, Downey M, Martin D, Miller S. McGlamry's comprehensive textbook of foot and ankle surgery. Lippincott: Williams and Wilkins; 2001.

Neuromotor Techniques, Physical Treatments and Orthoses in Spasticity

Alessandro Picelli, Elena Chemello and Nicola Smania

1 Introduction

Damage to the sensory-motor networks and descending tracts results in the positive and negative signs of upper motor neuron syndrome [1]. Spasticity, being a state of increased muscle tone with exaggerated reflexes, is considered a positive sign of upper motor neuron syndrome (other so-called positive consequences include clonus, spasms, co-contraction, extensor plantar response and associated reactions) [2]. Spasticity is clinically characterized by a velocity-dependent increase in resistance to passive movement [3]. It may interfere with motor function, leading to the need for pharmacological and non-pharmacological, rehabilitation interventions [4, 5].

The following are the main phenomena leading to disability in patients with spasticity: paresis (reduced voluntary recruitment of skeletal motor units), soft tissue contractures (muscle shortening and joint retraction) and muscle overactivity (reduced ability to relax muscles) [6, 7]. On this basis, motor impairment due to spasticity can be described in terms of a cycle of overactivity–contracture–overactivity that evolves in parallel with one of paresis–disuse–paresis [6–8]. Thus, in order to optimize motor recovery and function, both of these cycles need to be disrupted [8].

Accurate prognostic indicators would be helpful in order to achieve adequate planning of spasticity management. For example, in previous studies, an early

A. Picelli (✉) · E. Chemello · N. Smania
Department of Neurosciences, Biomedicine and Movement Sciences,
Neuromotor and Cognitive Rehabilitation Research Center, University of Verona,
P.le Ludovico Antonio Scuro 10, 37134 Verona, Italy
e-mail: alessandro.picelli@univr.it

G. Sandrini et al. (eds.), *Advanced Technologies for the Rehabilitation of Gait and Balance Disorders*, Biosystems & Biorobotics 19,
https://doi.org/10.1007/978-3-319-72736-3_32

increase in muscle tone, greater severity of initial paresis, the presence of hemi-hypesthesia, and a low Barthel Index score have been proposed as reliable predictors of post-stroke spasticity [8–12]. Furthermore, the topical distribution of the initial paresis and the location of the brain lesion have been found to relate to the development of spasticity in patients with stroke [13, 14].

2 The Approach to Spasticity Treatment

The presence of spasticity is not, in itself, an indication for treatment [15]. Indeed, it does not necessarily have a negative impact on patients' wellbeing, and may even aid in the performance of some functional tasks (e.g. increased knee extensor tone can be exploited in standing and transfers) [15, 16]. Thus, the most reasonable approach is to treat spasticity whenever it becomes disabling or problematical [15].

The treatment goals of spasticity management usually include: (1) drug potentiation, (2) restoration of biomechanics, (3) improvement of motor control, (4) strengthening of weak muscles, (5) integration of functional activities, and (6) improvement of endurance [17]. In particular, the aims for lower functioning patients tend to be passive, for example improved positioning, orthotic fit and compliance; decreased associated spasms, pain, caregiver burden and nursing care; and prevention of complications (e.g. contractures and learned nonuse of the paretic limb) [15]. Conversely, the aims for higher functioning patients tend to be active, such as improved prehension and grasp-release; improved reaching and overhead activities; reduced shoulder pain during movement; increased independence in activities of daily living; decreased time to accomplish activities of daily living; improved speed, balance, quality and safety of gait; prevention of long-term injury due to alterations of joint biomechanics; discontinuation of oral spasmolytic drugs to decrease the risk of adverse events; and reduction of the time spent on exercise programs [15].

3 Drug Potentiation

Botulinum toxin type A is a first-line treatment for spasticity in upper motor neuron syndrome [5, 18–21]. It acts in the cytosol of nerve endings and inhibits acetylcholine release at neuromuscular junctions by cleaving the synaptosomal-associated 25 kDa protein, which is required for vesicle docking and, consequently, neurotransmitter release [22, 23]. The binding and translocation processes of botulinum toxin type A have been reported to have a half time of approximately 12 and 5 min respectively [24].

In animal models, electrical stimulation was found to enhance the neuromuscular blockade effect of botulinum toxin type A by increasing and accelerating the uptake of the toxin at the motor nerve terminals [24–26]. In humans, despite a number of studies reporting that electrical stimulation may effectively enhance the blockade effect of botulinum toxin type A, there is no agreement as to the best stimulation procedure to couple with botulinum toxin for spasticity [27–41]. In particular, there has been considerable debate over several aspects of electrical stimulation: the timing of its administration (e.g. immediately after injection, the day of injection at a non-specified time, the day after injection); the frequency of sessions (e.g. once a day, twice a day, three times a day, six times a day, twice a week); and the duration of the treatment (e.g. one day, three days, five days, a week, two weeks) [27–31, 33–36, 39, 40]. Considering that cultured neuron models have shown that botulinum toxin type A is rapidly internalized via high-affinity receptor-mediated endocytosis (which mainly occurs a few minutes after toxin exposure) [42, 43], we suggest that low frequency electrical stimulation, aimed at boosting botulinum toxin type A internalization, should be delivered immediately after injection [32, 33, 39].

4 Restoration of Biomechanics

Muscle stretching is a common rehabilitation approach in the management of spasticity [4], and it may be classified into the following modalities: prolonged positioning; passive stretching; active stretching; isotonic stretching (the affected limb is held at maximal range of motion); and isokinetic stretching (involving continuous movement of the affected limb) [44]. The common goals of the above-mentioned stretching modalities are to improve the viscoelastic properties of muscles and tendons as well as to decrease motor neuron excitability [4, 44–46].

Stretching can be used with adjunct interventions such as taping, casting, splinting and orthotics [44]. In particular, adhesive taping in association with botulinum toxin type A was proposed as an effective means of reducing wrist and finger flexor spasticity [29, 47]. On the other hand, casting was found to give better results than taping after botulinum toxin type A injection for spastic equinus foot [48]. Considering the significantly better long-term effect on spasticity of delayed casting after botulinum toxin type A injection [49], it should be recommended to perform casting at the time when botulinum toxin takes full effect (generally considered to be 2 or 3 weeks after injection) [17]. Orthoses may be used in place of casting provided that they are flexible and the angle is changed regularly (rigid orthoses are not appropriate during active spasticity management as they may limit the range of motion available to the patient) [17]. From a functional point of view, ankle-foot orthoses have been reported to have beneficial effects on knee and ankle kinematics by preventing foot-drop in early stance, swing phase and toe-off, facilitating weight bearing on the paretic leg, and reducing the energy cost of walking [50].

5 Improvement of Motor Control

The rehabilitation approaches aimed at improving motor control in patients suffering from spasticity due to upper motor neuron syndrome usually include body weight-supported treadmill training, robot-assisted training, neurofacilitatory techniques and functional electrical stimulation [15].

Treadmill training (with or without body weight support) has been reported to improve gait ability in patients with stroke. Those who are able to walk appear to be the ones who benefit most from this type of intervention [51].

As regards robotic training, stroke patients who receive robot-assisted upper limb training after stroke have been found to obtain improved function and muscle strength of the affected upper limb, as well as improvements in their activities of daily living [52, 53]. Furthermore, people who undergo electromechanical-assisted gait training combined with physical therapy after stroke are more likely to achieve independent walking than those who receive overground gait training without these electromechanical devices. Specifically, patients in the first three months after stroke onset and those who are not able to walk seem to benefit most from this type of intervention [54].

Many neurofacilitatory techniques have been proposed for the management of spasticity [55]. One of the most widely applied methods is the Bobath approach, which is based on a hierarchical model of motor control in the nervous system [56]. This technique involves the use, by physical therapists, of reflex inhibitory positioning to normalize muscle tone [56, 57]. The Bobath method has been reported to have an effect on muscle tone as well as on the excitability of alpha motor neurons on the affected side in patients with stroke [57, 58]. Conversely, the motor relearning program proposed by Carr and Shepherd shifted the focus away from normalizing tone, concentrating, instead, on muscle strength improvement and task practice [55, 59]. Compared with the Bobath approach, this technique has been found to allow patients to leave hospital earlier, thanks to their significantly greater improvement in motor function [60].

Functional electrical stimulation is the use of electric current to activate muscles and nerves that are weak or paralyzed because of upper motor neuron damage [41]. It has been suggested to have direct effects on muscle tone reduction by stimulating antagonist muscles, in accordance with the reciprocal inhibition principle [41, 61, 62].

6 Strengthening of Weak Muscles

Muscle weakness (defined as the inability to generate normal levels of muscle force under a specific set of testing conditions) is a major factor contributing to disability in patients with upper motor neuron syndrome [4]. It is to be noted that there is no evidence supporting a relationship between muscle training and increased spasticity or decreased range of motion [44, 63–66].

Progressive resistance strength training is a widely used approach in patients with post-stroke spasticity. One of its key elements is that it allows patients, by completing a relatively small number of consecutive repetitions (usually less than 12), to develop sufficient resistance before the onset of fatigue (the amount of load should progressively increase as strength increases) [4, 63, 64]. Biofeedback is another approach that has been proposed to alleviate spasticity [44]. It allows people to use auditory or visual cues to control a particular muscle or muscle group and gain conscious control over them [4, 44].

Particular care and attention are warranted during muscle strengthening protocols in non-neurologically stable patients, post-surgical patients, patients with severe osteoporosis or acute joint injuries, patients with hemophilia or other blood disorders, and patients with severely limited articular range of motion [65].

7 Integration into Functional Activities

After achieving strength improvement it is fundamental to work on isolated motor control so as to exploit the new-found strength in functional activities, such as transfers, community ambulation, and specific fine motor activities, and, in so doing, help patients to meet their goals [17]. A number of strategies have been proposed to facilitate goal-directed activities.

Constraint-induced movement therapy is one of the most commonly used tools for recovering abilities in everyday activities [17]. It is a rehabilitation approach that involves forced use of, and intensive practice with, the affected arm by restraining the unaffected one [67]. In patients with stroke, specifically ones with some voluntary motor control of wrist and finger extensors, improvements after constraint-induced movement therapy have been suggested to be due mainly to adaptations, through learning, that optimize the use of intact end-effectors [68].

Occupational therapy, too, is an essential element in the rehabilitation of patients after stroke in order to improve personal abilities in activities of daily [69, 70]. It involves the use of specific goal-directed activities/interventions designed to achieve functional outcomes able to promote health and prevent injury or disability, as well as to develop, improve, sustain or restore the highest possible level of independence [70].

8 Improvement of Endurance

"Endurance typically improves when integration of improved motor control and functional activities has reached a level of daily practice independent of therapy" [17]. Some training strategies have been proposed to improve endurance in patients with upper motor neuron syndrome, such as treadmill training, aquatic training and circuit training [51, 71–73]. There is now considered to be sufficient evidence to incorporate cardiorespiratory training, involving walking, within post-stroke rehabilitation in order to improve speed, tolerance and independence during walking [72].

9 Physical Modalities in the Management of Spasticity

Some physical modalities have been reported to have some kind of antispastic effects. Such physical agents include (but are not limited to) extracorporeal shock wave therapy, therapeutic ultrasound, thermotherapy, cryotherapy, vibratory stimuli and transcutaneous electrical nerve stimulation [4, 17].

Shock waves are defined as a sequence of single sonic pulses characterized by high peak pressure (100 MPa), fast pressure rise (<10 ns) and short duration (10 μs) [74]. Extracorporeal shock wave therapy has been found to effectively reduce muscle tone and improve articular range of motion in patients with upper motor neuron syndrome, due to its purported neuromodulatory and non-neural rheological effects [74–76].

Thermal and mechanical effects of therapeutic ultrasound have been suggested to decrease spasticity by reducing the stretch sensitivity of muscle spindles as well as increasing local metabolism, circulation, extensibility of connective tissue and tissue regeneration [4]. To date there is conflicting evidence about the efficacy this physical modality in the management of spasticity [4, 77–81].

Thermotherapy has been reported to decrease spasticity and reduce spasms in patients with upper motor neuron syndrome [4, 82]. As regards local superficial heating modalities, hot temperature has been hypothesized to reduce the response of muscle spindles to stretch with a consequent greater extensibility of muscles under passive stretching [83]. On the other hand, it has also been suggested that the antispastic effects of global heating modalities rely on a decrease in gamma-afferent activity [84].

Local cryotherapy has been reported to temporarily decrease spasticity and clonus, mainly by reducing the sensitivity of the muscle spindle to stretch as well as increasing the pain threshold and consequently reducing the receptor sensitivity of low-threshold afferents [82, 85]. Considering the short duration of the treatment effect, local cooling of spastic muscles might be a useful tool for inhibiting muscle hypertonia and clonus during casting procedures [4].

Local application of vibratory stimuli as well as whole body vibration training have been found to be useful in order to reduce muscle tone in patients with upper motor neuron syndrome [4, 86–89]. In particular, local vibration is mainly used for inhibition of spasticity through facilitatory application over the antagonists, thus inducing reciprocal inhibition of the spastic muscle [87].

Transcutaneous electrical nerve stimulation applied on the common peroneal nerve, spinal dermatomes or over the region of the spastic muscles has been reported to reduce muscle tone in patients with upper motor neuron syndrome [4, 80]. Its anti-spastic effect has been suggested to be linked to decreased excitability of the motor neurons, and also to facilitation of cortical synaptic reorganization and motor output following the increased sensory input [90, 91].

10 Conclusions

The optimal combination of rehabilitation techniques and medical management may improve outcomes in spasticity treatment [4]. On the other hand, inappropriate management of spasticity may interfere with functional recovery and increase complications in patients with upper motor neuron syndrome [15].

Given that spasticity may lead to functional limitation and quality of life reduction in patients with upper motor neuron syndrome, its management should be guided by the potential impact on function and well-being [15, 92, 93]. Thus, considering that function depends not only on muscle tone but also on muscle strength, coordination, endurance and sensation, the management of spasticity should not focus exclusively on the management of difficulties with passive muscle stretch or loss of range of motion [4, 15].

References

1. Lundström E, Smits A, Terént A, Borg J. Time-course and determinants of spasticity during the first six months following first-ever stroke. J Rehabil Med. 2010;42:296–301.
2. Li S, Francisco GE. New insights into the pathophysiology of post-stroke spasticity. Front Hum Neurosci. 2015;9:192.
3. Lance JW. The control of muscle tone, reflexes and movement: Robert Wartenberg Lecture. Neurology. 1980;30:1303–13.
4. Smania N, Picelli A, Munari D, Geroin C, Ianes P, Waldner A, Gandolfi M. Rehabilitation procedures in the management of spasticity. Eur J Phys Rehabil Med. 2010;46:423–38.
5. Wissel J, Ward AB, Erztgaard P, Bensmail D, Hecht MJ, Lejeune TM, Schnider P, Altavista MC, Cavazza S, Deltombe T, Duarte E, Geurts AC, Gracies JM, Haboubi NH, Juan FJ, Kasch H, Kätterer C, Kirazli Y, Manganotti P, Parman Y, Paternostro-Sluga T, Petropoulou K, Prempeh R, Rousseaux M, Slawek J, Tieranta N. European consensus table on the use of botulinum toxin type A in adult spasticity. J Rehabil Med. 2009;41:13–25.
6. Gracies JM. Pathophysiology of spastic paresis. I: Paresis and soft tissue changes. Muscle Nerve. 2005;31:535–51.b.
7. Gracies JM. Pathophysiology of spastic paresis. II: Emergence of muscle overactivity. Muscle Nerve. 2005;31:552–71.
8. Wissel J, Verrier M, Simpson DM, Charles D, Guinto P, Papapetropoulos S, Sunnerhagen KS. Post-stroke spasticity: predictors of early development and considerations for therapeutic intervention. PM R. 2015;7:60–7.
9. Leathley MJ, Gregson JM, Moore AP, Smith TL, Sharma AK, Watkins CL. Predicting spasticity after stroke in those surviving to 12 months. Clin Rehabil. 2004;18:438–43.

10. Sommerfeld DK, Eek EU, Svensson AK, Holmqvist LW, von Arbin MH. Spasticity after stroke: its occurrence and association with motor impairments and activity limitations. Stroke. 2004;35:134–9.
11. Urban PP, Wolf T, Uebele M, Marx JJ, Vogt T, Stoeter P, Bauermann T, Weibrich C, Vucurevic GD, Schneider A, Wissel J. Occurence and clinical predictors of spasticity after ischemic stroke. Stroke. 2010;41:2016–20.
12. Wissel J, Schelosky LD, Scott J, Christe W, Faiss JH, Mueller J. Early development of spasticity following stroke: a prospective, observational trial. J Neurol. 2010;257:1067–72.
13. Picelli A, Tamburin S, Dambruoso F, Midiri A, Girardi P, Santamato A, Fiore P, Smania N. Topical distribution of initial paresis of the limbs to predict clinically relevant spasticity after ischemic stroke: a retrospective cohort study. Eur J Phys Rehabil Med. 2014;50:489–94.a.
14. Picelli A, Tamburin S, Gajofatto F, Zanette G, Praitano M, Saltuari L, Corradini C, Smania N. Association between severe upper limb spasticity and brain lesion location in stroke patients. Biomed Res Int. 2014;2014:162754.b.
15. Francisco GE, McGuire JR. Poststroke spasticity management. Stroke. 2012;43:3132–6.
16. Bethoux F. Spasticity management after stroke. Phys Med Rehabil Clin N Am. 2015;26:625–39.
17. Logan LR. Rehabilitation techniques to maximize spasticity management. Top Stroke Rehabil. 2011;18:203–11.
18. Esquenazi A, Novak I, Sheean G, Singer BJ, Ward AB. International consensus statement for the use of botulinum toxin treatment in adults and children with neurological impairments-introduction. Eur J Neurol. 2010;17:1–8.
19. Olver J, Esquenazi A, Fung VS, Singer BJ, Ward AB, Cerebral Palsy Institute. Botulinum toxin assessment, intervention and aftercare for lower limb disorders of movement and muscle tone in adults: international consensus statement. Eur J Neurol. 2010;17:57–73.
20. Sheean G, Lannin NA, Turner-Stokes L, Rawicki B, Snow BJ, Cerebral Palsy Institute. Botulinum toxin assessment, intervention and after-care for upper limb hypertonicity in adults: international consensus statement. Eur J Neurol. 2010;17:74–93.
21. Simon O, Yelnik AP. Managing spasticity with drugs. Eur J Phys Rehabil Med. 2010;46:401–10.
22. Esquenazi A, Albanese A, Chancellor MB, Elovic E, Segal KR, Simpson DM, Smith CP, Ward AB. Evidence-based review and assessment of botulinum neurotoxin for the treatment of adult spasticity in the upper motor neuron syndrome. Toxicon. 2013;67:115–28.
23. Simpson DM, Gracies JM, Graham HK, Miyasaki JM, Naumann M, Russman B, Simpson LL, So Y, Therapeutics and Technology Assessment Subcommittee of the American Academy of Neurology. Assessment: Botulinum neurotoxin for the treatment of spasticity (an evidence-based review): report of the Therapeutics and Technology Assessment Subcommittee of the American Academy of Neurology. Neurology. 2008;70:1691–8.
24. Simpson LL. Kinetic studies on the interaction between botulinum toxin type A and the cholinergic neuromuscular junction. J Pharmacol Exp Ther. 1980;212:16–21.
25. Black JD, Dolly JO. Interaction of ^{125}I-labeled botulinum neurotoxins with nerve terminals, II: autoradiographic evidence for its uptake into motor nerves by acceptor mediated endocytosis. J Cell Biol. 1986;103:535–44.
26. Hughes R, Whaler BC. Influence of nerve-ending activity and of drugs on the rate of paralysis of rat diaphragm preparations by Cl. botulinum type A toxin. J Physiol. 1962;160:221–33.
27. Baricich A, Carda S, Bertoni M, Maderna L, Cisari C. A single-blinded, randomized pilot study of botulinum toxin type A combined with non-pharmacological treatment for spastic foot. J Rehabil Med. 2008;40:870–2.
28. Bayram S, Sivrioglu K, Karli N, Ozcan O. Low-dose botulinum toxin with short-term electrical stimulation in poststroke spastic drop foot: a preliminary study. Am J Phys Med Rehabil. 2006;85:75–81.
29. Carda S, Molteni F. Taping versus electrical stimulation after botulinum toxin type A injection for wrist and finger spasticity. A case-control study. Clin Rehabil. 2005;19:621–6.

30. Detrembleur C, Lejeune TM, Renders A, Van Den Bergh PY. Botulinum toxin and short-term electrical stimulation in the treatment of equinus in cerebral palsy. Mov Disord. 2002;17:162–9.
31. Eleopra R, Tugnoli V, De Grandis D. The variability in the clinical effect induced by botulinum toxin type A: the role of muscle activity in humans. Mov Disord. 1997;12:89–94.
32. Franceschini M, Iocco M, Molteni F, Santamato A, Smania N, Italian Spasticity Study Group. Management of stroke patients submitted to botulinum toxin type A therapy: a Delphi survey of an Italian expert panel of specialist injectors. Eur J Phys Rehabil Med. 2014;50:525–33.
33. Frasson E, Priori A, Ruzzante B, Didonè G, Bertolasi L. Nerve stimulation boosts botulinum toxin action in spasticity. Mov Disord. 2005;20:624–9.
34. Hesse S, Jahnke MT, Luecke D, Mauritz KH. Short-term electrical stimulation enhances the effectiveness of Botulinum toxin in the treatment of lower limb spasticity in hemiparetic patients. Neurosci Lett. 1995;201:37–40.
35. Hesse S, Reiter F, Konrad M, Jahnke MT. Botulinum toxin type A and short-term electrical stimulation in the treatment of upper limb flexor spasticity after stroke: a randomized, double-blind, placebo-controlled trial. Clin Rehabil. 1998;12:381–8.
36. Kang BS, Bang MS, Jung SH. Effects of botulinum toxin A therapy with electrical stimulation on spastic calf muscles in children with cerebral palsy. Am J Phys Med Rehabil. 2007;86:901–6.
37. Kinnear BZ, Lannin NA, Cusick A, Harvey LA, Rawicki B. Rehabilitation therapies after botulinum toxin-A injection to manage limb spasticity: a systematic review. Phys Ther. 2014;94:1569–81.
38. Mudge A, Harvey LA, Lancaster A, Lowe K. Electrical stimulation following botulinum toxin A in children with spastic diplegia: a within-participant randomized pilot study. Phys Occup Ther Pediatr. 2015;35(4):342–53.
39. Picelli A, Smania N, Storti I, Munari D, Fontana C, Fiaschi A, Santilli V, Tamburin S. Immediate versus delayed electrical stimulation boosts botulinum toxin effect: a pilot study. Mov Disord. 2011;26:1784–5.
40. Rha DW, Yang EJ, Chung HI, Kim HB, Park CI, Park ES. Is electrical stimulation beneficial for improving the paralytic effect of botulinum toxin type A in children with spastic diplegic cerebral palsy? Yonsei Med J. 2008;49:545–52.
41. Wilkenfeld AJ. Review of electrical stimulation, botulinum toxin, and their combination for spastic drop foot. J Rehabil Res Dev. 2013;50:315–26.
42. Grumelli C, Verderio C, Pozzi D, Rossetto O, Montecucco C, Matteoli M. Internalization and mechanism of action of clostridial toxins in neurons. Neurotoxicology. 2005;26:761–7.
43. Keller JE, Cai F, Neale EA. Uptake of botulinum neurotoxin into cultured neurons. Biochemistry. 2004;43:526–32.
44. Sunnerhagen KS, Olver J, Francisco GE. Assessing and treating functional impairment in poststroke spasticity. Neurology. 2013;80:S35–44.
45. Picelli A, Bonetti P, Fontana C, Barausse M, Dambruoso F, Gajofatto F, Girardi P, Manca M, Gimigliano R, Smania N. Is spastic muscle echo intensity related to the response to botulinum toxin type A in patients with stroke? A cohort study. Arch Phys Med Rehabil. 2012;93:1253–8.
46. Picelli A, Tamburin S, Cavazza S, Scampoli C, Manca M, Cosma M, Berto G, Vallies G, Roncari L, Melotti C, Santilli V, Smania N. Relationship between ultrasonographic, electromyographic, and clinical parameters in adult stroke patients with spastic equinus: an observational study. Arch Phys Med Rehabil. 2014;95:1564–70.c.
47. Santamato A, Micello MF, Panza F, Fortunato F, Picelli A, Smania N, Logroscino G, Fiore P, Ranieri M. Adhesive taping vs. daily manual muscle stretching and splinting after botulinum toxin type A injection for wrist and fingers spastic overactivity in stroke patients: a randomized controlled trial. Clin Rehabil. 2015;29:50–8.

48. Carda S, Invernizzi M, Baricich A, Cisari C. Casting, taping or stretching after botulinum toxin type A for spastic equinus foot: a single-blind randomized trial on adult stroke patients. Clin Rehabil. 2011;25:1119–27.
49. Newman CJ, Kennedy A, Walsh M, O'Brien T, Lynch B, Hensey O. A pilot study of delayed versus immediate serial casting after botulinum toxin injection for partially reducible spastic equinus. J Pediatr Orthop. 2007;27:882–5.
50. Tyson SF, Sadeghi-Demneh E, Nester CJ. A systematic review and meta-analysis of the effect of an ankle-foot orthosis on gait biomechanics after stroke. Clin Rehabil. 2013;27:879–91.
51. Mehrholz J, Pohl M, Elsner B. Treadmill training and body weight support for walking after stroke. Cochrane Database Syst Rev. 2014;1:CD002840.
52. Kwakkel G, Kollen BJ, Krebs HI. Effects of robot-assisted therapy on upper limb recovery after stroke: a systematic review. Neurorehabil Neural Repair. 2008;22:111–21.
53. Mehrholz J, Pohl M, Platz T, Kugler J, Elsner B. Electromechanical and robot-assisted arm training for improving activities of daily living, arm function and arm muscle strength after stroke. Cochrane Database Syst Rev. 2015;11:CD006876.
54. Mehrholz J, Elsner B, Werner C, Kugler J, Pohl M. Electromechanical-assisted training for walking after stroke. Cochrane Database Syst Rev. 2013;7:CD006185.
55. Richardson D. Physical therapy in spasticity. Eur J Neurol. 2002;9:17–22.
56. Bobath B. Adult hemiplegia: evaluation and treatment. 3rd ed. London: Heinemann Medical Books; 1990.
57. Mikołajewska E. NDT-Bobath method in normalization of muscle tone in post-stroke patients. Adv Clin Exp Med. 2012;21:513–7.
58. Ansari NN, Naghdi S. The effect of Bobath approach on the excitability of the spinal alpha motor neurones in stroke patients with muscle spasticity. Electromyogr Clin Neurophysiol. 2007;47:29–36.
59. Carr JH, Shepherd RB. A motor relearning programme. London: William Heinemann; 1987.
60. Langhammer B, Stanghelle J. Bobath or motor relearning programme? A comparison of two different approaches of physiotherapy in stroke rehabilitation: a randomised controlled trial. Clin Rehab. 2000;14:361–9.
61. Alfieri V. Electrical treatment of spasticity. Reflex tonic activity in hemiplegic patients and selected specific electrostimulation. Scand J Rehabil Med. 1982;14:177–82.
62. Rossi PW. Electrical stimulation. In: Gelber D, Jeffery D, editors. Clinical evaluation and management of spasticity. New York: Humana Press; 2002.
63. Ada L, Dorsch S, Canning CG. Strengthening interventions increase strength and improve activity after stroke: a systematic review. Aust J Physiother. 2006;52:241–8.
64. Morris SL, Dodd KJ, Morris ME. Outcomes of progressive resistance strength training following stroke: a systematic review. Clin Rehabil. 2004;18:27–39.
65. Pak S, Patten C. Strengthening to promote functional recovery poststroke: an evidence-based review. Top Stroke Rehabil. 2008;15:177–99.
66. Picelli A, Chemello E, Castellazzi P, Roncari L, Waldner A, Saltuari L, Smania N. Combined effects of transcranial direct current stimulation (tDCS) and transcutaneous spinal direct current stimulation (tsDCS) on robot-assisted gait training in patients with chronic stroke: A pilot, double blind, randomized controlled trial. Restor Neurol Neurosci. 2015;33:357–68.
67. Corbetta D, Sirtori V, Castellini G, Moja L, Gatti R. Constraint-induced movement therapy for upper extremities in people with stroke. Cochrane Database Syst Rev. 2015;10: CD004433.
68. Kwakkel G, Veerbeek JM, van Wegen EE, Wolf SL. Constraint-induced movement therapy after stroke. Lancet Neurol. 2015;14:224–34.
69. Legg LA, Drummond AE, Langhorne P. Occupational therapy for patients with problems in activities of daily living after stroke. Cochrane Database Syst Rev. 2006;4:CD003585.
70. Legg L, Drummond A, Leonardi-Bee J, Gladman JR, Corr S, Donkervoort M, Edmans J, Gilbertson L, Jongbloed L, Logan P, Sackley C, Walker M, Langhorne P. Occupational therapy for patients with problems in personal activities of daily living after stroke: systematic review of randomised trials. BMJ. 2007;335:922.

71. Marinho-Buzelli AR, Bonnyman AM, Verrier MC. The effects of aquatic therapy on mobility of individuals with neurological diseases: a systematic review. Clin Rehabil. 2015;29:741–51.
72. Saunders DH, Sanderson M, Hayes S, Kilrane M, Greig CA, Brazzelli M, Mead GE. Physical fitness training for stroke patients. Cochrane Database Syst Rev. 2016;3:CD003316.
73. Wevers L, van de Port I, Vermue M, Mead G, Kwakkel G. Effects of task-oriented circuit class training on walking competency after stroke: a systematic review. Stroke. 2009;40:2450–9.
74. Manganotti P, Amelio E. Long-term effect of shock wave therapy on upper limb hypertonia in patients affected by stroke. Stroke. 2005;36:1967–71.
75. Picelli A, Marchina E, Gajofatto F, Pontillo A, Vangelista A, Filippini R, Baricich A, Cisari C, Smania N. Sonographic and clinical effects of botulinum toxin type A combined with extracorporeal shock wave therapy on spastic muscles of children with cerebral palsy. Dev Neurorehabil. 2017;20:160–4.
76. Santamato A, Notarnicola A, Panza F, Ranieri M, Micello MF, Manganotti P, Moretti B, Fortunato F, Filoni S, Fiore P. SBOTE study: extracorporeal shock wave therapy versus electrical stimulation after botulinum toxin type a injection for post-stroke spasticity-a prospective randomized trial. Ultrasound Med Biol. 2013;39:283–91.
77. Ansari NN, Adelmanesh F, Naghdi S, Tabtabaei A. The effect of physiotherapeutic ultrasound on muscle spasticity in patients with hemiplegia: a pilot study. Electromyogr Clin Neurophysiol. 2006;46:247–52.
78. Ansari NN, Naghdi S, Bagheri H, Ghassabi H. Therapeutic ultrasound in the treatment of ankle plantarflexor spasticity in a unilateral stroke population: a randomized, single-blind, placebo-controlled trial. Electromyogr Clin Neurophysiol. 2007;47:137–43.
79. Ansari NN, Naghdi S, Hasson S, Rastgoo M. Efficacy of therapeutic ultrasound and infrared in the management of muscle spasticity. Brain Inj. 2009;23:632–8.
80. Picelli A, Dambruoso F, Bronzato M, Barausse M, Gandolfi M, Smania N. Efficacy of therapeutic ultrasound and transcutaneous electrical nerve stimulation compared with botulinum toxin type A in the treatment of spastic equinus in adults with chronic stroke: a pilot randomized controlled trial. Top Stroke Rehabil. 2014;21:S8–16.a.
81. Sahin N, Ugurlu H, Karahan AY. Efficacy of therapeutic ultrasound in the treatment of spasticity: a randomized controlled study. NeuroRehabil. 2011;29:61–6.
82. Gracies JM. Physical modalities other than stretch in spastic hypertonia. Phys Med Rehabil Clin N Am. 2001;12:769–92.a.
83. Lee GP, Ng GY. Effects of stretching and heat treatment on hamstring extensibility in children with severe mental retardation and hypertonia. Clin Rehabil. 2008;22:771–9.
84. Matsumoto S, Kawahira K, Etoh S, Ikeda S, Tanaka N. Short-term effects of thermotherapy for spasticity on tibial nerve F-waves in post-stroke patients. Int J Biometeorol. 2006;50: 243–50.
85. Harlaar J, Ten Kate JJ, Prevo AJ, Vogelaar TW, Lankhorst GJ. The effect of cooling on muscle co-ordination in spasticity: assessment with the repetitive movement test. Disabil Rehabil. 2001;23:453–61.
86. Ahlborg L, Andersson C, Julin P. Whole-body vibration training compared with resistance training: effect on spasticity, muscle strength and motor performance in adults with cerebral palsy. J Rehabil Med. 2006;38:302–8.
87. Galea MP. Physical modalities in the treatment of neurological dysfunction. Clin Neurol Neurosurg. 2012;114:483–8.
88. Ness LL, Field-Fote EC. Effect of whole-body vibration on quadriceps spasticity in individuals with spastic hypertonia due to spinal cord injury. Restor Neurol Neurosci. 2009;27:621–31.
89. Noma T, Matsumoto S, Etoh S, Shimodozono M, Kawahira K. Anti-spastic effects of the direct application of vibratory stimuli to the spastic muscles of hemiplegic limbs in post-stroke patients. Brain Inj. 2009;23:623–31.

90. Ng SS, Hui-Chan CW. Transcutaneous electrical nerve stimulation combined with task-related training improves lower limb functions in subjects with chronic stroke. Stroke. 2007;38:2953–9.
91. Ng SS, Hui-Chan CW. Does the use of TENS increase the effectiveness of exercise for improving walking after stroke? A randomized controlled clinical trial. Clin Rehabil. 2009;23:1093–103.
92. Graham LA. Management of spasticity revisited. Age Ageing. 2013;42:435–41.
93. Nair KP, Marsden J. The management of spasticity in adults. BMJ. 2014;349:g4737.

Spinal Cord Stimulation as a Neuromodulatory Intervention for Altered Motor Control Following Spinal Cord Injury

Ursula S. Hofstoetter, Brigitta Freundl, Heinrich Binder and Karen Minassian

1 Controlling Spasticity After Spinal Cord Injury: Challenges and Pathways

Severe spinal cord injury (SCI) is a devastating event, which, apart from the obvious paresis or paralysis, causes manifold secondary complications impairing vital body functions caudal to the lesion. One major cause of disability stems from spasticity as one symptom of the upper motoneuron syndrome, with about 70% of individuals being affected one year after the injury [1, 8, 92].

Academically, spasticity is rather narrowly defined as a velocity-dependent form of hypertonia resulting from hyperexcitability of tonic stretch reflexes [57] as a consequence of the lesion-induced misbalance between inhibitory and excitatory inputs to spinal circuitry below the injury [55, 89]. Clinically, associated signs like spasms, clonus, resistance to passive movements, and the clasp-knife response are also commonly subsumed under the umbrella of spasticity [89]. Together, these symptoms often present a major hindrance in rehabilitation, further deteriorate residual motor performance, and negatively impact independence and quality of life [1, 78, 93]. Yet, certain aspects associated with spasticity may as well pose some benefit by increasing trunk stability, facilitating transfers, enabling some stepping movements, reducing the risk of deep venous thrombosis, and partially maintaining muscle bulk, thereby also protecting against pressure sore formation in wheelchair-bound individuals [1, 5, 78]. Any regimen applied with the aim to

U. S. Hofstoetter (✉) · K. Minassian
Center for Medical Physics and Biomedical Engineering, Medical University Vienna, Waehringer Guertel 18–20/4L, A-1090 Vienna, Austria
e-mail: ursula.hofstoetter@meduniwien.ac.at

B. Freundl · H. Binder
Neurological Center, Otto Wagner Hospital, Vienna, Austria

G. Sandrini et al. (eds.), *Advanced Technologies for the Rehabilitation of Gait and Balance Disorders*, Biosystems & Biorobotics 19,
https://doi.org/10.1007/978-3-319-72736-3_33

reduce spasticity therefore needs to carefully balance out between the need to alleviate its detrimental effects and the maintenance of its useful facets [1, 5].

Without doubt, successful management of spasticity has remained difficult and normally requires a multimodal approach, tailored to the individual clinical picture. Treatment modalities include physical therapy, oral medication, intrathecal drug delivery, and the application of Botulinum toxin (for a review see [5, 26, 98]). Surgical neuroablative approaches are often considered as last resort in the treatment of severe, resistant forms of spasticity [78]. Yet, some of the treatments used bear the risk of undesirable side effects, particularly weakness and fatigue that may be induced by antispasticity medication, the further deterioration of residual mobility, as well as permanent lesions within (previously undamaged) neural tissue caused by surgical methods [23, 78].

Neuromodulation techniques provide for an alternative, reversible, and adjustable concept for the treatment of diffuse spasticity and work through the modification of neural signal processing by targeted circuits within the central nervous system [40]. One method to modify the altered activity in the spared neural circuitry after SCI, aside from pharmacological approaches [73], is by electrical spinal cord stimulation (SCS). This chapter will trace the first applications of this technique from its early developments in the 1960s to its recent resurgence in neurorehabilitation and motor recovery after SCI, with a focus on practical aspects and clinical applications.

2 Epidural Spinal Cord Stimulation in Spinal Spasticity: The Early Period

The pioneering work on the nature and treatment of pain by Ronald Wall and colleagues in the 1960s [60, 98]; for a current review see [61] indirectly provided the scientific breeding ground for the later developments in the field of SCS. They postulated that (peripheral) stimulation of large-diameter cutaneous sensory fibers would reduce the perception of pain through the central inhibition of small-diameter fibers in the spinal cord circuitry involved in pain transmission. To control intractable, diffuse pain, Norman Shealy and co-workers demonstrated, first in cats, the particular effectiveness of concentrating the stimulation on the posterior columns of the spinal cord white matter, where the ascending continuations of cutaneous sensory fibers related to multiple dermatomes are closely assembled [87]. Shealy also conducted the first human application of SCS for pain relief in a cancer patient via a plate electrode surgically placed over the posterior columns at T3, leading to an immediate abolition of the pain [88]. Since then, and with technological advancements, SCS for pain control has become widely used [28]. In 1989, epidural SCS gained its approval by the U.S. Food and Drug Administration for the treatment of chronic intractable pain of the trunk and limbs and since then has developed into the most common of all neuromodulation therapies [52].

In fact, the application of epidural SCS in motor disorders is closely linked to its original use in pain conditions, as it followed from an unanticipated observation made in a patient with multiple sclerosis treated for pain [14]. In addition to relieving the pain, the stimulation, applied to the upper thoracic spinal cord, led to a considerable increase of the patient's sensory perception and voluntary motor control over the legs. Subsequent studies including numerous individuals with multiple sclerosis in whom pain was not a main complaint reproduced the positive impact of SCS on motor performance, taking the form of reduced spasticity and a feeling of lightness when moving the legs, increased endurance during ambulation, and the enabling of some voluntary movements in otherwise paralyzed limbs under SCS [13, 20, 25, 44, 90, 100]. Yet, not all patients benefitted equally from SCS, and in some individuals, no effects were achieved at all [45, 90, 91]. These inter-individual differences were attributed to the pathophysiological complexity of the disease itself as well as to the high variability of rostro-caudal stimulation sites employed across the different studies [23]; reviewed in [67, 68].

Despite this ambiguity, the positive results obtained in the patients with multiple sclerosis soon motivated first studies in SCI individuals [7, 23, 75, 79, 80, 91], which likewise produced positive yet variable outcomes (Fig. 1a). Richardson et al. [80] reported complete alleviation of spasticity in 6 individuals with severe thoracic SCI whose spasticity could not be controlled by other treatment modalities when applying SCS via epidural electrodes placed below the injury over the lumbar and sacral spinal roots at L1–L4 vertebral levels. On the other hand, Siegfried et al. [91] found no improvements in lower-limb spasticity in any of the 15 SCI individuals studied when treated by SCS. Notably, electrodes were always placed rostral to the level of severe SCI in their study. In a cohort of 59 SCI individuals, Dimitrijevic et al. [23] found a marked or moderate effect of SCS on spasticity in 37 patients, with only a marginal or no effect in the remaining 22 patients. Reduction of spasticity was generally achieved with electrode placements caudal to the injury level in the posterior epidural space. Yet, in severe cervical spinal cord lesions and with the electrodes placed immediately caudal to the injury, SCS failed to alleviate spasticity in the lower limbs, while in incomplete SCI, stimulation from similar sites produced considerable therapeutic effects. Dimitrijevic et al. [23] concluded that the effectiveness of SCS strongly depended on the specific rostro-caudal position of the electrodes with respect to the injury site and on the severity of the spinal cord lesion. Barolat et al. [7] studied the potential of SCS to control severe spasms in 16 SCI patients. The target placement of the electrodes was always caudal to the level of the lesion, ranging from T1–T6 levels depending on the individual distribution of spasticity, and in the posterior epidural space. Such electrode placement was achieved in 14 out of the 16 individuals tested and led to marked improvements of the spasms in terms of their severity, frequency, and duration in all 14 cases [7]. Specifically, with electrode placements at or rostral to T3, also spasms in the upper limbs were controlled by the stimulation. Pinter et al. [75] showed a considerable antispasticity effect in the lower limbs of 8 individuals with severe low-cervical to mid-thoracic lesions of the spinal cord when applying SCS from the posterior epidural space at vertebral levels of T11–L1, thereby specifically targeting the

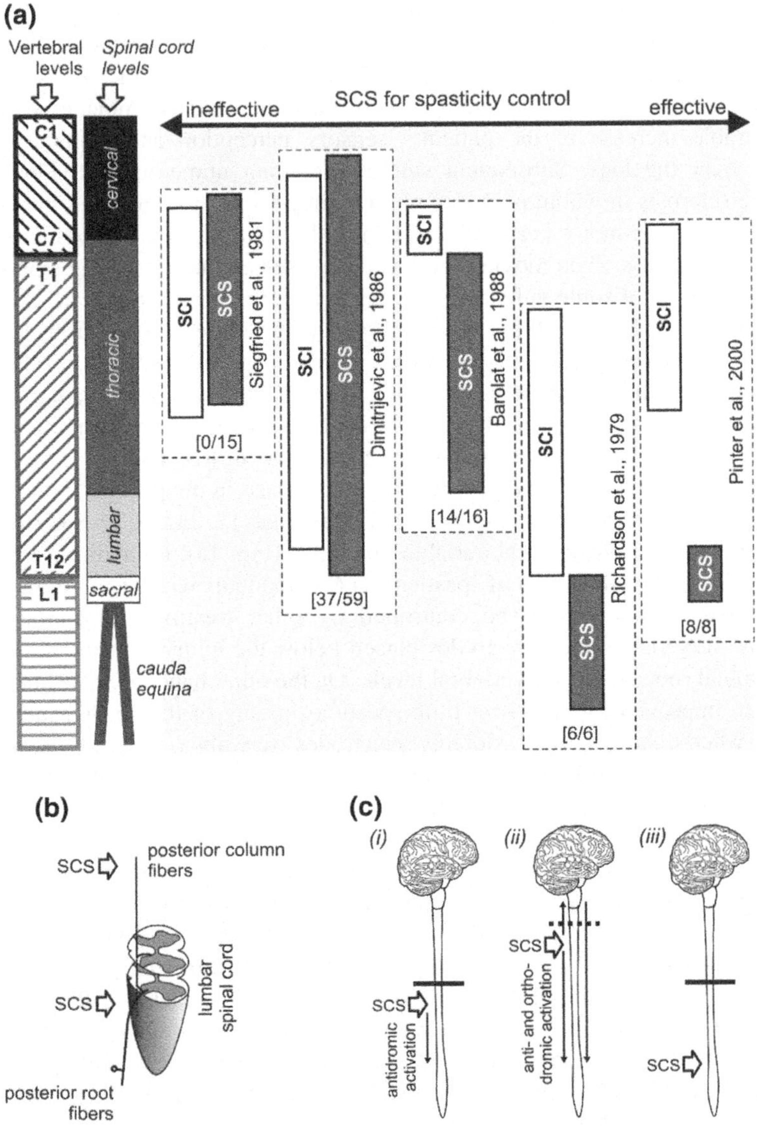

lumbar spinal cord. The effect was so pronounced that antispasticity medication could be completely discontinued in 7 of the patients and substantially reduced in the remaining subject. Across the various studies, the applied stimulation frequencies were within a range of 33–120 Hz and intensities were below the level causing muscle activity in the lower extremities and produced paraesthesias in individuals with sensory incomplete SCI. The stimulation was either continuously or intermittently applied for several hours per day via plate electrodes or percutaneous leads.

◂**Fig. 1** Epidural spinal cord stimulation (SCS) for spasticity control after spinal cord injury (SCI). **a** Studies conducted by various groups starting from the 1970s produced ambiguous results on the effectiveness of epidural SCS to reduce spasticity. The sketch on the left presents vertebral relative to spinal cord levels, white bars on the right depict ranges of SCI levels of the patients studied in the different studies, and black bars the respective rostro-caudal ranges of electrode positions. Studies are arranged from left to right according to the reported effectiveness of SCS to alleviate spasticity. Numbers in brackets are numbers of responders relative to the total numbers of SCI individuals included. **b** SCS can electrically activate large-to-medium-diameter sensory posterior root fibers or, given their functional integrity, their ascending continuations in the posterior columns of the spinal cord white matter, depending on the rostro-caudal electrode position. **c** The effectiveness of SCS to reduce lower-limb spasticity strongly depends on the rostro-caudal placement of the epidural electrode, the severity of SCI, and the neural mechanisms set into action by the stimulation. (i) SCS applied to the thoracic spinal cord caudal to a severe SCI activates the lumbar segmental circuitry via antidromic activation of posterior column fibers. (ii) In incomplete SCI, the stimulation may likely work through spinal-brainstem-spinal loops set into action by orthodromic conduction evoked within the posterior columns as well as through segmental spinal mechanisms following the antidromic posterior column activation. (iii) SCS over the lumbar spinal cord activates the local circuitry transsynaptically through the electrical stimulation of afferent fibers within the lumbar posterior roots

Barolat et al. [7] described an immediate amelioration of spasticity by the stimulation in most of the patients, but also found gradual decrease of spasticity occurring over several weeks in some of the individuals treated. In most subjects, there were carry-over effects after the stimulation had been turned off. The persistence of these effects was generally related to the duration of the stimulation, ranging from a few hours within the first weeks of stimulation to up to 5 days after several weeks of stimulation [7]. Accordingly, some patients adjusted their daily regimen of stimulation, and some could reduce its application to a few hours two or three times a week only, while maintaining the therapeutic effects [7]. Implantation as well as stimulation procedures were generally well accepted by the patients included in the various studies, and no adverse effects related to the stimulation were reported.

As suggested by Dimitrijevic et al. [23], the variability in the results produced by the different studies must be discussed in the light of the respective rostro-caudal stimulation sites employed, leading to the electrical activation of distinct neural structures, and in conjunction with the severity of the spinal cord lesions. At therapeutic intensities for the management of spasticity (see subsect. 3 of this chapter), the neural structures electrically stimulated through electrodes placed in the posterior epidural space are afferent fibers within the posterior roots or their rostral continuations within the posterior columns of the spinal cord white matter [41], also depending on the specific segmental electrode position. SCS targeted to the lumbar spinal cord predominantly activates large-to-medium-diameter afferents within the posterior roots [76] (Fig. 1b). Notably, of the afferent fibers originating from muscles, tendons, joints, and cutaneous tissues of the hip and lower limbs that enter the spinal cord via the lumbar and upper sacral posterior roots, only the ascending continuations of the cutaneous fibers are present also within the posterior columns with increasing distance to the lumbar spinal cord, since the other fiber types leave the posterior columns to ascend via alternative systems [19]. All other spinal neural structures are transsynaptically recruited through the SCS-induced sensory input [10, 62].

Following this line, three potential neural pathways by which the activity produced by SCS may reach (and modulate) the lumbar spinal circuitry involved in gating afferent input and regulating motoneuronal excitability associated with the lower limbs were suggested: first, via antidromic activation of the posterior column fibers when stimulation is directed to the thoracic spinal cord (Fig. 1c(i); [43]); second, via orthodromic conduction evoked within the posterior columns, leading to increased descending activation of spinal inhibitory circuitry through brainstem-spinal cord loops in incomplete SCI (Fig. 1c(ii); [23, 86]); and third, with SCS over the lumbar spinal cord, via orthodromic activation of afferent fibers within the lumbar and upper sacral posterior roots (Fig. 1c(iii); [62, 64, 71, 75, 76]).

These variable neural mechanisms set into action by the stimulation also provide a likely explanation for the lack of effectiveness in some patients versus the good results obtained in others (Fig. 1c). In the individuals with complete cervical SCI and the electrodes placed just caudal to the lesion zone, the functional integrity of the posterior columns at the stimulation site may too have been compromised by the injury or the effects would have required the stimulation of fiber types arising in the legs that are not present in the posterior columns at such distance from the lumbar spinal cord [68, 69]. Satisfactory results, on the other hand, were obtained with stimulation applied from same sites but in individuals with incomplete SCI. Apart from acting on lumbar spinal segmental circuity via antidromic posterior-column activation in these cases [23, 86], the stimulation likely also increased the descending activation of inhibitory spinal mechanisms through brainstem-spinal loops [23]; cf. [83].

3 Epidural Stimulation of the Lumbar Spinal Cord for the Control of Spasticity: Current Practice and Clinical Considerations

The various studies starting from the 1970s have taught that refractory forms of lower-limb spasticity may be alleviated by activating the lumbar spinal segmental circuitry involved in the regulation of afferent inputs and of the motoneuronal excitability associated with the legs and that this circuitry can—largely independently from the specific site and severity of SCI—be accessed with SCS specifically directed to the lumbar spinal cord [75]. Notably, despite the promising therapeutic outcomes achieved with epidural SCS in numerous patients suffering from various conditions [99], its application in motor disorders has remained off-label.

Practically, the stimulation is applied via a thin cylindrical lead with several electrodes on the distal end that is placed percutaneously and thus minimally invasive under fluoroscopic control into the posterior epidural space over the lumbar spinal cord. Alternatively, the stimulation may be delivered via a surgical paddle lead with electrodes arranged in arrays that require laminotomy or laminectomy, but at the same time allow for a more flexible control over the stimulation site employed [54]. On average, the rostro-caudal position of the electrodes corresponds to the T11 and T12 vertebral levels, but may be as caudal as the L1 vertebral level, as well [62, 71] (Fig. 2a). Stimulation from the targeted site allows for the activation of posterior-root afferents of several lumbar and upper sacral spinal cord levels bilaterally at the same time [62] (Fig. 2b). Consequently, at low stimulation frequencies (e.g., 2 or 5 Hz) and with adequate stimulation intensity, each stimulus pulse evokes twitch-contractions in multiple muscles of both legs [71] (Fig. 2c), so-called posterior root-muscle (PRM) reflexes termed according to their initiation and recording sites [62, 65]. With other words, from the targeted stimulation site over the lumbar spinal cord, PRM reflexes will be elicited in muscle groups with distinct segmental innervation (cf. Fig. 2b), and intraoperative surface-electromyographic recordings of such reflex responses hence serve as a physiological marker guiding the correct rostro-caudal placement of the epidural electrodes over the lumbar spinal cord [32, 38, 64, 71, 75]. In individuals with sensory incomplete SCI, the placement can be also guided by the elicitation of paraesthesias in the lower-limb dermatomes, when stimulation is applied at higher frequencies (e.g., 30 or 50 Hz), like in epidural SCS for pain control [54].

After its implantation in the lumbar epidural space, the electrode lead is normally externalized and connected to a test stimulator for a trial period of 1–2 weeks. During this period, various combinations of SCS parameter settings are systematically tested for their effectiveness in controlling lower-limb spasticity. The epidural lead carries several independent electrodes that can be set to "+", "–", and "off", allowing for different bi- (and multi-) polar electrode combinations. The selection of the active cathode also allows for shifting the active stimulation site along the extent of the multiple electrodes. Stimulation frequencies normally used for spasticity control are within a range of 50–100 Hz [75]. Therapeutic stimulation intensities are below the level evoking muscle twitches in the trunk, hip, or lower limbs and are generally within a range of 0.5–5 V with an impedance of 300–1000 Ω for a bipolar electrode configuration [75]. Individuals with incomplete SCI may perceive a non-painful tingling sensation (paraesthesias) in the lower-limb dermatomes during the stimulation. With the designated parameter settings, the effects of SCS on the patients' spasticity and residual motor control are thoroughly assessed clinically and neurophysiologically, also tailored to the patients' individual clinical picture of spasticity and needs, and comparing them to the corresponding assessments conducted before the implantation and with the stimulation turned off (Fig. 3). This trial procedure is necessary since there are still no generally accepted clinical or physiological markers to clearly identify in advance those patients who will benefit from epidural SCS. A more recently developed transcutaneous version of SCS may develop into an easy-to-apply and useful procedure, which could serve this purpose in the future (see Sect. 5 of this chapter). Given a positive evaluation by the patient, the attending neurologist, and the involved physiotherapists after the trial period, a programmable implantable pulse generator (IPG) is eventually placed subcutaneously in the abdominal wall [54] and connected to the epidural electrode lead, forming a closed system for chronic stimulation. The IPG is then set to run

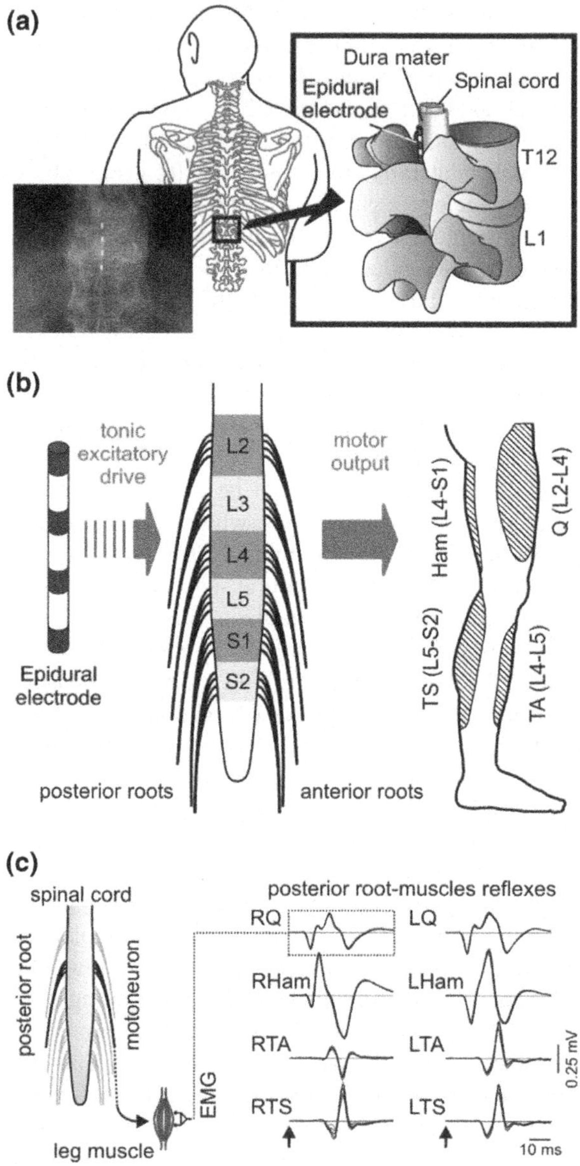

continuously with the determined frequency and electrode combination, which are typically only altered should the effect change over time, e.g. because of migration of the electrode lead [75] or carry-over effects emerging over time, allowing the patient to (temporarily) withdraw the stimulation or reduce the stimulation amplitudes [7]. The stimulation intensity is manually adjustable using a patient programmer. At the Neurological Center, Otto-Wagner-Hospital, Vienna, roughly 30

◀**Fig. 2** Epidural stimulation of the lumbar spinal cord. **a** X-ray and schematic sketch illustrate the placement of the epidural electrodes in the epidural space, inside the vertebral canal and outside the meninges covering the spinal cord, over the lumbar spinal cord corresponding on average to T11 and T12 vertebral levels. **b** Epidural stimulation of the lumbar spinal cord synchronously activates large-to-medium-diameter afferent fibers within the lumbar and upper sacral posterior roots bilaterally that are associated with muscle groups of the lower limbs. Sketch on the right depicts segmental innervation of quadriceps (Q), hamstrings (Ham), tibialis anterior (TA), and triceps surae (TS). **c** Stimulation of the lumbar spinal cord with above motor-threshold intensity elicits short-latency posterior root-muscle reflexes, i.e., reflexes initiated within posterior-root afferents and recorded via surface-electromyography (EMG), in multiple lower-limb muscle groups bilaterally. Stimulus-triggered, superimposed representation of 10 consecutive PRM reflexes elicited at 2 Hz in right (R) and left (L) Q, Ham, TA, and TS, black arrows indicate times of stimulus application

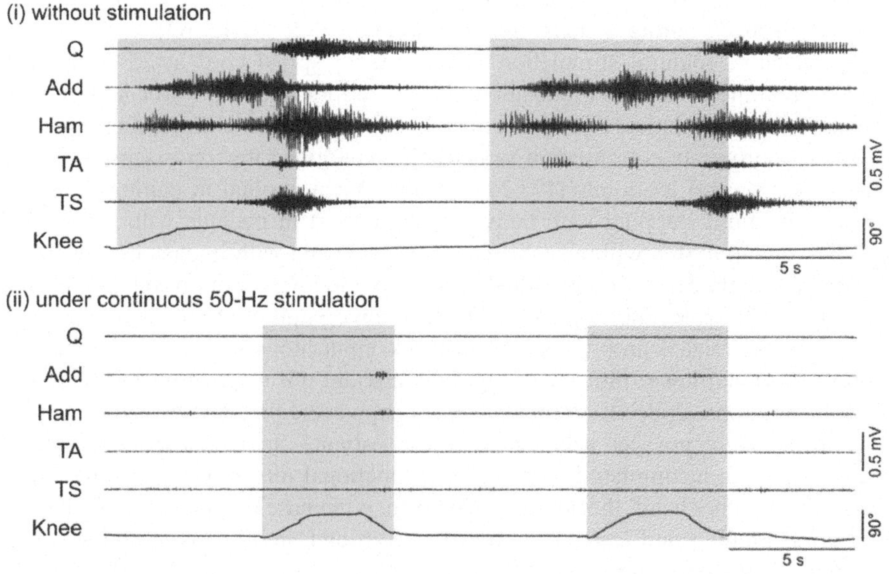

Fig. 3 Control of lower-limb spasticity by epidural stimulation targeting the lumbar spinal cord. Electromyographic (EMG) activity recorded in an individual with spinal spasticity during passive flexion and extension movements at hip and knee in the supine position (i) without stimulation and (ii) under continuous 50 Hz stimulation with sub-motor threshold intensity of 5 V using a bipolar electrode configuration with the cathode targeting the upper lumbar spinal cord segments, which corresponded in this subject to the 12th thoracic vertebral level as identified by X-ray. The stimulation suppresses lower-limb spasticity as reflected by complete attenuation of the EMG activity associated with the tonic stretch reflex recorded from quadriceps (Q), adductors (Add), hamstrings (Ham), tibialis anterior (TA), and triceps surae (TS). Shaded backgrounds mark the passive movement, shown are two repetitions of the same maneuver. Data derived from an individual with chronic motor complete spinal cord injury, American Spinal Injury Association Impairment Scale (AIS) grade B, neurological level of injury: C5–C6

individuals with chronic SCI have received devices for epidural lumbar SCS for spasticity control within the past 15–20 years.

4 The Recent Resurgence of Epidural Spinal Cord Stimulation: Inducing and Enabling Movement After Spinal Cord Injury

Apart from controlling severe forms of spasticity, which, by itself, allows the expression of some voluntary mobility in many cases, lumbar SCS with certain stimulation parameter settings may also *induce* [17, 24, 47, 62, 64, 77] or *enable* [4, 6, 32, 68, 69] movements in otherwise paralyzed legs, as well as facilitate the activity produced during assisted treadmill training [32, 33, 42, 63].

Specifically, epidural stimulation of the lumbar spinal cord at 25–50 Hz can induce rhythmic contraction-relaxation patterns across multiple lower-limb muscle groups in motor complete SCI individuals lying supine, and some of these patterns have the appropriate coordination to result in synergistic flexion-extension movements over several leg joints [17, 24, 47, 62]. When applied in conjunction with assisted treadmill stepping with body weight support in patients with severe SCI [32, 63], epidural SCS within such frequency range and with intensities close to or slightly above the level eliciting PRM reflexes in the lower limb muscle groups has an immediate augmentative effect on the electromyographic activity as produced by the gait-phase related proprioceptive feedback input alone [21, 59, 102], and can recruit additional lower-limb muscle groups that are not responding to the guided stepping motions alone. It should be noted, however, that independent stepping movements were not yet achieved in these patients. In wheel-chair dependent individuals with incomplete lesions but sub-functional motor strength in the lower limbs, on the other hand, the addition of SCS may increase the outcome of intensive locomotor training and lead to improved overground ambulation, walking speed, step length, and endurance [33, 42].

When applied at 5–16 Hz, epidural SCS can induce bilateral extension in the lower-limbs of (motor) complete SCI individuals [47]. In a recent study, SCS could induce full-weight bearing standing in four patients with (motor) complete SCI and after intensive training standing could be maintained for several minutes with minimal self-assistance for balance control under ongoing SCS [32, 77].

Much of the current resurgence of interest in epidural SCS in the rehabilitation of SCI is most probably attributable to the rediscovery of its *enabling* effects on otherwise ‘clinically silent’ translesional volitional motor control. Even in an SCI clinically classified as complete, some residual white matter tracts through the injury zone or propriospinal system bridging the lesion [27, 72] are generally still present [22, 48–50]. These surviving connections may provide for some—sub-clinical—excitatory [22] or inhibitory [12] brain/brainstem influence over the lumbar spinal circuitry despite the otherwise clearly perturbed neural signal transmission [68]. The SCS-evoked 'tonic' driving input increases the excitability of the lumbar spinal motor circuitry and thereby enhances its responsiveness to this otherwise insufficient supraspinal input, allowing for rudimentary volitional motor control over otherwise paralyzed legs (cf. [68]). First reported in the 1980s [6, 7], this therapeutic potential of SCS was recently revisited [4, 32]. Under SCS at 25 Hz or 30 Hz, four patients with clinically classified (motor) complete SCI could volitionally induce hip and knee flexion, dorsiflexion, and toe extension. After intense training, one patient maintained the regained voluntary control over leg flexion after SCS was turned off [4].

These recent studies on epidural SCS applied to augment residual motor control have fueled ambitious expectations on the level of functional recovery that may be achieved even after clinically complete SCI. In ensemble with current technological [11, 101] and pharmacological [29–31, 94] advancements, as well as the introduction of new training paradigms pursuing the principles of activity-dependent neuroplasticity [4, 46], epidural SCS may indeed be considered as high priority for imminent translation to individuals with severe SCI (cf. [68, 69]).

5 Transcutaneous Spinal Cord Stimulation: A Non-invasive Method to Activate the Lumbar Spinal Circuitry

The bilateral and synchronous activation of afferent fibers within multiple posterior roots and the resulting multisegmental driving input to the lumbar spinal circuitry produced with tonic stimulation was previously suggested to be the key to the observed neuromodulation effects of epidural lumbar SCS in SCI individuals [17, 38, 62, 64, 75]. With the development of a non-invasive, transcutaneous version of SCS, the stimulation of posterior root afferents has become possible from the body surface [65, 66]. The set-up originally described by Minassian et al. [65] utilizes self-adhesive transcutaneous electrical neural stimulation (TENS) electrodes placed over the T11 and T12 spinous processes, manually identified by palpation, as well as larger indifferent electrodes placed paraumbilically on the abdomen (Fig. 4a). Other electrode set-ups have been used as well [15, 18, 53, 84], and the exact dimensions and shapes of the surface electrodes are not decisive [66]. When using a stimulator delivering biphasic stimulus pulses, the electrodes are connected to the stimulator such that the paravertebral electrodes act as anode for the first and as cathode for the second pulse phase [36, 39]. In case of monophasic stimulus pulses, the paraspinal electrodes are connected to the negative output of the stimulator, and the abdominal electrodes to the positive output [70].

Despite the relatively distant stimulation and the non-focused electrical field produced, transcutaneous SCS indeed allows for the selective activation of large-to-medium-diameter afferent fibers within the lumbar and upper sacral posterior roots bilaterally [16, 56, 65]. This is possible because of tissue heterogeneities

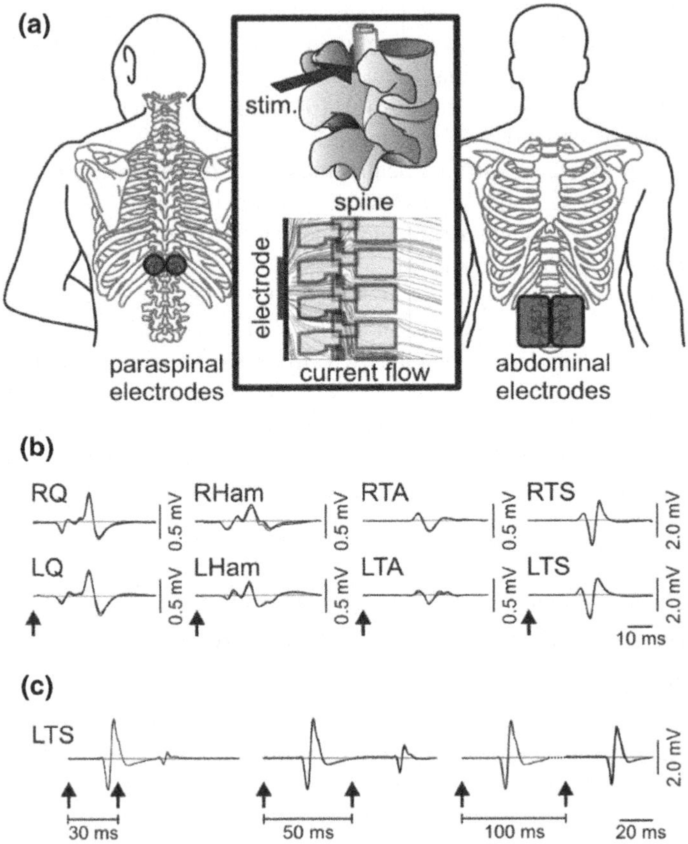

Fig. 4 Transcutaneous stimulation of the lumbar spinal cord. **a** Schematic sketch illustrates the placement of the paraspinal stimulating electrodes on the back at the level of the lumbar spinal cord corresponding on average to T11 and T12 vertebral levels and of the indifferent abdominal electrodes. Sketch in the middle depicts stimulation (stim.) through the better conductive elements (ligaments and discs) in-between the bony structures of the spine, along with a computer simulation of the current flow produced in a mid-sagittal plane. **b** Transcutaneous stimulation of the lumbar spinal cord elicits posterior root-muscle (PRM) reflexes in multiple lower-limb muscle groups bilaterally. Stimulus-triggered, superimposed representation of 3 consecutive PRM reflexes elicited in right (R) and left (L) quadriceps (Q), hamstrings (Ham), tibialis anterior (TA), and triceps surae (TS) of an individual with chronic incomplete spinal cord injury, American Spinal Injury Association Impairment Scale (AIS) grade C, neurological level of injury: C6. Black arrows indicate times of stimulus application (cf. Fig. 2c). **c** The stimulation of afferent fibers can be verified by testing the recovery cycle of the evoked responses using double-stimuli at varying interstimulus intervals. Shown are exemplary results of left triceps surae (LTS) at interstimulus intervals of 30, 50, and 100 ms derived from an individual with chronic incomplete spinal cord injury, AIS grade D, neurological level of injury: C5

between the paraspinal and abdominal electrodes as well as along the neural pathways of the roots [56]. First, at the level of the lower thoracic and upper lumbar spine, the posterior aspect of the vertebral canal is only partially shielded by bony structures. The transversal electrical resistance is substantially reduced by the ligaments and intervertebral discs that have considerably better electrical conductivities than bony structures, which allow the current flow produced by transcutaneous SCS to cross the vertebral canal and thecal sac [96]. Second, fibers within the lumbar and upper sacral posterior roots have particularly low excitation thresholds when entering the spinal cord *inter alia* due to the considerable change in electrical conductivities at the interface of the cerebrospinal fluid and the spinal cord [56, 76]. Further, myelinated afferent fibers with larger diameters corresponding to groups I [56, 65] and II [36, 39] have the lowest thresholds for electrical stimulation [16, 76], while thresholds considerably increase with decreasing fiber diameters [95, 97].

Like epidural SCS, transcutaneous stimulation of the lumbar spinal cord evokes PRM reflexes in multiple lower-limb muscles bilaterally [34, 56, 65] (Fig. 4b), which can serve as a means to neurophysiologically monitor the placement of the paraspinal electrodes over the lumbar spinal cord and to identify the immediately, electrically stimulated neural structures [36, 39]. The stimulation of afferent input structures to the lumbar spinal cord circuitry can be tested by applying double-stimuli at varying interstimulus intervals of e.g. 30, 50, and 100 ms to assess the recovery cycle of the evoked responses [36, 65, 81] (Fig. 4c). The presence of post-activation depression [74], as reflected by attenuated responses to the second stimulus pulse, verifies the transsynaptic and hence the reflex nature of the evoked responses [65, 81]. The stimulation of motor fibers in the anterior roots, on the other hand, would lead to the elicitation of two responses of similar amplitude even at such short interstimulus intervals.

Given the activation of the same neural input structures to the spinal cord as by epidural SCS, the transcutaneous technique may as well be used as a neuromodulation tool to modify altered activity of spinal circuits after SCI when used to apply 'tonic' stimulation [35–37, 39, 63, 66]. Additionally, as a non-invasive method, transcutaneous SCS can be employed to evoke 'test' PRM reflexes in neurophysiological studies of the organization of motor control and sensorimotor transmission at the level of the spinal cord, both in individuals with intact or altered central nervous system [2, 3, 15, 34, 65, 66, 81, 82], very similarly as in classical conditioning-test paradigms utilizing the H reflex [51, 85].

When applied for neuromodulation purposes, one has to consider though that unlike epidural stimulation, transcutaneous SCS is not suitable for permanent or chronic use. To be of therapeutic value, the induced effects therefore need to outlast the stimulation application or must stem from the intensification of the outcome obtained by other treatment modalities with which transcutaneous SCS is combined.

In the control of spinal spasticity specifically, a recent proof of concept study has demonstrated that a single 30 min session of transcutaneous SCS at 50 Hz and with an intensity producing paraesthesias but no muscle activity in the lower limbs temporarily alleviated various clinical signs of spasticity and enhanced voluntary

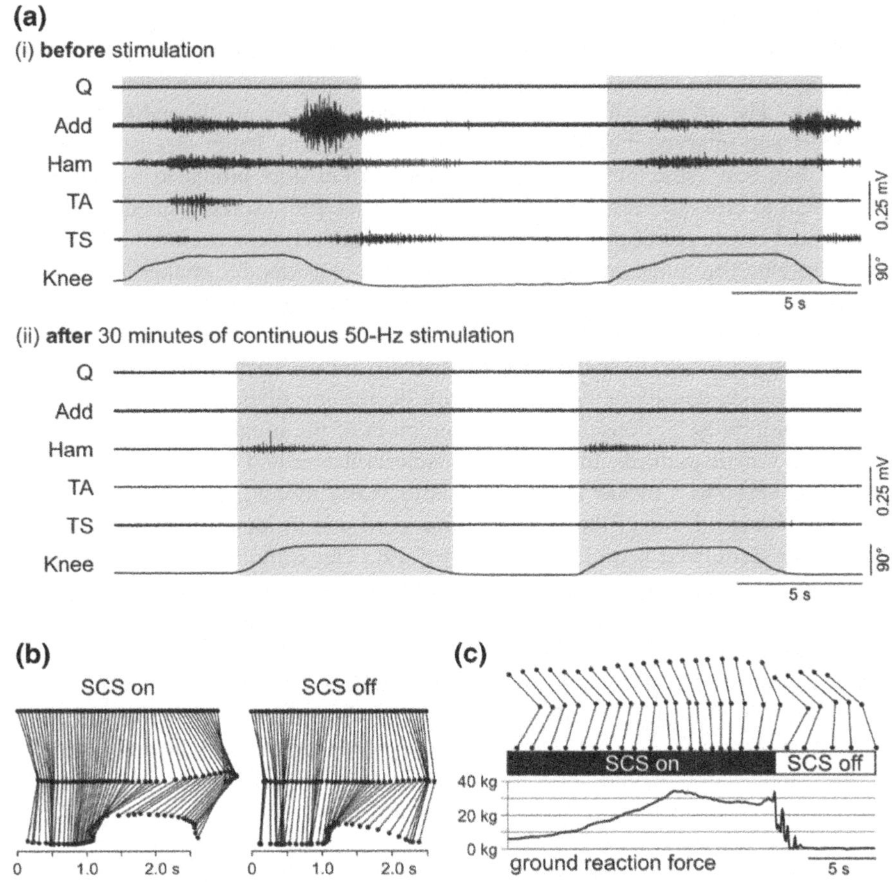

motor control of three individuals with incomplete SCI [36] (Fig. 5a). Preliminary results obtained in seven subjects with SCI of various severity further suggest the temporary persistence of these antispasticity effects for at least two hours after the stimulation [37]. In one of the patients, the effects of repetitive exposure to transcutaneous SCS over a period of six weeks was tested [37]. It was found that the stimulation-induced effects outlasted each stimulation session for at least 24 h and were progressively increasing over the six weeks. The effects could still be detected seven days after the last application of transcutaneous SCS [37]. The subject was later selected for implantation of an epidural system with which effective spasticity control was also achieved, suggesting that transcutaneous SCS may serve as a non-invasive trial procedure to identify responders to epidural SCS.

Transcutaneous SCS at around 30 Hz, i.e., within frequency ranges found to be effective in epidural SCS to promote locomotor-like activity, and with intensities below motor threshold for the lower limbs was found to facilitate residual voluntary locomotor control in ambulatory, motor incomplete SCI individuals actively

◂**Fig. 5** Applications of transcutaneous stimulation of the lumbar spinal cord in rehabilitation after spinal cord injury. **a** Control of lower-limb spasticity by transcutaneous stimulation of the lumbar spinal cord. Electromyographic (EMG) activity elicited by tonic stretch reflex in an individual with spinal spasticity during passive flexion and extension movements at hip and knee (i) *before* stimulation and (ii) *after* a 30 min session of tonic 50 Hz stimulation. The stimulation led to almost complete suppression of the EMG activity recorded from quadriceps (Q), adductors (Add), hamstrings (Ham), tibialis anterior (TA), and triceps surae (TS) and this effect outlasted the application of transcutaneous SCS for several hours. Shaded backgrounds mark the passive movement in the supine position, shown are two repetitions of the same maneuver. Data derived from an individual with chronic incomplete spinal cord injury (SCI), American Spinal Injury Association Impairment Scale (AIS) grade C, neurological level of injury: C6. **b** Transcutaneous stimulation at around 30 Hz and sub-motor threshold intensity can immediately modulate the walking capability of individuals with motor incomplete SCI. Displayed stick-figures were calculated on the basis of hip and knee goniometric data and averaged from 10 consecutive gait cycles *during* ongoing spinal cord stimulation (SCS on, left) and without stimulation (SCS off, right). The stimulation enhanced movement during swing and increased joint stability during stance. Note that all stepping movements were volitionally initiated and maintained by the subject, no EMG activity was produced by the stimulation in the absence of the voluntary attempt to step. Subject with incomplete SCI classified as AIS D, neurological level of injury: T9, stepping without manual assistance or body weight support, treadmill belt speed: 1.6 km/h. **c** Stimulation at around 15 Hz with an intensity above the motor threshold can generate standing-up and upright standing in individuals with severe SCI. Shown are stick-figures of one leg along with corresponding ground reaction forces. Starting from a supported sitting position in an overhead harness, the stimulation induced bilateral lower-limb extension, leading to an upright standing position with ground reaction forces of up to 40 kg per leg. Note that with increased loading of the legs, additional proprioceptive feedback input to the spinal cord was produced that further supported extension. The standing position was maintained until the stimulation was turned off (SCS off). Data derived from an individual with complete SCI classified as AIS A, neurological level of injury: T9

stepping on a treadmill [35, 39] (Fig. 5b). The effects included the step-phase appropriate augmentation of electromyographic activity in the lower limbs and changes in the gait kinematics as assessed by goniometric recordings from the hip and knee joints, mainly an augmented flexion movement during swing phase. Notably, the step-phase appropriate modulations occurred despite continuous administration of transcutaneous SCS during stepping with unchanged parameters throughout the gait cycles. Further, as soon as the treadmill belt was stopped and the subject stopped the active stepping, i.e., without the subjects' voluntary contribution, no electromyographic activity was produced in the lower limbs by the stimulation alone. It was hypothesized that the stimulation elevated the state of excitability of the lumbar locomotor circuitry, which in turn became more responsive to the voluntary commands to step through the surviving descending axons [39]. Considering the incomplete nature of the injuries, the stimulation could have modulated the activity of neural circuits rostral to the lesion via the partially functional posterior-column tracts as well. In individuals with (motor) complete SCI passively stepping on a treadmill using a robotic-driven gait orthosis, transcutaneous SCS at 30 Hz and with intensities above the motor threshold for the lower extremities considerably enhanced the motor output produced by the proprioceptive feedback input and recruited additional muscle groups [70] a finding reminiscent of that obtained with epidural SCS [32, 63].

Finally, transcutaneous SCS at around 15 Hz and with intensities above the lower-limb motor thresholds can induce standing in individuals with motor complete SCI (Fig. 5c). Two mechanisms thereby facilitate the extension movements of the legs generated by SCS: first, the progressive increase in lower-limb load when initiating the standing-up movement from a sitting position by manipulating body position leads to an increase in the proprioceptive feedback input to the spinal cord, which likely adds to the activation of the spinal circuitry; second, due to the rich connectivity of each group Ia muscle spindle fiber to a large proportion of its homonymous (and partially also heteronymous) motoneuron pools [9, 58], the activation of even a portion of the afferents within the posterior roots by transcutaneous SCS can effectively increase the motoneuronal excitability and recruitment.

6 Conclusions

Electrical SCS has been employed for the rehabilitation of various motor disorders for more than 40 years, but has not yet gained general acceptance and has been used in a few interested and specialized centers only. Recent high-profile studies that rediscovered the use of SCS as a neuro-augmentative tool have fueled a resurgence of interest in electrical neuromodulation of the spinal cord. Not only can SCS be tuned to effectively control diffuse and severe forms of spinal spasticity without further negatively impacting residual motor control in SCI individuals, it may indeed improve functional motor recovery even in patients with severe SCI. A wide spread use and eventual acceptance of SCS in clinical practice will essentially depend on a better understanding of its interaction with the neurophysiology of the targeted neural networks as well as the identification of markers that can distinguish responders from non-responders before implantation of an SCS system. The availability of transcutaneous SCS may facilitate these processes and by itself develop into a useful clinical tool for neuromodulation of altered motor control.

References

1. Adams MM, Hicks AL. Spasticity after spinal cord injury. Spinal Cord. 2005;43:577–86.
2. Andrews JC, Stein RB, Roy FD. Post-activation depression in the human soleus muscle using peripheral nerve and transcutaneous spinal stimulation. Neurosci Lett. 2015;589:144–9.
3. Andrews JC, Stein RB, Roy FD. Reduced postactivation depression of soleus H reflex and root evoked potential after transcranial magnetic stimulation. J Neurophysiol. 2015;114:485–92.
4. Angeli CA, Edgerton VR, Gerasimenko YP, et al. Altering spinal cord excitability enables voluntary movements after chronic complete paralysis in humans. Brain. 2014;137:1394–409.
5. Barnes MP. Management of spasticity. Age Ageing. 1998;27:239–45.

6. Barolat G, Myklebust JB, Wenninger W. Enhancement of voluntary motor function following spinal cord stimulation–case study. Appl Neurophysiol. 1986;49:307–14.
7. Barolat G, Myklebust JB, Wenninger W. Effects of spinal cord stimulation on spasticity and spasms secondary to myelopathy. Appl Neurophysiol. 1988;51:29–44.
8. Biering-Sørensen F, Nielsen JB, Klinge K. Spasticity-assessment: a review. Spinal Cord. 2006;44:708–22.
9. Brodal A. Neurological anatomy in relation to clinical medicine. 3rd ed. New York: Oxford University Press; 1981.
10. Capogrosso M, Wenger N, Raspopovic S, et al. A computational model for epidural electrical stimulation of spinal sensorimotor circuits. J Neurosci. 2013;33:19326–40.
11. Capogrosso M, Milekovic T, Borton D et al. A brain spinal interface to alleviate lower limb deficits after neuromotor disorders. In: Neurosci Meet Planner, Chicago, IL, Soc Neurosci; 2015. 428.08. http://www.abstractsonline.com/Plan/ViewAbstract.aspx?sKey=1cecc2a2-8e4f-4585-9cbe-268cd58172d4&cKey=04840ed1-447c-4af5-a45b-c0a96ed93dc5&mKey=d0ff4555-8574-4fbb-b9d4-04eec8ba0c84.
12. Cioni B, Dimitrijevic MR, McKay WB, Sherwood AM. Voluntary supraspinal suppression of spinal reflex activity in paralyzed muscles of spinal cord injury patients. Exp Neurol. 1986;93:574–83.
13. Cook AW. Electrical stimulation in multiple sclerosis. Hosp Pract. 1976;11:51–8.
14. Cook AW, Weinstein SP. Chronic dorsal column stimulation in multiple sclerosis. Preliminary report. N Y State J Med. 1973;73:2868–72.
15. Courtine G, Harkema SJ, Dy CJ, et al. Modulation of multisegmental monosynaptic responses in a variety of leg muscles during walking and running in humans. J Physiol. 2007;582:1125–39.
16. Danner SM, Hofstoetter US, Ladenbauer J, et al. Can the human lumbar posterior columns be stimulated by transcutaneous spinal cord stimulation? A modeling study. Artif Organs. 2011;35:257–62.
17. Danner SM, Hofstoetter US, Freundl B, et al. Human spinal locomotor control is based on flexibly organized burst generators. Brain. 2015;138:577–88.
18. Danner SM, Krenn M, Hofstoetter US, et al. Body position influences which neural structures are recruited by lumbar transcutaneous spinal cord stimulation. PLoS ONE. 2016;11:e0147479.
19. Davidoff RA. The dorsal columns. Neurology. 1989;39:1377–85.
20. Davis R, Emmonds SE. Spinal cord stimulation for multiple sclerosis: quantifiable benefits. Stereotact Funct Neurosurg. 1992;58:52–8.
21. Dietz V, Colombo G, Jensen L, Baumgartner L. Locomotor capacity of spinal cord in paraplegic patients. Ann Neurol. 1995;37:574–82.
22. Dimitrijevic MR, Dimitrijevic MM, Faganel J, et al. Suprasegmentally induced motor unit activity in paralyzed muscles of patients with established spinal cord injury. Ann Neurol. 1984;16:216–21.
23. Dimitrijevic MM, Dimitrijevic MR, Illis LS, et al. Spinal cord stimulation for the control of spasticity in patients with chronic spinal cord injury: I. Clinical observations. Cent Nerv Syst Trauma. 1986;3:129–44.
24. Dimitrijevic MR, Gerasimenko Y, Pinter MM. Evidence for a spinal central pattern generator in humans. Ann N Y Acad Sci. 1998;860:360–76.
25. Dooley DM, Sharkey J. Electrostimulation of the nervous system for patients with demyelinating and degenerative diseases of the nervous system and vascular diseases of the extremities. Appl Neurophysiol. 1977;40:208–17.
26. Elbasiouny SM, Moroz D, Bakr MM, et al. Management of spasticity after spinal cord injury: current techniques and future directions. Neurorehabil Neural Repair. 2010;24: 23–33.
27. Faganel J, Dimitrijevic MR. Study of propriospinal interneuron system in man. Cutaneous exteroceptive conditioning of stretch reflexes. J Neurol Sci. 1982;56:155–72.

28. Gildenberg P. Neuromodulation: a historical perspective. In: Krames E, Peckham P, Rezai A, editors. Neuromodulation. London: Elsevier-Academic Press; 2009. p. 9–20.
29. Guertin PA. Synergistic activation of the central pattern generator for locomotion by l-beta-3,4-dihydroxyphenylalanine and quipazine in adult paraplegic mice. Neurosci Lett. 2004;358:71–4.
30. Guertin PA. Central pattern generator for locomotion: anatomical, physiological, and pathophysiological considerations. Front Neurol. 2012;3:183.
31. Guertin PA. Preclinical evidence supporting the clinical development of central pattern generator-modulating therapies for chronic spinal cord-injured patients. Front Hum Neurosci. 2014;8:272.
32. Harkema S, Gerasimenko Y, Hodes J, et al. Effect of epidural stimulation of the lumbosacral spinal cord on voluntary movement, standing, and assisted stepping after motor complete paraplegia: a case study. Lancet. 2011;377:1938–47.
33. Herman R, He J, D'Luzansky S, et al. Spinal cord stimulation facilitates functional walking in a chronic, incomplete spinal cord injured. Spinal Cord. 2002;40:65–8.
34. Hofstoetter US, Minassian K, Hofer C, et al. Modification of reflex responses to lumbar posterior root stimulation by motor tasks in healthy subjects. Artif Organs. 2008;32:644–8.
35. Hofstoetter US, Hofer C, Kern H, et al. Effects of transcutaneous spinal cord stimulation on voluntary locomotor activity in an incomplete spinal cord injured individual. Biomed Tech (Berl). 2013. https://doi.org/10.1515/bmt-2013-4014.
36. Hofstoetter US, McKay WB, Tansey KE, et al. Modification of spasticity by transcutaneous spinal cord stimulation in individuals with incomplete spinal cord injury. J Spinal Cord Med. 2014;37:202–11.
37. Hofstoetter US, Krenn M, Danner SM et al. Short- and long-term effects of intermittent transcutaneous spinal cord stimulation on spinal spasticity and residual motor control. In: Neurosci Meet Planner, Washingotn, DC, Soc Neurosci; 2014b. 630.04. http://www.abstractsonline.com/Plan/ViewAbstract.aspx?sKey=d4a1ebd1-790a-474a-865c-6def8b901ee8&cKey=04026d5f-dacb-410d-b5f9-12ff12fd7243&mKey=54c85d94-6d69-4b09-afaa-502c0e680ca7.
38. Hofstoetter US, Danner SM, Freundl B, et al. Periodic modulation of repetitively elicited monosynaptic reflexes of the human lumbosacral spinal cord. J Neurophysiol. 2015;114:400–10.
39. Hofstoetter US, Krenn M, Danner SM, et al. Augmentation of voluntary locomotor activity by transcutaneous spinal cord stimulation in motor-incomplete spinal cord-injured individuals. Artif Organs. 2015;39:E176–86.
40. Holsheimer J. Concepts and methods in neuromodulation and functional electrical stimulation: an introduction. Neuromodulation. 1998;1:57–61.
41. Holsheimer J. Which neuronal elements are activated directly by spinal cord stimulation. Neuromodulation. 2002;5:25–31.
42. Huang H, He J, Herman R, et al. Modulation effects of epidural spinal cord stimulation on muscle activities during walking. IEEE Trans Neural Syst Rehabil Eng. 2006;14:14–23.
43. Hunter JP, Ashby P. Segmental effects of epidural spinal cord stimulation in humans. J Physiol. 1994;474:407–19.
44. Illis LS, Oygar AE, Sedgwick EM, et al. Dorsal-column stimulation in the rehabilitation of patients with multiple sclerosis. Lancet. 1976;1:1383–6.
45. Illis LS, Sedgwick EM, Tallis RC. Spinal cord stimulation in multiple sclerosis: clinical results. J Neurol Neurosurg Psychiatry. 1980;43:1–14.
46. Jackson A, Zimmermann JB. Neural interfaces for the brain and spinal cord—restoring motor function. Nat Rev Neurol. 2012;8:690–9.
47. Jilge B, Minassian K, Rattay F, et al. Initiating extension of the lower limbs in subjects with complete spinal cord injury by epidural lumbar cord stimulation. Exp Brain Res. 2004;154:308–26.
48. Kakulas BA. Pathology of spinal injuries. Cent Nerv Syst Trauma. 1984;1:117–29.

49. Kakulas A. The applied neurobiology of human spinal cord injury: a review. Paraplegia. 1988;26:371–9.
50. Kakulas BA, Kaelan C. The neuropathological foundations for the restorative neurology of spinal cord injury. Clin Neurol Neurosurg. 2015;129:S1–7.
51. Knikou M. The H-reflex as a probe: pathways and pitfalls. J Neurosci Methods. 2008;171: 1–12.
52. Krames E, Rezai A, Peckham P, et al. What is neuromodulation? In: Krames E, Peckham P, Rezai A, editors. neuromodulation. London: Elsevier-Academic Press; 2009. p. 3–8.
53. Krenn M, Hofstoetter US, Danner SM, et al. Multi-electrode array for transcutaneous lumbar posterior root stimulation. Artif Organs. 2015;39:834–40.
54. Kumar K, Lind G, Winter J, et al. Spinal cord stimulation: placement of surgical leads via laminotomy—techniques and benefits. In: Krames E, Peckham P, Rezai A, editors. Neuromodulation. London: Elsevier-Academic Press; 2009. p. 1005–11.
55. Kumru H, Murillo N, Samso JV, et al. Reduction of spasticity with repetitive transcranial magnetic stimulation in patients with spinal cord injury. Neurorehabil Neural Repair. 2010;24:435–41.
56. Ladenbauer J, Minassian K, Hofstoetter US, et al. Stimulation of the human lumbar spinal cord with implanted and surface electrodes: a computer simulation study. IEEE Trans Neural Syst Rehabil Eng. 2010;18:637–45.
57. Lance JW. The control of muscle tone, reflexes, and movement: Robert Wartenberg lecture. Neurology. 1980;30:1303–13.
58. Lloyd DPC. Reflex action in relation to pattern and peripheral source of afferent stimulation. J Neurophysiol. 1943;6:111–9.
59. Maegele M, Müller S, Wernig A, Edgerton VR, Harkema SJ. Recruitment of spinal motor pools during voluntary movements versus stepping after human spinal cord injury. J Neurotrauma. 2002;19:1217–29.
60. Melzack R, Wall PD. Pain mechanisms: a new theory. Science. 1965;150:971–9.
61. Mendell LM. Constructing and deconstructing the gate theory of pain. Pain. 2014;155: 210–6.
62. Minassian K, Jilge B, Rattay F, et al. Stepping-like movements in humans with complete spinal cord injury induced by epidural stimulation of the lumbar cord: electromyographic study of compound muscle action potentials. Spinal Cord. 2004;42:401–16.
63. Minassian K, Persy I, Rattay F, et al. Effect of peripheral afferent and central afferent input to the human lumbar spinal cord isolated from brain control. Biocybern Biomed Eng. 2005;25:11–29.
64. Minassian K, Persy I, Rattay F, et al. Human lumbar cord circuitries can be activated by extrinsic tonic input to generate locomotor-like activity. Hum Mov Sci. 2007;26:275–95.
65. Minassian K, Persy I, Rattay F. Posterior root-muscle reflexes elicited by transcutaneous stimulation of the human lumbosacral cord. Muscle Nerve. 2007;35:327–36.
66. Minassian K, Hofstoetter US, Rattay F. Transcutaneous lumbar posterior root stimulation for motor control studies and modification of motor activity after spinal cord injury. In: Dimitrijevic M, Kakulas B, McKay W, Vrbova G, editors. Restorative neurology of spinal cord injury. New York: Oxford University Press; 2011. p. 226–55.
67. Minassian K, Hofstoetter U, Tansey K et al. Neuromodulation of lower limb motor control in restorative neurology. Clin Neurol Neurosurg. 2012;114:489–497.
68. Minassian K, McKay WB, Binder H et al. Targeting lumbar spinal neural circuitry by Epidural stimulation to restore motor function after spinal cord injury. Neurotherapeutics. 2016a. https://doi.org/10.1007/s13311-016-0421-y.
69. Minassian K, Hofstoetter US. Spinal cord stimulation and augmentative control strategies for leg movement after spinal paralysis in humans. CNS Neurosci Ther CNS Neurosci Ther. 2016. https://doi.org/10.1111/cns.12530.
70. Minassian K, Hofstoetter US, Danner SM, et al. Spinal rhythm generation by step-induced feedback and transcutaneous posterior root stimulation in complete spinal cord-injured individuals. Neurorehabil Neural Repair. 2016;30:233–43.

71. Murg M, Binder H, Dimitrijevic MR. Epidural electric stimulation of posterior structures of the human lumbar spinal cord: 1. muscle twitches—a functional method to define the site of stimulation. Spinal Cord. 2000;38:394–402.
72. Nathan PW, Smith MC. Fasciculi proprii of the spinal cord in man. Brain. 1959;82:610–68.
73. Penn RD. Intrathecal drugs for spasticity. In: Lozano AM, Gildenberg PL, Tasker RR, editors. Textbook of stereotactic and functional neurosurgery. Berlin: Springer; 2009. p. 1973–81.
74. Pierrot-Deseilligny E, Burke D. The circuitry of the human spinal cord. Cambridge: Cambridge University Press; 2012.
75. Pinter MM, Gerstenbrand F, Dimitrijevic MR. Epidural electrical stimulation of posterior structures of the human lumbosacral cord: 3. Control of spasticity. Spinal Cord. 2000;38:524–31.
76. Rattay F, Minassian K, Dimitrijevic MR. Epidural electrical stimulation of posterior structures of the human lumbosacral cord: 2. quantitative analysis by computer modeling. Spinal Cord. 2000;38:473–89.
77. Rejc E, Angeli C, Harkema S. Effects of lumbosacral spinal cord epidural stimulation for standing after chronic complete paralysis in humans. PLoS ONE. 2015;10:e0133998.
78. Rekand T. Clinical assessment and management of spasticity: a review. Acta Neurol Scand Suppl. 2010;190:62–6.
79. Richardson RR, McLone DG. Percutaneous epidural neurostimulation for paraplegic spasticity. Surg Neurol. 1978;9:153–5.
80. Richardson RR, Cerullo LJ, McLone DG, et al. Percutaneous epidural neurostimulation in modulation of paraplegic spasticity. Six case reports. Acta Neurochir (Wien). 1979;49: 235–43.
81. Roy FD, Gibson G, Stein RB. Effect of percutaneous stimulation at different spinal levels on the activation of sensory and motor roots. Exp Brain Res. 2012;223:281–9.
82. Roy FD, Bosgra D, Stein RB. Interaction of transcutaneous spinal stimulation and transcranial magnetic stimulation in human leg muscles. Exp Brain Res. 2014;232:1717–28.
83. Saadé NE, Tabet MS, Atweh SF, et al. Modulation of segmental mechanisms by activation of a dorsal column brainstem spinal loop. Brain Res. 1984;310:180–4.
84. Sayenko DG, Atkinson DA, Dy CJ, et al. Spinal segment-specific transcutaneous stimulation differentially shapes activation pattern among motor pools in humans. J Appl Physiol. 2015;118:1364–74.
85. Schieppati M. The Hoffmann reflex: a means of assessing spinal reflex excitability and its descending control in man. Prog Neurobiol. 1987;28:345–76.
86. Sedgwick EM, Illis LS, Tallis RC, et al. Evoked potentials and contingent negative variation during treatment of multiple sclerosis with spinal cord stimulation. J Neurol Neurosurg Psychiatry. 1980;43:15–24.
87. Shealy CN, Taslitz N, Mortimer JT. Electrical inhibition of pain: experimental evaluation. Anesth Analg. 1967;46:299–305.
88. Shealy CN, Mortimer JT, Reswick JB. Electrical inhibition of pain by stimulation of the dorsal columns: preliminary clinical report. Anesth Analg. 1967;46:489–91.
89. Sheean G (2002) The pathophysiology of spasticity. Eur J Neurol. 2002; S1:3–9.
90. Siegfried J, Krainick JU, Haas H, et al. Electrical spinal cord stimulation for spastic movement disorders. Appl Neurophysiol. 1978;41:134–41.
91. Siegfried J, Lazorthes Y, Broggi G. Electrical spinal cord stimulation for spastic movement disorders. Appl Neurophysiol. 1981;44:77–92.
92. Singh A, Tetreault L, Kalsi-Ryan S. Global prevalence and incidence of traumatic spinal cord injury. Clin Epidemiol. 2014;6:309–31.
93. Sköld C, Levi R, Seiger A. Spasticity after traumatic spinal cord injury: nature, severity, and location. Arch Phys Med Rehabil. 1999;80:1548–57.
94. Steuer I, Rouleau P, Guertin PA. Pharmacological approaches to chronic spinal cord injury. Curr Pharm Des. 2013;19:4423–36.

95. Struijk JJ, Holsheimer J, Boom HB. Excitation of dorsal root fibers in spinal cord stimulation: a theoretical study. IEEE Trans Biomed Eng. 1993;40:632–9.
96. Szava Z, Danner SM, Minassian K. Transcutaneous electrical spinal cord stimulation: Biophysics of a new rehabilitation method after spinal cord injury. Müller, Saarbrücken: VDM Verlag Dr; 2011.
97. Veltink PH, Van Alsté JA, Boom HB. Influences of stimulation conditions on recruitment of myelinated nerve fibers: a model study. IEEE Trans Biomed Eng. 1988;35:917–24.
98. Wall PD, Sweet WH. Temporary abolition of pain in man. Science. 1967;155:108–9.
99. Waltz JM. Spinal cord stimulation: a quarter century of development and investigation. A review of its development and effectiveness in 1336 cases. Stereotact Funct Neurosurg. 1997;69:288–99.
100. Waltz JM. Chronic stimulation for motor disorders. In: Gindelberg PL, Tasker RR, editors. Textbook for stereotactic and functional neurosurgery. New York: McGraw-Hill; 1998. p. 1087–99.
101. Wenger N, Moraud EM, Raspopovic S et al. Closed-loop neuromodulation of spinal sensorimotor circuits controls refined locomotion after complete spinal cord injury. Sci Transl Med. 2014;6:255ra133.
102. Wernig A, Müller S. Laufband locomotion with body weight support improved walking in persons with severe spinal cord injuries. Paraplegia. 1992;30:229–38.

Functional Surgery and Early Rehabilitation Treatment in Hemiplegic Patients

Paolo Zerbinati, Erika Giannotti, Maria Longhi and Davide Mazzoli

1 Introduction

Advances in the therapy of patients with neurological disorders have resulted in a large and growing population of subjects with dysfunction and deformity of the extremities secondary to a central nervous system lesion (upper motor neuron syndrome, UMNS). Traumatic brain injuries (TBIs) and cerebral vascular accidents (CVAs), or strokes, can have profound effects both on the patient and on society. Stroke is currently the third leading cause of mortality and is a common cause of long-term disability, generating increasing annual healthcare costs. Approximately 60% of these patients survive, and half of them may have residual hemiparesis. Due to the central nervous system damage, stroke patients show muscle weakness, abnormal muscle tone, and disorders of balance and posture control, which lead to difficulty controlling movements, limb spasticity and limb deformities [1, 2]. Limb deformities are commonly the result of both static and dynamic phenomena. The former include heterotopic ossification, fracture malunion and soft tissue contractures, and the latter weakness, spasticity, rigidity and impaired motor control. In more than 80% of hemiplegic patients, equinovarus foot deformity (EVFD), resulting in abnormal walking patterns, is the main factor limiting post-stroke gait [3]. It usually results from spasticity of the plantar flexor and invertor muscles,

P. Zerbinati (✉)
Neuroorthopaedic Service, MultiMedica Santa Maria Hospital, Castellanza (VA), Italy
e-mail: paoloze@alice.it

E. Giannotti · M. Longhi · D. Mazzoli
Gait & Motion Analysis Laboratory, Sol et Salus Hospital, Rimini, Italy

E. Giannotti
Department of Orthopaedic Rehabilitation, University of Padova, Padua, Italy

D. Mazzoli
Gait & Motion Analysis Laboratory, Sol et Salus Hospital, Rimini, Italy

G. Sandrini et al. (eds.), *Advanced Technologies for the Rehabilitation of Gait and Balance Disorders*, Biosystems & Biorobotics 19,
https://doi.org/10.1007/978-3-319-72736-3_34

associated with a deficit of the dorsiflexors, their antagonists. Specifically, deformity of the foot can be seen in the presence of combined spasticity of several different muscles, including the gastrocnemius, soleus, tibialis anterior (TA), tibialis posterior (TP), flexor hallucis longus (FHL), and flexor digitorum longus (FDL), while associated weakness can be recorded in the peroneal muscles. Foot deformities interfere with toe clearance in the swing phase, with correct pre-positioning of the foot at the end of the swing phase, with loading of the stance leg, and with ankle stability during the stance phase [1]. Consequently, neurological patients with EVFD are often unable to walk unassisted, requiring either an orthotic device or crutches [4].

Different treatment options have been described for EVFD. These include non-surgical and surgical interventions. Non-surgical modalities include physical therapy with stretching, serial casting, orthoses, oral drug therapy for muscle relaxation and relief of spasms, phenol nerve blocks, and chemodenervation using botulinum toxin injections to reduce hypertonicity [5].

Surgical techniques for an EVFD include soft tissue release, tendon transfer and tendon lengthening. In the past, long-term treatment of chronic spastic contracture deformity was limited to medical and brace therapy, which was frequently ineffective. The consequence of this approach was that lower extremity contractures, spasticity, pain, gait instability and pressure sores reduced the patient's level of activity, quality of life, comfort, ambulatory status and ability to live outside a care facility [6].

Various surgical and non-surgical treatments have been described to treat this foot deformity. The traditional surgical approach consists of a combination of Achilles tendon lengthening with or without posterior ankle joint capsular release, various tendon transfer procedures, tendon lengthening or release procedures, calcaneal osteotomy, and hindfoot fusion. These reconstructive procedures typically require general anaesthesia, cessation of anti-coagulant medications, and a long postoperative course, during which there must be no weight bearing on the foot. Frequently, these patients find it physically impossible to comply with this latter requirement, and have to use a wheelchair. Indeed, crutches and other non-weight-bearing ambulatory aids will typically not be a practical option for stroke patients owing to their overall weakness, spasticity and contractures, which often affect the upper extremity.

Recently, minimally invasive soft tissue procedures were introduced for the correction of longstanding foot and ankle deformity; in stroke patients submitted to EVFD surgery, this approach was recently combined with early rehabilitation treatment characterised by immediate full weight bearing [7].

The positive effects of soft tissue surgery correction of EVFD have been documented [8, 9]. A recent review by Renzenbrink et al. [10] analysed the long-term effects of surgical intervention in EVFD. In all 15 studies included in the review, surgical correction of foot deformity was demonstrated to be safe, permanent and effective in improving walking ability and in diminishing the need for an orthosis. One of the most useful diagnostic studies available for preoperative planning is gait analysis combined with dynamic electromyography (dEMG) [11, 12]. Muscle activation patterns measured by dEMG during gait are used to distinguish between normal or pathological activity of lower limb muscles in stroke patients [7, 12]. In the study by Perry et al. TA, gastrocnemius, soleus, peroneus longus and brevis muscles were recorded with dEMG, while fine-wire electrodes were used for the TP, FDL and FHL [11]. In normal gait, the TA should be active in eccentric contraction during initial contact and loading and then again in concentric contraction during the mid- to late-swing phase. Muscles are expected to be quiescent between these two phases. Fifty percent of TBI patients were reported to show continuous activity in the TA throughout gait [13]. Examining 41 spastic equinovarus deformities, Fuller and colleagues [12] showed that supplementing a thorough clinical evaluation with preoperative instrumented gait analysis, including dEMG as a component, resulted in alteration of 64% of the predetermined surgical plans and increased inter-surgeon agreement to a significant degree.

Despite many good results, the scientific evidence in favour of soft tissue surgical correction of EVFD remains limited because the studies included in the review by Renzenbrink et al. [10] had a low level of evidence; the outcomes measured and preoperative planning were heterogeneous and the criteria used to select patients suitable for surgical treatment varied. In particular, the authors pointed out that pre-operative gait analysis, a fundamental tool in the decision-making process, is still not used in clinical practice in stroke patients.

The literature does not contain guidelines on specific post-operative rehabilitation treatments (start and duration of treatment, type of exercises). In particular, there is no agreement regarding the need for a period of immobilisation in a cast after surgery, and some authors suggest an immediate weight-bearing programme with a non-articulated ankle-foot orthosis (AFO) [14].

2 Surgical Indications

Indications for surgery include deformities failing to respond to multidisciplinary non-operative approaches. Patients should have reached a plateau of neurological improvement (typically 6 months following CVA and 18 months following TBI) [15]. Namdari and colleagues [16] investigated outcomes of split anterior tibialis tendon transfer (SPLATT) in a cohort of stroke patients with spastic equinovarus deformities. They reported that age and sex did not affect outcomes and all patients showed improvements, in spite of the wide range of intervals since stroke. Specific goals of surgery are to achieve a balanced and functional foot, minimization of bracing, pain relief, callus and ulcer prevention and easier hygiene [17]. Wheelchair-bound patients may qualify for surgery if the correction will produce a plantigrade foot that can more easily be placed on a wheelchair foot rest. Early in the course of spastic foot and ankle deformities, the equinus is dynamic and should generally be treated by balancing muscles through lengthening or transfer. Although static deformities have fixed capsules, ligaments, muscles and/or tendons, they may be treated as dynamic alterations after releasing the spastic structures.

Differentiating between a dynamic and a static deformity can be difficult, especially in the clinical setting. An intraoperative evaluation of the patient, performed under anaesthesia, can be compared with the preoperative evaluation and this can help to determine whether the deformity is dynamic or static.

3 Preoperative Evaluation

Preoperative assessment is useful for categorising patients into ambulatory and non-ambulatory groups. Both these groups can benefit from surgery to provide a plantigrade foot that allows better sitting balance and a more comfortable fit of a brace or shoe. It is also possible that improved brace wear and comfort may allow a non-ambulatory patient to walk.

When considering surgery, the various components of deformities must be carefully evaluated. Thorough clinical evaluation combined with instrumental evaluation (gait analysis and dEMG) is the most helpful approach [10, 12].

Clinically, the degree of dynamic deformity must be assessed and defined on the basis of fixed soft tissue and joint contractures, or bony deformities. Spasticity is dynamic, related to body position and movement, and affected by various stimuli. As far as possible, a patient should be examined in multiple positions and observed during various activities. Observing the foot position during transfers and while removing shoes and socks provides excellent input for the clinical assessment.

Physical examination should include both active and passive movements performed in a sitting position. Even a non-ambulatory patient should be observed in an upright position whenever possible because reflex leg extension can be evoked in standing.

The degree of muscle tone can be rated using the Modified Ashworth Scale (Table 1). The Modified Ashworth Scale is a practical clinical instrument for measuring spasticity and has been shown to be both reliable and repeatable [18, 19].

Table 1 Modified Ashworth Scale for grading spasticity

Grade	Description
0	No increase in muscle tone throughout flexion or extension movement
1	Slight increase in muscle tone manifested by a catch and release at the end of the range of motion when the limb is moved into flexion or extension
1+	Slight increase in muscle tone, manifested by a catch, followed by minimal resistance throughout the remainder (50%) of the range of motion
2	More marked increase in muscle tone through most of the range of motion, but the affected limb is easily moved
3	Considerable increase in muscle tone; passive movement is difficult
4	Affected limb is rigid in flexion and extension

Equinus foot is generally the result of abnormal activity of the gastrocnemius, soleus, FDL and FHL muscles. Comparison of ankle dorsiflexion with the knee extended and flexed is not a reliable method of distinguishing the relative dynamic (spastic) contributions of the gastrocnemius and soleus muscles, because knee extension triggers a mass pattern of activity in the entire leg, including the ankle plantar flexors and long toe flexor muscles [20]. When dealing with a static (non-spastic) equinus deformity, flexion of the knee resulting in improved ankle dorsiflexion can distinguish the different contributions of the gastrocnemius and soleus muscles to the contracture and consequently to the EVFD. In a clinical setting, it is often difficult to distinguish between dynamic and static components of equinus foot.

The final clinical evaluation is observation of the patient walking while barefoot. The velocity of ambulation can be calculated by timing the patient over a set distance. The Functional Ambulation Classification (FAC) (Table 2) is a validated and clinically useful classification of walking ability in stroke patients. It does not consider the need for bracing, shoe modifications, or upper extremity assistive devices, as many patients are unable to use such aids until their deformities have been corrected. The classification consists of six categories ranging from no ambulation to normal walking [21].

Gait analysis and dEMG have led to a better understanding of the aetiology of EVFD. Such testing is also important to supplement a comprehensive physical examination, with the purpose of identifying whether specific muscle groups are spastic and contribute to the deformity, and thereby guiding the treatment. Fuller and colleagues [12], in a prospective study, showed that gait analysis resulted in a refinement of the surgical planning in 64% of patients. The experience of the surgeon did not affect the impact of the gait analysis. Perry and colleagues [11], using dEMG, demonstrated that when varus deformity is observed in stroke patients, the TA muscle is active during 80% of the swing phase and during the entire stance phase. Additionally, the activity of the TP muscle was found to be variable, while the activity of the FHL muscle may be of critical importance in very

Table 2 Functional ambulation scale

Level	Status of ambulation
0	No ambulation
1	Non-functional ambulation
2	Household ambulation
3	Neighbourhood ambulation
4	Independent community ambulation
5	Normal ambulation

spastic feet because toe flexors contribute to ankle plantar flexion. In patients who have had a stroke or TBI, the TP is less commonly a contributor to varus deformity.

An improved understanding of the complex causes of deformity has resulted in the refinement and evolution of the corrective surgical procedures used. For instance, as the SPLATT procedure has evolved, additional interventions have been included in the surgical correction of deformities in order to maintain strength and optimise both the achievement and maintenance of a plantigrade foot. Spasticity of the extensor hallucis longus (EHL) muscle and resulting hyperextension deformity of the hallux are countered by an EHL transfer to the mid dorsum of the foot; this also provides the ankle with additional dorsiflexion force. Patients require lifelong muscle balancing of multiple muscle groups. As a result, the SPLATT procedure has become routinely combined with procedures such as Achilles tendon lengthening, TP lengthening, and assorted transfers and releases of intrinsic and extrinsic foot flexor and extensor tendons.

4 Equinus Deformity

The choice between Achilles tendon and gastrocnemius-soleus lengthening is made in the operating theatre. If the equinus deformity persists once the patient is under anaesthesia, this indicates the presence of a static contracture, which should be addressed through an Achilles tendon lengthening. However, if the equinus deformity corrects itself under anaesthesia, this means that the deformity is primarily dynamic, and should respond to lengthening at the muscle tendon junction. Great care must be taken not to over-lengthen and cause a calcaneal gait [5].

The procedure most commonly performed for Achilles contractures is percutaneous triple hemisection tenotomy (Hoke lengthening or tendo-Achilles lengthening, TAL) [9, 22].

In this procedure, transverse hemisections of the Achilles tendon are performed through three stab incisions starting in the midline while the foot is held in maximum dorsiflexion. Generally (for a varus deformity) the most distal and proximal incisions address the medial half of the Achilles, while the middle incision addresses the lateral half of the Achilles. The orientation of the hemisection can be reversed for a valgus deformity (Fig. 1).

If the deformity is determined to be primarily dynamic, a proximal gastrocnemius and soleus lengthening should be performed. In this procedure the junction between the gastrocnemius and soleus muscle bellies is identified in the midleg through a medial approach. The individual tendons overlying the respective muscle are then transected and lengthened along the belly with the foot in dorsiflexion [5]. These procedures are generally performed in association with other ones, which then dictate the postoperative course.

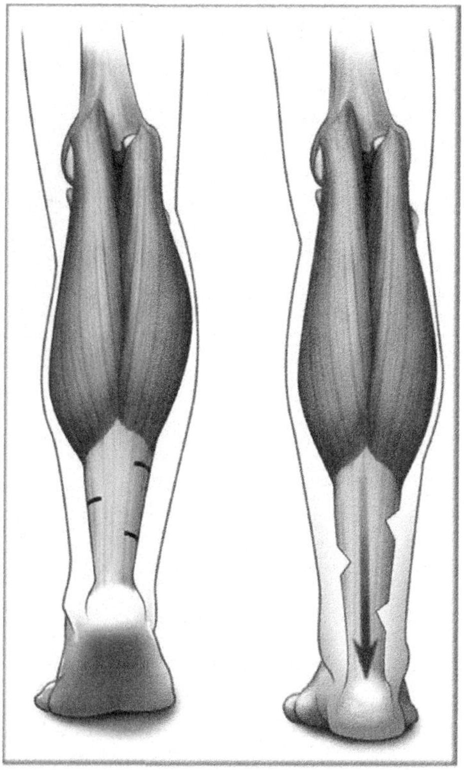

Fig. 1 The Hoke triple hemisection technique for lengthening of the Achilles tendon

5 Varus Deformity

SPLATT

The varus component of EVFD is most commonly secondary to an overactive TA muscle. Therefore, a useful and commonly used procedure to correct this portion of the deformity is SPLATT. In this procedure the lateral half of the TA tendon is transferred to the cuboid or lateral cuneiform to balance the foot in a neutral position. Originally devised by Garett and described by Hoffer for cerebral palsy, its indications have expanded to include any spastic varus or equinovarus deformity [23]. This procedure is indicated when there is dynamic varus or equinovarus in a patient over 4 years of age. It is often performed in association with a TAL and is one of the most common and successful tendon transfers known in orthopaedic surgery [2, 24]. A three-incision technique is used (Fig. 2). First, a medial incision overlying the insertion of the TA on the medial cuneiform is performed. The lateral half of the TA tendon is split longitudinally and transected at its insertion as far distally as possible. The second incision is made 8–10 cm proximal to the ankle joint just lateral to the tibial crest. The fascia overlying the TA is divided and the lateral half of the tendon is passed from distal to proximal. The final incision is

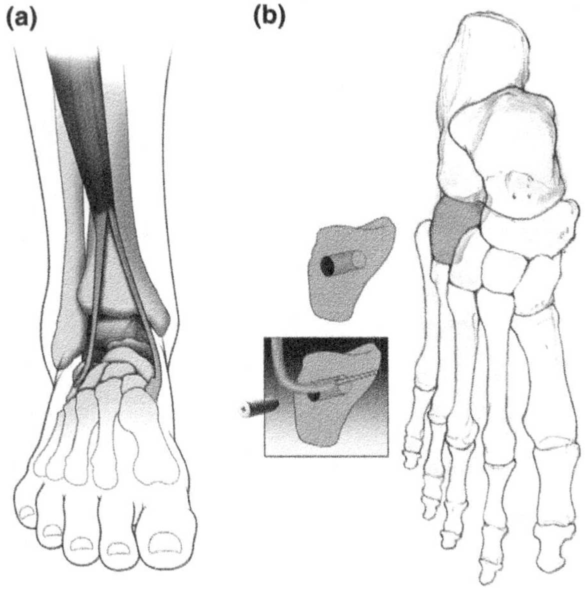

Fig. 2 SPLATT. **a** The completed SPLATT transfer. **b** The tunnel in the cuboid bone for the lateral arm of the tibialis anterior tendon. (From Keenan [5]; with permission)

made over the cuboid or lateral cuneiform, and the tendon is redirected in a subcutaneous fashion from proximal to distal. A bone tunnel is then created perpendicular to the surface and the tendon is passed through and secured with an interference screw [25].

Interference screw fixation has demonstrated strength to failure of 166N, 44N stronger than traditional fixation [26]. To avoid overcorrection or undercorrection, it is important to have the foot in a neutral position when balancing the tension of the transferred portion of the TA with the medial intact portion. However, some authors advocate transfer of the entire TA tendon, and a cadaver study has demonstrated that neither split nor whole tendon transfer led to overcorrection [26, 27].

6 Flexor Hallucis Longus (FHL) Transfer

As an alternative to the SPLATT procedure for spastic EVFD, the FHL can be transferred through the interosseous membrane and this procedure has given good results [28, 29]. It generally requires a long harvest of the FHL tendon from the midfoot, transfer from posterior to anterior through the interosseous membrane, and tenodesing of the FHL around the 3rd or 4th metatarsus.

7 Flexor Digitorum Longus (FDL) Transfer to the Calcaneus

Muscle overactivity or an exaggerated muscle response to a quick stretch stimulus should not be misinterpreted as strength. Spastic muscles are inherently weak muscles. Lengthening of the Achilles tendon or fractional lengthening of the proximal gastrocnemius and soleus muscles further compromises the plantar flexion strength of patients with UMNS. Transfer of the FDL to the calcaneus has been shown to increase calf strength and decrease the need for bracing during ambulation after surgery [30].

An incision is made on the medial border of the foot and the FHL and FDL tendons are dissected free and individually identified. A 3-cm longitudinal incision is made posterior to the medial malleolus, the FDL is identified, passed subcutaneously from the incision posterior to the medial malleolus to a 1-cm incision made over the medial calcaneus. A drill is used to create a bony tunnel through the calcaneus medially to laterally, and the FDL tendon is passed into the calcaneus and fixed with an interferential screw.

8 Toe Deformities

Flexion deformities of the toes are very common in spastic EVFD because of overactivity of the FHL, FDL and their associated brevis muscles. This spasticity can also contribute to the equinus component of the deformity, with the toe deformity unmasked or accentuated when the equinovarus position is corrected. 1-cm longitudinal plantar incisions are made over the proximal flexion creases. The tendon sheaths are opened, and both the short- and the long-flexor tendons are transected sharply using a scalpel [31].

Hyperextension of the hallux due to overactivity of the EHL is an underestimated deformity in spastic equinovarus patients [32]. This spastic movement can contribute to the varus foot deformity. When the hyperextended hallux is symptomatic, transferring the EHL tendon to the dorsum of the foot can correct this problem as well as improve ankle dorsiflexion force. The transfer is achieved through an incision over the dorsum of the hallux. The EHL tendon is transected, and the proximal tendon stump is then transferred around the 3rd or 4th metatarsus while the ankle is held in neutral position.

9 Fractional Lengthening of Tibialis Posterior Tendon

Fractional lengthening of the TP tendon is indicated when dynamic EMG shows continuous activity in this muscle; this is most commonly seen in cerebral palsy. Some spastic CVA and TBI patients also present TP spasticity that contributes to hindfoot varus, although in general the TA hyperactivity dominates. To achieve a fractional lengthening, an incision is made 2 cm above the medial malleolus posterior to the tibia. The myotendinous junction is incised with two to three incisions a few centimetres apart with manipulation of the foot to achieve correction. This incision is often performed in association with and before performing the SPLATT procedure [4].

10 Fixed Deformities

Severe and chronic fixed varus hindfoot deformities can result from a longstanding spastic condition particularly in younger patients with a developing skeleton. These patients usually have some degree of varus at the subtalar joint and secondary medial soft tissue contraction. Associated midfoot equinus and adduction is common and very important to recognize. In this situation, soft tissue procedures alone will not correct the fixed bone deformity. Midfoot arthrotomy may be required to address the different components of the deformity. The appropriate soft tissue procedures, among those previously described, should be considered, in combination with the bone correction, in particular a TAL, TP lengthening with talonavicular joint capsule and spring ligament release, and possibly SPLATT to help with dorsiflexion. In severe deformities a closing wedge can be performed through the joint by resecting bone from the lateral aspect of both the talus and the calcaneus. Standard screw fixation should be used. Alternatively, lateralizing calcaneal osteotomy of the tuberosity with or without a closing wedge may be performed [15].

11 Rehabilitation After Surgery

In a recent study Giannotti et al. [7] proposed a specific rehabilitation treatment (six days/week for a 4 week period, 90 min per session—Table 3) from the first day after EVFD. Each of the 24 sessions was conducted individually by a trained physiotherapist. Gait training was carried out for the first 20 days after surgery with a non-articulated AFO which was removed from day 20 to 30. The orthosis wearing protocol was: (1) 23 h per day for the first 14 days to protect the foot position (the orthosis was removed only for medical treatment, passive and active ankle mobilisation, muscle strengthening and stretching exercises); (2) 12 h per day from

Table 3 Rehabilitation treatment

Patient education (10 min)
Information about exercises by the physiotherapist
Warm-up (20 min)
Respiratory exercises (2 series of 10 repetitions)
Chest and shoulder stretching exercises (2 series of 10 repetitions)
Spine and upper limb stretching exercises (2 series of 10 repetitions)
Main period (40 min)
Passive and active mobilisation of lower limbs: (a) coxo-femoral: add/abduction (AB-AD), intra-extra rotation (IR-ER) and flexo-extension (F-E); (b) knee: F-E;(c) ankle*: dorsiflexion-plantar flexion, AB-AD, IR-ER (2 series of 10 repetitions)
Muscle strengthening for lower limbs[a]: quadriceps, hamstring, tibialis anterior (TA), extensor hallucis longus (EHL), extensor digitorum longus (EDL), soleus (SOL), gastrocnemius medialis and lateralis (GM-GL) (2 series of 10 repetitions)
Stretching exercises* for lower limbs, in particular: quadriceps, hamstring, TA, EHL, EDL, SOL, GM-GL (2 repetitions for 30 s)
Gait training: for the first 20 days after surgery patients used an articulated ankle-foot orthosis, which was removed from day 20 to 30 (10 min)
Cooling down (20 min)
Respiratory exercises (2 series of 10 repetitions)
Training with exercise bikes (10 min)

[a]Note for transfer surgery: avoid stretching the transferred muscles; strengthening is allowed but only with active exercises

day 15 to 20 (the orthosis was worn only at night). This non-articulated AFO, in which ankle was placed in neutral position, allowed full weight bearing during the first 14 days after surgery. From day 15 to day 30 patients maintained full weight bearing in their footwear.

Strengthening and stretching exercises must be done with great caution after surgical tendon transfer. The physiotherapist must take into account the osseointegration time and the suture healing time (osseointegration with interference screws requires at least 30–40 days, while tendon sutures take at least 3 weeks to heal). Therefore, in the early rehabilitation period it is better to avoid stretching exercises involving transferred muscles; only active strengthening exercises are allowed.

12 Discussion

Spastic foot deformities are caused by selectively increased muscle tone that disturbs the physiological agonist-antagonist balance of the lower extremity musculature.

It is important to employ a systematic approach to the evaluation, diagnosis and treatment of limb dysfunction in order to maximize function [3, 10, 12]. Orthopaedic surgery can contribute to the restoration of function in many patients.

A retrospective analysis conducted in 47 stroke patients showed improvements in balance and foot clearance during gait, and recovery of neutral heel foot-ground contact and of ankle DF during stance and swing at one month after EVFD surgery combined with early rehabilitation treatment; there were no complications related to the early mobilisation and weight bearing [7].

Due to the significant results obtained, this combined treatment could be proposed as an adjunctive treatment in the multidisciplinary management of patients with EVFD following stroke.

Furthermore, cases where an orthosis is still necessary after EVFD surgical correction, it will be lighter and more flexible and the patients will be able to walk with more stability.

Moreover, early surgical treatment has proved to be more cost-efficient because it reduced the need for physical rehabilitation or the use of orthoses. In a study by Reddy et al. [6], 19 out of 29 patients interrupted their physical therapy after surgical treatment and 17 patients abandoned the use of orthoses, while a more recent study showed that 44% of the patients removed their orthosis and 48% started walking without any aid week after surgery [33]. Despite the well-documented success of functional surgery in stroke patients, the importance of the timing of surgery needs to be better recognised in clinical practice, especially from the perspective of the costs of managing patients with EVFD after stroke.

Although the scientific literature does not specify when is right time to intervene surgically after stroke, it is important to consider functional surgery as therapeutic option that may be used before deformities become structured, thereby avoiding the need for more aggressive surgery and longer immobilisation time post-surgery.

References

1. Keenan MA, Mayer NH, Esquenazi A, et al. A neuro-orthopaedic approach to the management of common patterns of upper motoneuron dysfunction after brain injury. J Neuro Rehabil. 1999;I2:119–43.
2. Banks HH. The management of spastic deformities of the foot and ankle. Clin Orthop Relat Res. 1977;122:70–6.
3. Lin PY, Yang YR, Cheng SJ, Wang RY. The relation between ankle impairments and gait velocity and symmetry in people with stroke. Arch Phys Med Rehabil. 2006;87:562–8.
4. Keenan MA, Creighton J, GarlandDE, et al. Surgical correction of spastic equinovarus deformity in the adult head trauma patient. Foot Ankle. 1984;5:35–41.
5. Keenan MA. The management of spastic equinovarus deformity following stroke and head injury. Foot Ankle Clin. 2011;16(3):499–514.
6. Reddy S, Kusuma S, Hosalkar H, et al. Surgery can reduce the nonoperative care associated with an equinovarus foot deformity. Clin Orthop Relat Res. 2008;466:1683–7.
7. Giannotti E, Merlo A, Zerbinati P, Longhi M, Prati P, Masiero S, Mazzoli D. Early rehabilitation treatment combined with equinovarus foot deformity surgical correction in stroke patients: safety and changes in gait parameter. Eur J Phys Rehabil Med. 2016;52 (3):296–303.

8. Waters RL, Frazier J, Garland DE, et al. Electromyographic gait analysis before and after operative treatment for hemiplegic equinus and equinovarus deformity. J Bone Joint Surg. 1982;64:284–8.
9. Redfern JC, Thordason DB. Achilles lengthening/posterior tibial tenotomy with immediate weightbearing for patients with significant comorbidities. Foot Ankle Int. 2008;29:325–8.
10. Renzenbrink GJ, Buurke JH, Nene AV, Geurts AC, Kwakkel G, Rietman JS. Improving walking capacity by surgical correction of equinovarus foot deformity in adult patients with stroke or traumatic brain injury: a systematic review. J Rehabil Med. 2012;44:614–23.
11. Perry J, Waters R, Perrin T. Electromyographic analysis of equinovarus following stroke. Clin Orthop Relat Res. 1978;131:4753.
12. Fuller DA, Keenan MAE, Esquenazi A, et al. The impact of instrumented gait analysis on surgical planning: treatment of spastic equinovarus deformity of the foot and ankle. Foot Ankle Int. 2002;23(8):738–43.
13. Perry J. Gait analysis: normal and pathological function. Edited by SLACK Incorporated. Thorofare, NJ 1992.
14. Bofelli TJ, Collier RC. Minimally invasive soft tissue release of foot and ankle contracture secondary to stroke. J Foot Ankle Surg. 2014;53(3):369–75.
15. Lawrence SJ, Botte MJ. Management of the adult, spastic, equinovarus foot deformity. Foot Ankle Int. 1994;15:340–6.
16. Namdari S, Park M, Baldwin K, et al. Correcting spastic equinovarus post-cerebro-vascular accident: do age, sex, and timing matter? Foot Ankle Int. 2009;30(10):923–7.
17. Keenan MAE, Lee G. Orthopaedic management of lower extremity dysfunction following stroke or brain injury. In: Chapman M, editor. Chapman's operative orthopaedics. Philadelphia: Lippincott Williams and Wilkins; 2001. p. 3201–43.
18. Lee KC, Carson L, Kinnin E, et al. The Ashworth scale: a reliable and reproducible method of measuring spasticity. J Neurol Rehabil. 1989;3:205–9.
19. Bohannon RW, Smith MB. Interrater reliability of modified Ashworth scale of muscle spasticity. Phys Ther. 1987;67(2):206–7.
20. Pinzur MS, Sherman R, DiMonte-Levine P, et al. Adult-onset hemiplegia: changes in gait after muscle-balancing procedures to correct the equinus deformity. J Bone Joint Surg. 1986;68:1249–57.
21. Viosca E, Martinez JL, Almagro PL, et al. Proposal and validation of a new functional ambulation classification scale for clinical use. Arch Phys Med Rehabil. 2005;86:1234–8.
22. Hoke M. An operation for the correction of extremely relaxed flat feet. J Bone Joint Surg Br. 1931;13:773–83.
23. Hoffer MM, Reiswig JA, Garret AM, et al. The split anterior tibial tendon transfer in the treatment of spastic varus hindfoot in childhood. Orthop Clin North Am. 1974;5:31–8.
24. Edwards P, Hsu J. SPLATT combined with tendo Achilles lengthening for spastic equinovarus in adults: results and predictors of surgical outcome. Foot Ankle. 1993;14:335–8.
25. Barnes MJ, Herring JA. Combined split anterior tibial-tendon transfer and intramuscular lengthening of the posterior tibial tendon. Results in patients who have a varus deformity of the foot due to spastic cerebral palsy. J Bone Joint Surg [Am]. 1991;73:734–8.
26. Fuller DA, McCarthy JJ, Keenan MA. The use of the absorbable interference screw for a split anterior tibial tendon (SPLATT) transfer procedure. Orthopedics. 2004;27:372–4.
27. Hosalkar H, Goebel J, Reddy S, et al. Fixation techniques for split anterior tibialis transfer in spastic equinovarus feet. Clin Orthop Relat Res. 2008;466:2500–6.
28. Morita S, Yamamoto H, Furuya K. Anterior transfer of the toe flexors for equinovarus deformity due to hemiplegia. J Bone Joint Surg Br. 1994;76(3):447–9.
29. Ono K, Hiroshima K, Tada K, et al. Anterior transfer of the toe flexors for equinovarus deformity of the foot. Int Orthop. 1980;4:225–9.
30. Keenan MA, Lee GA, Tuckman AS, et al. Improving calf muscle strength in patients with spastic equinovarus deformity by transfer of the long toe flexors to the Os calcis. J Head Trauma Rehabil. 1999;14:163–75.

31. Carda S, Bertoni M, Zerbinati P, Rossini M, Magoni L, Molteni F. Gait changes after tendon functional surgery for equinovarus foot in patients with stroke. Am J Phys Med Rehabil. 2009;88:292–301.
32. Carda S, Molteni F, Bertoni M, Zerbinati P, Invernizzi M, Cisari C. Extensor hallucis longus transfer as an alternative to split transfer of the tibialis anterior tendon to correct equinovarus foot in hemiplegic patients without overactivity of tibialis anterior. J Bone Joint Surg Br. 2010;92(9):1262–6.
33. Vogt JK, Bach G, Cantini B, Perrin S. Split anterior tibial tendon transfer for varus equinus spastic foot deformity. Initial clinical findings correlate with functional results: a series of 132 operated feet. Foot and Ankle Surgery. 2011;17(3):178–81.

The manufacturer's authorised representative in the EU is Springer Nature Customer Service Centre GmbH, Europaplatz 3, 69115 Heidelberg, Germany. If you have any concerns regarding our products, please contact ProductSafety@springernature.com

Printed and bound by CPI Group (UK) Ltd, Croydon, CR0 4YY
30/09/2026
02225229-0018